Knee Joint Arthroplasty

Wooshin Cho

Knee Joint Arthroplasty

Springer

Wooshin Cho
Department of Orthopedic Surgery
ASAN Medical Center
University of Ulsan
College of Medicine
Seoul
Korea, Republic of South Korea

ISBN 978-3-642-39388-4 ISBN 978-3-642-39389-1 (eBook)
DOI 10.1007/978-3-642-39389-1
Springer Heidelberg New York Dordrecht London

Library of Congress Control Number: 2013950313

Printed on acid-free paper

Springer is part of Springer Science+Business Media (www.springer.com)

Preface

When I first ventured the field of arthroplasty, I was under the impression that the operation can be performed by simply following the manuals provided by the manufacturers. However, as my apprehension regarding the knee joint arthroplasty increased, I realized that I cannot always only follow the manuals in order to achieve good results and that the entire process starting from patient selection to postoperative treatment is not easy.

After an experience of more than 6,000 cases of knee arthroplasty in the last 20 years, I came to believe that arthroplasty is an interesting and highly gratifying operation that requires deep contemplation.

During this time, I wandered a lot academically. I was unsure of my own beliefs whenever others shared their opinion with me. There must have been some truth in their opinion, but I always felt that the actual truth was hidden somewhere which I must explore.

Of course, there could be more than one truth and numerous academic theories. Even then, I was surprised to see that the relatively widely accepted theories did not stand true practically. I am certain that many other surgeons must have experienced these problems which I was confronted with.

I am well aware that my arguments must have evidence-based academic background. However, it was sometimes difficult to prove certain theories due to the numerous variables and I was also confronted with several obstacles to present my opinion which was different from the preexisting theory. Nevertheless, I could not keep everything to myself. I just wanted to share my opinion with the other surgeons. This was the first motivational factor for writing this book.

As my experience increased, I realized that I should always keep thinking about the operative procedures, I should not overlook any of the operation findings, and I should be able to feel even the smallest difference during the operation in order to achieve better results. However, this was not described in any other book as it was not easy to express this in words. Also, I have developed a few surgical tips throughout these years and I thought that it would be valuable to share them with the other surgeons. This was the second motivational factor for writing this book.

For a carpenter to build a good house, a good design and good materials are needed, and it should be built using good tools. In arthroplasty, the tools used for the operation should ensure convenience, accuracy, and reproducibility, but many surgical instruments lack these properties. I have modified the existing surgical instruments and have also invented some new surgical instruments. Although these surgical instruments have undergone many trials and errors, some of the surgical instruments that I have invented are still very useful. I wanted to share the information regarding these surgical tools with the other surgeons. This was the third motivational factor for writing this book.

These motivational factors gave me the energy to write this book. I have reviewed about 1,500 articles and 5–6 textbooks in about 3 years and have exerted my opinion to publish the Korean version of "Knee Joint Arthroplasty" in 2004.

Seeing the enthusiasm of my readers, I felt that it was my responsibility to revise the first edition, and I published the second edition in 2007. With encouragement from the Korean readers and a few colleagues, I planned to publish the English version and I have also added new concepts and theories in the second edition of the Korean version.

It is not easy for a person to write a book all by himself, and there may be some shortcomings. First, there may be a lack of in-depth knowledge. Since my knowledge is limited, I have tried to read and refer to as many articles as possible. Second, my perspectives on the contents may be biased. I believe that this part has improved to a great extent in comparison with the first and second editions of the Korean version. Third, some of the descriptions may be inaccurate. I promise to keep making corrections.

On the other hand, there are some benefits as well. The descriptions are well organized and consistent, making it easier for the readers to read and comprehend.

Since English is not my native language, some of the expressions may sound awkward for the English readers. This was the biggest obstacle for me in writing the English version. I have tried to use the appropriate expressions at most places, but I do agree that some of the expressions are still strange. I hope that my readers will point out these mistakes so that I can publish a much better written book next time.

This book consists of ten chapters that are arranged in the order of management of the patients. Each chapter provides theoretical information as well as surgical tips, and the main points have been emphasized in italics. I have described my thoughts and have given tips in the boxes of "Author's Opinion" and "Author's Method" after describing certain theories or techniques. Although some of the readers may not agree with my thoughts, my comments would help my readers summarize and apprehend the concepts and techniques of the knee joint arthroplasty.

I hope to interact with many more surgeons through this book and contribute to the academic foundation and surgical advancement of knee joint arthroplasty.

Finally, many people have helped me publish this book.

First, I would like to give my appreciation to my wife and my three daughters who have supported me throughout.

Second, I would like to thank the prior Dean and Professor Key Yong, Kim who guided me to become an orthopedic surgeon.

Third, I would like to thank Professor Yoon Seok Yeom, who will succeed this book after me, and Doctor Young Sun Yoon, Seongeun Byun, and Kunal Dhurve who have helped me arrange the contents of this book.

Finally, I would also like to thank the officials at the Department of Orthopedic Surgery, Asan Medical Center and officials of Springer Korea.

Seoul, South Korea Wooshin Cho

Contents

1 Patient Selection

Here, I have used the term "patient selection" instead of the medical term "indication" because total knee arthroplasty (TKA) is an elective and is not an emergency or lifesaving procedure. Hence the patient's physical condition and their socioeconomic status should be considered while planning the operation.

The success of the TKA is closely related to the patient's satisfaction, which is reflected mainly by the relief of pain and improvement of function as well as psychological relief which is manifested by improvement in the quality of life. Even though the operation is successful, the knee joint function cannot return to normal. Oriental patients experience many instances of inconveniences as they are required to kneel down frequently due to their traditional lifestyle. In some patients, pain may persist to a greater or lesser extent even after arthroplasty. Also, TKA cannot be successful in all cases. If the operation fails, the condition of the knee joint would be worse than that before the operation. Even if the operation is successful, since the artificial joint does not assimilate into the human body, a revision surgery is needed after a certain period of time.

Therefore, it is desirable to carefully consider the advantages and drawbacks of TKA before taking the decision to perform the operation.

1.1 Social Conditions

Social conditions generally include the patients' family, surroundings, and patients' activities.

In most of the oriental societies, the patients live together with their children, although this tradition is changing gradually. Even when the patients live apart from their children, most of the families start living together again when their parents are seriously ill.

Many problems may develop within the family, in case the patient is unable to walk. In such a situation, it is desirable to perform arthroplasty in order to regain mobility as early as possible. In fact, family satisfaction is greater than patient satisfaction if the operation is successful. This indicates that the life of the family members of the patient becomes better as a result of freedom from caregiving, while the patients themselves continue to have difficulty while performing the activities of daily living such as kneeling down and sitting on the floor, despite of being able to walk without pain. Total knee arthroplasty can be delayed if the family members are affectionate towards the patients.

Therefore, *the family's attitude towards the patient, patient's activity level, and patient's motivation to modify their lifestyle are important factors to be considered while deciding to perform the operation.*

1.2 Economic Conditions

Economic conditions also have a considerable impact on patient satisfaction. In case of elderly patients, high hospitalization costs can lead to an increase in the patient's anxiety level, thereby resulting in a poor prognosis. If the patient's socioeconomic condition is not good, he/she may need to return to work after the operation. Therefore, total knee arthroplasty is indicated in the patients who have the ability to pay the hospitalization charges without much difficulty and *who can make a living without doing any laborious work after the surgery.*

1.3 Psychological Conditions

Although psychological conditions are easily overlooked, *they are closely related to the patient's perception of pain.* The patient's psychological condition also affects the postoperative rehabilitation. If patient motivation is poor and the patient is not willing to follow the surgeon's instructions, the results of TKA may not be satisfactory. The patients who lack *motivation*, have been forced to undergo an operation by the family, are stubborn or dependent, and are accustomed to complain about minor discomforts have a lower level of satisfaction after the surgery. The patients who have a rigid

W. Cho, *Knee Joint Arthroplasty*,
DOI 10.1007/978-3-642-39389-1_1,

mindset towards the outcome of TKA or are oversensitive to pain also show poor results.

The patient's expectations should not be too high. If the patients expect that their knee joint function will return to normal and they can get involved in vigorous sports activities and laborious work, the decision to perform a TKA should be reconsidered. Scott et al. and Noble et al. reported that postoperative patient satisfaction is primarily dependent not on the knee joint function but on the patients' expectations. Hepinstall et al. suggested that high, unrealistic expectations of TKA are common and should be moderated to maintain patient satisfaction. Culliton et al. reported that preoperative expectations did not correlate with postoperative satisfaction. However, postoperative satisfaction was predicted by how well preoperative expectations were met after surgery. Therefore, patient education program for managing expectations should be established on the other hand Gandhi et al. reported that although young, male, and low-BMI patients have higher expectations from TKA, they get better pain relief.

If the patient seems to suffer from a *psychological disorder or depression*, it is recommended to consult a psychiatrist prior to the operation so as to assess whether the patient's *psychological* condition can be optimized with medications. Ellis et al. reported that psychopathology such as presence of somatization, depression, and/or a panic or anxiety disorder showed significantly higher levels of perception disability even though these patients still benefit with same degree of improvement in function. They recommended routine assessment for psychological distress prior to TKA. However, in contrast to the general assumption that the prognosis would be worse in patients with a psychological disorder, Riddle et al. and Lingard and Riddle reported that postoperative pain is not related to the presence of psychological disorders. Brander et al. also reported that the presence of psychological disorders affects the prognosis, but only until postoperative 1 year, and it has no effect on the prognosis thereafter.

Dementia is not a contraindication for TKA, but a patient suffering from dementia *is not a good candidate* for TKA as his/her behavior can be quite erratic.

1.4 Indication

An indication refers to the physical condition. The indication should be decided according to the age of the patient, patient's physical condition, and condition of the knee joint.

1.4.1 Age

Age is a very important factor in deciding the indication, since we must take into account both the patients' activity level and implant survival. If the patients are young, there is a higher possibility of the need of revision surgery because young patients are more active and they live longer than the duration of implant survival. Revision TKA is technically more difficult than primary TKA, and the prognosis is not as good as that of primary TKA. So, it is desirable that the patients benefit from the TKA throughout their life without requiring revision TKA. However, *developments in implants and surgical techniques for primary and revision TKA and prolonged life span have resulted in widening of the indications based on the patient age.*

TKA is not indicated in teenagers because they are skeletally immature.

In the 3rd–5th decade of life, TKA can be indicated for ankylosed knees, far advanced secondary OA, or rheumatoid arthritis. It is not appropriate to expect the young patients to tolerate the extreme pain just because they are young. TKA can be of great help to the patients who have been suffering from uncontrolled pain and who are bedridden due to polyarthritis.

In the 6th decade of life, if the pain and functional disturbance is not very severe, the conservative treatment should be tried or joint-conserving operations such as chondroplasty, high tibial osteotomy, and unicondylar arthroplasty can be performed. Of course, *TKA is indicated for advanced osteoarthritis and rheumatoid arthritis in this age group.* Crowder et al. reported that they achieved good clinical results in the patients of rheumatoid arthritis who were younger than 55 years of age. A few surgeons recommend arthrodesis of the knee in the younger age group, but I have an opposite opinion taking two aspects into consideration. The first aspect is that the handicap associated with an ankylosed knee is much more than that with the ankylotic hip with respect to walking the stairs, voiding, getting into a car, and performing the activities of daily living. And hence the patient is likely to be isolated from the society and can lose his/her financial independence. The second aspect is that it is much easier to perform arthrodesis for failed TKA than for failed THA. If a TKA fails, arthrodesis of the knee joint can be performed more easily afterwards.

However, performing TKA in the young patients with severe arthritis is quite different from converting the ankylosed joint to a mobile joint. In other words, *if a young patient has severe pain and functional disturbance and he does not engage in laborious work, TKA may be considered instead of knee fusion, whereas if the joint is ankylosed in a young laborer, it is better not to convert the ankylosed joint to a mobile joint.*

The most appropriate age for TKA is around 65 years. At this age, the patient does not engage in laborious work, and he/she may not need to undergo a revision operation since the average life span is around 80 years. Also, the patient's physical condition is relatively good at this age, and the risk of operation is not very high. When 5 years are added or subtracted from this age of 65 years, the patients in the age group of 60–70 years are a good indication for TKA according to the knee joint condition.

Between 70 and 80 years of age, TKA can be considered in patients having moderate pain and moderately advanced osteoarthritis. Osteoarthritis will progress in the near future, and passing the time away by attempting conservative treatments and waiting for an absolute indication will make the situation more difficult for performing an operation as the patient gets older.

It is not recommended to perform TKA in young patients, but also many problems may occur when TKA is performed *in patients who are too old*. When the patient is too old, the risk of operation increases, and the prognosis may not be as good due to comorbidity and muscle weakness. If some unfavorable events occur, the result may be worse than that without the operation. *When the patient's age is more than 80 years, the decision of performing an operation should be made very carefully*, and it may be better not to perform a TKA unless the patient is really healthy, although there are also some reports suggesting that there is no difference in the outcomes and morbidity after TKA in the patients more than 80 years of age. Alfonso et al. reported through the survey of 25 TKAs performed in patients more than 90 years of age that the pain was decreased and life span was extended as compared to that in the population belonging to the same age group who did not undergo a TKA. However, they experienced operation-related complications in 80 % of the cases and medical comorbidities in 56 % of cases.

Briefly, TKA is contraindicated in skeletally immature patients, but operation can be performed in patients less than 60 years of age if the symptoms are severe, and the best age for TKA is 60–70 years. TKA can be considered in moderately advanced osteoarthritis in 70–80-year-old patients. Patients more than 90 years of age should undergo TKA only in extremely exceptional cases. However, surgeons *should take into account the chronological age as well as the physiological age*. This should be done since some patients look healthier than their chronological age and vice versa.

1.4.2 Physical Conditions

1.4.2.1 General Conditions

Patient's general condition is likely to worsen postoperatively due to anorexia, insomnia, and voiding difficulties. Poor general condition of the patient has an adverse effect on wound healing and muscle strength which leads to a poor prognosis, and fatal results may occur due to comorbidity.

Most of the patients have hypertension, diabetes mellitus (DM), cardiopulmonary, renal, and other endocrine disorders. Hypertension, DM and other endocrine disorders are not a contraindication for TKA as they can be controlled perioperatively. The presence of cardiovascular and renal disorders is closely related with patient's capacity to endure the operation and their postoperative activity level. Meding et al. screened 1,438 patients preoperatively and reported that 8.3 % of the patients had cardiovascular problems, 7.2 % had chronic obstructive pulmonary disease, 56 % had hypertension, 37 % had gastrointestinal problems, and 12 % had DM. Among them, 2.5 % of patients were not suitable for the operation. Huddleston et al. reported that cardiovascular problems occurred in 3.9 % of patients among 2,033 TKA patients. Memtsoudis et al. reported fatal results in patients who underwent revision, who were old, and in patients with comorbidities and dementia. The most common causes of death were pulmonary embolism and cerebrovascular accident. Lingard and Riddle and Long et al. demonstrated, through the survey of the patients, that *the better the patient's preoperative physical condition, the better the prognosis and the higher the patient satisfaction*.

1.4.2.2 Obesity

Patients with obesity have a higher incidence of osteoarthritis. The patients whose body mass index (BMI) is over 25 are categorized as obese. *Obesity by itself cannot be a contraindication for TKA, but experience of the surgeon is needed to achieve a better result of TKA in morbidly obese patients*. I personally believe that the more the patient is obese, the more difficult is the surgical performance. According to the annual report of 2005, about 24 % of the whole population in the United States can be categorized as obese. Fehring et al. reported that about 52 % of their TKA patients were obese. The surgical performance and prognosis of TKA may be adversely affected when BMI is above 30, or body weight is more than 200 lb or 100 kg.

It is generally agreed that *obesity increases the complications such as wound problems, patellofemoral maltracking, and wear and loosening resulting in decreased implant survival rate*. Foran et al. reported worse clinical results and also reported that the incidence of revision was increased due to wear and loosening in obese patients. Kerkhoffs et al. reviewed 15,276 patients and reported the result of meta-analysis that deep infection occurred more often and revision rate was increased in patients whose BMI is more than 30. Dewan et al. stated that the morbidly obese patients whose BMI was over 40 showed muscle weakness and extensor mechanism dysfunction postoperatively. Gadinsky et al. found that patients with higher BMI had lower preoperative and postoperative ROM. However, Amin et al. and Bastis et al. reported that obesity had no adverse effect on the knee joint function and did not lead to an increase in the complications at the midterm follow-up of TKA.

1.4.2.3 Neuromuscular Conditions

In the presence of paralysis of the opposite lower limb, the indication for TKA is decided on the basis of how severe is the pain in the knee joint that needs to be operated, how much is the strength of muscle power in both lower limbs, and whether the patient can at least walk with crutches preoperatively. Generally, *arthroplasty may be indicated when the muscular strength of the limb to be operated upon is greater than grade IV.*

Parkinson's disease is a relative contraindication since there is motor incoordination and muscle tremor along with affective disorder, and it is a progressive disease.

The most difficult patient to decide operation is the one who has a minor or latent cerebrovascular lesion which cannot be detected by the symptoms and on physical examination. So, in case of any doubt, a preoperative work-up should be performed for detecting cerebrovascular lesion in the patients who have a history of cardiovascular problems or if the patient is very old.

1.4.2.4 Spinal Conditions

Patients with osteoarthritis often have accompanying spinal stenosis. Even if they do not feel any pain in the back, it might have been masked since they have more pain in the knees and they may experience back pain when the knee pain disappears.

A coexisting spinal stenosis may require an operative intervention as well. Surgeons should decide *the priority of the operation* that is to be performed first, since the physiological stress is increased if two major operations are performed within a short time span. *Motor power and the severity of pain is the determining factor for deciding which operation between the spinal operation and TKA is to be performed first. If there is accompanying motor weakness, it is strongly recommended to perform the spinal operation first.* If the pain intensity is nearly the same at both the sites, it is recommended to perform the spinal operation first. This is because the patient satisfaction is decreased when the back problem persists, no matter how successful the TKA is. When TKA is being planned, it is indicated only when the muscle power is at least greater than grade IV.

1.4.2.5 Hip or Other Joint Conditions

In the presence of a disorder of the hip joint, the priority of which operation should be performed first may be determined on the basis of pain intensity and condition of the hip joint. *In case there is accompanying ankylosis or motion limitation of the hip joint, it is desirable to perform the hip operation first* because an ankylotic and deformed hip makes the TKA operation more difficult and alters the biomechanics of the knee joint resulting in early failure of TKA.

When the opposite limb is amputated or there is accompanying muscle weakness and deformity due to poliomyelitis sequelae, indication should be determined very carefully since increased load on the operated knee can lead to early wear and loosening.

1.4.2.6 Vascular Conditions

Vascular conditions, although often neglected, should also be taken into consideration. When the patients have varices or when there is a history of frequent swelling of the lower limbs, there is a higher possibility of swelling and DVT postoperatively.

In case of arterial insufficiency, ischemic symptoms are often masked as the activity of the patients with osteoarthritis is low. Indication for TKA is determined after a careful work-up for the detection of vascular lesion. TKA is contraindicated in arterial insufficiency such as atherosclerosis or diabetes vasculopathy as severe ischemic pain or necrosis of the limb may develop.

1.4.3 Knee Joint Conditions

Knee joint condition is the most important factor in deciding the indication for TKA. This includes the symptoms, functions, and disease entity along with its severity.

1.4.3.1 Symptoms

The most important symptom is pain. Although pain is patient-specific, TKA is indicated when pain is noted while resting, there is sleep disturbance due to the pain, medications provide only transient pain relief, or in cases when the patient cannot take analgesics due to gastrointestinal or other medical problems. TKA is also indicated in patients in whom a joint-preserving operation such as chondroplasty or high tibial osteotomy has failed or is likely to fail. Cross et al. reviewed several literatures and stated that *the first indication for TKA is pain that cannot be controlled with medications.*

Since the arthritic changes on the X-ray do not always correlate with the pain intensity, it is recommended to delay the operation if the pain is not severe even though severe arthritic changes are seen on the X-ray. In such a situation, physiotherapy, limitation of activity, and medications should be tried. If the pain subsides by the above methods, or the patients are not willing to restrict their activity, it means that they are not ready to undergo TKA.

1.4.3.2 Functions

Functions are represented by the ability to walk, walking the stairs, or performing activities of daily living. If the patient cannot walk even one block, TKA is recommended. TKA is also considered when the patient needs to use a cane for walking and has a waddling or lurching gait. TKA is helpful to the patient who cannot stand for a short period of time for performing activities of daily living and cannot walk the stairs.

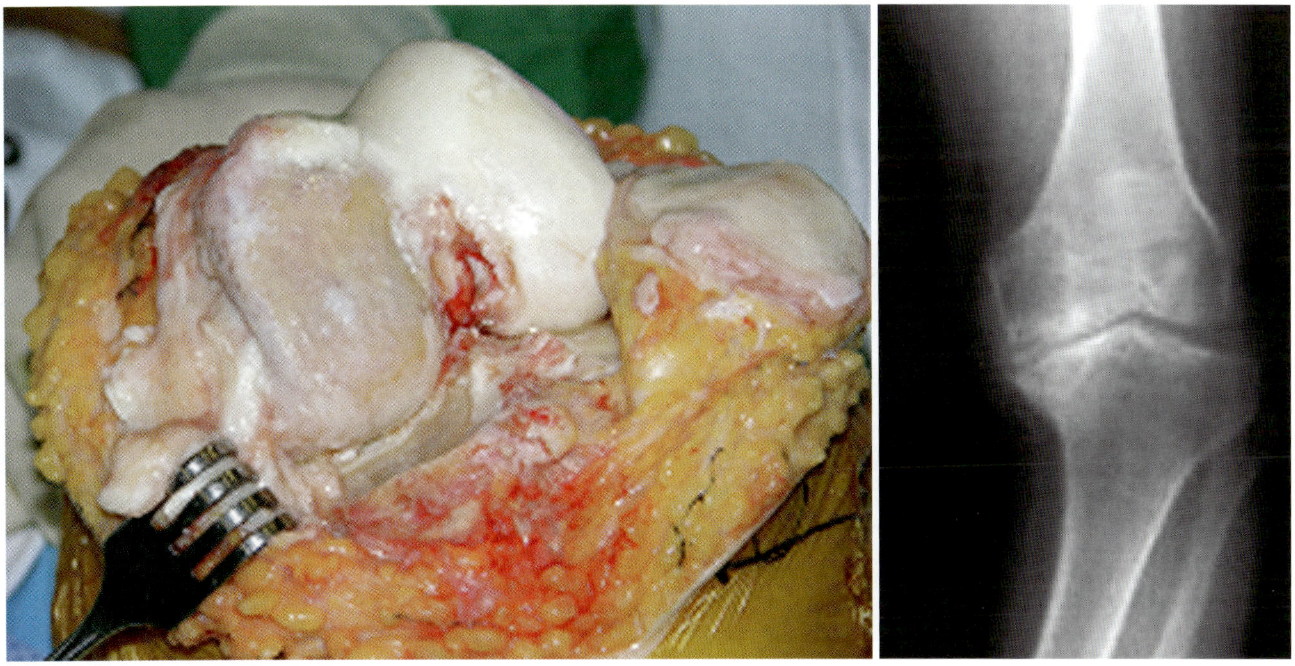

Fig. 1.1 Advanced osteoarthritis. Operative findings and X-ray of the knee joint

1.4.3.3 Causative Disease

The most common indication for TKA is osteoarthritis, followed by rheumatoid or other inflammatory arthritis, osteonecrosis, and ankylosed knee in that order.

Osteoarthritis (OA)

Advanced osteoarthritis is the best indication for TKA. When the pain due to the osteoarthritis does not respond to other treatment methods, it can be a good *indication* for TKA. The severity of osteoarthritis is divided into four grades: mild, moderate, advanced, and far advanced according to the X-ray findings of joint space narrowing, joint line irregularity, subchondral sclerosis, spur formation, cystic changes, deformity, and bone defect. According to the Kellgren–Lawrence classification, grade III is moderate osteoarthritis and grade IV is advanced osteoarthritis (Fig. 1.1).

It is inappropriate to perform TKA in patients whose *X-ray shows minimal osteoarthritis* or minimal to moderate osteoarthritis. *The symptoms in these patients can be controlled by other conservative treatments, and pain may be originating from causes other than the osteoarthritic lesion.* When the patient complains of severe pain with minimal osteoarthritic changes on the X-ray, surgeons should search for other causes of pain with the help of MRI or arthroscopic surgery, even in the elderly patients. On MRI, a meniscal or ligament lesion, a synovial lesion, and a small osteochondral lesion can be detected, and these lesions are not an indication for TKA.

Of course, the surgeon can find severe osteoarthritic changes during the operation even though there are minimal osteoarthritic changes on the X-ray. *In order not to miss the changes of advanced osteoarthritis, Rosenberg view which is the P–A view of the knee in 45° flexion is recommended* (Fig.1.2).

Secondary osteoarthritis, unlike primary osteoarthritis, occurs in relatively younger patients, and the symptoms may not be as severe as that perceived from the X-ray (Fig. 1.3). Since the prognosis of TKA for secondary osteoarthritis is not as good as that for primary osteoarthritis, the indication for TKA should be considered carefully. In particular, TKA for secondary osteoarthritis due to infection sequelae or traumatic arthritis is likely to reactivate the infection, and the previous operation of the knee joint can cause skin necrosis after TKA. Saleh et al. reported TKA failure in one-third of patients who had undergone open reduction and internal fixation of the tibial plateau fracture earlier.

Rheumatoid Arthritis (RA)

Rheumatoid arthritis is also a good indication for TKA. Although it occurs at a relatively younger age, it is associated with marked pain and functional disturbance.

In RA, the clinical courses including duration of morbidity, response to medication, joint deformity, and activity level are more important decisive factors for the indication for TKA rather than the X-ray findings alone (Fig 1.4).

Clinically, severe and intractable pain which does not respond to medications and marked functional disturbance are good indications for TKA. TKA is necessary in the

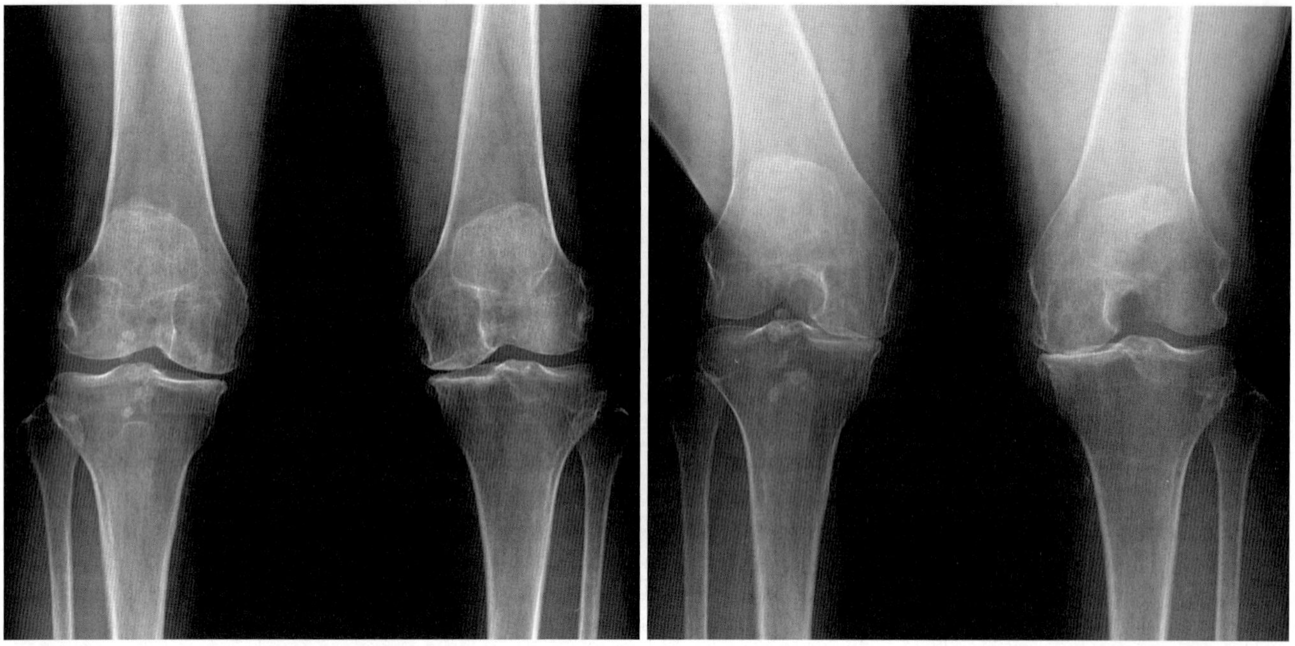

Fig. 1.2 Difference between the standing X-ray and the Rosenberg view. *Left* image shows the standing X-ray, and *right* image shows the Rosenberg view of the same patient. Arthritic changes are more prominent on the Rosenberg view

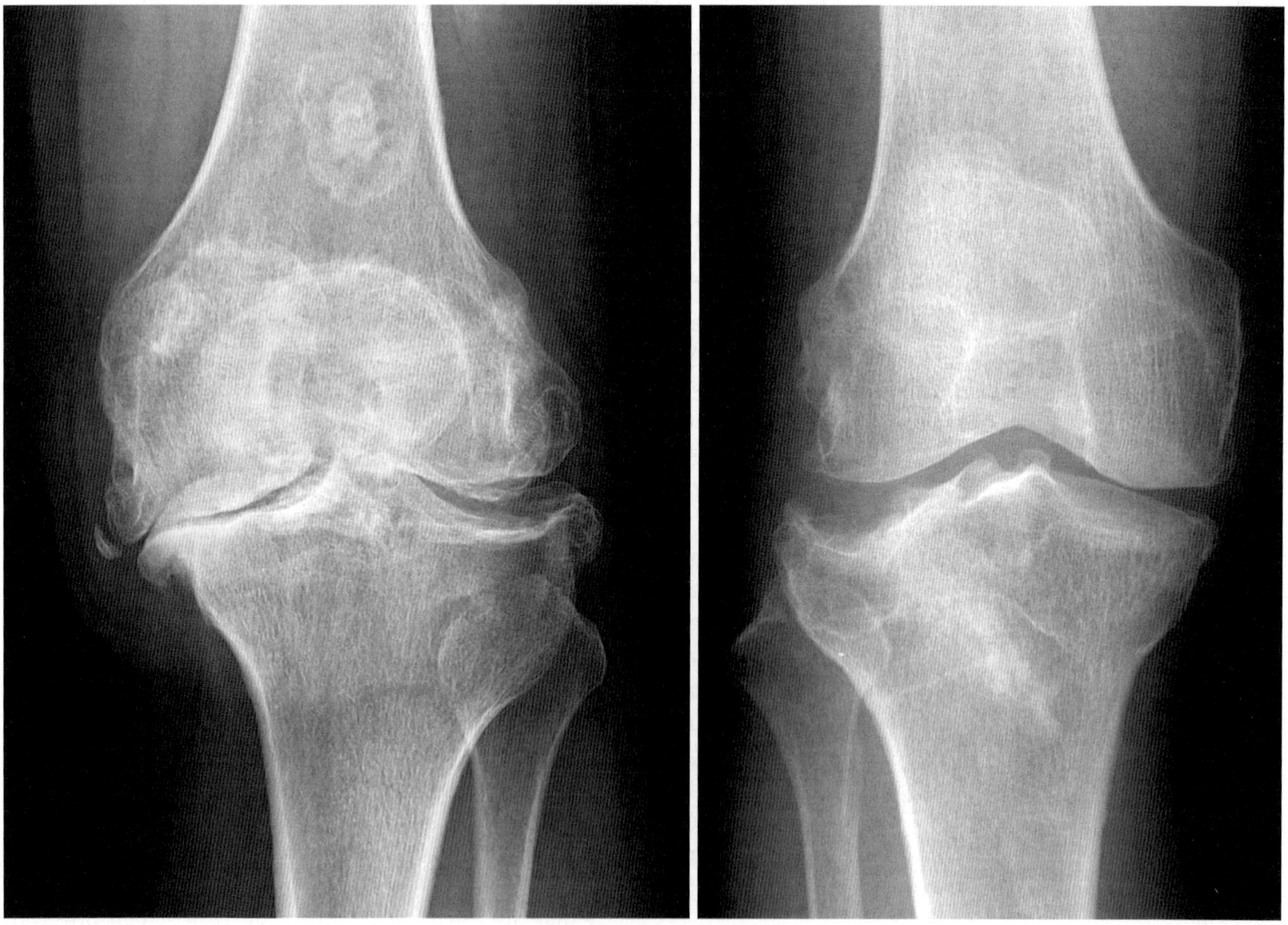

Fig. 1.3 Secondary osteoarthritis of the knee joint. *Left* X-ray shows secondary osteoarthritis probably due to sequelae of pyogenic arthritis. *Right* X-ray shows traumatic arthritis due to tibial plateau fracture

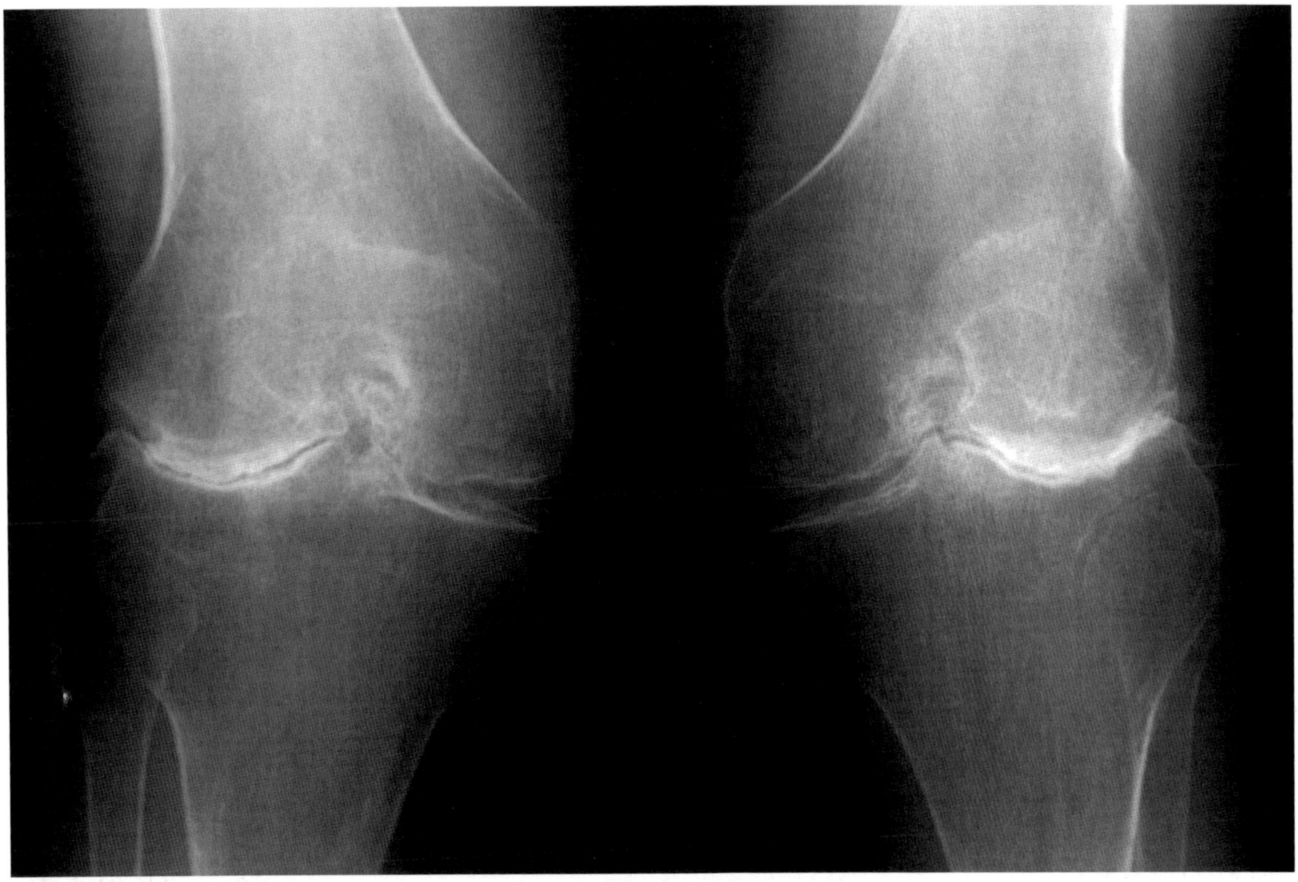

Fig 1.4 X-ray findings in rheumatoid arthritis

presence of severe bony destruction, huge cyst, a marked deformity, and joint space narrowing or ankylosis of the knee joint on the X-ray.

As RA involves multiple joints, the decision regarding operation of *which joint is to be performed first should be made carefully*. With respect to the pain, operation of the more painful joint should be performed first. But if motion limitation is noted in the hip joint, performance of THA should take precedence.

When the inflammatory reaction is severe, it is better to wait until the acute symptoms subside with medications.

In inflammatory arthritis mimicking rheumatoid arthritis, the principle is same as that in RA.

Osteonecrosis

Symptoms and signs *of osteonecrosis are severe pain with articular collapse or extensive bone necrosis. Articular fragmentation involving more than 1/2 of the articular surface is an indication for TKA*. If the lesion involves less than 1/2 of the articular surface, clinical observation is needed with administering medications. X-ray findings in osteonecrosis are somewhat different from those in osteoarthritis. In osteonecrosis, there is mixed radiolucency and sclerosis in the epi- and metaphyseal area. Like in hip osteonecrosis, MRI is of a great help to know the extent and patterns of the osteonecrosis.

Spontaneous osteonecrosis of the knee (SPONK) should be differentiated from true osteonecrosis. The site of involvement, pattern, and pathologic findings in SPONK are different from those in true osteonecrosis (Fig 1.5). Since the SPONK lesion is confined to the epiphysis, it can be a good indication for unicondylar arthroplasty or TKA (Fig 1.6).

It is important to know the causes of osteonecrosis since the progression of osteonecrosis may vary according to its causes. Mont et al. experienced failure of TKA in about half of the 31 patients with steroid-induced osteonecrosis. They reported that the causes of TKA failure were loosening in 11 cases and infection in 3 cases.

Ankylosis

It is desirable to leave the ankylosed knee untreated in young active laborers. In non-laborers, conversion to TKA is indicated in cases of noninfectious ankylosis, ankylosis with a good bone stock, muscle and skin condition, and the ankylosed knee in which the extensor mechanism is preserved (Fig 1.7). This is because the handicap associated with an ankylosed knee is so severe that difficulties and inconveniences could occur during activities of daily living. An operation can be performed to convert an ankylotic knee with absent patella into a mobile joint, but this should be reserved for the highly experienced surgeons.

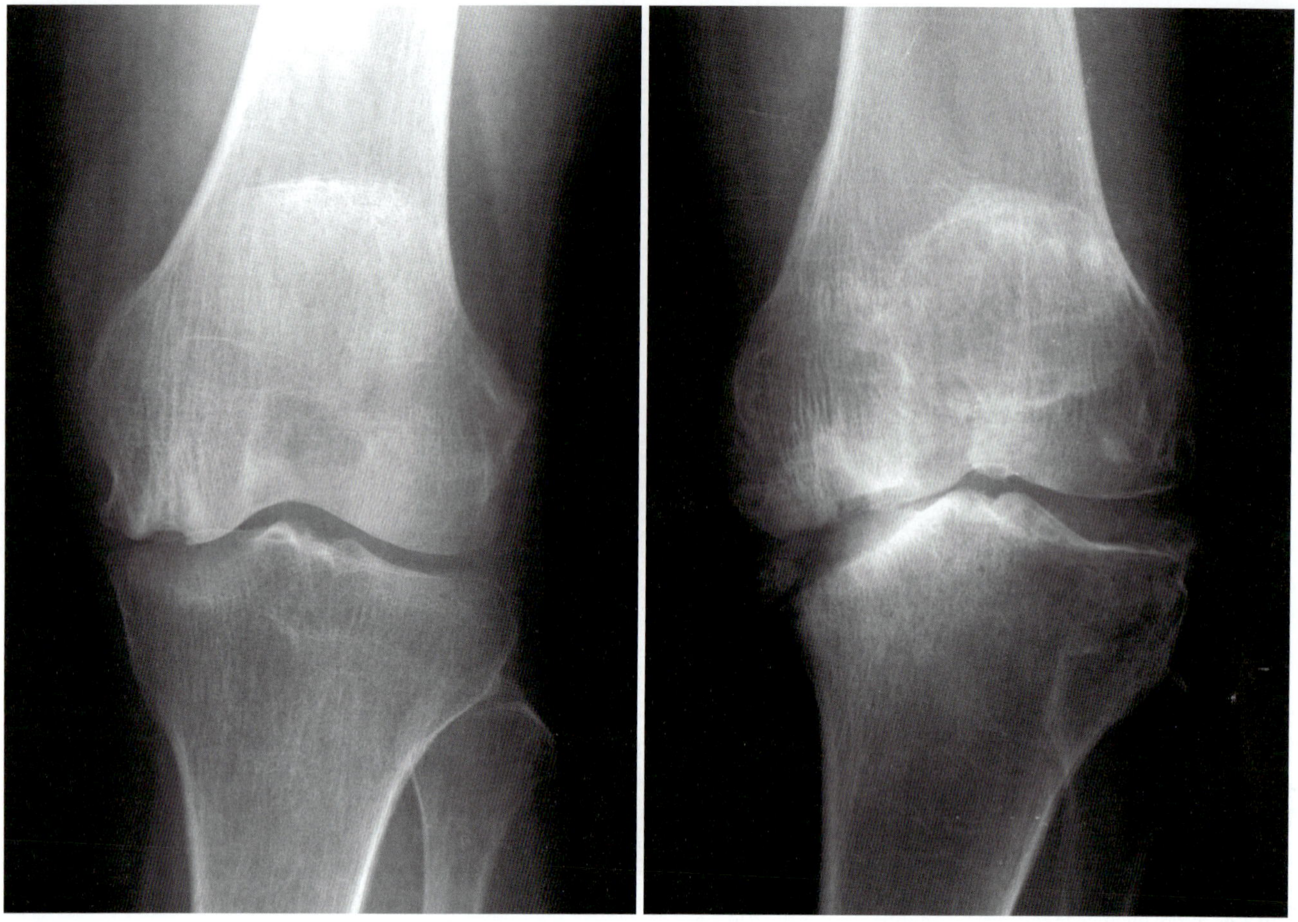

Fig 1.5 X-ray of the SPONK lesion and osteonecrosis. *Left*: SPONK lesion, *right*: Osteonecrosis

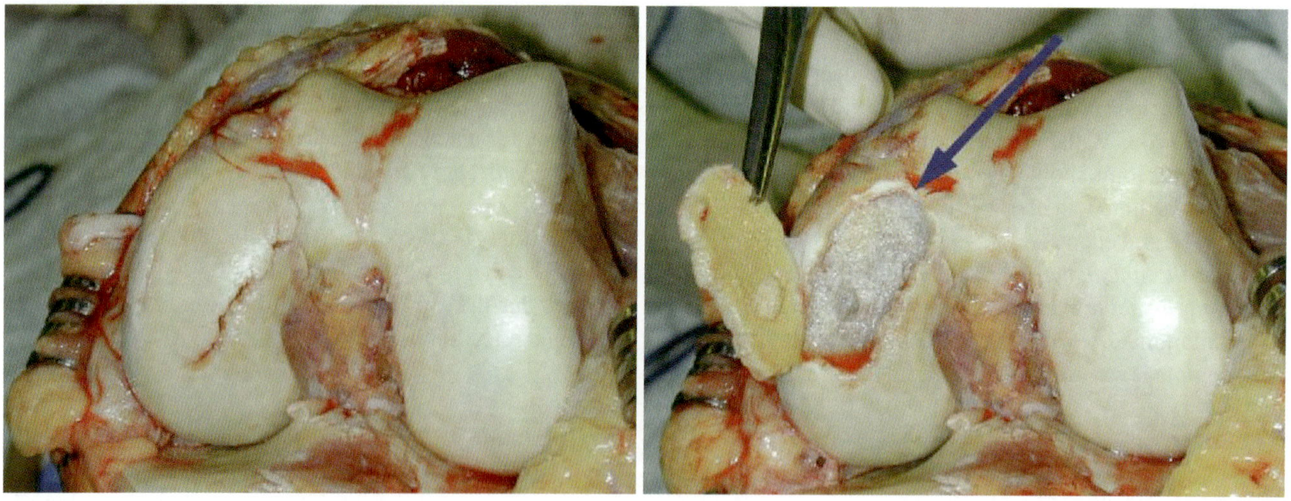

Fig 1.6 Operative findings of the SPONK lesion

Charcot Joint

Charcot joint is a relative contraindication for TKA. This is because the patients can feel little pain despite severe destruction of the joint on the X-ray, the operation is difficult, the joint protection ability is decreased, the prognosis is poor, and revision is much more difficult (Fig 1.8). I have an experience of five cases of TKA for Charcot joint with poor results at long-term follow-up except for one case. Hence, the *indication for TKA is limited to the patients who cannot walk even with brace fitting*.

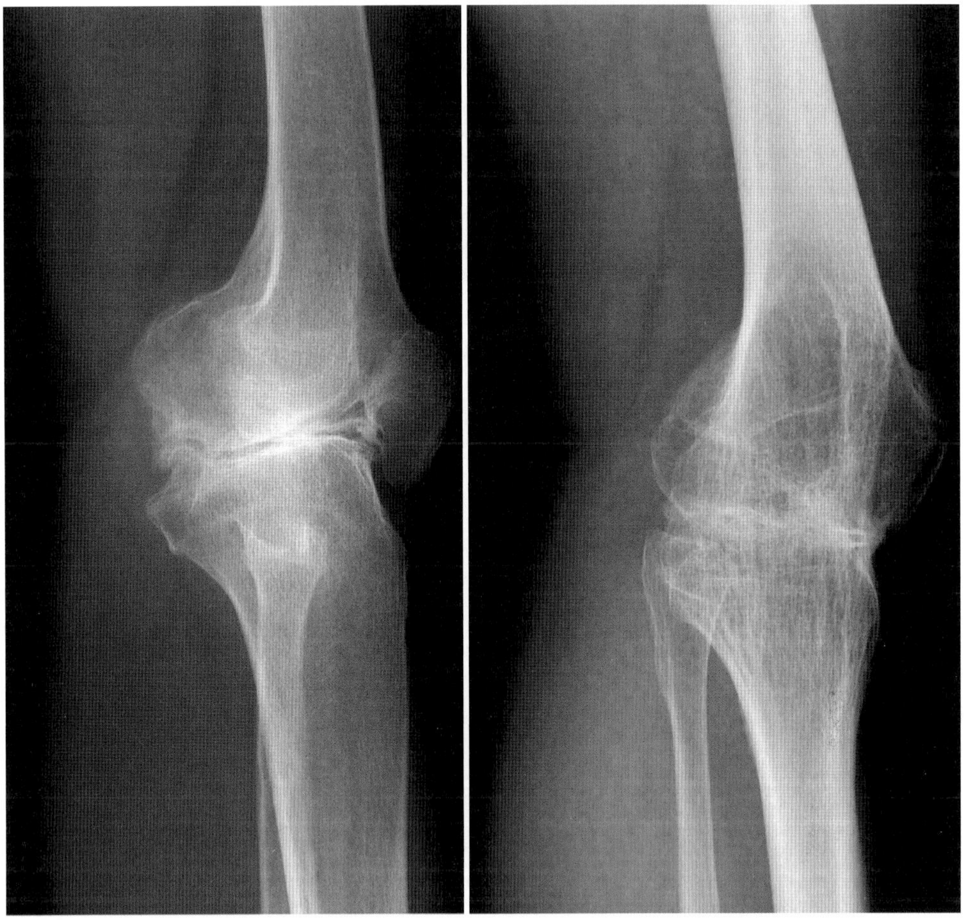

Fig 1.7 Ankylosed knee. *Left*: X-ray shows ankylosed knee with patella baja. *Right*: X-ray shows ankylosed knee with an absent patella. These are relative contraindications for TKA

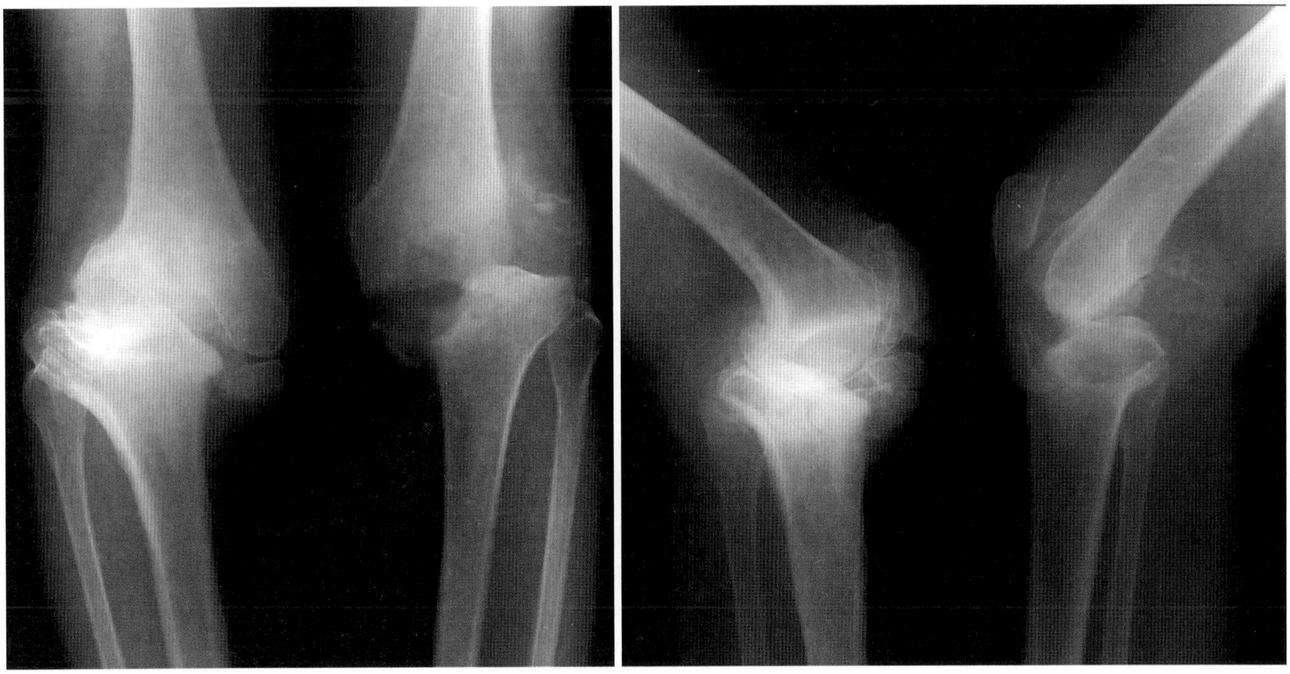

Fig 1.8 X-ray findings in Charcot joint. Bone destruction and joint instability are severe

1.4.4 Surgeon's Experience

Despite of careful patient selection and good if the implant choice, there is a *high probability of failure of TKA operation is not performed well due to lack of surgeon's experience in TKA*. Manley et al. compared the results of TKA between the less-experienced surgeons (25↓/year) and the more-experienced surgeons (200↑/year). They reported that there was no difference in the results of TKA between the less-experienced surgeons and the more-experienced surgeons at the short-term follow-up, but there was an increased risk of revision in the cases operated by the less-experienced surgeons at the mid-term and long-term follow-up. Hence, an operation beyond the surgeon's ability cannot be a good indication for TKA.

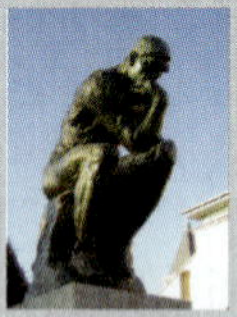

Author's Opinion

I decide the indication considering the patient's age, symptoms, and functional disturbance in combination with the X-ray findings. Pain and function are well expressed on the HSS score. In conclusion, *indication is determined according to the patient's age, HSS score, and X-ray findings*.

Age is divided into less than 60 years, between 60 and 70 years, between 70 and 80 years, and above 80 years. HSS score is divided into categories of less than 50, between 50 and 60, and more than 60. X-ray findings are also divided into moderately advanced OA, advanced OA, and far advanced OA.

In the less than 60 years age group, I perform TKA when the HSS score is less than 50, and the X-ray findings are indicative of far advanced osteoarthritis. When the patient fulfills one of the two criteria, I try the conservative treatment first.

In the 60–70 years age group, either one of the two criteria, HSS score less than 50 or far advanced osteoarthritis, can be a good indication. Also, I perform TKA in this age group when the HSS score is between 50 and 60, and the X-ray findings are indicative of advanced OA. In cases with moderately advanced osteoarthritis or the HSS score of more than 60, the decision of whether or not to perform the operation is made according to the socioeconomic condition of the patient.

In the 70–80 years age group, when the HSS score is between 50 and 60 and the X-ray findings are indicative of moderately advanced osteoarthritis, or the HSS score is more than 60 and the X-ray findings are indicative of advanced osteoarthritis, I perform TKA. In a patient with a HSS score of more than 60 and the X-ray findings indicative of moderately advanced osteoarthritis, conservative treatment can be tried first. This is because osteoarthritis is likely to progress, and performing TKA at a later date is difficult due to the comorbidities, and the appropriate timing of the operation is missed.

In an exceptional case of a healthy-looking patient more than 80 years of age, I also perform TKA when the X-ray findings are indicative of far advanced osteoarthritis (Table 1.1).

For making a quick decision, I established a database of my own modalities of treatment.

Table 1.1 Author's age-based treatment modalities for osteoarthritis

		X-ray		
Age↓	HSS	Far advanced OA	Advanced OA	Moderately advanced OA
60↓	50↓	TKA	CFT	Con
	50–60	CFT	Con	Con
	60↑	Con	Con	Con
60–70	50↓	TKA	TKA	TKA
	50–60	TKA	TKA	CFT
	60↑	TKA	CFT	Con
70–80	50↓	TKA	TKA	TKA
	50–60	TKA	TKA	TKA
	60↑	TKA	TKA	CFT
80↑	50↓	CFT	Con	Con
	50–60	Con	Con	Con
	60↑	Con	Con	Con

TKA total knee arthroplasty, *CFT* conservative treatment followed by TKA, *Con* conservative treatment

1.5 Contraindications

Active infection is an absolute contraindication for TKA, and if there is any suspicion of infection, TKA should be postponed.

If the patients have a history of recent acupuncture and moxibustion or operation, surgeon should be confident that the surgical site is free from infection. Prior arthroscopic surgery is not an important factor, but any other operation of the knee joint in which the incision is different from that in TKA, it is better to delay the operation for a while. In pyogenic arthritis, it is also recommended to delay the operation for about 6 months after the laboratory results for infection have subsided to the normal range. In case of tuberculous arthritis, primarily debridement and curettage should be performed, and after 4–6 weeks of medication, TKA can be performed in the second stage.

TKA is contraindicated in the patients with poor general condition, who lack motivation, are young laborers, are skeletally immature, and who are expected to have difficulties in walking despite of undergoing TKA.

Conditions such as *dementia, neuropathic joint, Parkinson's disease, extensor insufficiency, vascular disease of the limb, psoriasis, morbid obesity, and history of osteomyelitis are all relative contraindications for TKA.*

Bibliography

Aglietti P, Windsor RE, Buzzi R, et al. Arthroplasty for the stiff or ankylosed knee. J Arthroplasty. 1989;4:1–5.

Alfonso DT, Howell RD, Strauss EJ, et al. Total hip and knee arthroplasty in nonagenarians. J Arthroplasty. 2007;22:807–11.

Amin AK, Patton JT, Cook RE, et al. Does obesity influence the clinical outcome at five years following total knee replacement for osteoarthritis? J Bone Joint Surg Br. 2006;88-B:335–40.

Batsis JA, Naessens JM, Keegan MT, et al. Body mass index and the impact on hospital resource use in patients undergoing total knee arthroplasty. J Arthroplasty. 2010;25:1250–7.

Biau D, Mullins MM, Judet T, et al. Is anyone too old for a total knee replacement? Clin Orthop. 2006;448:180–4.

Bourne R, Mukhi S, Zhu N, et al. Role of obesity on the risk for total hip or knee arthroplasty. Clin Orthop. 2007;465:185–8.

Brander V, Gondek S, Martin E, et al. Pain and depression influence outcome 5 years after knee replacement surgery. Clin Orthop. 2007;464:21–6.

Cross 3rd WW, Saleh KJ, Wilt TJ, et al. Agreement about indications for total knee arthroplasty. Clin Orthop. 2006;446:34–9.

Crowder AR, Duffy GP, Trousdale RT. Long-term results of total knee arthroplasty in young patients with rheumatoid arthritis. J Arthroplasty. 2005;20 Suppl 3:12–6.

Culliton SE, Bryant DM, Overend TJ, et al. The relationship between expectations in patients undergoing primary total knee arthroplasty. J Arthroplasty. 2012;27:490–2.

Della Valle CJ, Rosenberg AG. Indications for total knee arthroplasty. In: Callahan JJ, editor. The adult knee. 1st ed. Philadelphia, PA: Lippincott Williams & Wilkins; 2003. p. 1047–58.

Dewan A, Bertolusso R, Karastinos A, et al. Implant durability and knee function after total knee arthroplasty in the morbidly obese patient. J Arthroplasty. 2009;24:89–94.

Diduch DR, Insall JN, Scott WN, et al. Total knee replacement in young, active patients. J Bone Joint Surg Am. 1997;79-A:571–82.

Ellis EB, Howard KJ, Khaleel MA, et al. Effect of psychopathology on patient-perceived outcomes of total knee arthroplasty within an indigent population. J Bone Joint Surg Am. 2012;94-A:e84(1–8).

Fehring TK, Odum SM, Griffin WL, et al. The obesity epidemic: its effect on total joint arthroplasty. J Arthroplasty. 2007;22:71–6.

Foran JR, Mont MA, Etienne G, et al. The outcome of total knee arthroplasty in obese patients. J Bone Joint Surg Am. 2004;86-A:1609–15.

Foran JR, Mont MA, Rajadhyaksha AD, et al. Total knee arthroplasty in obese patients: a comparison with a matched control group. J Arthroplasty. 2004;19:817–24.

Gandhi R, Davey JR, Mahomed N. Patient expectations predict greater pain relief with joint arthroplasty. J Arthroplasty. 2009;24:716–21.

Gadinsky NE, Ehrhardt JK, Urband C, et al. Effect of body mass index on range of motion and manipulation after total knee arthroplasty. J Arthroplasty. 2011;26:1194–7.

Harwin SF. Indications and patient selection. In: Scuderi GR, editor. Surgical techniques in total knee arthroplasty. 1st ed. New York, NY: Springer; 2002. p. 3–8.

Hepinstall MS, Rutledge JR, Bornstein LJ, et al. Factors that impact expectations before total knee arthroplasty. J Arthroplasty. 2011;26:870–6.

Hernandez-Vaquero D, Fernandez-Carreira JM, Perez-Hernandez D, et al. Total knee arthroplasty in the elderly. Is there an age limit? J Arthroplasty. 2006;21:358–61.

Huddleston JI, Maloney WJ, Wang Y, et al. Adverse events after total knee arthroplasty: a national Medicare study. J Arthroplasty. 2009;24:95–100.

Kerkhoffs GM, Servien E, Dunn W, et al. The influence of obesity on the complication rate and outcome of total knee arthroplasty: a meta-analysis and systemic literature review. J Bone Joint Surg Am. 2012;94-A:1839–44.

Leclere LE, Sechriest 2nd VF, Holley KG, et al. Tuberculous arthritis of the knee treated with two-stage total knee arthroplasty. A case report. J Bone Joint Surg Am. 2009;91-A:186–91.

Lingard EA, Katz JN, Wright EA, et al. Predicting the outcome of total knee arthroplasty. J Bone Joint Surg Am. 2004;86-A:2179–86.

Lingard EA, Riddle DL. Impact of psychological distress on pain and function following knee arthroplasty. J Bone Joint Surg Am. 2007;89-A:1161–9.

Long MJ, McQueen DA, Bangalore VG, et al. Using self-assessed health to predict patient outcomes after total knee arthroplasty. Clin Orthop. 2005;434:189–92.

Lotke PA. Primary total knees. Standard principles and techniques. In: Lotke PA, editor. Master techniques in orthopedic surgery. Knee arthroplasty. 1st ed. New York, NY: Raven; 1995. p. 65–6.

Manley M, Ong K, Lau E, et al. Total knee arthroplasty survivorship in the United States Medicare population: effect of hospital and surgeon procedure volume. J Arthroplasty. 2009;24:1061–7.

Meding JB, Klay M, Healy A, et al. The prescreening history and physical in elective total joint arthroplasty. J Arthroplasty. 2007;22:21–3.

Memtsoudis SG, Della Valle AG, Besculides MC, et al. Risk factors for perioperative mortality after lower extremity arthroplasty: a population-based study of 6,901,324 patient discharges. J Arthroplasty. 2010;25:19–26.

Mont MA, Mathur SK, Krackow KA, et al. Cementless total knee arthroplasty in obese patients. A comparison with a matched control group. J Arthroplasty. 1996;11:153–6.

Mont MA, Myers TH, Krackow KA, et al. Total knee arthroplasty for corticosteroid associated avascular necrosis of the knee. Clin Orthop. 1997;338:124–30.

Noble PC, Conditt MA, Cook KF, et al. Patient expectations affect satisfaction with total knee arthroplasty. Clin Orthop. 2006; 452:35–43.

Pagnano MW, McLamb LA, Trousdale RT. Total knee arthroplasty for patients 90 years of age and older. Clin Orthop. 2004;418:179–83.

Perka C, Arnold U, Buttgereit F. Influencing factors on perioperative morbidity in knee arthroplasty. Clin Orthop. 2003;378:183–9.

Riddle DL, Wade JB, Jiranek WA, et al. Preoperative pain catastrophizing predicts pain outcome after knee arthroplasty. Clin Orthop. 2010;468:798–806.

Robertsson O, Dunbar M, Pehrsson T, et al. Patient satisfaction after knee arthroplasty. A report on 27,372 knees operated on between 1981 and 1995 in Sweden. Acta Orthop Scand. 2000;71:262–7.

Saleh KJ, Sherman P, Katkin P, et al. Total knee arthroplasty after open reduction and internal fixation of fractures of the tibial plateau: a minimum five-year follow-up study. J Bone Joint Surg Am. 2001;83-A:1144–8.

Scott CE, Howie CR, MacDonald D, et al. Predicting dissatisfaction following total knee replacement: a prospective study of 1217 patients. J Bone Joint Surg Br. 2010;92-B:1253–8.

Scott W, Alpert SW, Koval KJ, et al. Neuropathic arthropathy: a review of current knowledge. J Am Acad Orthop Surg. 1996;4:100–8.

Soudry M, Binazzi R, Johanson NA, et al. Total knee arthroplasty in Charcot and Charcot-like joints. Clin Orthop. 1986;208:199–204.

Stern H, Insall JN. Total knee arthroplasty in obese patients. J Bone Joint Surg Am. 1990;72-A:1400–4.

Vince KG, Insall JN, Bannerman CE. Total knee arthroplasty in the patient with Parkinson's disease. J Bone Joint Surg Br. 1989;71-B:51–4.

2 Implant Selection

Most of the surgeons would agree that the surgical technique itself is the most important prognostic factor for TKA. However, there may be some flaws in the designs or the materials used in TKA prosthesis which can lead to a poor prognosis and early TKA failure. Even if these prostheses do not have any problem, the operation can be difficult and outcomes can be poor if an inappropriate implant is selected for the patient.

It was a general and traditional concept to adopt a graduated system for implant selection, and the selection of prosthesis was made gradually based on the severity of the lesion. For example, a unicondylar prosthesis was used in single-compartment arthritis, whereas a hinged prosthesis was used in the most severely degenerated and deformed knees. But with the development of implants and surgical techniques, implant selection is now done according to the surgeon's choice if arthritic change, deformity, or instability is not extreme.

No matter which type of prostheses is used, *the material should have certain strength and should offer biocompatibility and durability. Also, the implants should be designed such that they are compatible with the mechanics of artificial joint and should allow the performance of the operation with ease.* If possible, the implants should provide various options for their use in special situations and they should cause little problems during revision surgery.

It is difficult to know at a glance which implant satisfies all these requirements since the implants show quite different results in the in vitro and in vivo studies. Generally, it is recommended to select those implants that have *sound theoretical background, provide good long-term clinical results, and are familiar to the surgeon.*

Here, I would like to provide information on the materials and designs of implants, bone cement, and surgical instruments used in TKA.

2.1 Material

Materials include metals for the femoral and tibial components, recently developed ceramics, polyethylene (PE) for the patella and spacers, and bone cement for fixation. These materials are produced through sufficient testing in each manufacturer's laboratory. *However, even if the materials have been proved to be excellent in an in vitro study, quite different outcomes can be resulted clinically after application of the implant to the patients.* Barrack stated that it is important to understand the properties of these materials because the laboratory results do not always correspond to the clinical results.

2.1.1 Metal

The metals which are used in prostheses should be biocompatible, should have enough strength to endure the load, and should not corrode under physiological conditions. Most of the metals used in the human body are alloys. These are iron-based stainless steel alloy, cobalt chrome-based alloy, titanium-based alloy, zirconium-based alloy, and tantalum.

The properties of metals such as strength, durability, and biocompatibility are determined according to their composition and structure. These properties can be changed by various manufacturing processes applied to the metal.

Metal is a kind of crystal and is formed into various alloys to improve its natural properties. Alloys can be made by adding very small interstitial atoms (C, O, N, etc.) or little larger substitutional atoms (Mn, Al, V, etc.) to the basic metal. Application of heat to disperse the substitutional atoms uniformly is called precipitation hardening. *Metal can be processed through hot working and cold working. Hot working alters its shape and solidifies the internal bonding by*

W. Cho, *Knee Joint Arthroplasty*,
DOI 10.1007/978-3-642-39389-1_2, © Springer-Verlag Berlin Heidelberg 2014

Table 2.1 Changes in properties according to the metal grain or crystal size

	Increase in metal grain or crystal size
Ductility	↑
Toughness	↓
Strength	↓
Young's modulus	↓
Tensile strength	↓

reducing grain sizes. The outcomes vary according to the temperature and time. *Cold working reduces dislocation of metal crystals by strengthening the bonding between crystals, thereby improving yield strength and reducing ductility* (Table 2.1).

Strength is also affected by the method in which implants are fabricated. *Most implants used in orthopedic surgery are fabricated by casting, machining, or forging*. Since casting may not ensure an even grain size, it can decrease the strength of the implant. Even in the best implant material, the Young's modulus can be changed if the metal has defects during the manufacturing or fabrication, and even a 0.2 % of defect in the metal can affect its strength.

Fatigue and corrosion is closely related with durability. Fatigue strength is the break point of the material at which cracks develop under repeated constant impact of 10^7 cycles. Fatigue strength is closely related to how the metal is used (strength and direction of force) and defects in the metal, along with property of the metal. *Corrosion is oxidative degradation of the metal and is caused by the electrochemical dissolution phenomenon and wear, or the synergy of both. It is rapidly accelerated when the metal breaks. The corrosion of the metal inserted into the human body has two effects: first, it reduces the implant strength, and second, the materials or ions generated by corrosion induce bone loss and inflammatory reactions* around the implants. Corrosion may occur focally or on the whole metal surface. When exposed to air or saline, *a very thin 2–10 nm passive film is formed on the outermost surface of the metal by oxidation of metal elements*. This passive film serves as the barrier that prevents corrosion and release of metal ions. Stainless steel forms FeO, Fe_2O_3, and Cr_2O_3 (if there is Cr), while cobalt chromium forms Cr_2O_3 and titanium forms TiO_2. *The strength of this passive film and the bonding of this film with the main metal greatly affect the extent of corrosion*. In order to reduce corrosion, metal is dipped in aqueous nitrogen or the surface is treated during manufacturing in order to increase the strength of this passive film.

Biocompatibility is affected by either the wear particles or materials generated by corrosion or both. These materials either spread to the entire body through the blood circulation *to cause tissue damage or immune reaction or are deposited focally to evoke inflammatory reactions, tissue destruction, and tumor formation*. These reactions are different according to the type of the metal, duration of exposure, and amount and size of wear particles.

2.1.1.1 Stainless Steel

Stainless steel is an iron-based alloy and is of many types according to the strengthening method used by addition of nitrogen or manganese, or according to the manufacturing process. It is mainly used in the plate and screws for fracture treatment. In the past, *stainless steel has also been used in artificial joints, but it is no longer used for this purpose since it is not as reliable as cobalt chromium or titanium*.

2.1.1.2 Cobalt Chromium

This alloy is very strong and resistant to corrosion but tends to lose its strength as the grain size becomes irregular when the implants are made by casting. It has low ductility and strong resistance to wear, but this means that it is hard to machine during the fabrication process. Molybdenum (Mo), carbon, nickel, silicon, or iron is added to this metal to strengthen its properties. Vitallium contains Mo; addition of 2–3 % Mo reduces pitting and corrosion.

2.1.1.3 Titanium

Pure titanium is only used to obtain porous coating since it has low strength. Currently aluminum–vanadium–titanium ($Ti–Al_6–V_4$) alloy is generally applied to the human body in the orthopedic field because *it has excellent biocompatibility as it does not evoke inflammatory and toxic reactions, and it is strong and has high fatigue strength*. Its elastic modulus is about half of that of cobalt chromium and this helps in distributing the load imposed on the implants to the bones so as to reduce bony resorption caused by stress shielding. However, titanium alloy has a *poor mechanism of passive film formation that prevents corrosion in the body compared to that with cobalt chromium. It is no more used in the femoral component of knee joints, as it causes wear problems when articulated with PE.*

2.1.1.4 Zirconium

Zirconium is a metal similar to titanium. Zirconium alloy containing 2.5 % niobium (Zr-2.5Nb) has fatigue strength similar to that of cobalt chromium. When the oxygen diffusion method is applied to zirconium, its surface gets transformed into approximately 5 μm thickness of zirconia (OxZr), which is ceramic in nature. In other words, the main part remains metallic in nature, while the surface changes into a ceramic component which reduces surface wear. Hence, surface fragmentation develops when it is sterilized by heating.

This ceramic has superior abrasive/adhesive wear performance than other metals. It is reported that zirconia can reduce the abrasive/adhesive PE wear by 40–90 % compared to cobalt chromium. Ezzet et al. reported that an oxidized zirconium femoral component could significantly reduce PE

Table 2.2 Comparison of properties of the materials used in the tibial and femoral components

	Stainless steel	Cobalt chromium	Ti–Al_6–V_4	Ceramics
Corrosion resistance	4th	3rd	2nd	1st
Young's modulus	3rd	2nd	4th	1st
Yield strength	2nd	1st	2nd	4th
Ductility	1st	2nd	3rd	4th
Hardness	3rd	2nd	4th	1st

1st (=highest) > 2nd > 3rd > 4th (=lowest)
Yield strength of stainless steel and Ti–Al_6–V_4 is similar

wear under simulated conditions of athletically active patients with modestly malaligned TKA prostheses. *But wear of the knee joint is mainly the delamination wear, which is different from the abrasive/adhesive wear. Thus it is uncertain whether zirconia reduces the wear rate in the knee joint.* Hui et al. reported no significant differences in the clinical, subjective, and radiographic outcomes with the use of zirconia femoral components. In a 5-year follow-up study, Kim also reported that there were no differences in size, weight, and shape of wear particles between cobalt chrome and zirconia. However, there were no adverse effects associated with the use of oxidized zirconium femoral implants.

2.1.1.5 Tantalum

It is a kind of biomaterial that offers several potential advantages over commonly used metals in the human body, including low stiffness, high porosity, and high coefficient of friction. Tantalum surface also has the effect to increase host white blood cell activation and lower bacterial adherence.

The elastic modulus of this metal is similar to that of the bone. Bony ingrowth occurs when 80 % porosity is maintained. It is mainly used as trabecular system in a contained defect and in prefixed tibial plate with PE.

2.1.1.6 Interaction Between Metals

When two different implants are used in the same site, if possible, the same metals should be used so as to reduce galvanic corrosion. Galvanic corrosion occurs due to electrochemical shift between metals. *Galvanic corrosion is more prominent between stainless steel and cobalt chromium, and between stainless steel and titanium. It is minimal between cobalt chromium and titanium.*

2.1.2 Ceramic

Ceramic has a stable surface and its wear is less as it has a low coefficient of friction. *Ceramics used in the human body are the oxidative form of aluminum (OxAl) or zirconium (OxZr) derivatives. Ceramic is chemically stable as it does not undergo oxidative degeneration. Ceramic has good biocompatibility and excellent strength and is particularly resistant to corrosion and fatigue. Also, its elastic modulus is close to that of bones, so load transmission to the bones is more gradual than that of metals.* The zirconia-based ceramic is less brittle and less stiff than the alumina-based ceramic. Another benefit is that the bone can grow into the surface pores of the ceramic. Due to these benefits, it has been used in the hip joint prosthesis since the 1960s.

However, it is difficult to use ceramic in the knee joint prosthesis because the knee joint has more complex biomechanics and structural congruency than the hip joint. *And ceramic has to be fixed without bone cement.* As a result, it causes problems of *migration* into the acetabulum in the hip joint, and same problems occur *in the tibial side*. Onishi reported that when ceramic was used in the knee joint, *the major cause of failure was loosening of the tibial component*, not due to the chemical reaction but due to the mechanical factors. Therefore, in order to ensure stable fixation, fabrication of a metal-backed ceramic is currently under investigation.

Ceramic is strong against primary compressive forces but is weak against tensile and shear forces. Also, it is brittle due to low ductility. When a cyclic force is applied, it can undergo a microfracture. Moreover, it may be hard to achieve homogeneity during fabrication, since it is difficult to control the grain size. The ceramic may pose problems during sterilization as it is weak against heat. Although it does not cause much wear if it articulates with PE, the zirconia–zirconia articulation dramatically increases the wear (Table 2.2).

2.1.3 Polyethylene (Ultrahigh Molecular Weight Polyethylene: UHMWPE, PE)

2.1.3.1 History

Various materials have been used since artificial joints were introduced in the late nineteenth century. Hey-Groves used ivory in the femoral head prosthesis in 1922. Judet used synthetic polymer for the first time in 1936, but it caused problems of wear and loosening. In 1958, Charnley used polytetrafluoroethylene (PTFE; known as Teflon, but not strictly Teflon), but it was replaced with HMWPE (high molecular weight polyethylene) due to its weakness against creep deformity and abrasive wear. Currently, UHMWPE (ultra HMWPE) is used. Other similar products include polyacetal and polyester. Polyacetal was used in the early products as it has high yield strength and is easy to

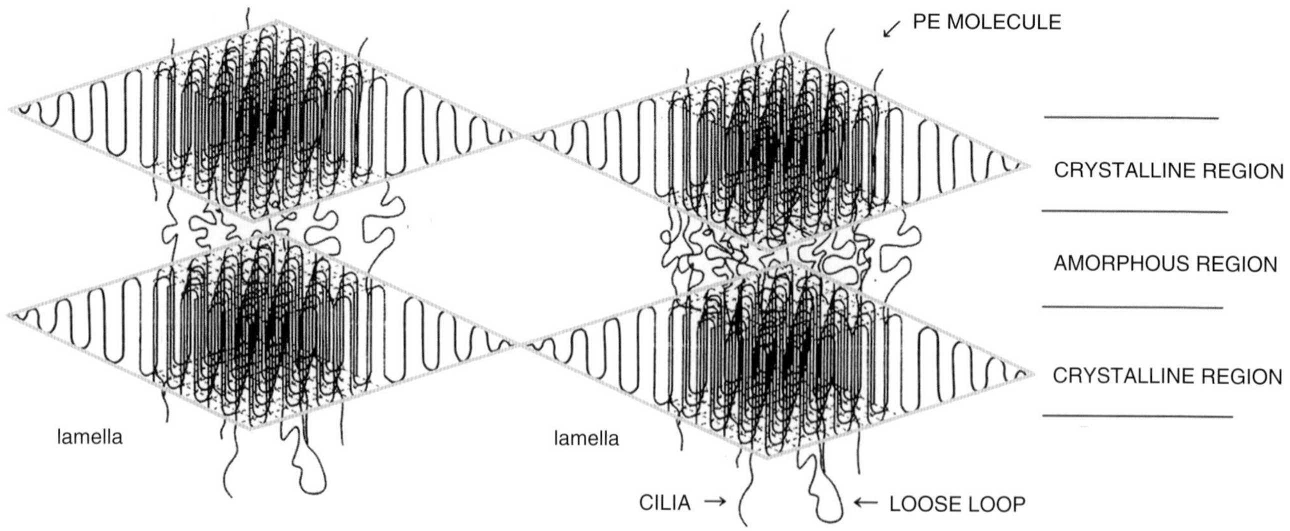

Fig. 2.1 Schematic figure of polyethylene

manufacture, but it is only used in trials currently due to its high failure rate. Polyester is not used now because it causes bone resorption.

2.1.3.2 Polyethylene (PE) in TKA

In TKA, PE is used as a spacer between the tibia and femur and as a patellar component. The mechanical strength of PE is weaker than that of metal or ceramic, but *PE has the advantage of high corrosion resistance, high elasticity, and flexibility*, which make it possible to make various forms of PE. Good PE should be easy to manufacture, inexpensive, not easily damaged, durable, and biocompatible.

The most common complication of recent artificial implants is the wear, and a lot of research have been undergoing to reduce the wear of PE. *The factors that affect long-term implant survival and good performance of PE include molecular weight, manufacturing process, sterilizing method, cross-linking, and the properties of materials articulating with PE.*

Properties

The properties of PE are closely related to its molecular weight which is correlated with the number of branches of ethylene radicals (C_2H_4). *The molecular weight of PE is calculated by multiplication of the number of ethylene radicals.*

UHMWPE is produced by polymerization of ethylene and its *molecular weight is 2–6 million*, which is much higher than the molecular weight of high-density polyethylene (50,000–200,000). *Due to its high molecular weight, UHMWPE has an excellent impact strength, toughness, and resistance to abrasion wear*. Hence, it is used in the site where a high abrasion resistance is required such as the bottoms of the skis or snow mobiles.

Properties of PE are also affected by its structure. *PE is a form of semicrystalline polymer, meaning that it has crystals and amorphous component*. PE originally has longer chains and can hardly form crystals. Its crystal content is determined by its molecular weight and the manufacturing temperature. Synthetic PE generally contains 58–75 % of crystals and its crystallization is altered when it is heated beyond its melting point. This crystal is the smallest structural unit of PE and gathers to form a lamella of about 10 nm in size, which determines the properties of PE (Fig. 2.1).

With high crystallization, its elastic modulus and yield strength increase along with an improvement in resistance to creep deformity and fatigue strength. Hence, many attempts have been made to improve its crystallization. One of them has been the addition of carbon. This type of PE has improved resistance against compressive and tensile forces and has higher creep resistance. However it is no longer used in artificial joints because it is difficult to mold, has low fatigue resistance, and has a high probability of surface damage. A product called Hylamer was introduced that improved crystallization using a completely different method, and improved the elastic modulus by 375 % and tensile yield strength by 30 %. However, this product had a limited commercial use because it easily underwent oxidative degradation under gamma radiation sterilization, and caused eccentric wear and rim fracture due to the design problem. Recently, vitamin E-containing PE has been introduced to prevent oxidative degradation. Haider et al. reported that the vitamin E-stabilized material had minimal changes and exhibited 73 % to 86 % reduction in wear for both CR and PS TKA prostheses.

Manufacturing

When ethylene is polymerized, it turns into a fine granular white powder. Small amounts of titanium chloride ($TiCl_4$) and aluminum are added during the polymerization process.

Four to six bar pressure is imposed at 66–80 °C to maximize the molecular weight and any particles larger than 500 μm are filtered out.

There are three methods to produce polyethylene. First is the direct molding method, which comprises of adding powder into a mold and applying pressure to it. The advantage of this method is that it is possible to make complex shapes of PE in one step and create a very smooth surface. The drawback of this method is that it is expensive due to the time-consuming process and the properties of PE can be affected by the molding conditions. Second is the ram-extruding method. Powder is poured into a cylinder and heat is applied. After that, PE is pushed out to produce a cylindrical PE of 1–6 in. in diameter, which is carved into the desired shape. Third is making compression-molded PE sheets of about 8 × 8 × 8 cm in size and then modifying them into the desired shape by machining (Fig. 2.2). But the products obtained by machining may have surface irregularities.

Recently, the annealing or remelting process has been added to the process of manufacturing PE in order to reduce

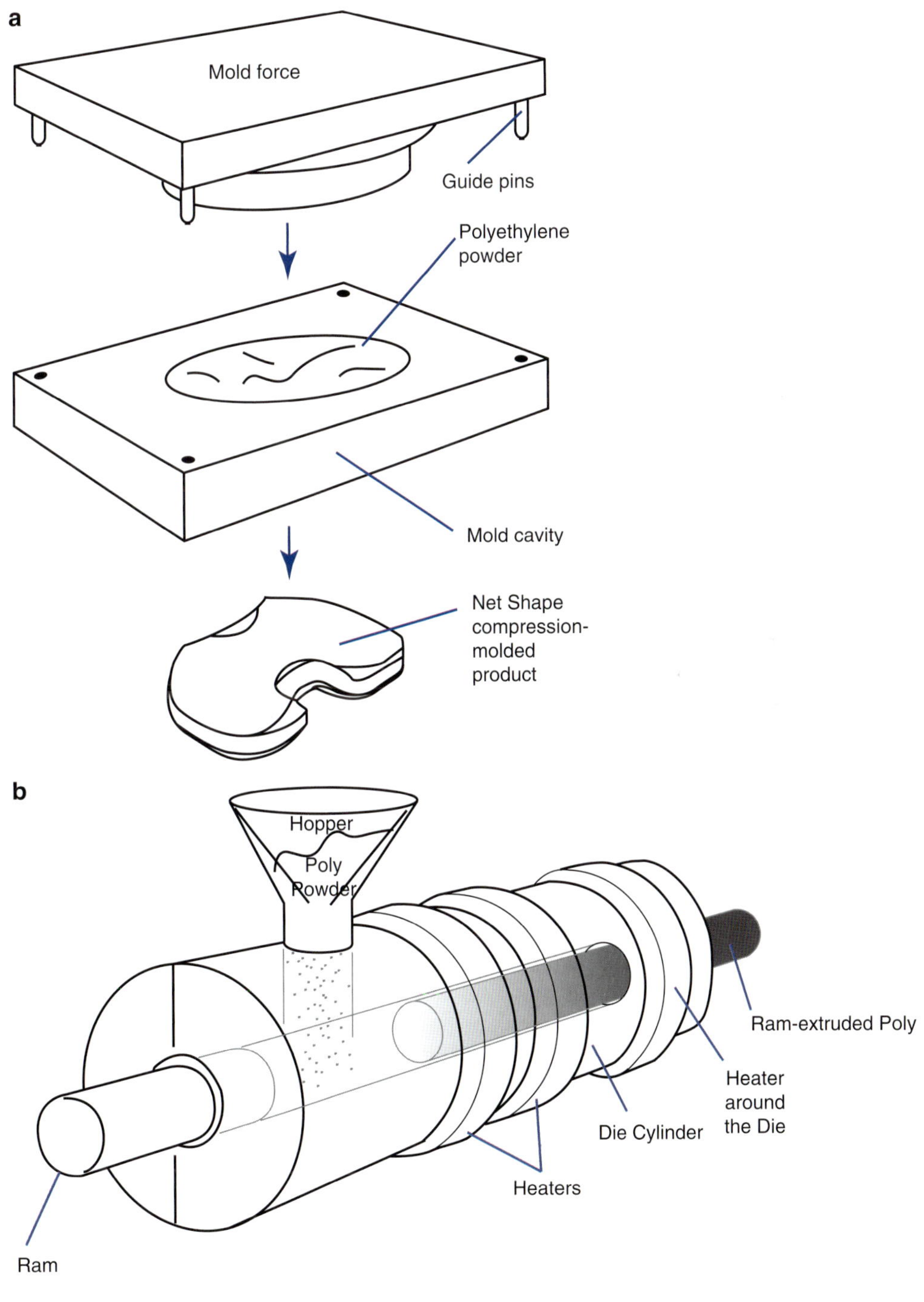

Fig. 2.2 Manufacturing of polyethylene (Courtesy of Zimmer, Warsaw, IN). (**a**) Direct molding (net shape), (**b**) Ram extrusion, (**c**) Compression-molded sheet machined into final parts

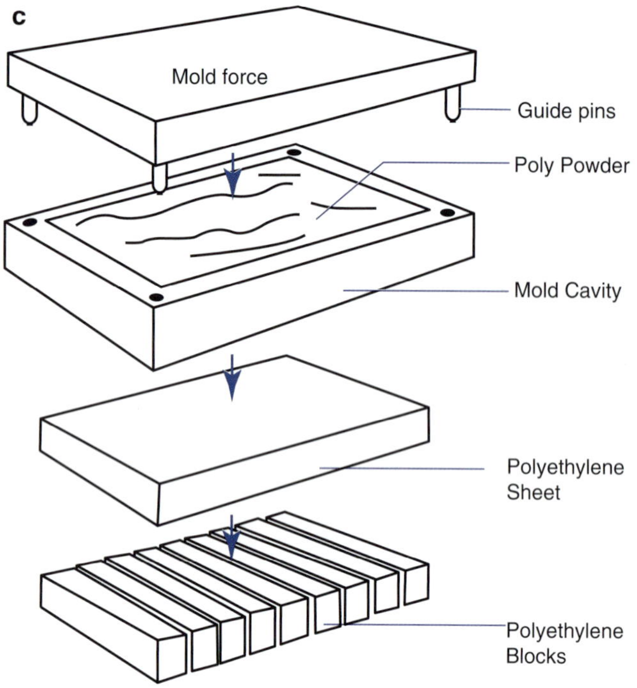

Fig. 2.2 (continued)

the surface wear, improve the resistance to fatigue, and decrease oxidation. *Annealing process involves heating the PE at a temperature below its melting point. With this process, the crystallinity and properties of PE are maintained, while the defect of PE is decreased. Remelting process involves heating beyond the melting point (135–138 °C) of PE.* The properties of PE can be changed by the remelting process. *This process reduces the free radicals which are related to oxidative degradation.*

Cross-linking of the PE unit can occur by changes in the amount and method of irradiation and by remelting process. When cross-linking occurs, the properties of PE change and it becomes more stiff and more resistant to the surface wear. Recently, *the 3rd generation of highly cross-linked PE (HXPE or X3) has been introduced. Its superiority has been proven in the laboratory tests and in the hip joint prosthesis. However, more experimental studies and more observations are needed for its clinical application in the knee joint prosthesis.*

Sterilization and Storage

The properties of PE change according to the method of sterilization and storage. Oxidation occurs during these procedures and long-term survival of PE is affected by oxidative degradation.

If PE is irradiated by gamma rays, the stable polymers become oxidized and *carbon is transformed into the reactive form.*

This reactive form undergoes one of the following three processes:

1. *Recombination* to return to its original state
2. *Chain scission* is that the chain breaks to *degrade into high-density polyethylene* with reduced molecular weight and elastic modulus and increase the wear rate
3. *Cross-linking*, in which two polymer chains undergo chemical bonding (Fig. 2.3)

These three processes are affected by the amount of irradiation and the presence of oxygen during sterilization. When PE is irradiated with 3.0 Mrad in the presence of oxygen, cross-linking does not occur and the quality of PE is degraded. When PE is irradiated with 4.0 Mrad in vacuum, cross-linking occurs. Also, when PE is irradiated with 5.0–10.0 Mrad, cross-linking does not occur, but the strength improves. Therefore, most of the manufacturers have used a different method of sterilization to reduce the degradation of PE. They sterilize PE either in vacuum or in argon gas during gamma radiation. Either EO gas (ethylene oxide) or gas plasma sterilization method is also used. MacDonald examined retrieved 20 EO gas sterilized PE and reported that the PE remained stable with respect to both oxidative and mechanical properties for up to 10 years in vivo, and there was no evidence of delamination. However, Medel et al. reported that gamma sterilization in inert gas did not provide PE with a significant improvement in terms of wear resistance as compared with gamma sterilization in air, except for a lower incidence of delamination. However, EO gas sterilization is not effective for metal-backed implants since the penetration of EO gas to the metal is weak. In the gas plasma sterilization method, microenergy and gas are used. According to McNulty et al., this method does not break the polymer chains or generate free radicals that cause PE oxidation. However, *gamma irradiation under vacuum is still the most popular method of sterilization.*

After storage for a long duration, a white line is formed at about 1–2 mm from the surface of PE and this is a type of aggregation of the fracture line. This white line is *closely related to the exposure time to the air* and it is a common finding in case of PE that has been *stored on a shelf for more than 4 years.* Generally, the white line is known to indicate degradation of the quality of products, but some surgeons state that it does not affect the survival of PE implants or incidence of osteolysis in the hip joint. However, Barrack emphasized that this *white line can be critical for the knee joints*, since PE in the knee joint prosthesis is mostly under shear force as opposed to that in the acetabular cups of the hip joints. Also, oxidative degradation can occur in vivo as time elapses.

Cross-Linking

Cross-linking occurs when the amount of gamma radiation is increased to a little higher level than what is needed for

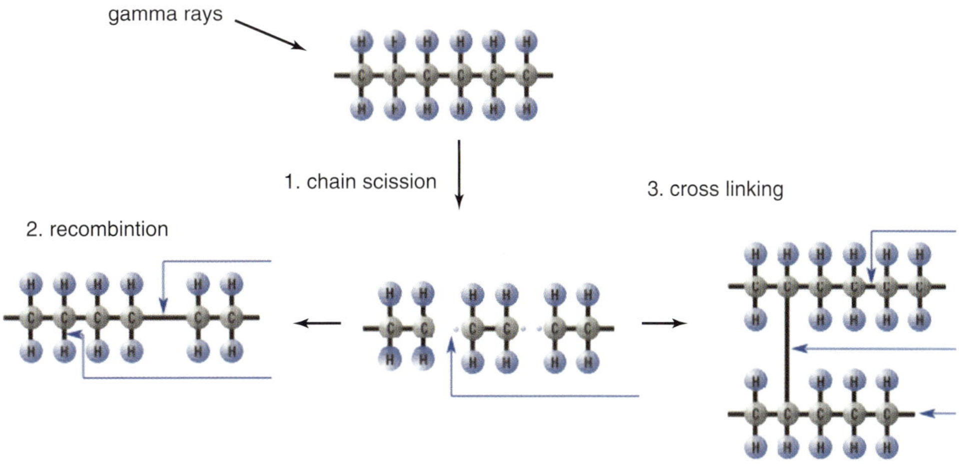

Fig. 2.3 Changes after irradiation of PE

sterilization in oxygen-free condition and thermal stabilization is applied afterwards. More cross-linking makes the PE stiffer and more resistant to abrasive/adhesive wear, but resistance to fatigue failure decreases due to the reduction in elastic modularity.

In the laboratory, *the wear decreases dramatically*, resistance to fatigue crack propagation and ultimate tensile strength increases, and fracture toughness improves as well. But, *a strong resistance to wear means that the size of the wear particles becomes smaller, and these smaller particles are more likely to cause inflammatory reaction and osteolysis*.

In the hip joint prosthesis, cross-linked PE has been used for the acetabular cups with promising results, but *it has not been proven that this PE has a longer survival rate than the conventional PE in the knee joint*. TKA is different from THA in several aspects; the hip joint is a ball-and-socket joint in which the forces are distributed evenly to cause abrasive/adhesive wear, whereas *wear of the knee joints is mainly pitting and delamination wear due to eccentric forces and repeated trauma. A stiff cross-linked PE can be more problematic in the knee joint prosthesis*. Furthermore, the incidence of loosening of the knee joint prosthesis is increased and a fracture may occur at the post of the PS type or lugs of the patella. Therefore, its use in the knee joint prosthesis is limited to the mobile-bearing joint, and further observation is needed in the fixed-bearing joint.

2.1.4 Bone Cement (Polymethylmethacrylate, PMMA)

Bone cement is the most frequently used material to fix the prosthesis to the bone. It was applied in cranioplasty and for replacement of the head of the femur by Judet. Charnley used polymethylmethacrylate, which has been used in temporary dentures, to fix the femoral stems into the bone marrow cavity.

2.1.4.1 Role of Bone Cement and Its Relevant Theories

The primary purpose of using bone cement is to enhance stability of the implants by increasing the bone–implant contact area and to absorb shock by evenly distributing the load. When the implants are not securely fixed to the bones, they can become loose. Loosening can occur either between the cement and the bone or between the cement and the implant, but it can sometimes occur at both the interfaces.

The factors that are involved in loosening are penetration of cement into the bones, the strength of bone cement, the bonding strength between cement and implants, and the forces transmitted to the implants. The bonding strength is affected by the properties of bone cement, the timing of cementing, the pressure applied to fix the cement, the presence of a foreign body, and the quality of the bone.

The bonding strength between cement and bone is dependent on the micro-interlock obtained by cement penetration into the bone. Miller et al. stated that bonding strength of low-viscosity cement is inferior. If the implant is not securely fixed to the bone, it will cause loosening or accelerate loosening by causing a fracture at the bone–cement interface.

With respect to stability between bone cement and implants, many authors believe that *bone cement enhances stability of the implants by positioning the implants in the right location rather than a glue action*. Jasty et al. reported the results of a retrieval study of THA which indicates that the first step in loosening is the separation between the implants and bone cement at an early postoperative period and followed by slowly progresses to a fracture at the bone–cement interface and loosening between the bone cement and the bone in that order. Fornasier and Cameron reported five cases of hip retrieval study which demonstrated that the loosening

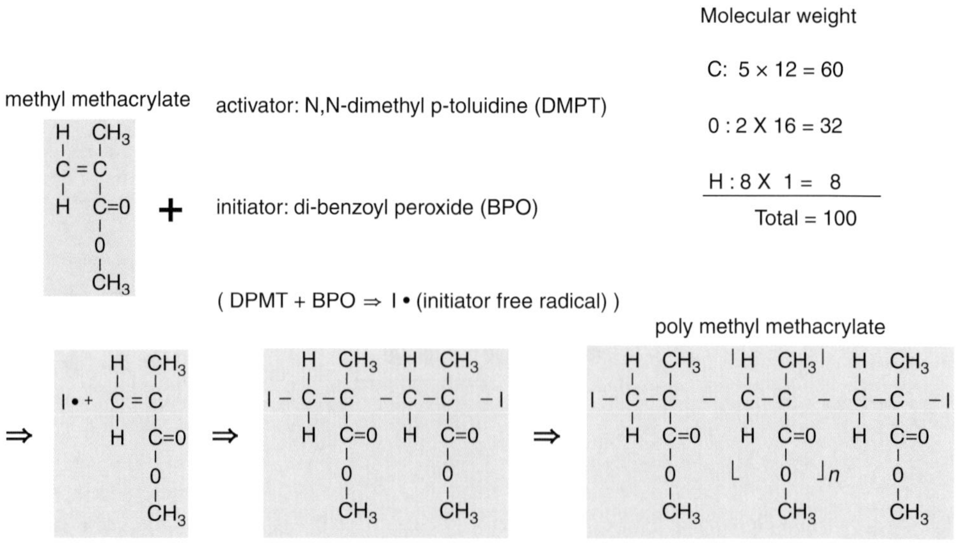

Fig. 2.4 Basic structure of methylmethacrylate and illustration of its activation

occurred between the bone cement and implants in all cases, and the gap was filled with fibrous membranes. They assumed that the gaps are created by hammering during the curing stage of bone cement, the stem returns to its original size from its expanded size due to the heat generated during the setting of cement, or there is a decrease in bone cement volume by about 2 % after curing.

On the other hand, Davis and Harris emphasized the *glue action of bone cement* and Ahmed et al. stated that the implants begin to move when they lose their bonding with the bone cement. Bonding force is related to the properties of cement, surface treatment of implants, timing of cementing, and curing temperature. Cho et al. reported the results of bonding strength of CMW (DePuy Ltd. Blackpool, UK) and Simplex P (Stryker-Howmedica-Osteonics, Allendale, NJ) cement to the implants in an in vitro study, which suggested that *bonding strength between implant and cement was markedly decreased at 5–6 min after mixing of the polymer and monomer*. Pittman et al. reported that bonding is weaker when the surface is smooth and *it is stronger when* the surface *is precoated or roughly finished*. In comparison between titanium and cobalt chrome, titanium provided stronger bonds, but the difference was not statistically significant.

Bone cement volume decreases after curing, and bonding strength between the bone cement and implants decreases. So, the greater the change in bone cement volume, the greater the decrease in bonding strength.

A composite unit of bone cement and implants is formed as a result of this bond which enhances the strength of implants. However, it has to be reconsidered whether stronger bonds between the bone cement and implant are clinically desirable, because a stronger bond increases the stress between the cement and the bone causing the cement to loosen from the bones.

Stability is also affected by the forces applied to the implants. It is known that *stability of cemented implants is the strongest against compressive force followed by that against shear force and tensile force in that order.*

2.1.4.2 Composition

PMMA is a type of polymer similar to PE, polyvinyl chloride (PVC), and polystyrene. It comprises of a *series of carbon units whose molecular weight is 100* and has chains with variable lengths (Fig. 2.4).

The length of the chain varies according to the manufacturing process and the amount of initiator and activator included in bone cement. It is known that with a longer length of the chain, the *PMMA molecular weight increases, the properties of bone cement improve, and the viscosity of PMMA increases.*

The bone cement packet contains prepolymerized solid particles (so-called polymer) in powder form and liquid monomer. This powder contains copolymer and dibenzoyl peroxide (BPO, BP), which is the initiator. Liquid monomer contains hydroquinone that prevents the monomer from being converted into polymers, along with activator N, N-dimethyl-p-toluidine (DMPT). Each product of prepolymerized powder varies in the grain size, molecular weight, and chain length. When polymerization occurs, PMMA size becomes between 30 and 150 nm and *molecular weight becomes between 20,000 and 2,000,000 with an average molecular weight of 170,000.*

Barium sulfate ($BaSO_4$) or zirconium oxide (ZrO_2) may be added to allow better visualization on X-ray.

2.1.4.3 Heat Generation

When the polymer in powder form is mixed with the monomer in liquid form, the activator (DMPT) in the liquid and the initiator (BPO) in the powder are mixed together to generate free radical initiators (I∘), which convert the double bonds of carbon in methylmethacrylate into single bonds for polymerization with the monomers. This process of *polym-*

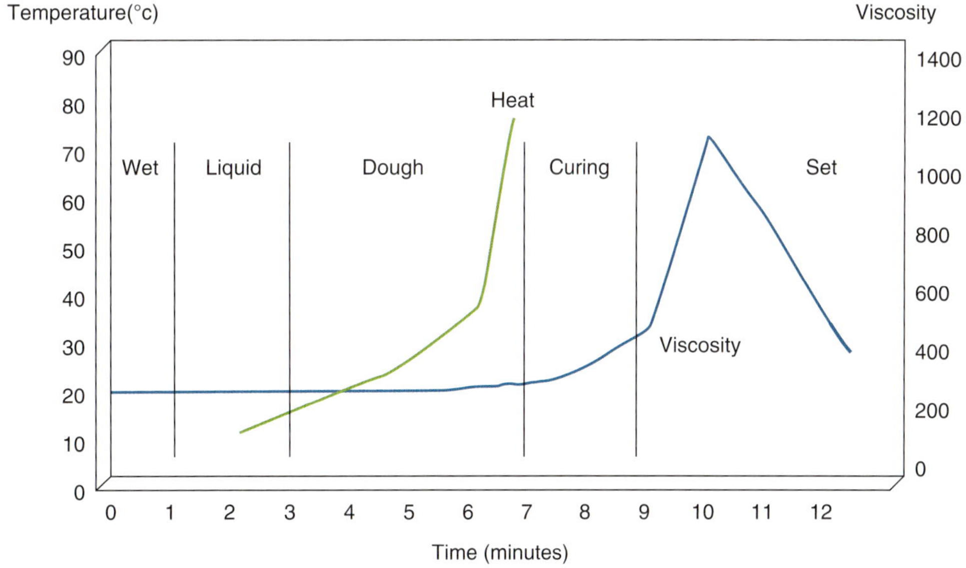

Fig. 2.5 Relationship between heat and viscosity according to the time sequence during polymerization of bone cement (CMW)

erization generates heat. About 130 cal of heat is generated per 1 g of monomer; and about 2,600 cal of heat is generated per 20 g of liquid monomers.

Heat generation during the operation varies according to the type of bone cement, dispersion of heat to the surrounding tissues, the amount and the thickness of bone cement, and the initial temperature (before mixing). In the laboratory, an average 66–82.5 °C of heat was generated. *The temperature reaches 60 °C with the use of 3 mm thick cement and 107 °C with the use of 10 mm thick cement*. However, *in the operation field, a temperature of 40–43 °C is generated* since the metal implants diffuse the heat, the bones are wet, there is blood, and saline is used to cool down the temperature. *This temperature is lower than 56 °C at which protein denaturation occurs and is lower than 47 °C at which thermal necrosis of the bones occurs.*

2.1.4.4 Stages of Cementing

The stages of cementing can be divided according to the time sequence after mixing. When the powder and the liquid are mixed, the powder and the liquid first form lumps (*wetting stage*). *Wetting of the prepolymeric powder with the liquid monomers generates free radical initiators by the action of BPO and DMPT.*

After the wetting stage, the mixture enters the *liquid stage*. The cement is in a homogeneous liquid form with a relatively low viscosity. In this stage, the mixture can be poured and easily transferred to a cement gun.

Chemical reaction for polymerization begins at this stage and the mixture reaches the *dough stage*. In this stage, polymers with chains of various lengths are formed in the mixture. In the dough stage, the mixture does not form strings or adhere to surgical gloves, and the polymerized cement volume increases slightly and it generates heat. As polymerization progresses, the mixture undergoes curing (*curing stage*), and finally, complete setting (*setting stage*) takes place.

The amount of polymers formed is affected by several factors including the ratio of liquid and powder, the concentrations of BPO and DMPT, grain size, and temperature during mixing. However, it is known that about 1.4 % of monomers remain in the cement even at 4 months after setting, and bone cement becomes even harder as the amount of monomers decreases.

Temperature plays an important role in the speed of polymerization. High temperature accelerates the speed of polymerization. Therefore, it is recommended to cool down the temperature so as to extend the setting time. The setting time is also delayed by about 1 min when humidity is increased by 20 %. On the other hand, the setting time is shortened by vacuum mixing.

The 3–7 min of the dough stage is actually very important in cementing technique and the method of cementing differs according to the viscosity of cement. CMW®-1 (DePuy Ltd., Blackpool, UK) has the highest viscosity, followed by Palacos® (Heraeus Medical, Wehrheim, Germany), Simplex P® (Stryker-Howmedica-Osteonics, Allendale, NJ), and LVC® (Zimmer, Inc., Warsaw, Indiana). Therefore, it is easier to use CMW® and Palacos® with the hands, but not with the cement gun. On the other hand, LVC® has a very low viscosity and is suitable for use with the cement gun. Simplex P® has medium viscosity and may be used with the cement gun (Fig. 2.5).

2.1.4.5 Strength

The strength of bone cement varies according to the molecular weight, grain size, the ratio of polymers and monomers, method of sterilization, defects and void in bone cement, and foreign materials (barium, antibiotics, etc.) in bone cement.

The strength of bone cement increases with an increase in the molecular weight. In terms of the method of sterilization,

Table 2.3 Factors affecting the strength of bone cement

Condition	Cement strength
Moisture content	3–10 % ↓
Inclusion of blood or tissue (depending on the amount)	Up to 70 % ↓
Antibiotic inclusion	10–15 % ↓ (1:1), 40–60 % ↓ (1:2)
Radiopaque fillers	5 % ↓
Vacuum mixing	10–25 % ↑
Hand mixing	Up to 21 % ↓
Pressurization delay	Up to 40 % ↓
Environmental temperature (body temperature)	10 % ↓ at body temperature than at room temperature

gamma radiation lowers the molecular weight and the strength of bone cement is decreased, whereas EO gas does not alter the strength of bone cement.

Vacuum mixing is recommended to increase the strength of bone cement, while the strength of bone cement is decreased by hand mixing since about 10 % of air is mixed during hand mixing. However, Rimnac et al. reported that there was no clinically significant difference in the strength of bone cement when compared between the hand-mixing and vacuum-mixing methods.

Air content decreases in lower viscosity bone cement. Since LVC has a lower viscosity, it has the potential to increase its strength by decreasing the air content; however, it naturally has low strength due to low molecular weight (Table 2.3).

The strength of bone cement can be decreased by mixing it with the other materials. Antibiotic-loaded cement is frequently used to prevent or to control the infection. If antibiotics are added in the ratio of 1:1, the cement strength decreases by about 10–15 % with little adverse effects. When antibiotics are mixed in the ratio of 1:2 (one pack cement: two packs or vials of antibiotics), the strength decreases by about 40–60 %.

Creep is another problem associated with the use of bone cement. When bone cement is under a force that is greater than its elastic strain, cement creep occurs and leads to implant subsidence.

2.2 Design

2.2.1 Introduction

There are *some guidelines* that need to be respected *for designing TKA prostheses*. In 1913, Freeman and colleagues outlined the following objectives of designing the prosthesis. First, a salvage procedure should be readily available. To achieve this, *the bone should be preserved as much as possible* so as to leave broad, flat cancellous bones. Second, the chances of *loosening should be minimized*. In order to do so, the tibial and femoral components should be incompletely constrained in relation to each other. Any hyperextension-limiting mechanism should be progressive and not sudden. The prosthetic component should be fitted to the bone by a means which allows dissipation of the loads over the largest possible area of the bone–prosthesis interface. Third, the *rate of production of wear debris should be minimized*. In order to do so, the friction between the components should be minimized and the debris produced should be as innocuous as possible. Fourth, *possibility of infection should be decreased by reducing the dead space*. Fifth, *the consequence of infection should be minimized by avoiding the use of long intramedullary stems and intramedullary cement*. Sixth, *a standard surgical technique* should be available. Seventh, the prosthesis should *allow knee joint motion from 5° of hyperextension to at least 90° of flexion*. Eighth, *some freedom of rotation should be resisted*. And finally, *excessive movements in any direction should be resisted* by the soft tissues, particularly by the collateral ligaments. By following these guidelines, knee joint function can be preserved as much as possible and the survival of TKA can be extended by reducing the complications.

The design of the knee prosthesis is largely based on two concepts: the first is the design focused on anatomy and the second is the design focused on function. In the anatomical design, the normal anatomy is preserved as much as possible and the prosthesis is designed similar to the anatomy of the knee joint. In the functional design, an attempt is made to improve function by preserving kinematics of the artificial knee joint. This can be achieved by simplification of biomechanics of the knee joint and by sacrificing some of the anatomy. However, the current prostheses are designed considering the concept of both the anatomy and function.

In order to improve the knee joint function, the key factor to be considered in TKA prosthesis is "to what extent the anatomy should be reflected on the design." The anatomy cannot be ignored, but every knee joint is different and the anatomy of the knee joint is altered during the operation. Since the anatomy of the knee joint is already altered due to the operation, the changes in biomechanics of the knee joint should also be considered. As the anterior cruciate ligament (ACL) or both the anterior and posterior cruciate ligaments (ACL and PCL) and both menisci are already removed during the operation, the kinematics of the artificial knee joint is quite different from those of normal joint, for example, the four-bar linkage concept does no longer exist.

Therefore, *the most desirable prosthesis design for knee joints is the design in which the changes in the geometry and biomechanics of the knee joint are taken into consideration, and at the same time, it should also be compatible with the altered knee joint mechanics and should be more forgiving*.

However, there has been a recent resurgence in the trend to preserve normal knee kinematics in TKA prosthesis design in an attempt to improve function and lessen anterior knee pain. One of the most important anatomical structures of physiological kinematics is both the cruciate ligaments. Based on this concept, there are some prostheses which retain both the cruciate ligaments.

2.2.2 Anatomy and Biomechanics

In the past, the anatomical and biomechanical studies concerning the design of artificial joints were accomplished with primitive biomechanical studies under static conditions, cadaveric structural study, and gait analysis. But these methods were not accurate as they did not provide dynamic information regarding biomechanics and only provided indirect and two-plane information. Currently, with the advancements in electronic technology and computer system, more accurate and detailed information can be obtained through fluoroscopy, CT, MRI, stereoscopic study, etc.

The biomechanical study of TKA is mostly concerning A–P translation, rotation, flexion–extension motion, and condylar lift-off. Since these motions are interrelated with each other, it is very difficult to interpret the results when all of them are considered together, as there can be countless combinations. Furthermore, the results of this mechanical study can be changed according to the status of weight bearing. When the knee joint is not loaded with the weight, it follows the path of least resistance of motion. When the knee joint is loaded with the weight, its motion is affected by muscle interactions, soft tissue tension, soft tissue impingement, and articular congruity.

The A–P translation is often expressed *as rollback and it greatly affects the ROM. It is known that normal translation is about 19.2 mm on the lateral side and 3.4 mm on the medial side*. This is different from the traditional concept which implies that the degree of translation is uniform on both the sides. There are other reports suggesting that the rollback is less on the medial side before 120° of flexion as described above, but the rollback is equal on both the sides between 9 and 10 mm after 120° of flexion. The amount of rollback varies according to the existence of cruciate ligaments. The rollback clearly decreases even when only the ACL is removed. Therefore, *not only the PCL but also the ACL is involved in rollback* and this is one of the reasons why the range of motion after TKA becomes less than that in the normal joints. The theory that only the PCL is involved in rollback could have been derived from the studies which are focused on the role of the PCL, because the ACL is removed in all the cases during arthroplasty and there is a need for comparing the CR and PS type of implants. However, rollback does not occur in all cases and the so-called *paradoxical rollback*, in which the femoral part is pushed forward, may occur due to the design defect or surgical failure. *When paradoxical rollback occurs, soft tissue impingement develops, and the patellofemoral mechanism becomes overstuffed causing a reduction in flexion motion and provokes rapid increase in the PE wear.*

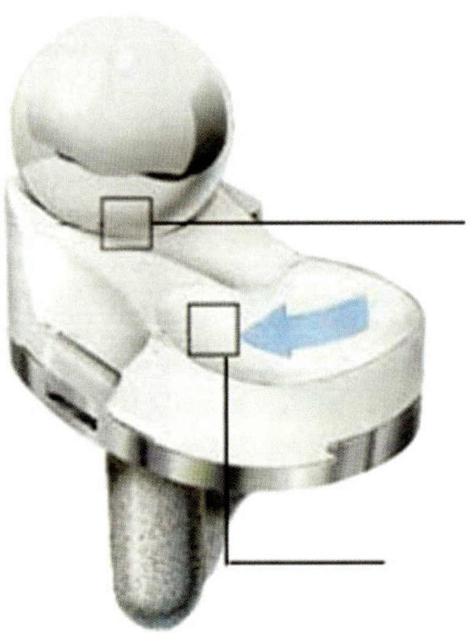

Fig. 2.6 Movement of contact surface of the tibial implant and the femoral implant (ADVANCE, Wright Medical Technology, Arlington, TN)

In flexion–extension motion, the axis of motion is known to have a J-shaped inconsistent center, but the current theory that it is fixed around the transepicondylar axis is more convincing. Rolling and sliding occur during flexion. *Rolling occurs during the first 20–30° of flexion and then sliding occurs thereafter in a 1:2 ratio*. This has a critical impact on the range of motion and PE wear.

In the rotational motion, the tibia rotates internally by about 5.7° when the knee is bent during normal walking and displays up to 15° of internal rotation in maximum flexion when the weight is not loaded. The pattern of rotation on the medial side is similar to that in the ball-and-socket type of joint and that on the lateral side is just like two round boards articulating along the medial axis. However, as has already been mentioned regarding the rollback, the medial condyle moves about 3 mm in physiological state and the medial plateau translates a little back and forth (Fig. 2.6). The degree of rotation after TKA is less than normal, no matter whether or not the PCL is present. In a *mobile-bearing joint, it is known that the mechanism of rotation is similar to that in a normal joint, but the mechanism of rotation in a fixed-bearing joint is different from that in a normal joint*. However, these biomechanics are more complex when rollback and rotation are considered in combination, and *the biomechanics clearly vary greatly from product to product when the PCL has been removed.*

Condylar lift-off also affects the survival of the prosthesis (Fig. 2.7). When it occurs, stress concentration develops at

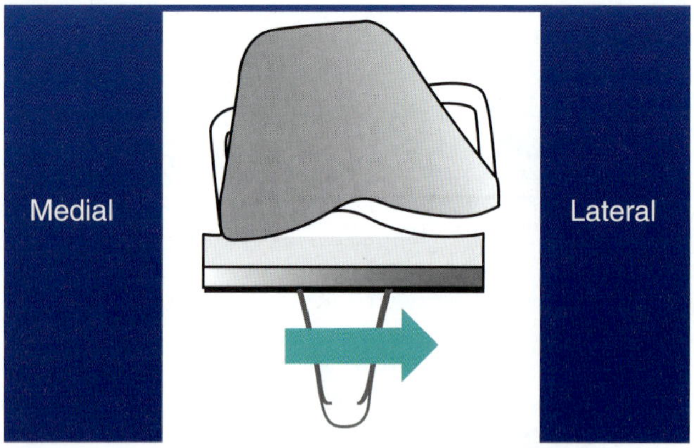

Fig. 2.7 Condylar lift-off

the compressed site inducing early wear. Condylar lift-off generally occurs on the lateral side at maximum flexion, but it occasionally occurs on the medial side. Condylar lift-off *is significantly influenced by the existence of cruciate ligaments* and is related to the attachment site of the cruciate ligaments to the femur. The ACL attaches to the inner side of the lateral condyle, so it acts as the checkrein for lateral lift, whereas the PCL attaches to the inner side of the medial condyle and prevents lifting of the medial condyle. Therefore, lift-off generally occurs at the lateral condyle when the PCL is retained.

In addition to these biomechanical studies, a simulator is used mainly for the study of survival of the implant. This simulator is designed to produce mechanics similar to that of the knee joint. The data obtained from the simulator are design specific and may be different according to design of the simulator.

In spite of these experimental studies, the clinical results may be somewhat different from the in vitro data. *Hence, the implant design should follow the clinical results based on the laboratory experiment.*

Banks et al. used the image-based measurement technique and reported the results of a few mechanical studies of TKA. The results of their study were different from the preexisting theories in several aspects. First, because the femur is bent forward and the tibia is sloped posteriorly, a usual osteotomy would cause an average 9.5° of knee hyperextension compared to the anatomical axis of the tibia and the femur in the sagittal plane. This is in stark contrast with the basic concept of conventional TKA. Hyperextension causes many problems such as anterior impingement when the knee is fully extended and excessive stress on the post in the PS type of implant. Moreover the results of mechanical studies of TKA may be different from the real situation because nearly all the current prostheses have been designed, assuming that the alignment of implants is identical to the alignment of bones in the sagittal plane. Second, it is true that femoral rollback increases the amount of flexion. However, in the dynamic study of walking, the femur would translate forward in flexion and backward in extension when the ACL was sacrificed and meniscectomy was done. In case of the CR type of implant, if the flexion gap is too wide, a paradoxical rollback would occur that could cause reduction in flexion motion. Third, posterior condylar geometry is closely related to the range of flexion. The range of flexion increases with an increased posterior condylar offset (the maximal distance between the posterior femoral cortex and the posterior condyle of implant: Fig. 2.8); when posterior condylar offset increased, the flexion angle increased. Unlike the assumption that using a smaller implant in the anterior referencing system would widen the flexion gap and increase the range of flexion, it would decrease the posterior condylar offset to decrease the range of flexion. Fourth, in the fixed-bearing type of implant, the tibia rotates internally with the rotational axis along the medial condyle during flexion as has been shown on biomechanical study. Whereas in the mobile-bearing type of implant, the medial femoral condyle would be pushed forward and may not act as the axis of rotation.

2.2.3 Factors to Be Considered in Implant Design

Most implant designs focus on the structural congruency, motion constraint between the components and the method of fixation. All these factors are mutually related in various aspects.

2.2.3.1 Congruency Between Components

Congruency is closely related to wear and loosening, which are the most critical complications of TKA. With good congruency between components, for example, *a round PE would increase the contact surface area reducing stress on the PE and decreasing the incidence of wear, while stress between the bone and the prosthesis interface would increase the incidence of loosening as a result.* With lower congruency between components, for example, *a flat PE would decrease the incidence of loosening at first, but wear would be accelerated and wear particles may cause osteolysis and further loosening (Fig. 2.9).*

Historically, the first modern prosthesis designs of TKA were focused on the stability of implants through increasing congruency, but many problems associated with loosening occurred. In order to solve this problem, congruency was reduced thereafter by sacrificing some amount of stability. However, a reduced congruency increased the incidence of wear and wear particles further accelerated loosening. Currently, most of the designs focus on maintaining the appropriate structural congruency.

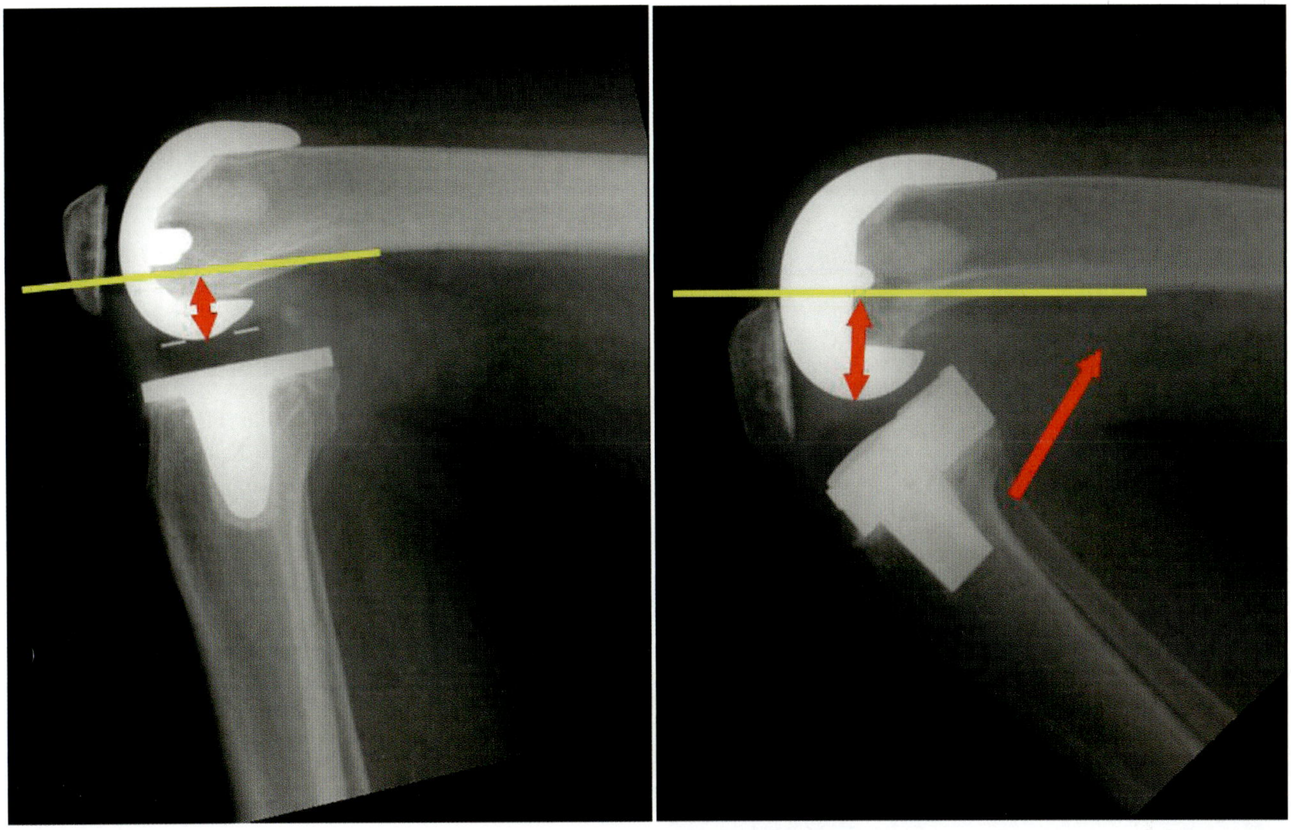

Fig. 2.8 Posterior condylar offset (*Left*: short offset, *Right*: long offset)

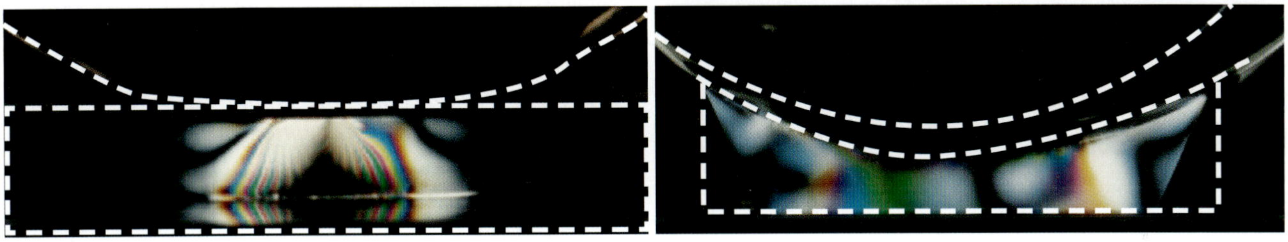

Fig. 2.9 Effect of congruency of TKA design. The *left image* shows lower congruency and the *right image* shows higher congruency. The load is evenly distributed in the right side. Stress is broadly dispersed in higher congruency (Right)

2.2.3.2 Motion Constraint Between the Components

Motion between components needs to be balanced with stability. Generally, increased motion of implants reduces the stability whereas an increase in stability decreases the range of motion.

The implants of artificial knee joint are classified into unconstrained, semiconstrained, and constrained designs according to the amount of motion restriction between each component. There is neither unconstrained nor constrained type of implant in a strict sense, but *the unconstrained type* of implant allows for more motion between the femoral and tibial components, and *the mobile-bearing joint is included in this category*. On the other hand, *any implant that strictly restricts valgus–varus motion could be classified as a constrained type* of implant. The constrained type of implant generally provides varus–valgus constraint and a few allow some rotational motion. *Most of the prostheses which are not included in the unconstrained and constrained categories are classified as the semiconstrained type* of implants.

The selection of implants according to motion constraint must be based on the condition of the knee joints. Generally, it is desirable to choose a design that allows less motion constraint and provides an appropriate level of stability. If an implant constrains motion to a great extent, it can increase the incidence of loosening. Whereas when instability is overlooked and an implant that allows less motion constraint is used, giving way or dislocation may develop.

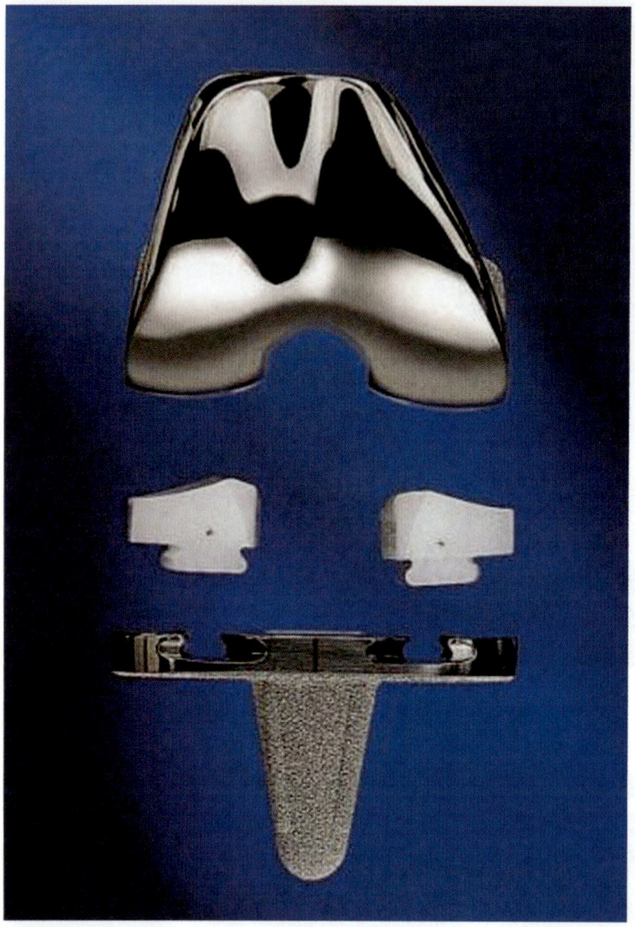

Fig. 2.10 Early form of the LCS meniscal-bearing joint (DePuy, Warsaw, IN)

Unconstrained Type

In TKA, the unconstrained type allows for motion between the PE and tibial components. *Mobile-bearing joint* is included in this category of implants, which allows A–P translation and rotation of PE placed on the tibial plate.

History

The first mobile-bearing joint was the Oxford Knee which was introduced by O'Connor as a concept of compartment replacement in the 1970s. In the Oxford Knee, the femoral condyle was designed in a spherical shape so as to retain both the cruciate ligaments.

Following this, the most popular mobile-bearing LCS (low-contact stress) New Jersey Knee was developed (Fig. 2.10).

Theoretical Background

The theoretical background of mobile-bearing joint is *to reduce the wear and loosening*, which are the most common complications affecting the survival of TKA. *Wear can be reduced by increasing conformity* to broaden the contact surface between the femur and PE. But the resultant decrease in motion between the femoral component and PE imposes *an excessive stress at the implant–bone interface that accelerates loosening* of the components. *If the PE is designed to move, stress at the implant–bone interface would be lowered, thereby decreasing the incidence of loosening* (Fig. 2.11).

However, in a mobile-bearing joint, there is a possibility of dislocation due to excessive motion of PE and breakage of PE due to increased conformity. Stability of the implants is a key factor in preventing dislocation of the mobile-bearing joint, and it relies on articulating geometry and ligament balance.

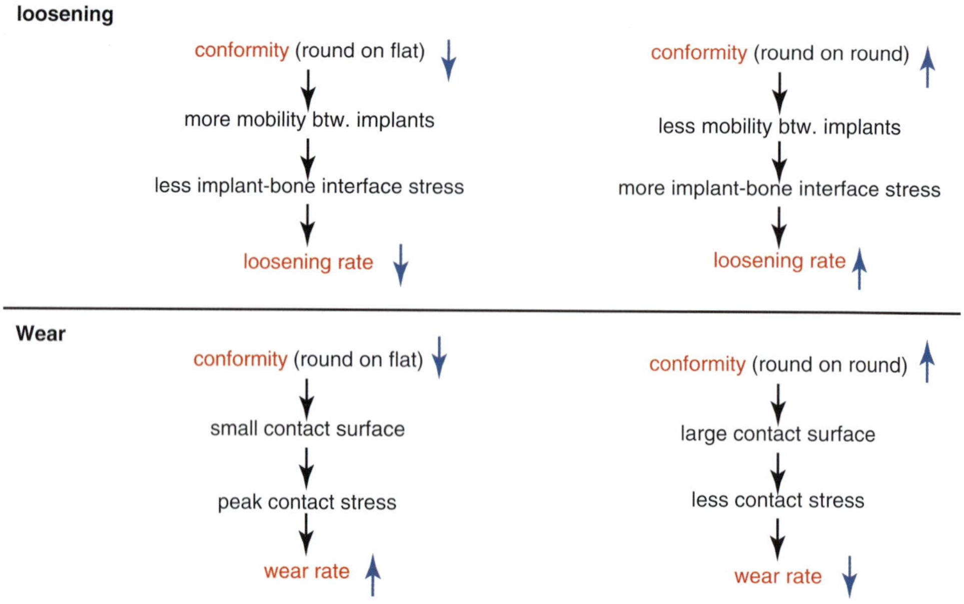

Fig. 2.11 Relationship between conformity and wear/loosening

To increase stability, there are some differences and modifications of design in mobile-bearing joint. Considering the pattern of articulation, *single-radius design of femoral component is often used to increase the stability*. A large single radius can push the bearing component too far back to cause dislocation in flexion/extension. So, *the radius of the posterior condyle is decreased to align the anatomical axis with the axis of implants* in the sagittal plane so that the anatomical axis can be at the center of the bearing component in flexion/extension (Fig. 2.12). The tibial component is also designed to control A–P translation to prevent the PE from translating too far back so as to reduce the incidence of dislocation. The ligament balance greatly affects the stability of mobile-bearing joint, so the earliest form of mobile-bearing joint was designed to retain both the cruciate ligaments. After a while, the ACL-sacrificing and both ACL- and PCL-sacrificing implants were introduced. In case both the anterior and PCLs are sacrificed, only axial rotation is permitted so that the bearing component is stabilized at the center. The patella component is designed to ensure stability and to improve tracking by its anatomical shape.

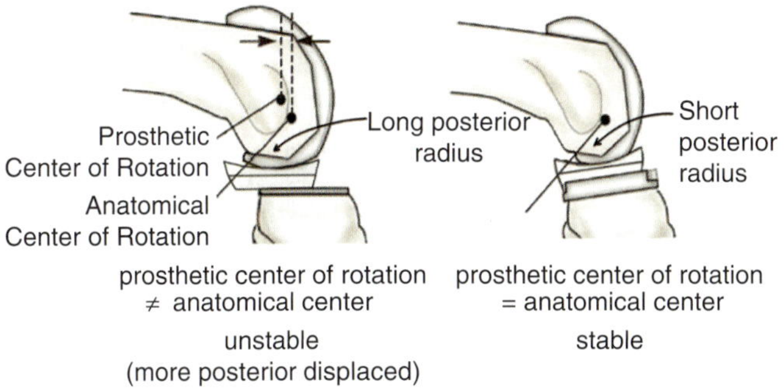

Fig. 2.12 Comparison of the femoral implants according to the radius of the lateral condyle in single-radius femoral implants. The *left image* shows a larger radius and the *right image* shows a smaller radius (reducing the radius of the posterior condyle can align the axis of flexion and extension of artificial joint to the real knee joint as much as possible so as to decrease lateral dislocation)

Breakage of PE occurred frequently when a sharp edge for increased conformity was combined with malrotation, when condylar lift-off developed or when a PE defect was noted. Therefore, the overall implant design has gradually improved. The more improved designs have edges that are not too sharp and excessive motion is constrained so as to reduce the condylar lift-off.

Types

Mobile-bearing joint is classified according to the method of PCL treatment into posterior cruciate-retaining (PCR), posterior cruciate-sacrificing (PCS), and posterior cruciate-stabilized (PS) type.

The first design of PCR implant had two separate bearing components (Fig. 2.13), but the current design has one meniscal bearing. It is designed to move anteroposteriorly and rotation is controlled to a small extent (Fig. 2.14). This movement is similar to the normal meniscal movement so as to facilitate load distribution and more flexion. The PCS type allows for rotation only (Fig. 2.15). The PCS type was modified into the PS type by the addition of cam and post mechanism.

Advantages of a Mobile-Bearing Joint

Menchetti and Walker found in a study of mobile-bearing joint using the Oxford jig that *it reduces the wear by uniformly reducing stress on the PE*, and Sharma et al. also reported almost similar results in an in vivo study. Many authors have reported an average wear rate of 0.09–0.36 mm/yr in mobile-bearing TKA, which was comparable with the wear rate of 0.20 mm/year in THA. Based on a retrieval study, Ho et al. reported that the wear was less in the mobile-bearing joint.

The greatest advantage of mobile-bearing joint is that the malrotation can be corrected automatically and normal knee joint biomechanics can be maintained by the free motion of the bearing component. In normal knees, the tibia rotates externally during the last phase of extension of the knee joint, and a mobile-bearing joint enables smooth rotation similar

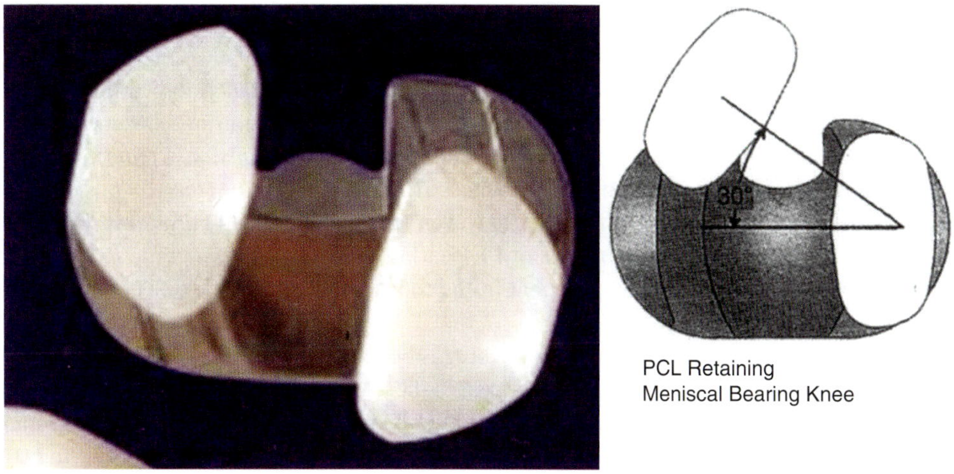

Fig. 2.13 Earlier form of meniscal-bearing knee that retains the posterior cruciate ligament in the LCS prosthesis (DePuy, Warsaw, IN)

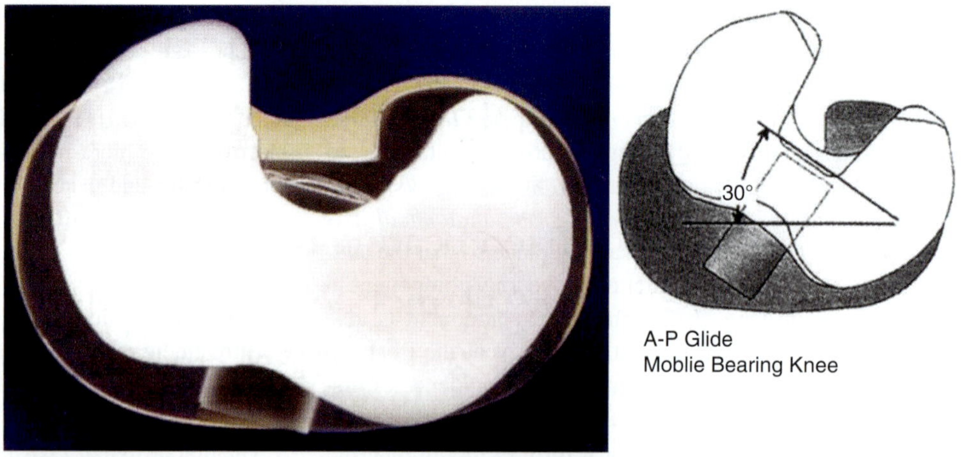

Fig. 2.14 The current A–P glide design of knee prosthesis (DePuy, Warsaw, IN)

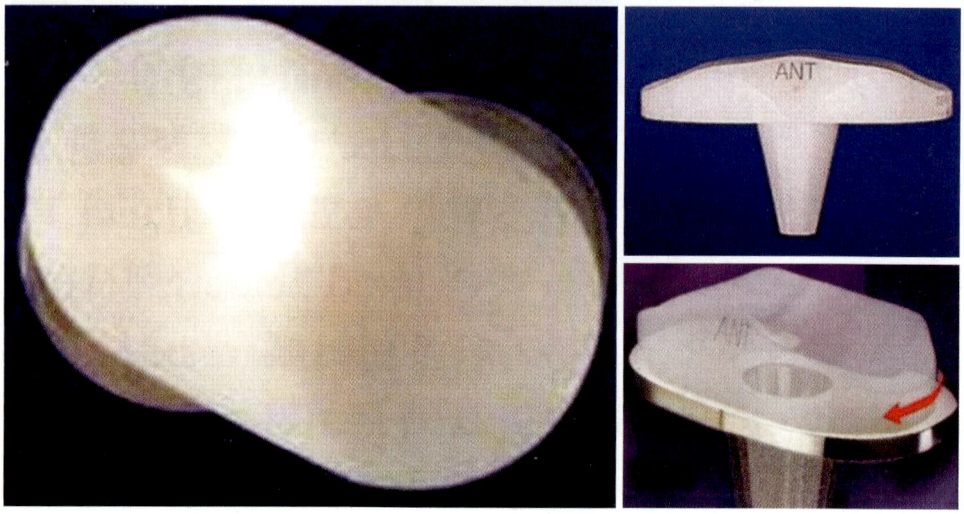

Fig. 2.15 Posterior cruciate-sacrificing LCS prosthesis (DePuy, Warsaw, IN)

to that in the normal knees (Fig. 2.16). However, a fixed-bearing joint does not allow tibial rotation biomechanically.

When there is malrotation, an excessive force is imposed on the PE and it causes rotational or mediolateral imbalance. A rotating platform design, through a rotation of the bearing, provides for greater self-correction of the component malalignment and allows better centralization of the extensor mechanism. When the tibial component was malrotated in the fixed-bearing joint, Matsuda et al. proved that stress on the PE was increased, whereas stress on the PE in the mobile-bearing joint was maintained constantly since malrotation could be corrected automatically (Fig. 2.17). These effects also decrease the stress between the implants and bone interface, thereby reducing the incidence of loosening. All rotating platform knee designs, however, are not the same kinematically. The kinematics of PE-bearing rotation is design specific and is quite different from products to products.

Sawaguchi et al. reported that patellar tracking is better in mobile-bearing joint, while Cho et al. reported that there was no difference in patellar tracking between mobile-bearing joint and fixed-bearing joint.

Disadvantages of a Mobile-Bearing Joint

The stability of mobile-bearing joint depends on the function of the surrounding ligaments. If these ligaments are not balanced, they cause instability. *So, careful ligament balancing during the operation is required for a mobile-bearing joint.* For this purpose, osteotomy is performed first in the tibia and the gap technique is used for femoral osteotomy.

Stiehl et al. reported the results of the mechanism of *femoral rollback* stating that 5.8 mm of rollback occurs in 0–30° flexion in the normal knee joints, whereas the PCR-type mobile-bearing joint shows excessive rollback of about 9.2 mm in the same range of flexion, *and the tibial portion is translated anteriorly in 60–90° flexion.* If tension on the PCL increases, posterior soft tissue impingement occurs causing *paradoxical anterior translation instead of rollback even though the flexion range is increased.* This may cause limited flexion and disturbance of the extensor mechanism of quadriceps muscles.

Condylar lift-off may also occur on both the sides, thereby increasing the wear rate.

There was a report stating that the peak stress on the mobile-bearing joint in 60° flexion was nearly the same as that on the fixed-bearing joint, which was quite different from the theoretical advantages of the mobile-bearing joint.

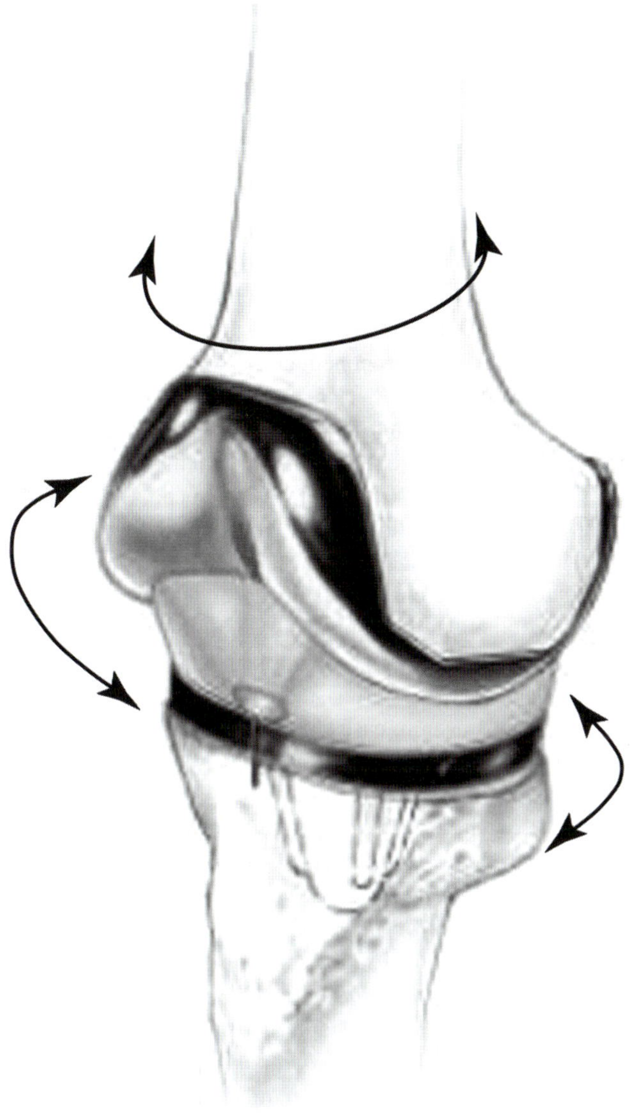

Fig. 2.16 Direction of motion of the mobile bearing knee prosthesis. It shows action similar to the native knee joint biomechanics in flexion–extension, axial rotation, and anterior–posterior translation

Wear can be divided into articular wear and undersurface wear according to the site, and *both surface wear may increase in the mobile-bearing joint*. Regarding the pattern of wear, Collier et al. reported that the LCS mobile-bearing prosthesis mostly showed burnishing which was a kind of abrasive/adhesive wear, whereas the fixed-bearing prosthesis mostly showed cracking and delamination wear. Kelly et al. reported that each bearing surface in mobile-bearing TKA was damaged to a similar extent as that in a fixed-bearing implant. Lu et al. reported that the articular surface wear was reduced, but the undersurface wear was increased. However, Barrack stated that the tibial component of mobile-bearing joint had good surface treatment causing less wear than that in the fixed-bearing joints.

Also, there are concerns regarding the wear particles that are generated in mobile-bearing joint. *The wear particles are smaller and these smaller wear particles are more likely to cause osteolysis than the larger particles*. In addition, polyethylene wear particles can get caught between the components and can cause problems such as third-body wear.

Another criticism is that little rotation of bearing actually occurs as shown in some kinematic studies. Wasielewski et al. reported that rotation was the best in the PS type of mobile-bearing prosthesis and it was only an average of 3.8° and reverse rotation to biomechanics also occurred in 17–32 % of cases. McEwan et al. reported that *the screw home movement was variable, and it was not a physiological movement in the mobile-bearing joint*.

Results

Good to excellent results have been reported by many authors. Kaper et al. reported a 94 % satisfaction rate during the midterm follow-up at 5 years or more, and Buechel et al. reported a 95 % or higher satisfaction rate during the long-term follow-up at 10 years or more and a 10-year survival rate of 97 %. Sorrels et al. reported excellent outcomes with a 13-year survivorship of 93 %. Carothers et al. reported the results of an average 8.6-year follow-up through meta-analysis of 3,506 cases of mobile-bearing TKA, which

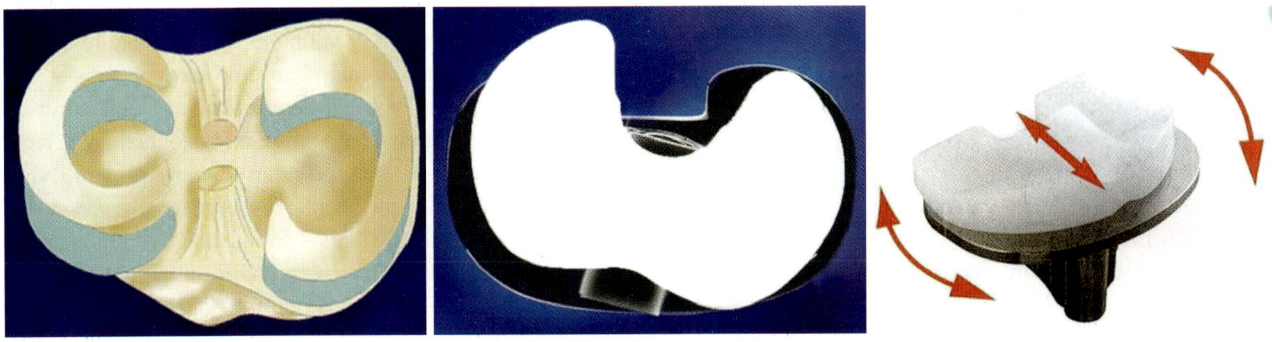

Fig. 2.17 How rotation is automatically corrected in mobile bearing knee prosthesis (DePuy, Warsaw, IN)

demonstrated that excellent results were obtained, and loosening and bearing instability were uncommon. However, *comparing the fixed-bearing and mobile-bearing joint*, Evans et al., Cho et al., Aglietti et al., and Mahoney et al. reported that *no difference was found in the clinical results or survival rate between mobile- and fixed-bearing joints. But these results were quite different among the implants used, especially in the mobile-bearing joint.*

By comparing between the PCR and PCS type of prosthesis, Stiehl et al. demonstrated that the PCR type showed better functional results, whereas the PCS type showed a better survival rate. Kim et al. reported that the PCS type is superior in terms of the ROM and patient satisfaction. In comparison between the cemented and cementless type of prosthesis, Hartford et al. reported a higher incidence of loosening in the cementless type.

In terms of complications, spinout is a specific complication to the mobile-bearing joint, and its incidence was reported to be between 0.5 % and 9.3 %.

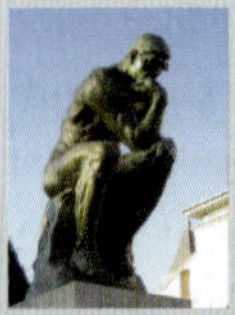

Author's Opinion

The concept of mobile-bearing knee joint is theoretically very sound and postoperative patient satisfaction is also very high. Some surgeons complain that it is difficult to perform the operation, but once accustomed to handle this system, it takes a shorter time than that for the fixed-bearing joint.

The key point of the operation is to balance the soft tissues. In this respect, *I would recommend not to use a mobile-bearing joint in cases with severe deformity and an unstable joint.*

In my opinion, selecting the right size of implant is also very important for ensuring stability. If the implant is too small, the joint space is widened causing dislocation of the implant.

I believe that proper selection of the size of the implant and a successful operation would help to ensure joint stability, increase the ROM, and reduce the incidence of wear and loosening, especially in the relatively younger patients.

Semiconstrained Type

Semiconstrained types are all fixed-bearing joints and are *currently the most commonly used type of implants.* Semiconstrained implants vary in shape and size based on how well they reflect the anatomy and biomechanics of the knee joint and how much stability and ROM of the knee joint can be achieved.

TKA implants have developed a lot so as to improve motion, stability, and survival, based on the anatomy and biomechanics of the knee joint. Constrained implants were developed early in the history of evolution of TKA and were followed by development of semiconstrained type of implants.

The most epoch-making event was the development of PCL-substituting type of implants. Most of the earlier semiconstrained implants were designed such that the ACL could be removed, but the PCL should be retained (so-called cruciate-retaining (CR) type). Soon thereafter, Total Condylar Knee prosthesis was developed for use in cases when the PCL was missing or weak. The term "total condylar" means that one component covers both the condyles of each bone. Total Condylar Knee prosthesis has two components covering the femur and the tibia respectively, and the basic concept is surface replacement. To achieve implant stability, the posterior lip of the PE was enhanced. But it caused limited motion and dislocation. To solve these problems, posterior-stabilized knee prosthesis was developed in 1978, and it showed good clinical results despite the fact that many were worried about the poor results initially. Since then, the PCL-substituting (PS) type of implants has been developed by modification of posterior-stabilized knee and is used by many surgeons even in cases which there were no problems with the PCL (Fig. 2.18).

Posterior Cruciate-Retaining Type (CR Type)

Posterior cruciate-retaining type of implant was developed to maintain the normal kinetics of the knee joint as much as possible by preserving the kinematic function of the PCL. The function of the PCL is to allow femoral rollback, improve the mechanical efficiency of the extensor mechanism, act as the axis of rotation, increase anteroposterior and varus–valgus stability of the knee joint, and contribute to proprioception. Besides, the PCL can reduce stress between the components and between the component and the bone by transferring the load to a functional ligament, thereby decreasing the wear and loosening.

In terms of joint line, the CR type is better for maintaining the joint line than the PS type. Maintenance of the anatomical joint line is potentially valuable because patellofemoral dysfunction remains the main cause of many unsatisfactory TKAs. Mihalko et al. proved the presence of mechanoreceptors within the ligament by immunohistochemistry techniques using S100 protein and neurofilament protein (NFP) and stated that the proprioception was better by preserving the PCL. Zhang and Mihalko found positive stained elements with both S100 protein and NFP immunohistochemical staining form the specimen of PCL in 5 CR-type retrievals, which had been in place 5–12 years. Another

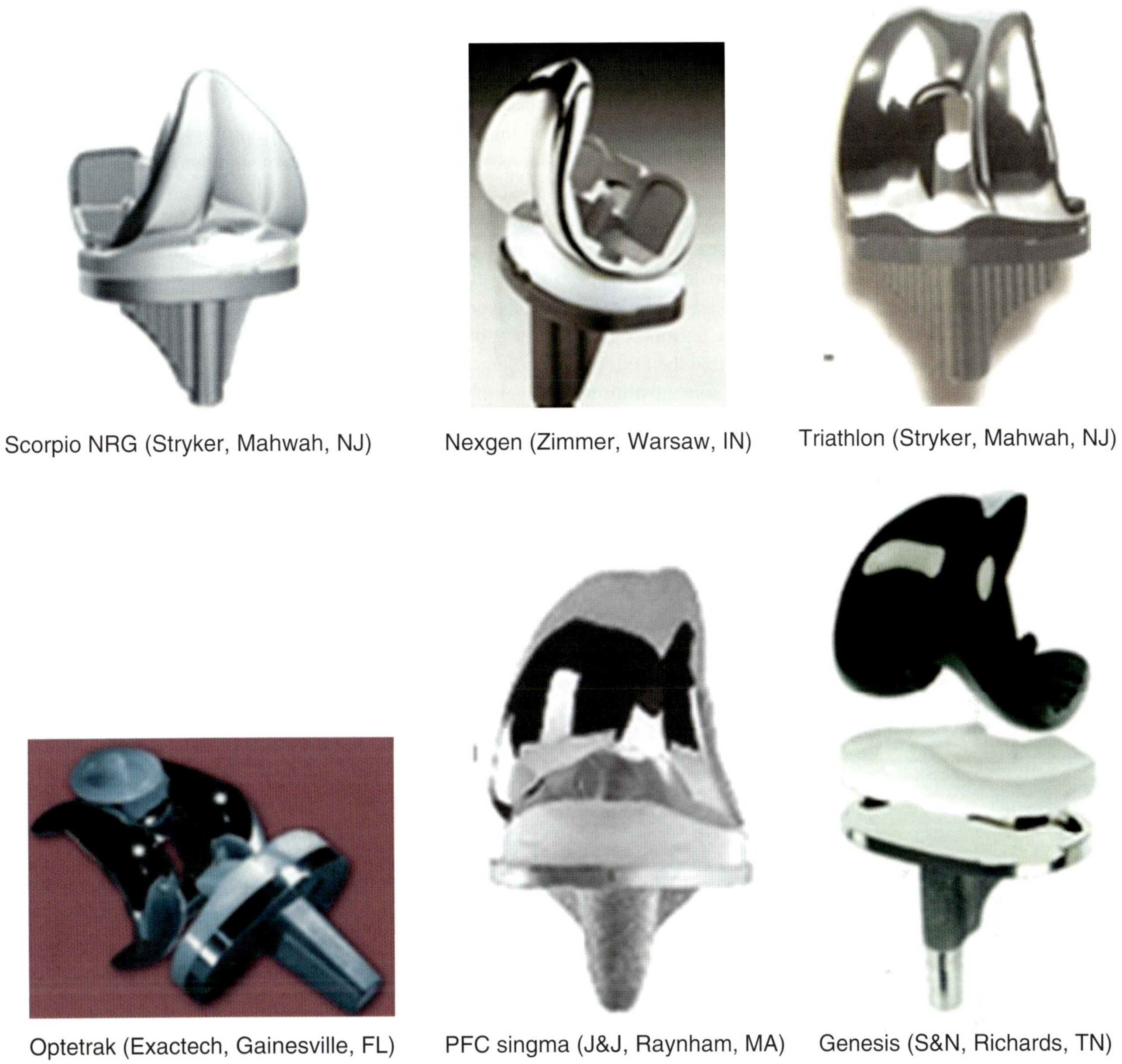

Fig. 2.18 Various kinds of semiconstrained type of implants

advantage of the CR type in comparison to the PS type is that more bone is preserved in the CR type.

However, there are many surgeons who are not in favor of the use of the CR type. Fluoroscopic studies by Stiehl et al. and Dennis et al. have demonstrated that the CR prostheses do not replicate the kinematics of the normal knee joint. Instead, paradoxical roll-forward occurs due to improper tensioning of the PCL in many cases. Hence, *maintaining the appropriate tension of the PCL is important*. If the PCL is too tight, it causes excessive rollback to increase the wear of the posterior portion. This movement is demonstrated in the "slide-back" test, which is tested by pushing the tibia posteriorly. If the PCL is too loose, it causes roll-forward to increase the wear of the anterior portion and the result is the same as that with the use of early type of Total Condylar Knee prosthesis. Therefore, the *CR type is recommended only when the PCL is functioning normally and in the absence of severe deformity, bone loss, or instability*.

The PE had to be flat for the CR type to induce rollback and to prevent impingement between the PE and the PCL, but a flat PE accelerated the wear and caused poor patellofemoral alignment (Fig. 2.19). Currently, the designs have evolved and a flat PE is not used even in the CR type. In other words, PE is designed to be round in shape to maintain the appropriate tension so that the PCL can adjust to this change of the PE. Some other problems noted with the past implant designs and materials have been corrected and improved. These include improvement in the patellofemoral mechanism, modularity, locking mechanism between PE and tibial plate, the back side wear, and improvement in manufacturing and sterilization of PE.

Posterior Cruciate-Sacrificing Type

History and Terminology of Posterior Cruciate-Sacrificing Type The implants used when the PCL has been removed can be called Posterior Cruciate Sacrificing (PCS), posterior cruciate-stabilizing, or posterior cruciate-substituting prostheses. These terms are used interchangeably although they have a little different meaning. It is necessary to define these terminologies.

PCS type of prosthesis literally indicates that the PCL has been sacrificed. It can be divided into the non-substituting and substituting type according to the functional restoration of PCL after removal of the PCL.

Types of Posterior Cruciate-Sacrificing Design

Posterior Cruciate Sacrificing-Non-substituting (PCS) Type This type of prosthesis has no cam and post mechanism

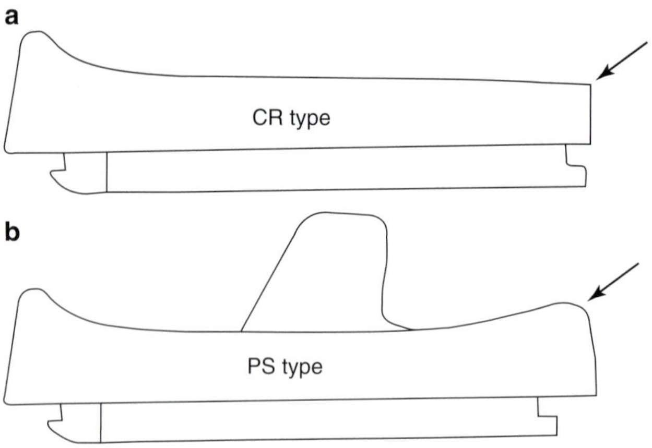

Fig. 2.19 Difference in the shape of the PE in CR and PS type. (**a**) Posterior end of PE (*arrow*) is flat to accommodate posterior cruciate ligament, (**b**) PS type has rounded posterior end (*arrow*) for better conformity

after sacrificing the PCL. Total condylar type of implant was developed in 1973 and it was the first non-substituting type and first patellar resurfacing type of implant. So, it can be classified as PCS non-substituting type of implant. This type of implant was designed to improve the A–P stability by increasing articular conformity, and the collateral ligaments played an important role in the overall implant stability. However, it could not induce femoral rollback during flexion motion and the range of motion was not more than 90°. Also, subluxation or dislocation occurred easily with the use of this type of implant due to instability when the ligaments were not balanced.

Soon after this, Total Condylar Knee prosthesis II was developed with a central post to increase the posterior stability. It improved the posterior stability, but it did not have the function to substitute the rollback mechanism. Therefore, it was called the posterior-stabilized type of prosthesis, but not the posterior-substituting type of prosthesis.

Recently, a new PCL-sacrificing non-substituting type of prosthesis, called *ultracongruent deep-dished prosthesis with an anterior buildup*, was introduced. In this design, posterior instability was reduced utilizing deep-dished, highly congruent PE with an anterior lip. The anterior portion has been built up to 12.5 mm, and the null point or resting position of the femur on the tibia is located posterior to the midline by 4–6 mm and the overall design mimics a ball-and-socket joint (Fig. 2.20).

In comparison to the posterior-substituting type, this design has several advantages: first, it can be used regardless of PCL sacrificing or not; second, the anterior build up maintains the tibial and femoral anteroposterior relationship throughout the arc of motion; third, bone loss is less than that in the PS type; fourth, there are less chances of development of patellar clunk syndrome; and finally, of course, there is not post wear and breakage.

This design can be used as an alternative in difficult revision cases of CR type of prosthesis, in which longer operation time is required when femoral component is well fixed but the

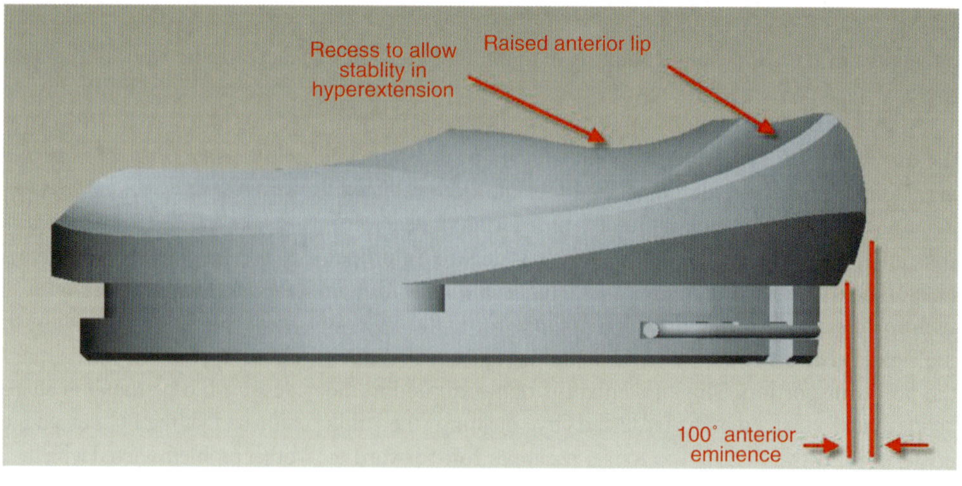

Fig. 2.20 Ultracongruent deep-dished prosthesis with an anterior buildup. The null point or femoral resting point is 4–6 mm posterior to the midline (Triathlon CS, Stryker, Mahwah, NJ)

PCL is degenerated or attenuated. There is no need to remove femoral component, as this PE can be replaced regardless of the PCL condition.

The disadvantage of this design is that it has less rotational motion during early flexion, thereby transmitting greater shear stress to the tibial component–bone interface and causing *early loosening*. The kinematic study has also demonstrated that *more quadriceps power is needed to extend the knee* due to insufficient pulling of the tibia posteriorly.

Posterior Cruciate-Substituting Type (PS Type) Soon after the Total Condylar Knee prosthesis was introduced, the Hospital for Special Surgery (HSS) developed the PCL-substituting type of prosthesis by *adding a post on the PE and a cam on the femoral component* so as to overcome the defect of Total Condylar Knee prosthesis and named it as Insall–Burstein posterior-stabilizing (IBPS) type of prosthesis. The terms "posterior-stabilizing type" and "posterior-substituting type" are often used in reference to the same concept, and both the terms have been used interchangeably, but the term posterior-stabilizing type should be used only for the Insall–Burstein posterior-stabilized (IBPS) or I–B II posterior-stabilized type as initially named by the HSS (Fig. 2.21).

The IBPS type of prosthesis has an improved design in several aspects and the ideas have been derived from the experience of failure of the hinged prosthesis. *The main concept of this design is to provide a substitute to the primary role of the PCL: rollback and posterior stability.* In the IBPS type of prosthesis, cam action starts from 70° of flexion, which means that the cam and the post do not come in contact until 70° of flexion so as not to disturb level walking. In other words, this means that the rollback does not occur until this flexion angle. The IBPS type of prosthesis becomes slightly lax in flexion, but it can prevent posterior dislocation and allows flexion up to an average of 115°.

The IBPS type became the standard model of the posterior cruciate-substituting type of prosthesis. Post and cam are attached to the CR type of implant to substitute the function of the PCL through the modification of posterior-stabilized knee joint in almost all products. Therefore, the PS type of implant means the posterior cruciate-substituting type in general and the mechanism and function of substitution vary slightly from product to product.

Theoretical Background of the PS Type Those who are in favor of using the PS type of prosthesis state that *the function of the retained PCL is not reliable and this inadvertently results in the use of the CR type of prosthesis in PCL-deficient patients*. It has been reported that the PCL was abnormal and weak even though it looked healthy to the naked eye. In the presence of severe degenerative arthritis, mucoid degeneration developed in the PCL and the normal tension was maintained in only 10–30 % of the PCL. Dennis et al. reported that when the PCL was retained since it looked healthy during the operation in patients with degenerative arthritis, functional loss of the PCL developed progressively showing roll-forward over time. In case of rheumatoid arthritis, Laskin reported functional loss of the PCL over time as it is surrounded by the synovial membrane. Shannon et al. also found loss of insertion site of the PCL on MRI in the patient whose PCL was preserved. In order to maintain an adequate PCL tension, the implants and surgical techniques should be completely compatible with the anatomy. But this is almost impossible and even the most experienced surgeon cannot guarantee a well-functioning PCL.

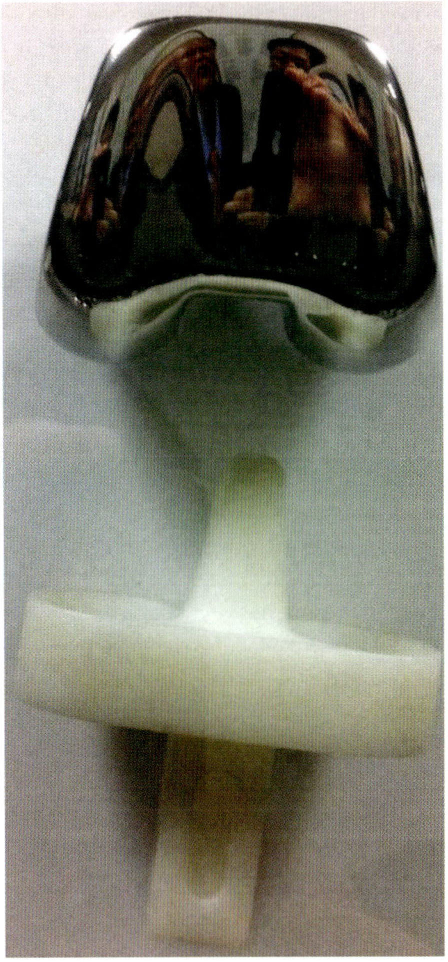

Fig. 2.21 The Insall–Burstein posterior-stabilized (IBPS) type of prosthesis

Advantages of the PS Type There are *many advantages* of the PS type. First, it is *easier to perform the operation with the use of the PS type*. It provides a better operation field and there is no need to protect the PCL. Second, *correction of the deformity is easier with the use of the PS type*. It facilitates release of soft tissue during correction of flexion deformity. Third, *it is not necessary to balance the PCL, so lesser osteotomy is required on the tibial side*, which results in fixation of the prosthesis on the stronger bone. Fourth, *PE conformity can be increased so as to reduce wear*. Fifth, according to Stiehl et al., *the kinetics of knee joint is shown to be improved* on fluoroscopic study.

Some surgeons were worried about the decrease of femoral rollback, but Dennis et al., Victor et al., and Yoshia et al. demonstrated that the PS type induces a uniform rollback, whereas the CR type often showed paradoxical rollback in which the femur is translated forward on flexion. With respect to the rollback, however, the femur rolls back on the tibia and its external rotation during flexion motion results in more rollback on the lateral side. In order to achieve this biomechanics, asymmetric cam–post mechanism is under investigation.

With respect to the contact between the femoral and tibial components, Incavo et al. reported that the PS type showed a more constant contact between the femoral and tibial components than the CR type.

Victor et al. performed an in vivo kinematic study and reported that the PS type was better than the CR type in terms of the rollback, rotation, and ROM, and these results were related with balancing during the operation.

Disadvantages of the PS Type However, sacrificing the PCL may result in the following drawbacks:

1. *More widening of the flexion gap than that of the extension gap to cause gap discrepancy*.
2. *Elevation of the joint line* due to increase in the flexion and extension gaps.
3. *Blockage of extension due to soft tissue impingement* between the notch and the post.
4. *Increase in the incidence of patellar clunk syndrome*.
5. *Removal of more bones, which causes an increase in the incidence of fracture*.
6. Increase in the backside wear of the PE.
7. Increase in the incidence of loosening due to increase in the shear force.
8. Development of a fracture and wear of the post if rotational alignment is poor.
9. *More chances of condylar lift-off*.
10. Dislocation may develop.
11. Decrease in proprioception.

Patellar clunk syndrome occurs occasionally because the PS type requires more box cutting and the *notch portion of the femur is extended more proximally than that in the CR type*, causing irritation of the quadriceps tendon during extension and flexion of the knee joint.

If more bones are removed with the use of the PS type, patients with severe osteoporosis can develop a fracture and bone loss becomes more serious in case of revision.

Dislocation of joints occurs more frequently with the use of the CR type, but only a few are reported because it can be easily reduced. As deep flexion can be achieved, there were cases of dislocation with the use of the PS type.

Currently, many surgeons are concerned about the wear and breakage of the post of the PS type. With respect to the design, post wear is closely related to the location and contact surface of the post. The post fracture and dislocation is described in Chap. 8.

Improving the Drawbacks of the PS Type Posterior cruciate-substituting type has been continuously undergoing improvement in order to overcome these drawbacks. The current products have:

1. Improved A–P stability
2. Increased range of motion
3. Reduced force imposed on the patellofemoral joint in extension to improve patellofemoral function
4. Reduced anterior impingement
5. Adjusted length of the notch to reduce the incidence of patellar clunk syndrome
6. Broadened contact surface and change in the position of the post to reduce the stress on the post

Indications for the PS Type As of now, whenever the use of a semiconstrained type is indicated, *the surgeons can choose either the PS type or the CR type. However, even those who prefer to use the CR type agree that the PS type should be used when there are severe degenerative changes in the PCL, the patient has a severe deformity, rheumatoid arthritis is progressing, or the PCL is damaged during the operation*.

Laskin emphasized that the PS type must be used in the patients with a varus deformity greater than 15°. He experienced increased radiolucent lines between the cement and the bone, and revision was required in more cases with use of the CR type. But, Scott and Volatile stated that only 1–2 % of patients fall into this category.

Comparison of the Results Between the CR Type and the PS Type

Surgeons who prefer the CR type emphasize, on the basis of the results of walking analysis, that the CR type showed better performance, especially in terms of going up and down the stairs as well as better patient satisfaction, higher functional scores, more ROM, and higher survival rate. Heck et al. analyzed 53,750 TKA patients and reported that the implant survival rate was better in the CR type than in the PS type. Conditt et al. also compared both the CR and PS types and reported that the clinical score was not different between the two, but the CR type showed better results in squatting and gardening. Abdel et al. reported the 15-year survival rate for 5,389 CR type of prosthesis and 2,728 PS type of prosthesis, which suggested that the CR type showed a significantly improved survival in comparison with the PS type.

Those who prefer the PS type state that it has better motion, shows equally good performance in terms of going up and down the stairs, and has a longer survival than the CR type, and the wear and loosening is lesser. With regard to the proprioception, Simmons et al. stated that there is no difference between the two types. Many surgeons were worried about poor prognosis of the posterior-stabilized type when it was first introduced, but more than 90 % of patients using the PS type showed excellent or good results, and Vince et al. reported that its 10-year survival rate was approximately 92–95 %.

An objective comparison showed that the *results between the CR and PS types were similar in terms of function, range of motion, wear, loosening, and survival rate, but the PS type seemed to be slightly better.*

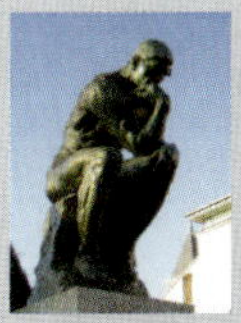

Author's Method

Based on my experience, at times I was not certain whether or not the PCL was in its normal condition during the operation. When CR type was used, recession of the PCL was often needed so as to loosen the tension when it was too tight.

It is a generally accepted concept that the operation for correcting the deformity is easier to perform and is more convenient with the use of the PS type, but this is not always the case because of the possibility of flexion and extension gap discrepancy after sacrificing the PCL. Therefore, more caution is required in PS type than that with the use of the CR type when deciding the size and soft tissue balancing.

In the past, I used the CR type predominantly, but the PS type has been used until now in most of the patients ever since a few cases of hyperextension were experienced in patients who received TKA with the CR type.

Constrained Type

Constrained prostheses have developed since the early history of TKA. The Guepar prosthesis is the first model of the modern constrained type. *The constrained type has valgus–varus stability* by the virtue of the implant itself. It has been used in *cases of severe deformity and in cases of instability which cannot be corrected with the usual semiconstrained type, revision TKA, and tumor surgery.*

The constrained type has *two subtypes, the VVC (varus–valgus control) type and the linked type.*

The VVC type has a deeper box portion on the femoral side and a longer and rectangular post than the PS type, and the interval between the box and the post is very narrow. This limits the gross varus–valgus and rotational motion, except for about of 1–2° of varus–valgus and slight rotational motion (Fig. 2.22).

Among the linked types, Endo-Model (Link, Hamburg, Germany) and MUTARS system (Implantcast, Buxtehude, Germany) allow for rotation, but the Kotz system (Howmedica, Kiel, Germany) does not allow rotation. A big discrepancy between the flexion and extension gap may cause dislocation of the VVC type even though the stability is improved. *The linked type of prosthesis increases the stability to a great extent, but the incidence of loosening increases as well.* Therefore, it is very important to align the limb when using the constrained type.

Newer design of the rotating hinge knee (Zimmer, Warsaw, IN; Fig. 2.22) was developed to reduce the risk of loosening and improve the kinematics through the incorporation of rotating bearings that eliminated the rotational constraint of the earlier prostheses. Despite of the theoretical advantages, these designs did not provide better results than the older non rotating hinge prostheses.

It requires more time for performing the operation using the constrained type and it is more costly since the *extension stem has to be used* to reduce loosening.

2.2.3.3 Designs According to the Fixation Methods

The methods of fixation of prosthesis include the cement fixation method, press-fit method, and cementless biologic method. Cemented THA in younger patients demonstrated unsatisfactory results in long-term follow-up. In an effort to improve the long-term results of THA, cementless biologic fixation was offered as a potential solution. The cementless method for biological fixation through bone ingrowth has been developed due to the so-called *cement disease which is caused by changes in the strength of the cement and foreign body reaction* after a long-term use. The success of cementless THA in younger patients led to increased interest in cementless TKA. Cement can be used in the cementless

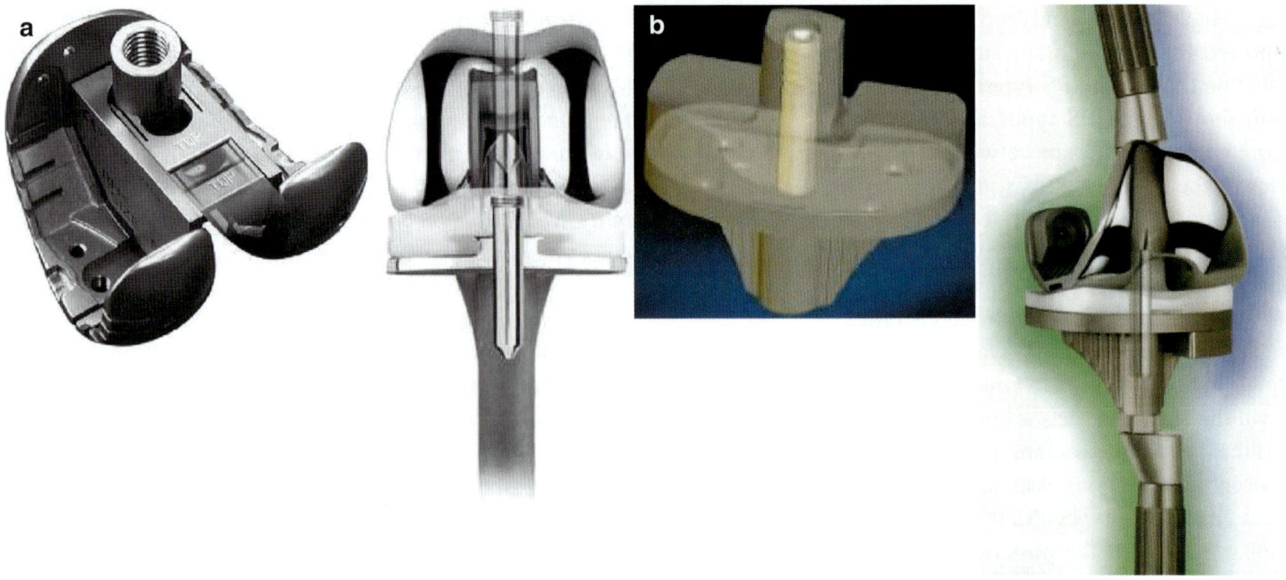

Fig. 2.22 Valgus–varus constrained prostheses. (**a**) Rotating hinge knee (Zimmer, Warsaw, IN), (**b**) Scorpio TS (Stryker, Mahwah, NJ)

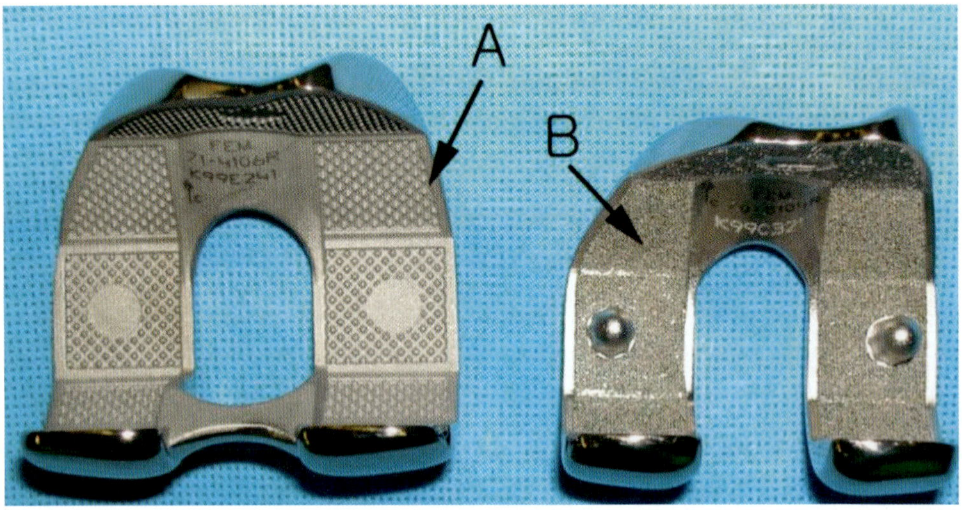

Fig. 2.23 Comparison between the cement and cementless implants. The *left figure* is the cement type with indentation pockets (*Arrow A*) to reinforce fixation with cement, and the *right figure* is the cementless type of implant with porous coating (*Arrow B*)

type, but the cement type has indentation pockets with thicker edges for more effective cement fixation (Fig. 2.23).

Cement Type

Cement type is the *most popular fixation method* and there are many clinical results of its application in TKA and THA. The 10-year survival rate of the cement type of knee prosthesis has been reported to be more than 95 %. *Its advantage is that early weight bearing is possible due to initial rigid fixation*. This is a great benefit for the elderly patients or patients with polyarthralgia. Another advantage is that *it can be applied in any patient and to any implant*. It is also beneficial since *it is easy and convenient to perform the operation*. Cement-type designs offer the benefit that slight incongruities of the bone–prosthesis interface can be overcome with the cement, whereas cementless prostheses require almost perfect contact following osteotomy.

Cementless Type

Since loosening is likely to develop in active patients when the implant is fixed with cement, a more durable fixation method was researched. In fact, good clinical results could be obtained with the current cement type of prosthesis owing to the development of implant design. In the past, failure rate was reported to be 20 % at the 5-year follow-up and the incidence of loosening was much higher in young active patients.

The theoretical background of this design is that when pores of a certain size are made using metal beads or mesh on the surface where the implant comes in contact with the bone, the bone would grow into these pores, thereby reinforcing the fixation.

The advantages of the cementless type are that the fixation is permanent, more bones are preserved, and no problems are caused due to bone cement. Other purported advantages are shorter operation time, decreased chances of third-body PE wear due to the cement debris, and easier revision surgery.

The prerequisites for the cementless type of fixation are that the component should have compressive force, chance of sinking or lift-off should be prevented by using the stem or screw fixation for an extra support, and there should be *no motion of the implant itself* such as bending due to a high elastic modulus, although micromotion in the implant cannot be prevented.

There are *a few factors that are needed to induce bone ingrowth.* First, the *pore size should be between 50 and 400 μm.* Bobyn et al. found that bone ingrowth did not occur or was incomplete when the pore size was less than 50 μm, and fibrous ingrowth occurred and it weakened the fixation when the pore size was greater than 400 μm. Second, bone ingrowth is affected by *the material of the pore surface.* Titanium induces more than double bone ingrowth than cobalt chromium and is mostly composed of mineral components. When the surface is treated with hydroxyapatite, it allows good bone ingrowth, but it has some problems due to the very few mineral components. However, Akizuki et al. demonstrated good bone ingrowth in all portions and achieved satisfactory clinical results by applying hydroxyapatite–tricalcium phosphate. Third, *implants must be securely fixed and should be in close contact with bones.* Nilsson et al. reported that there will be no bone ingrowth if the gap is wider than 50 μm. Hence, osteotomy must be done accurately. If the surface of osteotomy is irregular, contact between the implant and the bone becomes loose, and malalignment or instability may induce failure of bony ingrowth and provoke early loosening due to lift-off or sinking down by uneven distribution of the load. *To achieve rigid fixation, a minimally constrained type of prosthesis is recommended, extension stem is used for achieving more stable fixation,* and an asymmetric tibial component is beneficial. *Screw fixation* may be used for more rigid initial fixation, but it is not used currently since the *PE wear particles* penetrate into the cancellous bone *through the screw holes causing osteolysis.* Also, a stress-shielding effect occurs when the lug portion is treated with Porocoat. *For the stability of prosthesis in early stage* when bone ingrowth is taking place, *weight bearing needs to be restricted.*

In the cementless type, fixation is determined by the reliability of the bone ingrowth. Clinically, the *tibial portion is relatively unstable and bone ingrowth occurs insufficiently* in many cases. According to Hungerford and Kenna, about 40 % of bone ingrowth occurred in the tibial side, and only about half of them showed enough bone ingrowth to endure walking. Cook et al. also reported that 10 % of patients did not show any bone ingrowth, and in about 1/3 of the remaining cases, only fibrous tissues grew into the pores. However, these results vary from implant to implant.

The cementless type has a porous surface which interferes with clear visualization of the radiolucent lines, and if sclerosis of the bone increases beneath the implant, it may be misunderstood that the bone is consolidating. It must be remembered that the *radiolucent lines seen under the cement type rarely indicate progression of osteolysis, but they are likely to progress in the cementless type* because it indicates that bone ingrowth has not occurred.

Component breakage due to weakening of the main metal strength is another complication of the cementless type.

Controversies

There are many controversies concerning the cement type and the cementless type. Those who are *in favor of using the cement type* for all components state that *it is easier to perform an operation using the cement type and a strong initial fixation can be achieved so that the patients can start walking from the early postoperative period.* They emphasize that only a thin layer of cement is used for TKA and there is almost no cement extrusion outside the implant, and hence cement disease is not a big problem in the knee joints. Furthermore, *cement blocks the PE particles from penetrating into the cancellous bones, thereby reducing the risk of osteolysis.* And loosening does not occur primarily due to cement but occurs due to the bone as the strength of cement is greater than that of the bone.

If alignment is good and stability is achieved, the cement type offers many advantages. Fehring et al. reported that the cement type is much better than the cementless type in terms of clinical scores, pain-free period, and early revision rate. They emphasized that cement causes much lesser problems in the knee joints than those in the hip joints, because the prosthesis is under compressive force in the knee joint, whereas it is subjected to variable forces in hip replacement.

Basset et al. reported that they experienced almost no radiolucent lines with the cement type and Rand reported that the cementless type showed poorer clinical results due to problems with fixation, and more radiolucent lines were seen than those seen with the cement type, leading to progression of malalignment. Park et al. reported the results of a prospective comparative 13.6-year follow-up study which demonstrated that there were no advantages of the cementless type over the cement type. Duffy et al. reported 10-year survival rates of 94 % and 72 % for the cement and cementless type, respectively, and Illgen et al. reported a 10-year survival rate of 95 % for hybrid fixation. Furthermore, a longer operation time is required for cementless fixation than for cement fixation as accurate osteotomy and tight fitting of prosthesis are mandatory and the difficulties associated with revision of failed cementless implant are similar to those associated with revision of failed cemented implant.

On the other hand, *those who prefer using the cementless fixation* state that it requires a shorter operation time and it is easier to perform revision surgery. They also state that *it offers a strong and permanent fixation, more bones are preserved, and it does not cause cement disease* once bone ingrowth has occurred. McCaskie et al. reported a comparative study of the cement type and the cementless type, which demonstrated that there was no difference in the clinical results between the two types of fixation. However, much less radiolucent lines were seen in the cementless type. Regner et al. also reported a 5-year follow-up study which demonstrated that the cementless type with porous coating and hydroxyapatite coating achieved equivalent or better stability compared to the cement type.

As there is a high incidence of loosening of the tibial component, a hybrid technique, consisting of cement fixation of the tibial component and cementless fixation of the femoral component, is another option. But some surgeons state that the incidence of loosening around the femoral component is not less than that around the tibial component. Many retrieval studies support this finding and this is because the loosening on the femoral side is very difficult to detect on X-ray if the X-ray projection is not correct.

Patient Selection

Cementless type is recommended for the younger and more active patients. Although some surgeons recommend the use of the cementless type in elderly patients, it is not appropriate to use it in patients with severe osteoporosis or in the elderly. Elderly patients need early weight bearing and poor bone quality is associated with unacceptably large micromovement of the implant. Bone strength is a major factor in preventing subsidence and micromotion of the implant.

It is also controversial whether to use the cement type or cementless type in inflammatory diseases such as rheumatoid arthritis. In general, it is not recommended to use the cementless type in patients with inflammatory disease as most of them have accompanying osteopenia.

2.3 Design of Each Component

2.3.1 Femur

The design of femoral implants varies according to the overall shape, the method of fixation, CR or PS type, and the motion constraint.

2.3.1.1 Shape

The factors to be taken into consideration for the shape of the femoral component in coronal plane are the A–P length–width ratio, symmetricity of both condyles, shape of the cam, the length and width of the notch portion, shape and radius of the posterior condyle, and the depth and direction of the patellar groove. In the sagittal plane, each product differs according to the slope of the anterior flange, symmetricity of the condyles, and length and radius of the posterior condyle. Although the design is based on the anatomy and biomechanics of the knee joint, it should actually reflect the changes in the anatomy and biomechanics of the knee joint.

In the symmetric type, all parts or only the part which articulates with the PE can be symmetrical. If all parts are symmetrical, it is cheaper to fabricate and store the products, but this type is not used currently. In most of the symmetric types, only the joint part is symmetrical, so the anterior flanges and patellofemoral grooves are asymmetrical.

Ratio of A–P Length and Width

The ratio of the A–P length and width varies slightly between the prostheses. *The A–P length is related to the flexion gap and the width is related to coverage of the bone.*

If the size is chosen with the priority to the width, a flexion and extension gap discrepancy may develop. Whereas, when the implant size is chosen just according to the A–P length, the implant may overhang or underhang. *Overhang of the implant causes pain and motion limitation and underhang of the implant causes more bleeding, stress concentration, and instability.* So, the ratio of A–P length and width is a critical factor to be considered while designing the component.

It is known that this ratio is different between men and women and between races. Anatomically, *the width is narrower, anterior femoral condylar projection is lower, and patellar groove is more oblique in women than in men.* Certain prostheses are designed to reflect the femoral anatomical characteristics in women and are termed the Gender Knee prostheses (Zimmer, Warsaw, IN). But there are also anatomical differences in the geometry of the knee joint among women as well. Dargel et al. reported the morphometric data obtained from 60 human cadavers which demonstrated that male knees were significantly larger than female knees, but matched-pair analysis did not prove the difference in the A–P length–width ratio between men and women. Kim et al. also reported the results of the gender-specific prostheses, which suggested that they were not always necessary and smaller prostheses were inserted in 90 % of the patients when gender-specific prosthesis was used. Johnson et al. reported similar results which suggested that there is no difference in the outcome of patients with a gender-specific knee arthroplasty versus a unisex arthroplasty.

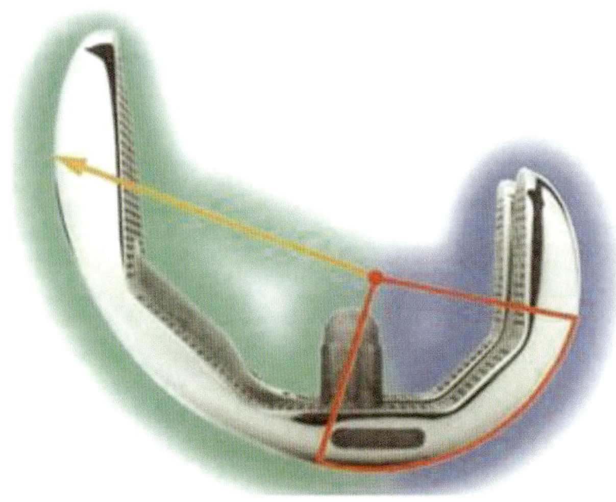

Single axis design (Scorpio, Mahwah,NJ)

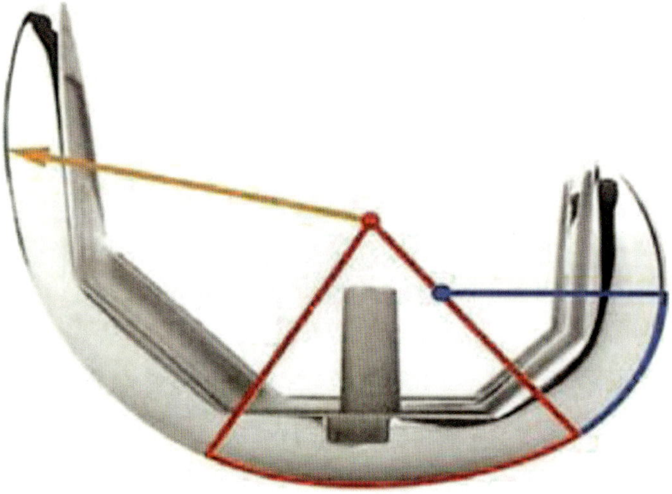

Multiple axis design (Zimmer, Warsaw, IN)

Fig. 2.24 Symmetric and asymmetric femoral component {NexGen (Zimmer, Warsaw, IN)}

Patellar Groove

Patella-friendly designs are developed *such that the patellar groove is oblique, deeper, and shifted laterally and the lateral portion is enhanced* for better alignment of the patella. The current patella-friendly design has reduced the incidence of patellar fracture, avascular necrosis, and lateral retinacular release as well. Yoshii et al. used an experimental model and demonstrated that specific changes in the femoral design, including deepening and distal extension of trochlear groove, resulted in an improvement in patellar tracking compared to that with a conventional femoral component.

Deepening the patellar groove has a major impact on the overall shape because the amount of osteotomy has to be increased or the implants should be thinner and the chamfer portion of implant needs to be reinforced to resist the bending force.

Axis of Motion

The radius and shape of the condyle are related to the PE design and constitute the most important characteristics of the femoral component.

A symmetric design means that the medial and lateral condyles are symmetric in the sagittal planes. One of the advantages of a symmetric design is that it has a longer extensor moment arm which helps to improve the quadriceps function and to reduce anterior knee pain. *In the asymmetric type, the radius of the medial and lateral condyle and the shape of the distal and posterior condyle are different* (Fig. 2.24). Mostly the radius of the lateral condyle is larger than that of the medial condyle, so the flexion–extension axis and axis of rotational motion change (multiple axis) during extension and flexion (Fig. 2.25).

Surgeons who are not in favor of a symmetric design state that the knee joint is asymmetric anatomically and biomechanically, and the center of motion on flexion and extension is not constant but shows a J shape. The J-curve motion is known to occur after 30–40° of flexion.

On the other hand, surgeons who are in favor of symmetric design state that the artificial joints should be designed according to the mechanics of artificial joints, not according to the biomechanics of human joints. *More recent studies showed a constant axis during flexion and extension motion rather than the J-shaped axis* (single axis).

The asymmetric design theoretically facilitates rollback and improves flexion, but the decreasing radius of curvature reduces the contact area of the articulating femur as the knee flexes, which may lead to an increase in PE stresses. *Decreasing the radius of medial condyle results in decreasing tension on the medial collateral ligament as the knee flexes, which results in mid-flexion instability*. However, *it has not yet been established as to which of these two designs is better*.

There is a design that has a *ball-shaped medial femoral condyle, so-called Medial Pivot Knee (ADVANCE; Wright Arlington, TN)*, based on the concept *that biomechanically the axis of rotation is on the medial condyle*. Some suggest that rollback of the medial condyle occurs to a lesser extent or may not occur at all, but biomechanically there is no problem in flexion motion as the motion increases through the lateral condylar rollback (Fig. 2.26). Blaha stated that A–P stability is important when walking and that the Medial Pivot Knee implant offers better stability than that with the CR and PS types of other implants in which there is anterior translation of the femur during the stance phase. However, it should be pointed out that medial pivoting does not occur when the cruciate ligament is sacrificed. *Clinical results of Medial Pivot Knee reported by the surgeons are quite the opposite, demonstrating both the good and poor results*.

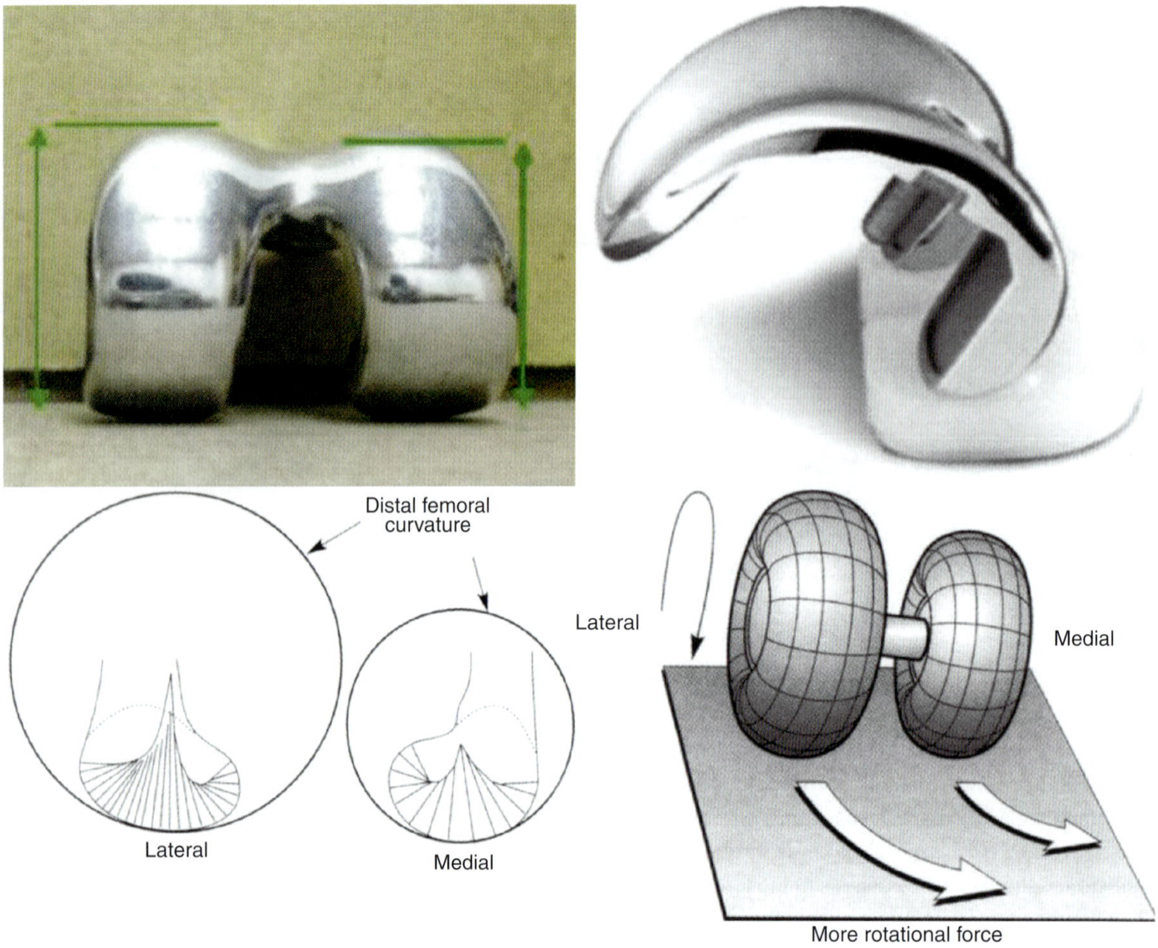

Fig. 2.25 Comparison of single-axis design and multiple-axis design. It is classified into single axis and multiple axis according to the movement of the center of axis in flexion and extension

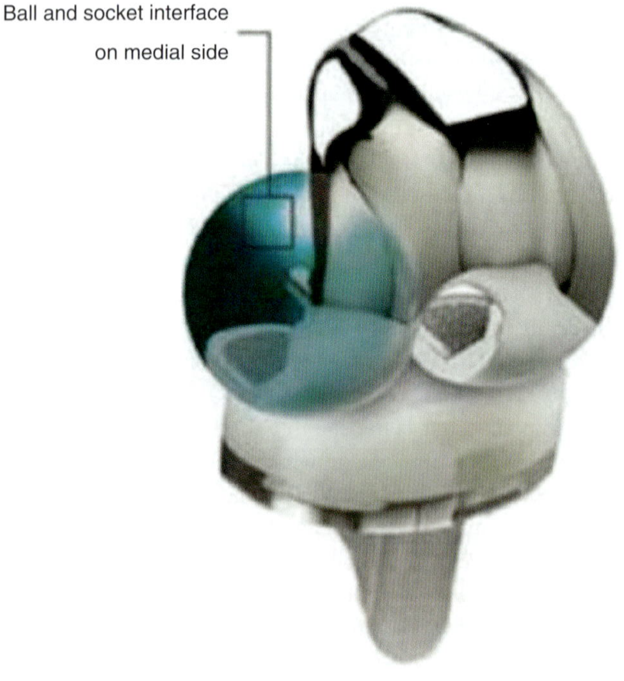

Fig. 2.26 Medial Pivot Knee implant (ADVANCE: Wright Medical Technology, Arlington, TN)

2.3.1.2 PS Type

PS type has an *oval-shaped cam in the cross section of the femur to achieve smooth femoral rollback*. Most of this rollback mechanism is designed to occur when the knee is flexed by 60–70°, but in some designs the rollback starts from 20 to 30° of flexion. Early engagement causes some discomfort in early flexion and late engagement increases the jump distance effectively as the cam rides down from the post (Fig. 2.27).

Currently, the notch portion has been shortened in the PS type to reduce the incidence of patellar clunk syndrome. Frye et al. reported that femoral component with a deep trochlear groove and smooth transition of the intercondylar box appears to accommodate better and reduces peripatellar fibrous nodule.

PS type can be classified into *open-box type, semi-open-box type, and closed-box type* according to the design of the notch portion. The open-box type exposes the bones in the notch area (Fig. 2.28, Left). In the open-box type, more time is required for cementing because the cement needs to be removed meticulously so that it does not come in contact with the post of the PE. However, a large osteotomy is not required and *IM nailing can be performed through the opening in the case of periprosthetic fracture*. In the *closed-box type*, the notch area is covered by the metal and it is *opposite*

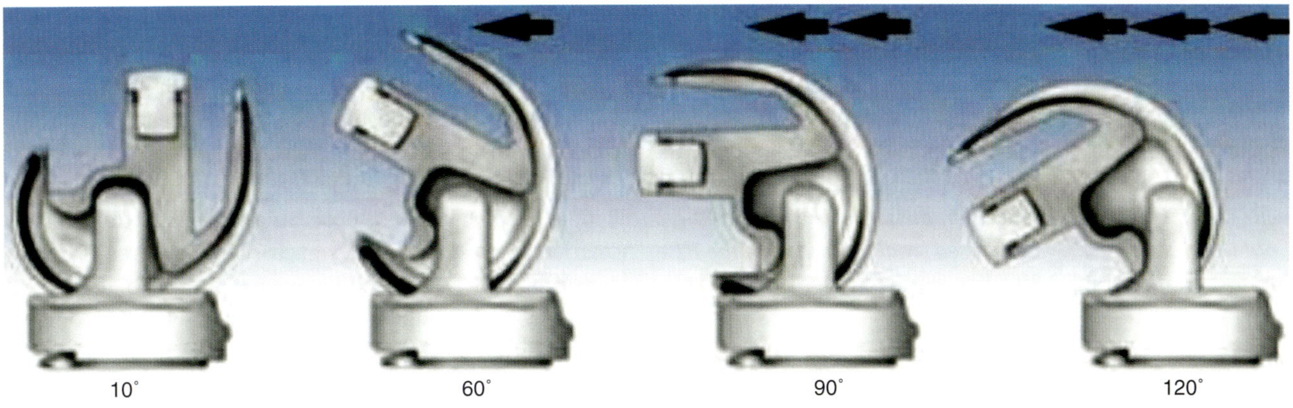

Fig. 2.27 How the cam effect occurs (Duracon: Stryker, Mahwah, NJ)

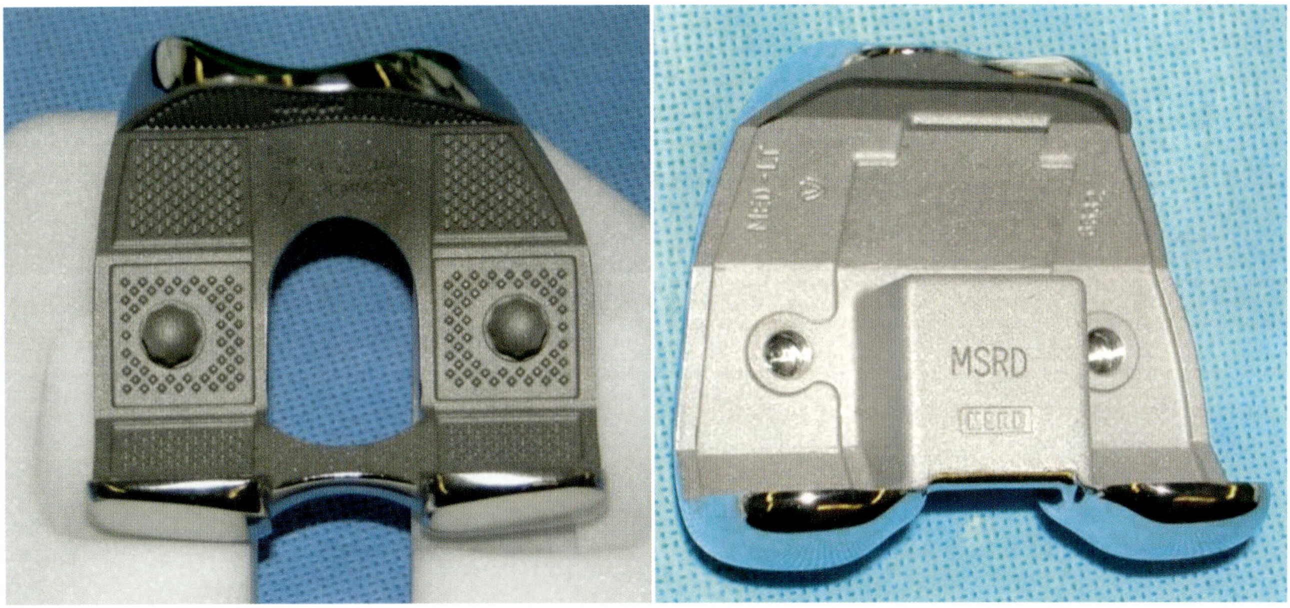

Fig. 2.28 *Left*. Open-box type of PS prosthesis (Scorpio: Stryker, Mahwah, NJ). *Right*. Closed-box type of PS prosthesis (Duracon: Stryker, Mahwah, NJ)

to the open-box type in terms of the advantages and disadvantages (Fig. 2.28, Right).

The semi-open-box type has walls on both the sides and the medullary canal is exposed. In the closed-box type and semi-open-box type, burst fracture can occur during insertion of the prosthesis, if the osteotomy is inadequate at the box area.

2.3.2 Tibia

Tibial implants are also designed according to the overall shape, shape of the stem, and fixation method of the PE to the tibial plate.

2.3.2.1 Shape

The overall shape of tibial implants varies according to the symmetricity of the medial and lateral plateau and the ratio of A–P length and width. Cho et al. reported that the medial plateau is about 4 mm larger than the lateral plateau in width in elderly Korean patients and that the A–P length–width ratio between the prostheses is significantly different. Because of this size discrepancy between the medial and lateral tibial plateaus, *some prostheses are designed asymmetrically* (Fig. 2.29).

In the symmetric designs, the size of the left and right side of the tibial component is the same and coverage of the medial condyle is usually inadequate. If a larger implant is used for better coverage of the medial condyle, the lateral side of the prosthesis overhangs and the fixation of the tibial component in the externally rotated position is restricted.

Provided that all other conditions are the same, the asymmetrical design is thought to be better, but it is more expensive and more caution is required when inserting the PE.

Because, although the implant is asymmetrical, the PE is symmetrical and the PE sometimes does not engage correctly in one side and can be broken during its insertion.

Some designs have screw holes on the surface in order to fix the tibial plate to the bone or to fix the metal augment. It is better not to have *screw holes* because they *cause cold wear of the PE which is placed on the top of the tibial plate. Cold wear is a type of wear caused by deformation of the PE due to pressure* (Fig. 2.30). If the screw holes are needed, they should not be in the center where the PE is compressed more during weight bearing.

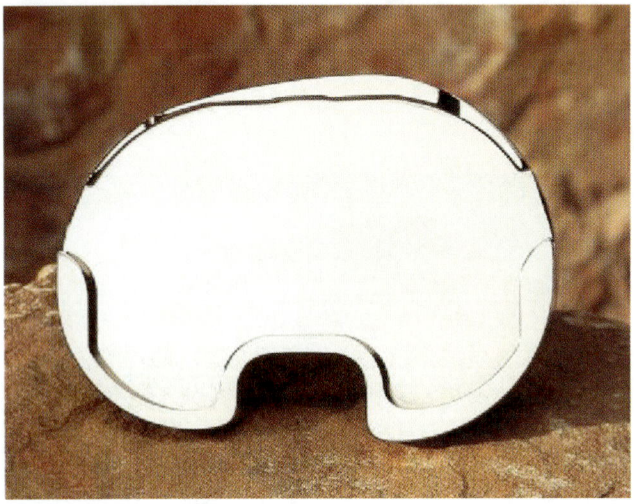

Fig. 2.29 Asymmetric tibial implant (Genesis II: S&N, Richards, TN)

Therefore, primary prosthesis and revision prosthesis are designed separately, and the primary prosthesis should not have any screw holes

When a size discrepancy is noted between the femur and the tibia, it is hard to choose an appropriate tibial plate. A particular prosthesis is designed such that three different sizes of the PE can be used in one size of the tibial plate by altering the edges of the tibial plate so that the PE is compatible with different sizes of the femur (Fig. 2.31).

2.3.2.2 Fixation Method

Surface fixation or a short lug was used in the past, but currently a keel or stem is used to reinforce the fixation. The stem is available in various forms: column, cone, cruciform, I-beam shape, and so on (Fig. 2.32). The length of the stem is different in each prosthesis and some prostheses have an off-center stem considering the anatomy of the tibial condyle.

In some of the cementless types of tibial components, screws were used to reinforce fixation, but they are not used currently because the wear particles flow into the cancellous bones through the screw holes causing osteolysis.

The posterior slope of the proximal tibia can be given by the implant itself or can be incorporated during tibial osteotomy. *Each of the prostheses has the most ideal posterior*

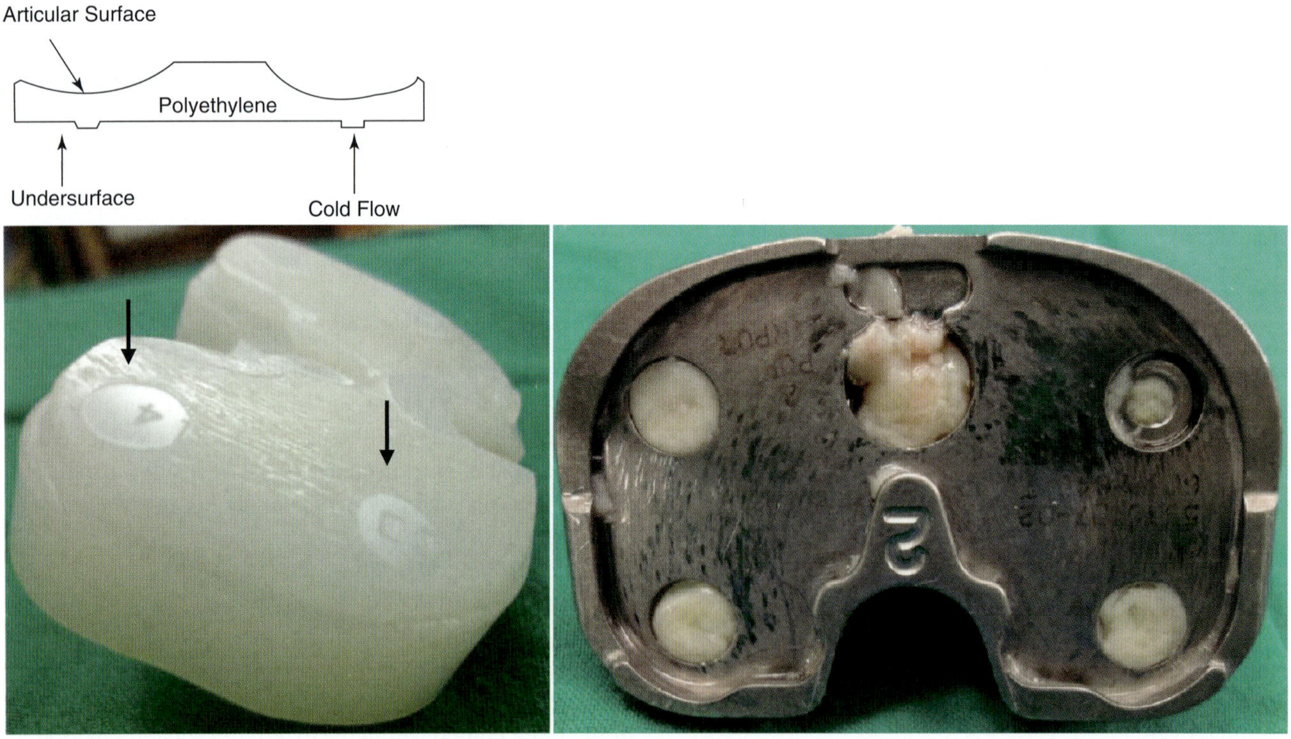

Fig. 2.30 Schematic drawings of cold wear (*top*) and deformation of PE as a result of long-standing pressure (*arrows; bottom, left*). The deformation is symmetrical to holes on the tibial component (*bottom, right*)

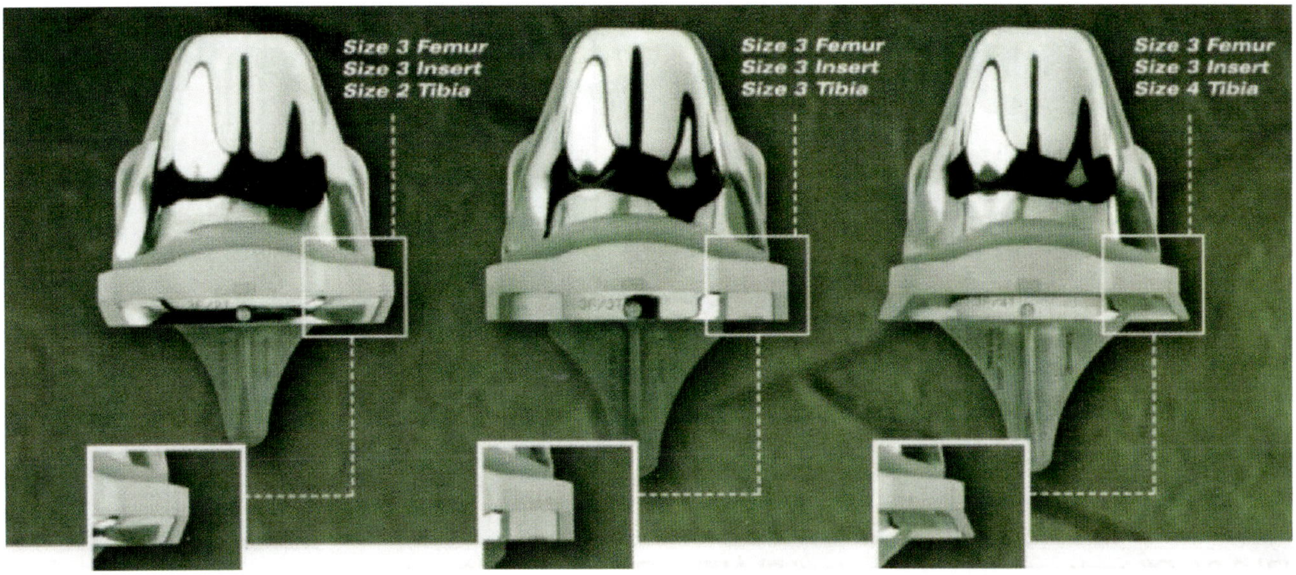

Fig. 2.31 Versatile PE (Optetrak: Exactech, Gainesville, FL). Three sizes of PE can be used in one size of the tibial plate

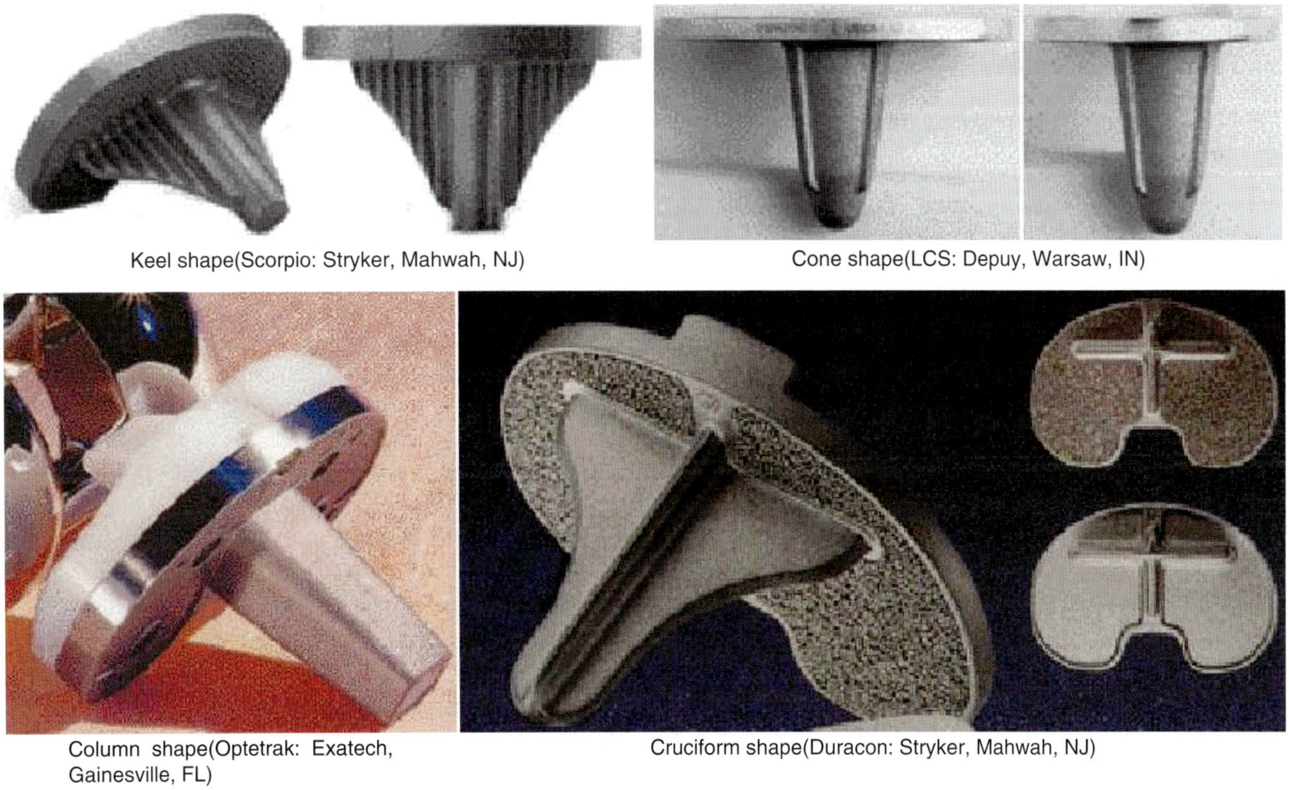

Fig. 2.32 Various shapes of the tibial stem

slope, and hence it is desirable to know the recommended slope before the operation. The slope can be 0° or 3–5° in primary prosthesis. But for most of the revision implants, it is set at 0° because a stem extension may sometimes be needed. *In the PS type, an excessive posterior slope induces stress concentration to the post, thereby causing early post wear and breakage. Most of the PS types have been designed to have less than 7° of posterior slope.*

2.3.2.3 PE Fixation onto the Tibial Plate

The advantages of metal-backed PE are that it ensures even distribution of load on the tibia, prevents the deformation

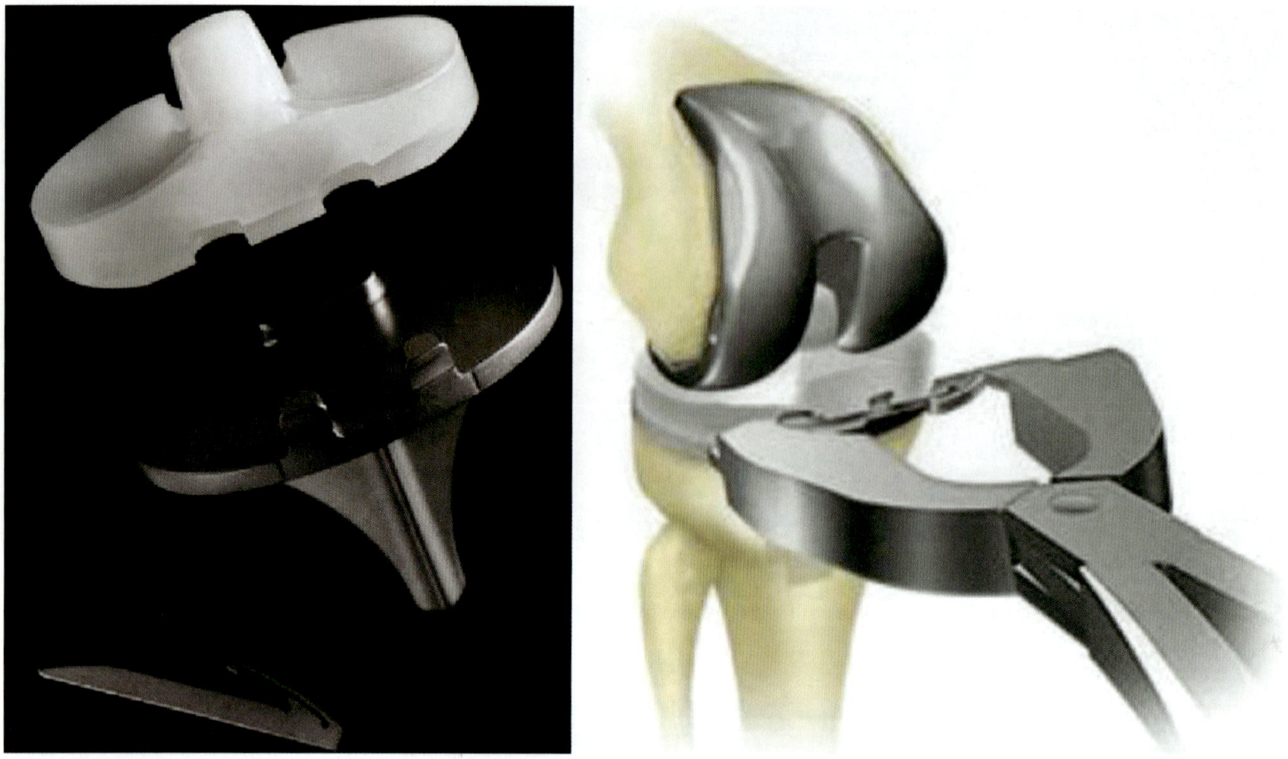

Fig. 2.33 PE fixation for the tongue type (Vanguard: Biomet, Warsaw, IN)

of PE, and allows for the use of PE of different thicknesses, and there is ease of potential revision and optimization of soft tissue balance. Hence, it is known as the most ideal form till now. *But metal-backed PE has a disadvantage that the PE has to be thinner or a larger osteotomy is required.*

Based on the method of fixation of PE onto the tibial implants, there are 3 types of *metal-backed PE*. The snap-fit type has a groove along the edge of the tibial plate and the PE is fixed onto the groove with a little pressure. There are some modified designs which have grooves on the PE anteriorly and posteriorly so as to enhance the fitting to the edges. This type improves the fixation, but the PE can be damaged when it is not inserted properly. The tongue type uses a metal lock for the fixation of PE (Fig. 2.33).

When thicker PE is used in constrained implants, metal screws or metal bars are used to fix the PE onto the base plate. However, Cho et al. experienced screw migration in the screw fixation type (Fig. 2.34).

Park et al. reported that *micromotion between the PE and the tibial implant could not be prevented no matter how solid the fixation was. So in the current implants, the surface of the tibial plate is made smooth or polished.* Berry et al. reported that the polished CoCr tibial tray showed less undersurface wear of the PE than that of rough titanium tray.

The all-poly tibial components which have been used in the past have become an issue again. Early (first generation) TKA implant designs included the all-poly tibial component, and their results were unsatisfactory over time. However, the current all-poly tibial component designs have demonstrated comparable long-term results in terms of both durability and function. *If the thickness of the PE is greater than 10 mm, it allows for even distribution of load just like that in the metal-backed PE. But, it is generally accepted that all-poly tibial components induce excessive load on the tibia.* Faris et al. stated that all-poly tibial components would show very different results according to the design. However, Dalury et al. reported the results of all-poly tibial components stating that the clinical results were excellent and the 7-year survival rate was 99.4 %. Bettinson et al. also reported that the 10-year survival rate was 97 % and Voight et al. similarly reported that the less expensive all-poly tibial components showed equivalent results to those obtained with cemented metal-backed tibial components.

There are some disadvantages of the all-poly tibial components. Specifically, there is a lack of modularity (which limits the intraoperative options), only cement-type implants are available in most of cases, they do not allow for liner insert removal for irrigation and debridement in cases of acute infection, they do not allow for late liner exchange, there is a potential difficulty for the removal of posteriorly extruded cement, and all-poly tibial components cannot be used in patients with severe deformities and bony defects.

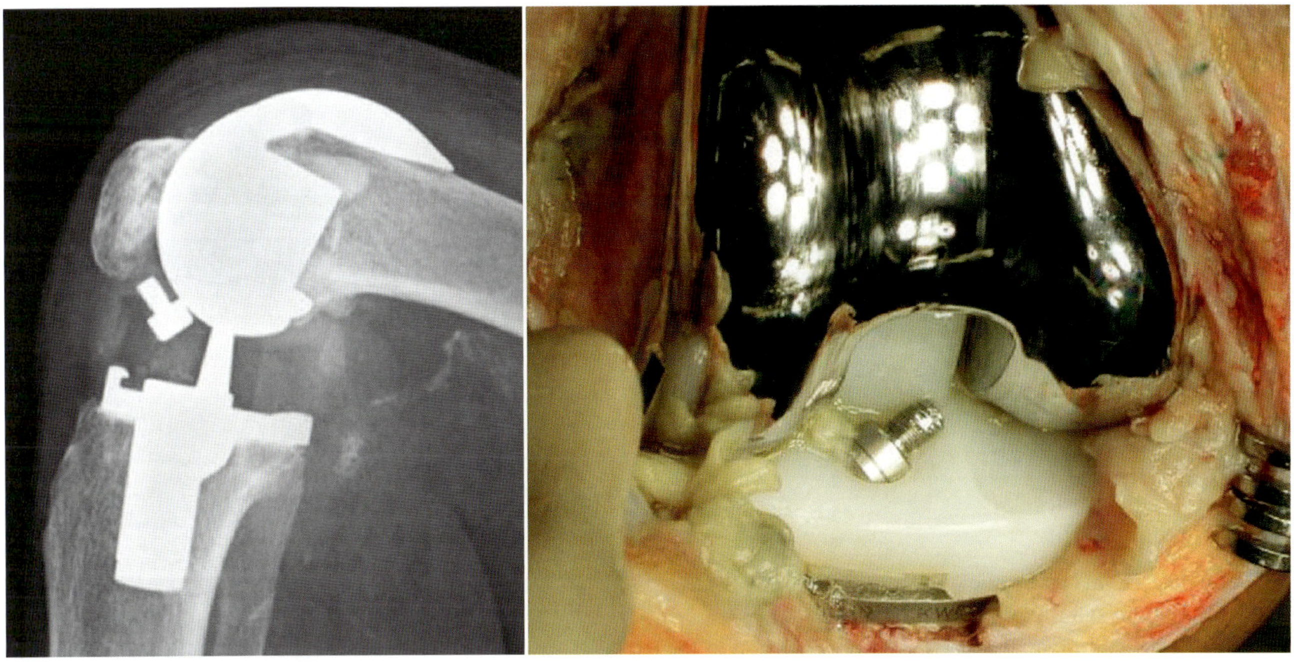

Fig. 2.34 Screw migration from the tibial plate

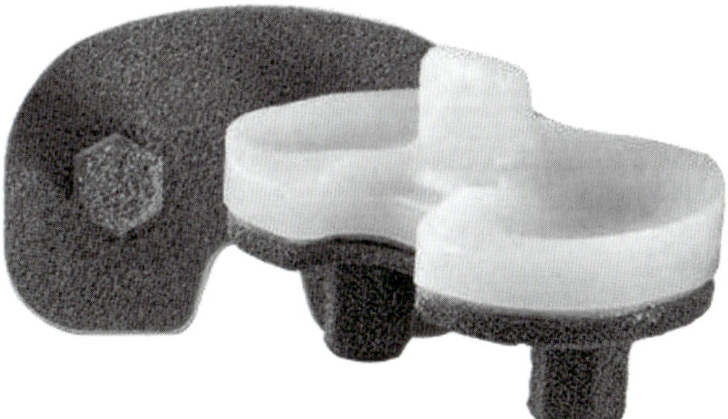

Fig. 2.35 Porous tantalum: PE unit (Zimmer, Warsaw, IN)

The prosthesis in which *the porous tantalum is prefixed (tantalum monoblock) to the PE* has also been introduced (Fig. 2.35). Kamath et al. achieved promising clinical and radiological results in younger patients at a minimum 5-year follow-up using uncemented tantalum monoblock.

In the mobile-bearing joints, there are two types of tibial plates for axial rotation. One has a cone-shaped stem into which the cone-shaped spacer is fitted, and the other has a trunnion over the tibial plate along which the mobile bearing rotates.

The surface of the tibial plate of mobile-bearing joints is polished so as to reduce undersurface wear, and in some designs, the margin of tibial plate is enhanced in order to reduce excessive motion.

2.3.3 Spacer (Polyethylene)

Spacer is a piece that is placed between the tibia and the femur. It is sometimes called the PE because most of the spacers are made of polyethylene. Since the patellar component is also made of PE, it is more appropriate to name the PE between the tibia and the femur as spacer.

Spacer is designed to fit the shapes of the femur and tibia and is closely related to the motion, stability, and wear which are directly related to the clinical outcome and to the survival of TKA.

The shape of the spacer varies greatly, mostly according to the degree of conformity, PCL retention or substitution, method of fixation onto the base plate, and constraint between the implants.

If the shape is too flat, it has low conformity and the incidence of wear is increased. If conformity is too high, the incidence of loosening is increased. If the edge is made too sharp so as to increase the conformity, it may cause an edge fracture, thereby accelerating further wear.

For better flexion motion, the current PE has a curved track instead of the straight track so as to allow femoral rotation during flexion, and the posterior portion is made smooth (posterior release) in some prostheses.

In the PS type, motion is determined by the size, length, location, and shape of the post. If the post is round and short, the motion is increased and the stability is decreased. If the length of the post is long and the post is located posteriorly, it reduces posterior dislocation of the joints. If it is rectangular and long and there is a little interval between the femur

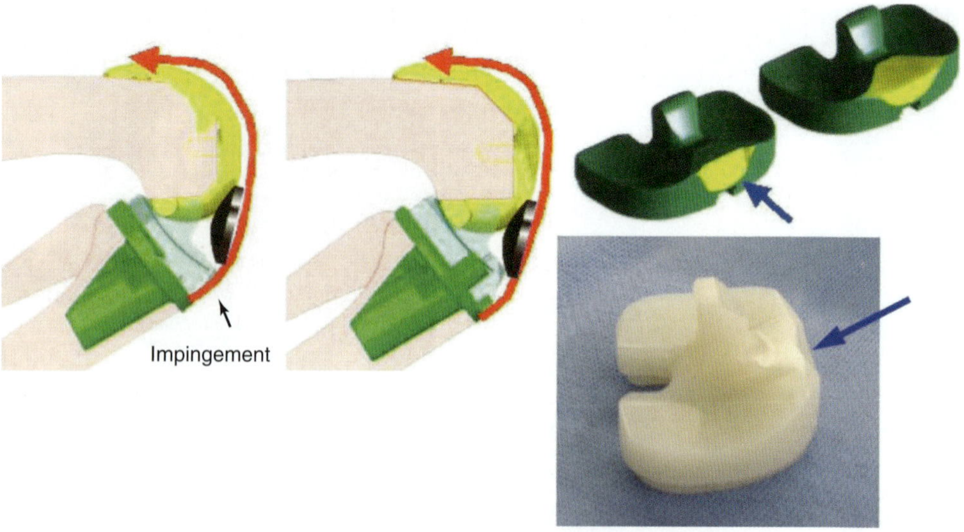

Fig. 2.36 Beveled PE (Optetrak: Exactech, Gainesville, FL, and NexGen: Zimmer, Warsaw, IN)

and the post, it becomes the constrained type with less motion and more stability.

In ultrahigh congruent designs, the anterior portion of the PE is elevated instead of the post so as to enhance the A–P stability.

Impingement can occur between the patella and the PE due to patella baja. *The current trend is to use the beveled type of PE in which the front of the PE is not cut vertically but diagonally* (Fig. 2.36).

In mobile-bearing joints, the CR type allows the PE to rotate and move forward/backward, whereas the PS type allows for rotation only.

The size of the PE is designed to fit in the tibial implants and its thickness varies between prostheses, and the surgeon can choose the thickness of the PE according to the flexion and extension gap. Thickness is closely related to the wear, and Bartel et al. found that *wear occurs rapidly when the thickness of the PE is less than 6 mm*. Most of the times, as the thinnest portion of the PE is thinner by more than 2 mm than the registered thickness of the PE, *any spacer thinner than 9 mm should not be used. PE must not be too thick either*, because it can alter the kinetics of the knee joint if it is too thick.

2.3.4 Patella

With respect to the patellar design, it should be remembered that *patellar tracking, contact area, and pressure distribution are significantly different between the native and prosthetic knees*.

The configuration and mechanical features to be considered in the patellar component design should include the functional range of motion in multiaxial planes, stability, fixation method, dimensions, load transfer areas, and materials. A successful patellofemoral articulation must be designed to function and endure high-stress conditions over a long period of time.

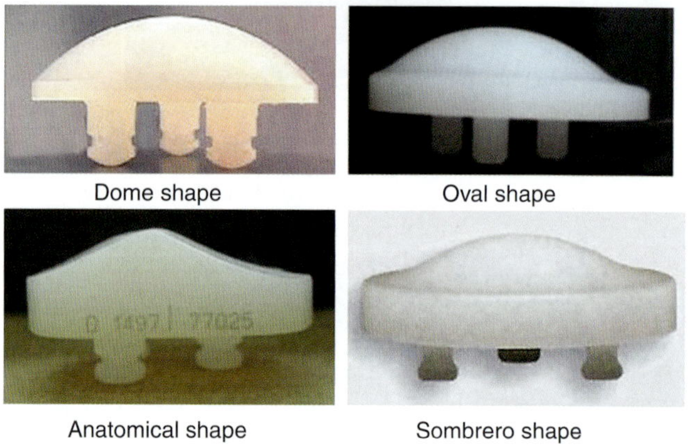

Fig. 2.37 Various shapes of patella component (Courtesy of Scorpio, Duracon, Sulzer Medica, DePuy)

The type of patellar implant varies according to the shape, fixation method, site of implantation, composition, and mobility.

2.3.4.1 Shape

The patellar implant is classified into the dome type, oval type, and anatomical type according to its shape, and each shape may have sharp and thin edges or may be of the sombrero type. *Sombrero (Mexican or Spanish hat) type, in which the edges are thickened, is designed to fit into the femoral groove and is theoretically strong against wear* because it distributes the stress uniformly (Fig. 2.37). Hsu and Walker found on a wear simulation test that increasing the conformity in the frontal plane increases the survival of the component by more than 20 times.

It is easy to perform operation with the dome type because it has no axis of rotation for tracking. Tracking of the oval type is known to be better than that of the dome type, but tracking of the oval type can be worse if the axis of rotation is not aligned. *The anatomical type is theoretically the best model for tracking* as it is designed based on the anatomy; *however it requires more accurate matching of the size and*

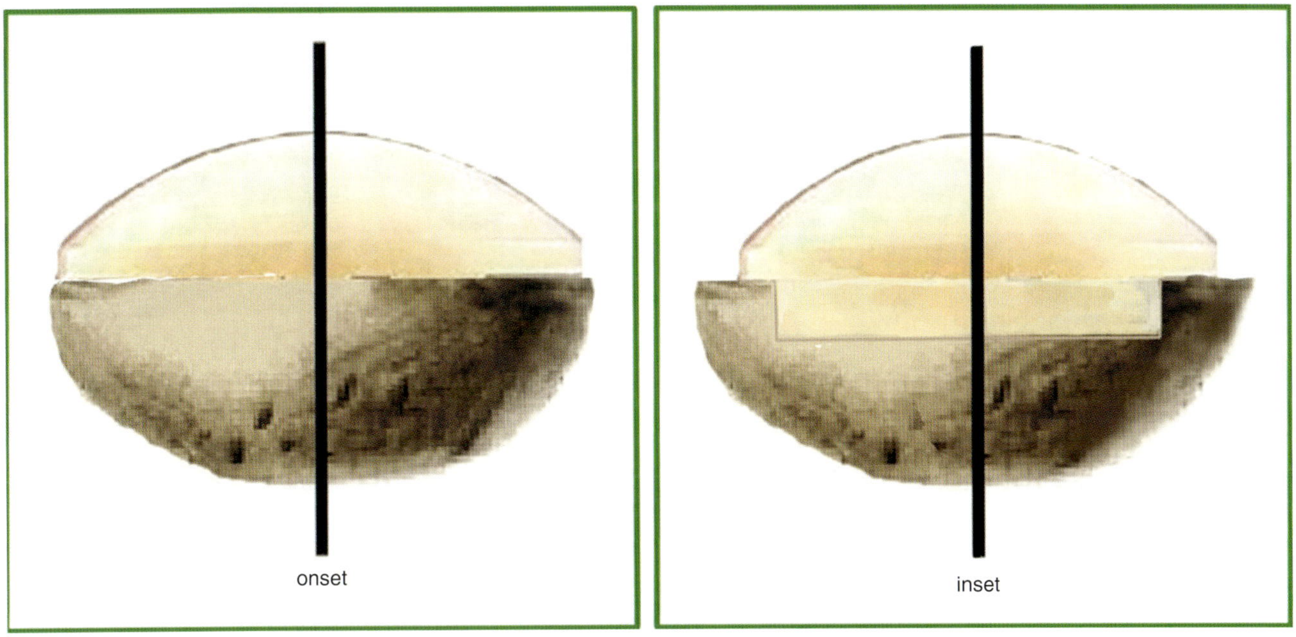

Fig. 2.38 Onset and inset patellar implant

axis. In other words, the dome-shaped components are easy to use, but it is more likely to develop maltracking and wear. However, the anatomically shaped patellar prostheses are more sensitive to malpositioning and hence implantation of anatomically shaped patellar prostheses needs careful surgical technique.

2.3.4.2 Composition

In the past, metal-backed patella was used, but it inevitably decreased the thickness of the PE, thereby increasing the PE wear. Therefore, the patella which is used currently is made of all poly.

2.3.4.3 Fixation Method

Patellar component has lugs to promote the fixation and are mostly fixed with bone cement. The design has evolved from one lug in the center to three lugs. The three-lug design reinforces the fixation, preserves more blood flow, and reduces the incidence of patellar fracture, but it increases the incidence of loosening due to the breakage of lugs.

2.3.4.4 Design According to the Site of Implantation

According to the site of the patellar component implantation, there is *an onset patellar implant* that is placed over the bone and *an inset patellar implant* that is implanted into a trough made in the bone. The onset patellar implant is the standard type.

The inset patellar implant was developed by Freeman et al. to improve the extensor mechanics, to increase the thickness of the PE, and for use even when there is bone erosion or bone loss. It has been suggested that the *inset patellar implant provides greater composite (implant + patella) strength and may decrease the amount of patellar tilt and shift*. But it is not widely used other than in patellofemoral arthroplasty because it is more complex to use, *there may be some problems related to the articular surface that has not been replaced*, and it increases the risk of patellar fracture (Fig. 2.38). With respect to the results, Rand et al. reported that there was no difference in anterior knee pain and going up and down the stairs between the onset patellar implant and the inset patellar implant. Even though tracking of the inset patellar implant is better, the radiolucent lines are more frequently observed with this implant. However, Ezzet et al. reported that tracking of the inset patellar implant is poorer than that of the onset patellar implant in flexion.

2.3.5 Size Matching

The results of TKA would be better when the sizes of the femur and PE, femur and patella, and femur and tibia are well matched, although it is not definite as to which size provides the best fit. But different sizes of implants may have to be used inevitably when the sizes of femoral and tibial bones are significantly different.

In such a case, the compatibility between the sizes should be considered so as to choose the allowable sizes. Matching a smaller femur with a larger tibia requires that the intercondylar distance between the femoral runners and PE should be constant and the PE surface should be almost flat. *For each implant, a combination of sizes has been recommended and most of them are compatible with one size up and one size down.*

In the components with the same serial number system, the same number of prostheses should be used with each other. Whereas the components with different serial number

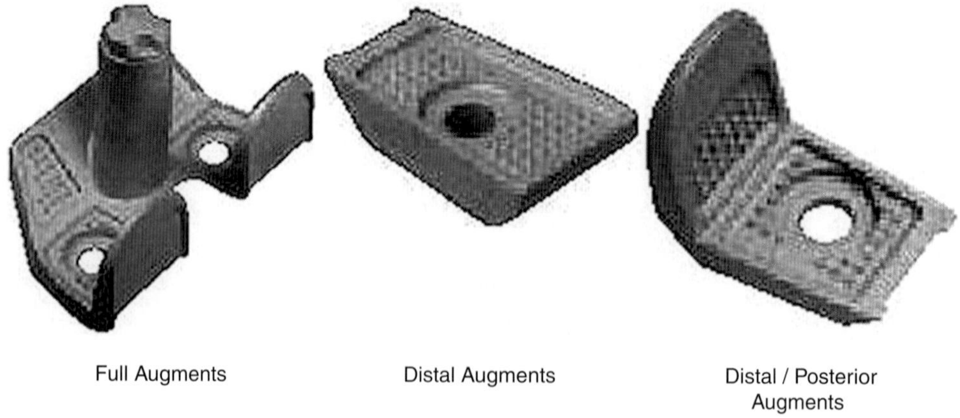

Fig. 2.39 Various shapes of femoral metal augments

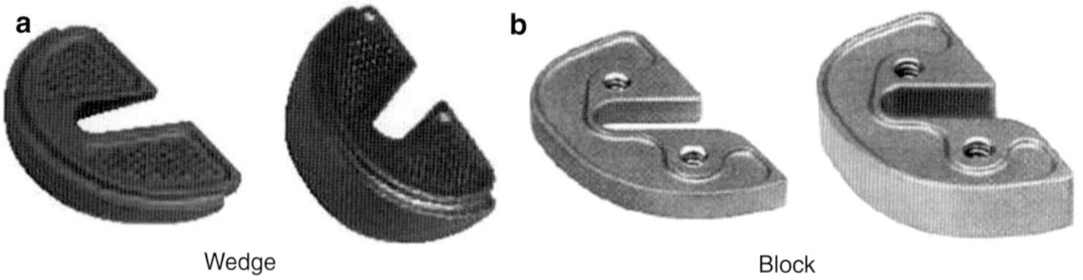

Fig. 2.40 Wedge (**a**) and block (**b**) type of tibial metal augment

system, the size selection is more forgiving. For example, if the femoral implants are numbered as A, B, C and the PE is also numbered as A, B, C, it is better to use the implants with the same serial number. Berend et al. reported through a mechanical study using AGC Knee (Anatomical Graduated Component: Biomet, Warsaw, Indiana) that if the femoral component was two sizes up, edge loading on the tibial component was increased by up to 126 %, which was one of the causes of failure of TKA. Although, it is often advertised by manufacturers that their components are compatible with components of all sizes, it is difficult to accept this claim, and hence it is desirable to select implants of similar sizes, if possible.

2.3.6 Options

In usual primary TKA, no optional components are needed. However, in revision cases with a severe bone defect or instability, some additional surgical procedures or some optional components are needed to fill the bone defect, to correct alignment, and to improve implant stability.

2.3.6.1 Metal Augment

If there is a severe bone defect, it is desirable to reconstruct the defect than to resect more bone up to the defect site and use a thicker PE. If osteotomy is done up to the level of the tibial defect, a smaller implant is required and more cancellous bone is removed which weakens the bone that support the implant. In the femur, the joint line will be elevated if the bone defect is not reconstructed.

The most biological way for *reconstruction of bone defect is bone grafting, but many surgeons prefer metal augmentation* if possible, *because it is easier to reconstruct the bone defect with metal augment and it allows for early weight bearing.*

A femoral metal augment is available for the anterior, distal, and posterior portions, and some augments comprise of all three portions in a single unit (Fig. 2.39). The metal augment is stronger when it is made as a single unit, so it is better to use one-unit augment if needed. However, too much bone removal may be required when using a one-unit augment.

Tibial metal augments are of the block type or wedge type (Fig. 2.40). With the use of the wedge-type metal augment, more bones can be preserved as most of the bone defects are wedge shaped, but it is a little more difficult to perform osteotomy and the metal augment is under shear force, thereby causing loosening more frequently than that with the use of the block-type metal augment. So *the block-type tibial metal augment is the most commonly used and it has shown better mechanical performance than the wedge-type tibial metal augment.*

Metal augments have different thicknesses according to the products, but they generally are up to 10 mm in thickness. Bone cement or screws are used for fixation to the main component. Screw fixation, although mechanically stable, creates the possibility of metallic debris formation by micromotion. Cement may not serve as the ideal bonding material between the main component and the metal augment, as the bonding strength is weak. Hence, a combined method is recommended.

2.3.6.2 Choren (Correction by Height and Orientation Renovation) Pad

I designed 2 mm and 3 mm metal augments *to correct the flexion–extension gap discrepancy, varus–valgus malalignment and femoral malrotation*. When these pads are applied to both the sides of the distal portion of the femoral component, they can decrease the extension gap. When the pad is applied to one side of the distal femoral component or underneath of the one side of the tibial component, it can correct varus or valgus malalignment without additional bone resection. Using these pads on both the posterior sides of the femoral condyle decreases the flexion gap. Malrotation of the femoral component can be corrected when the Choren pad is applied to one side of the posterior femoral condyles (Fig. 2.41).

2.3.6.3 Trabecular System

A metal trabecular system, which is biomechanically similar to the trabecular bone, has been developed for use in a severe cavitary bone defect (Fig. 2.42). This is made of porous tantalum and has high capability of biologic bone ingrowth. There are femoral, tibial, and patellar trabecular system. Size and shape of system is different according to the size and shape of defect where it is used. The advantages of this system are that large cavitary defect can be filled with one unit of this system and good bone ingrowth can be achieved. Lachiewicz et al. reported that the use of tantalum cones in revision TKA is a promising technique with a low rate of infection and component loosening. The drawbacks are that it is surgically demanding to implant and hard to remove during revision surgery.

2.3.6.4 Extension Stem

If a bone defect is too large such that the stability of implants is at a risk, or if the constrained type of implant is used, it is necessary to attach an extension stem to reinforce the fixation.

Extension stem is a part of the modular system. Hence, the diameter and length of an extension stem may be adjusted according to the size and length of each bone. The extension stem may not be straight or may be adjusted off-center in cases in which bones are severely deformed or when the bone loss is not consistent (Fig. 2.43).

Some surgeons are worried about the adverse effects of the use of extension stem on the host bone such as stress shielding, but it is reported that this does not result in severe osteoporosis. *End-of-stem pain* may develop at the area of the stem tip. It occurs *more commonly with the use of stiff cobalt chromium stem. The incidence of end-of-stem pain is decreased with the use of titanium stem and slotted or fluted stem.*

If an extension stem is used on the femoral side, more bones need to be resected at the notch area than that in the PS type, and the angle of the stem is set at 5–7° according to the prosthesis. When an extension stem is used on the tibial side, the angle between the main unit and extension stem is mostly 90° in the coronal and sagittal planes.

2.3.6.5 Custom-Made Prosthesis

Although custom-made prosthesis is not an optional component, it may be needed in special situation such as when the bone loss is very severe and the bone is too small. The prosthesis is custom made based on the anatomical data of patients and the opinions of the surgeon. However, manufacturing of the custom-made prosthesis is too time-consuming and costly. This is not used frequently with the development of the modular type of prosthesis. *Theoretically, custom-made prosthesis offers many benefits, but it can lead to worse results if something goes wrong during the operation.*

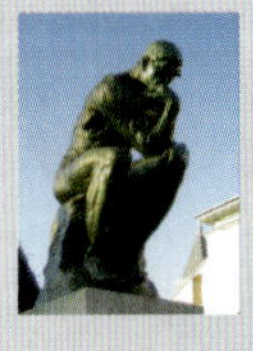

Author's Opinion

While using an extension stem on the femoral side, the femoral component tends to be inserted in some degree of anterior angulation. To avoid this, I would use an offset stem, use a larger implant and cementing on the anterior side, or insert the femoral component in some degree of anterior angulation.

I think this occurs not because of size mismatching, but because of improper location of the femoral stem. Most of the extension stem axes do not match with femoral medullary axis. The anatomical axis of distal femur in the sagittal plane falls at the center of the anterior half of the femoral condyle, but the axis of extension stem is located a little lower than medullary axis in some of the prostheses. Even if we insert the correct size of femoral component, the axis of extension stem becomes a little lower than the medullary axis resulting in anterior angulation of the implant.

I think the implant design should be modified such that the location of the extension stem axis on the femoral component is a little more anterior in sagittal plane.

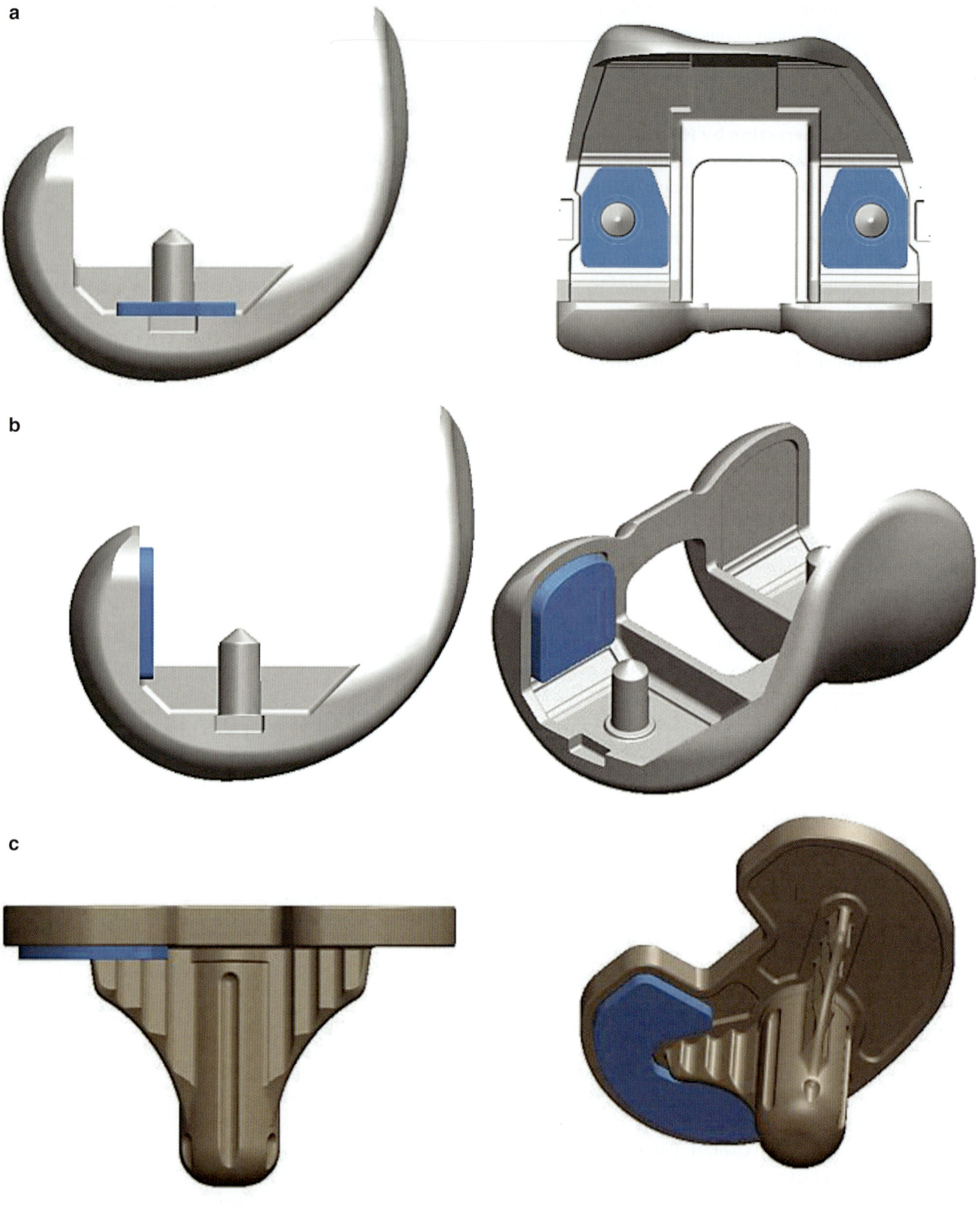

Fig. 2.41 Choren pad. (**a**) femoral distal pad, (**b**) femoral posterior pad, (**c**) tibial pad (Corentec, Seoul, Korea)

2.3.7 Design to Increase Knee Flexion

The ability to bend the knee joint to a greater degree is desirable, especially in Orientals whose traditional lifestyle needs high-flexion activities such as sitting on the floor and squatting.

Two aspects should be considered in high-flexion knee designs: how to increase flexion and how to do so without an increase the complication rate. To increase knee flexion, it is required to improve the rollback, prevent impingement, decrease the posterior radius of the femoral condyle, and increase the rotation according to the biomechanics of the knee joint. These are determined mainly by the design of the femoral implants and the PE because the PE comes in contact with the femoral implants.

Flexion can be increased by improving the rollback. The PS type is mostly designed to allow for the cam effect from 70° of knee flexion. Flexion can be increased if the cam action starts earlier at an angle lesser than 70°. The other way to achieve more rollback is to place the post on the posterior side. However, if the post is placed too posteriorly, it can cause roll-off and dislocation. *Flexion can be increased due to the increase in the rollback, if the posterior radius is smaller than the distal radius.*

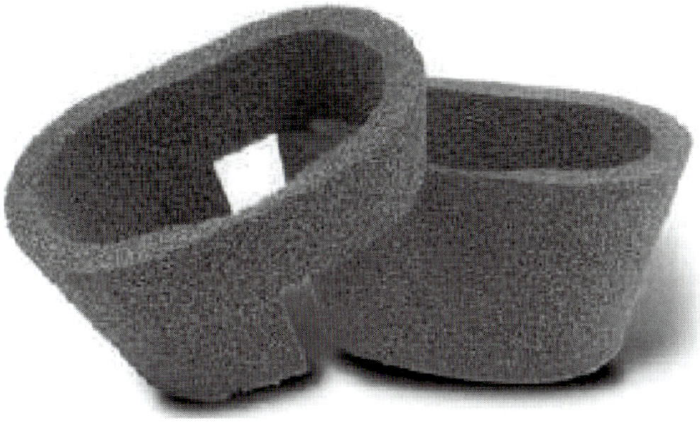

Fig. 2.42 Trabecular metal augment (Zimmer, Warsaw, IN)

To reduce impingement, the impingement angle should be large. Impingement angle is the flexion angle at which the posterior femoral cortex meets the tibial PE, and it is closely related to the posterior condylar offset. *Posterior condylar offset refers to the distance between the posterior cortex of the femur and the posterior condylar portion of the implant* (Fig. 2.8). If the posterior condylar offset is large, soft tissue impingement is reduced, thereby increasing knee flexion. Massin et al. reported that flexion is decreased by 10° when the posterior condylar offset is reduced by 3 mm. However Ishii et al. found that the medial posterior condylar offset was significantly larger before surgery and the lateral posterior condylar offset was significantly larger after surgery. Therefore, correct recognition of the condyle which reflects the ROM may be difficult using conventional X-ray.

If rotation is limited, flexion is also limited. Therefore, in some designs, femoral implants of different shapes were made for the medial and lateral condyles, and the end of the posterior condyle flared out to increase axial rotation. The shape of the PE articulating with the femoral condyle is also changed into a curved shape to achieve better rotation (Fig. 2.44).

Making the posterior margin of the PE smooth (posterior release) is another option for increasing flexion motion. However, it may cause an increase in posterior instability.

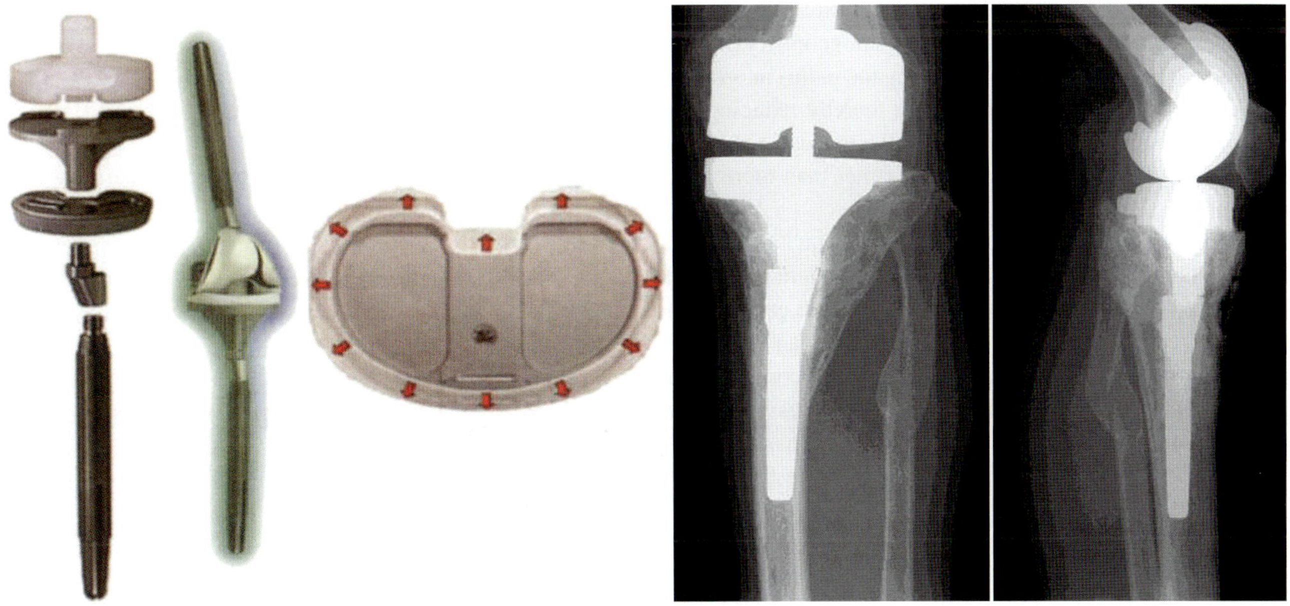

Fig. 2.43 Offset stem (stem extension) and its application in arthroplasty

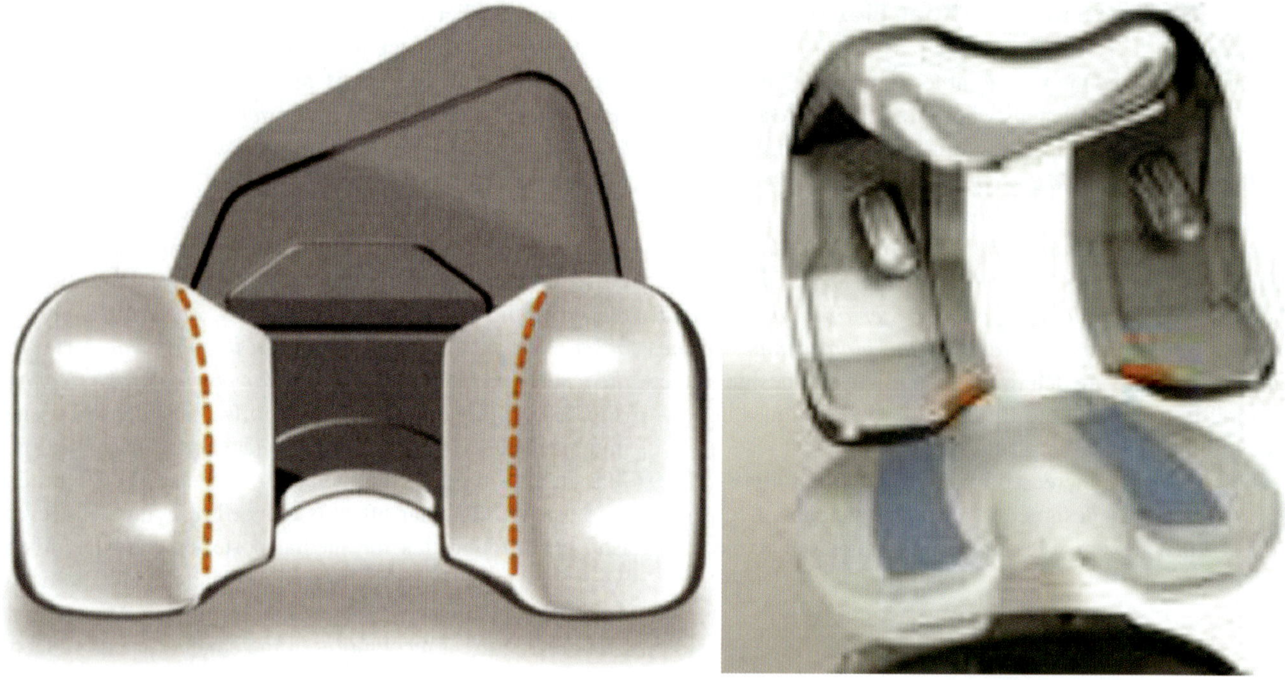

Fig. 2.44 The posterior side of the condyle flared out to achieve more rotation and the articular surface of the PE is curved so as to increase rotation (Stryker, Mahwah, NJ)

Achieving better flexion is desirable, but it should not cause instability or any other complications, such as wear or loosening. When flexion is increased, four factors affect the survival of implants. First, the vertical compression increases. Second, stress on the posterior part of the PE increases. Third, the forces imposed on the patella increase. Fourth, the forces imposed on the PCL (CR type) or post (PS type) increase. Therefore, it is not only important to increase flexion, but it is also important to decrease the wear and loosening caused by the increase in the stress. High-flex design has improved posterior condylar geometry of the femoral component instead of reducing the radius in order to improve contact area in high flexion, thereby reducing the risk of PE wear. In this sense, high-flexion design should consider possible complications first rather than more flexion motion.

There were also some reports suggesting that high-flexion knee designs showed abnormal kinematic pattern compared to that in the conventional prosthesis. Shimizu et al. found that post–cam engagement occurred significantly earlier under non-weight-bearing than weight-bearing conditions in high-flexion posterior-stabilized total knee design. Early engagement of the femoral cam puts the cam at risk of jumping the tibial post, particularly if there is instability in mid-flexion.

The clinical results of high-flexion knee prosthesis still need further observation. Kim et al. and McCalden et al. reported that there was no difference in the ROM and clinical results between the conventional and high-flexion knee designs. Ritter et al. and Kim et al. reported that the postoperative range of motion is related more to the preoperative range of motion, surgical techniques, and lifestyle rather than to the use of high-flexion knee implants. Han et al. reported that they experienced early loosening in 38 % of cases with high-flexion knee prostheses.

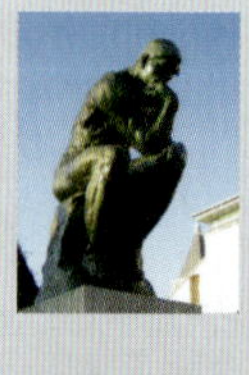

Author's Opinion

When the flexion motion increases, the patient's satisfaction increases as they feel more comfortable. Even though high-flexion knee prosthesis is used, if the preoperative ROM is limited or surgical procedure is not performed well, the ROM does not increase as much as expected.

High-flexion activity, such as squatting, increases the stress on the prosthesis resulting in early failure of TKA. It is recommended to use a high-flexion knee design with the understanding that it is not to create high flexion but to accommodate high flexion.

One particular prosthesis has been reported to have a high complication rate, but this may be confined to that prosthesis only.

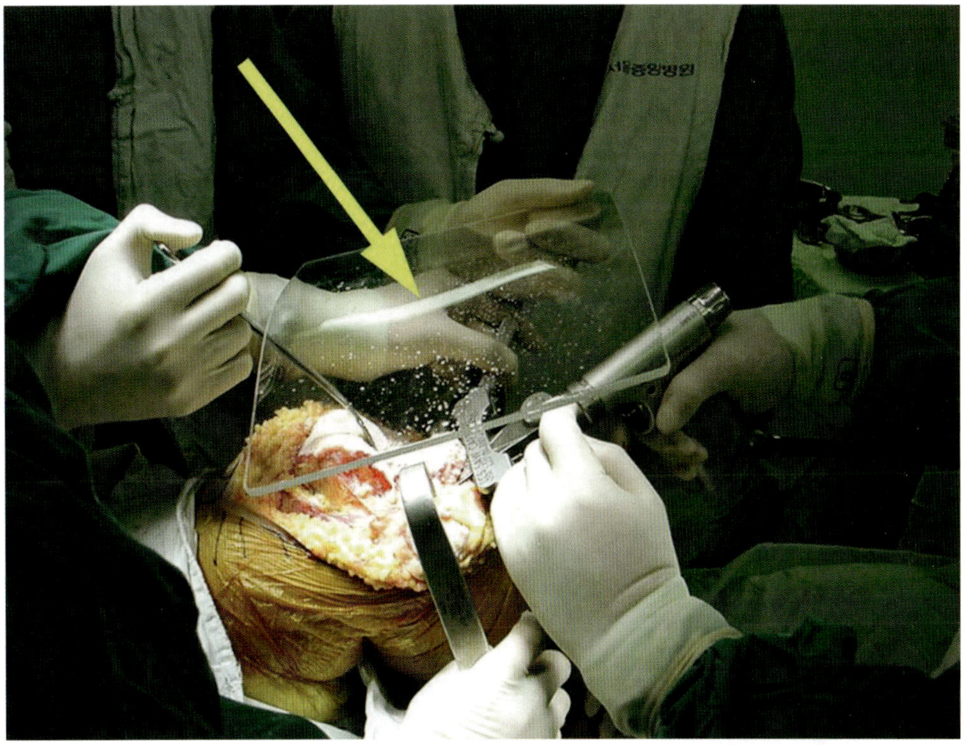

Fig. 2.45 Use of a plastic cover

2.4 Surgical Instruments

In order to build a good house, a good design, materials, techniques, and tools are needed. If arthroplasty is compared with building a house, tools can be regarded as the surgical instruments.

It is not recommended to use surgical instruments that require too much energy to handle because the accuracy is decreased and they may cause an injury to the tissues. If the surgical instruments are too complicated to use and the anatomical characteristics cannot be comprehended, they would interfere with the surgical procedures. If the surgical instruments are not fixed firmly on the hard or soft bones during osteotomy, the osteotomy procedure may go wrong.

Good surgical instruments are those that provide comprehensive coverage of the anatomy during the surgical procedure, are easy to handle, and are accurate.

2.4.1 Surgical Instruments for Use in TKA

2.4.1.1 Plastic Cover

Infection is the most critical complication following arthroplasty. While sawing or inserting the trials or implants, bone particles or liquid can splash on the face or head of the surgical team members and drop down on the operation field. This may be a source of infection.

In order to prevent contamination, all attendants in the operation theatre should wear a body exhaust suit or space suit that protects the body from exposure. But it is not always available as it is expensive. A clear plastic cover can be used to prevent contamination without interference of the surgical view (Fig. 2.45).

2.4.1.2 Retractor

Retractor is needed not only to ensure better exposure but also to protect important tissues. A good retractor can increase accuracy of the operation, protect the important tissues, and save time.

It is desirable to prepare a special retractor designed for TKA in addition to the usual retractor.

The first type is the S-shaped retractor, which is convenient to use during osteotomy as it safely retracts the collateral ligaments and protects the posterior soft tissues (Fig. 2.46).

The second type is a U-shaped patellar retractor. When performing TKA, the most difficult task for the assistant is patellar retraction. Patella has the tendency to return to its original position from the everted state. Even when a sharp retractor is used, it can slip and increase the risk of injury to the articular surface or the patellar PE.

Patellar retractor is designed to retract the patella efficiently so as to provide a good operation field when performing osteotomy of the tibia, inserting implants, or removing extruded bone cement (Fig. 2.47).

2.4.1.3 Plateau Cover

In addition to the retractor, it is recommended to have a plateau cover to protect the tibial plateau during femoral

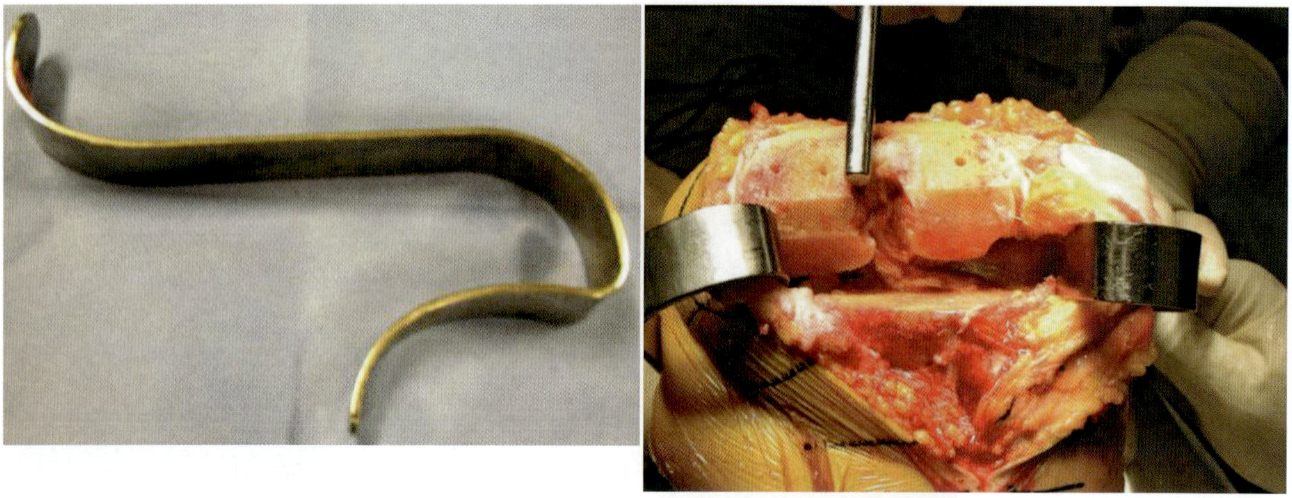

Fig. 2.46 S-shaped retractor used for total knee replacement and its method of use

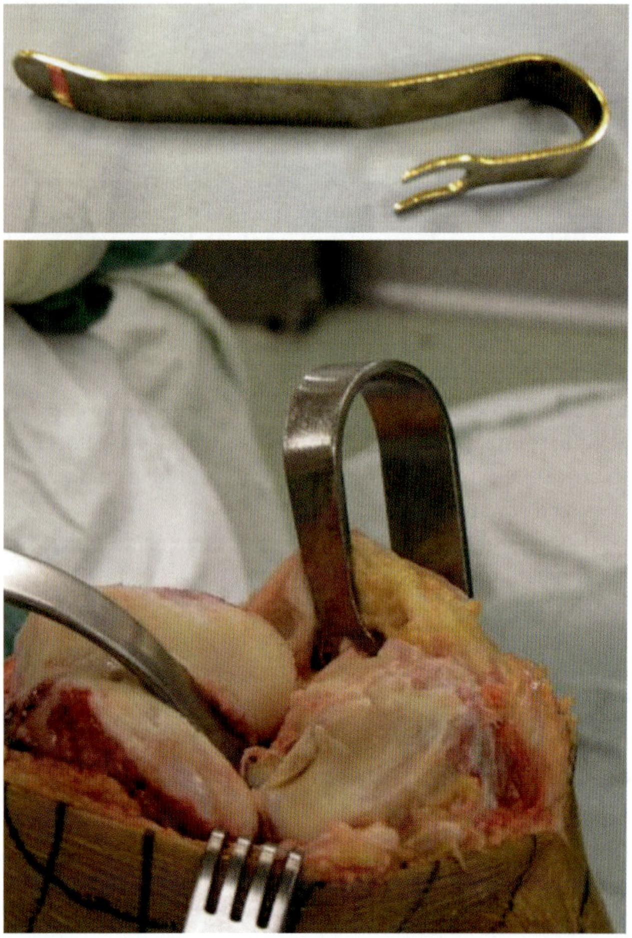

Fig. 2.47 Patellar retractor and its method of use

osteotomy. When performing osteotomy of the femur for the PS type, the tibial plateau may be damaged during femoral box cutting.

I have designed the following instrument to prevent this type of damage. It is a stainless steel plate similar to the shape of the tibial plateau. I place this instrument on the tibial plateau and perform box cutting, and thus the tibial plateau can be protected from damage (Fig. 2.48).

2.4.1.4 Patellar Tendon Protector

If patellar eversion is difficult as in revision cases or in case of severe osteoporosis, forceful eversion of the patella may cause the patellar tendon to be stripped off. A staple or K-wire is applied in advance to prevent this occurrence, but it may not provide sufficient protection or tearing of the patellar tendon can occur.

Therefore, it is important to use an instrument designed to protect the patellar tendon from stripping or tear (Fig. 2.49).

Currently, I use a retrieved miniplate and fix it with smooth head pins for this purpose, since more time is needed for insertion of the patella tendon protector and the pins for fixation are too long. The miniplate is flexible and it is easier to handle (Fig. 2.50).

2.4.1.5 Femoral Lifter

Lifting the thigh with the hands is not effective while removing the osteophyte in the posterior portion of the femoral condyle or while working on the posterior soft tissues.

The femoral lifter is an L-shaped instrument and is designed such that a rod can be inserted into the femoral medullary canal for lifting the thigh up (Fig. 2.51).

2.4.1.6 Lamina Spreader

This is the modified form of the lamina spreader that is used in spine surgery. The lamina spreader is used to check the gap and tension in extension and flexion state after osteotomy, and it is used as a retractor while clearing the posterior soft tissues (Fig. 2.52).

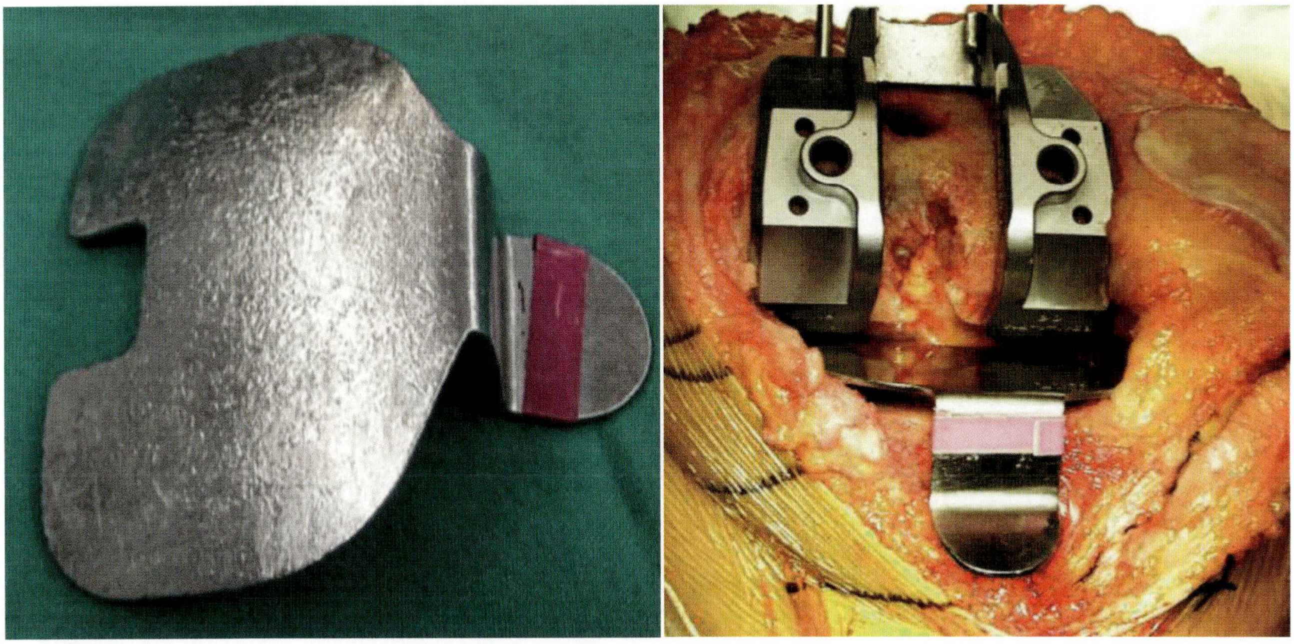

Fig. 2.48 Plateau cover and its method of use

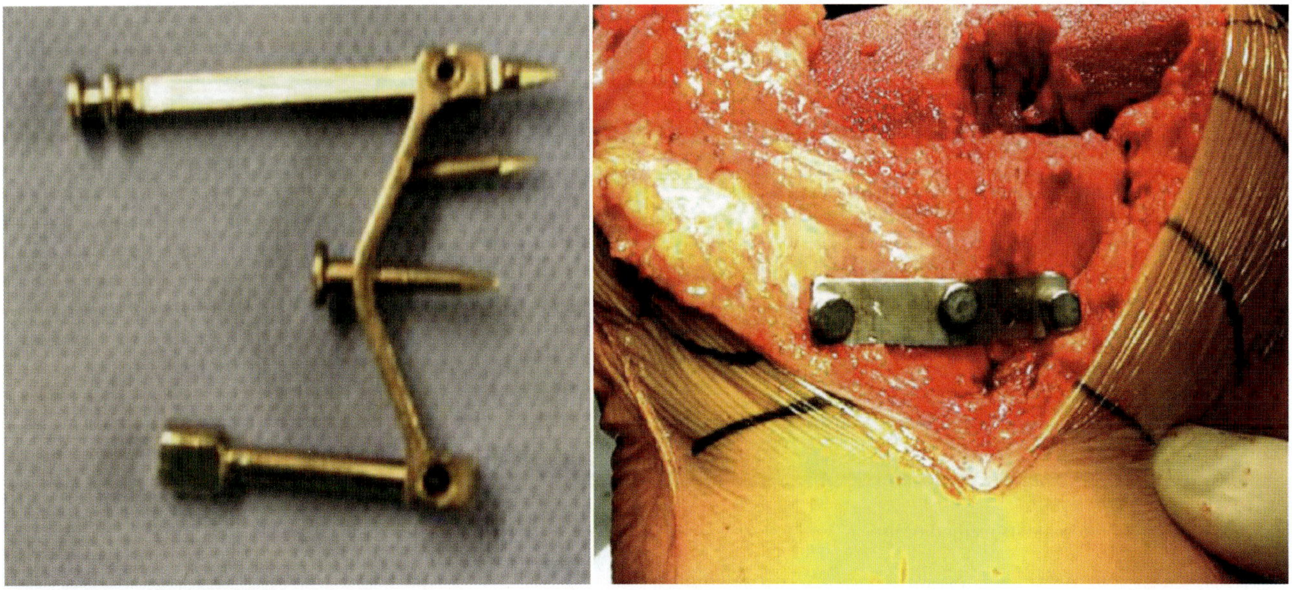

Fig. 2.49 Patellar tendon protector and its method of use

2.4.1.7 Bifacial Hammer

Hammer must not be too heavy. It is desirable to have metal on one side and plastic on the other side. When doing cementing for fixation, it is convenient to use a plastic hammer instead of a metal impactor at first. A bifacial hammer is also used for inserting the PE (Fig. 2.53).

2.4.1.8 Pin Extractor

When working on the hard bones, the surgeon attempts not to insert the pin deep enough because it becomes difficult to remove it. However, this causes movement of the instruments during sawing and the accuracy is reduced.

With the use of the slot type of pin extractor, it is possible to save time and efforts while extracting the pins (Fig. 2.54).

2.4.1.9 Lewin Clamp

Instruments can be used for patellar osteotomy, but most of them would slip during the osteotomy. Two towel clips have been used to hold the patella when performing the osteotomy manually, but towel clips have to be held with both the hands.

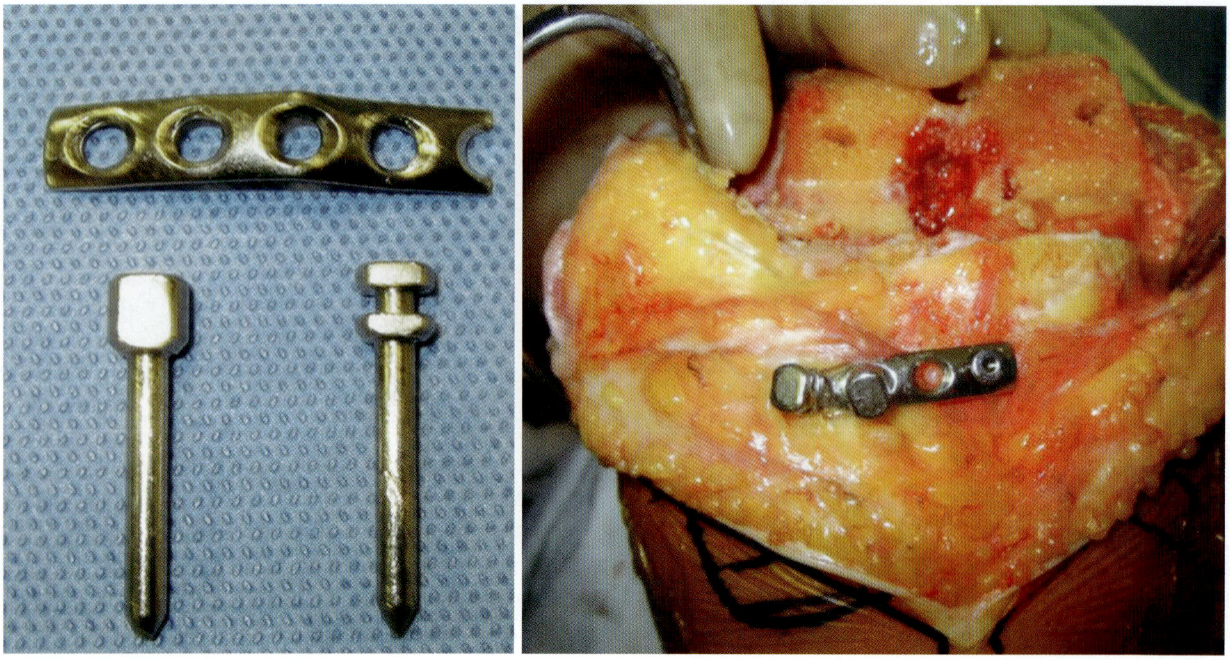

Fig. 2.50 Miniplate and its method of use

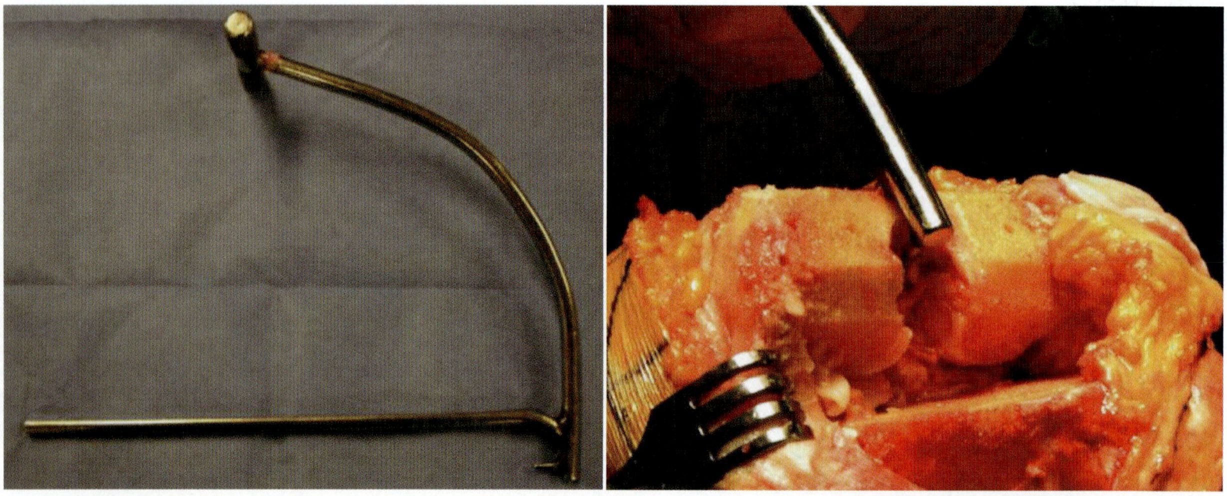

Fig. 2.51 Femoral lifter and its method of use

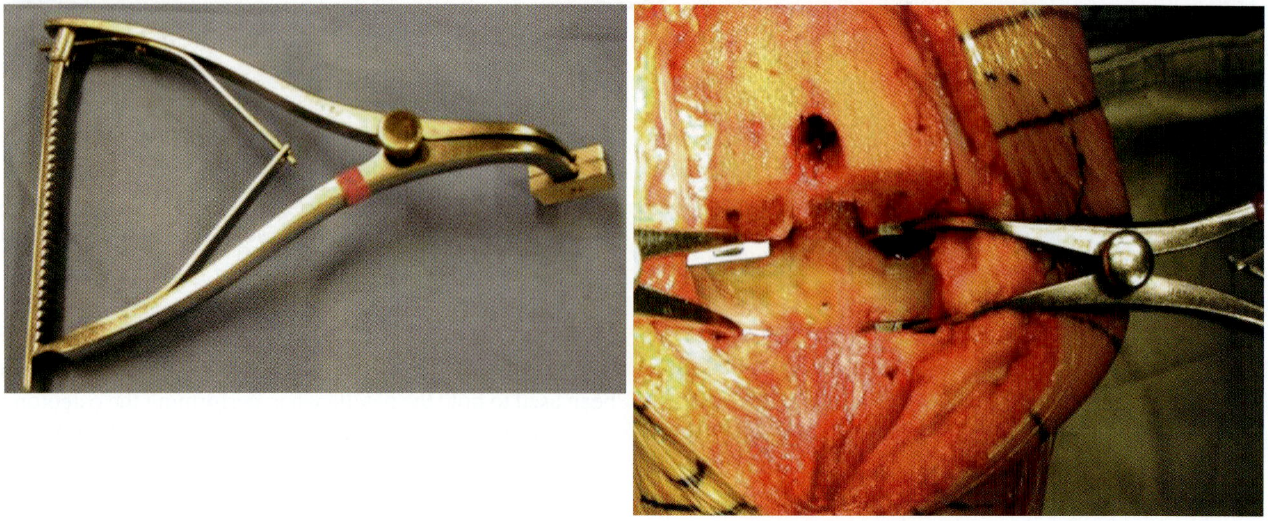

Fig. 2.52 Lamina spreader and its method of use

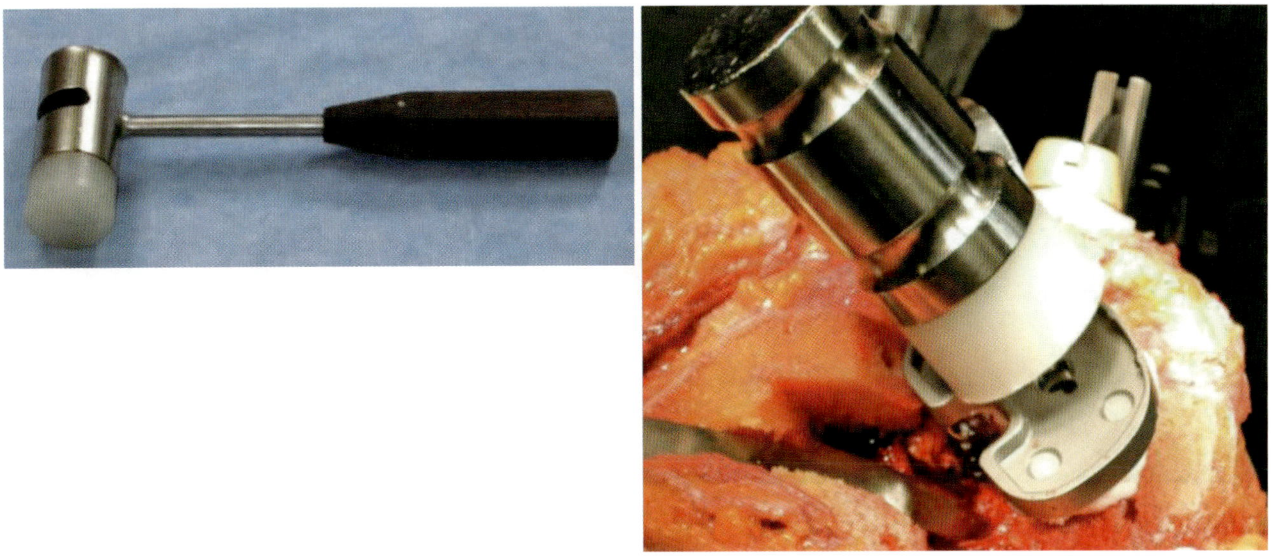

Fig. 2.53 Bifacial hammer. It has metal component on one side and plastic component on the other side

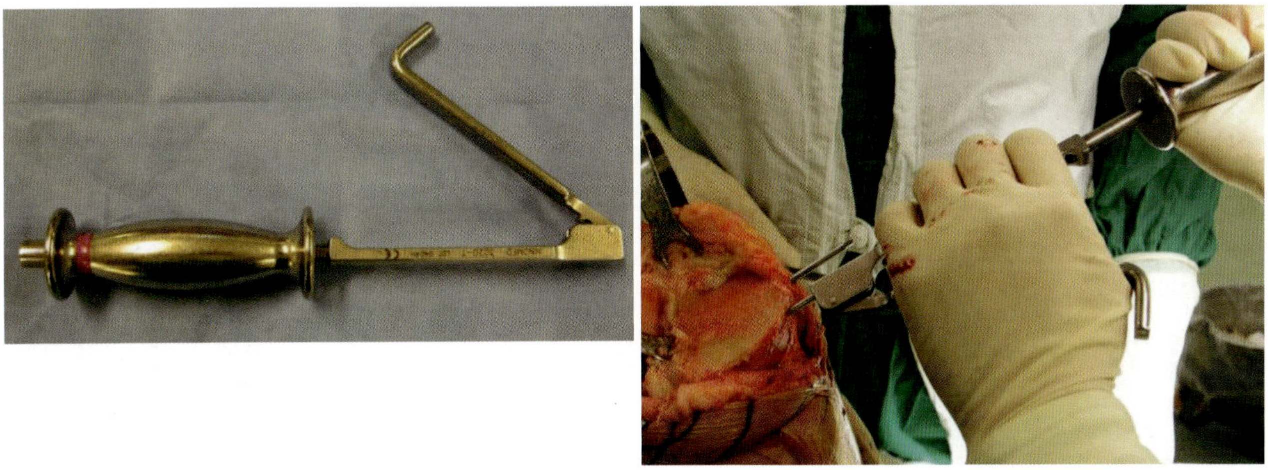

Fig. 2.54 Pin extractor and its method of use

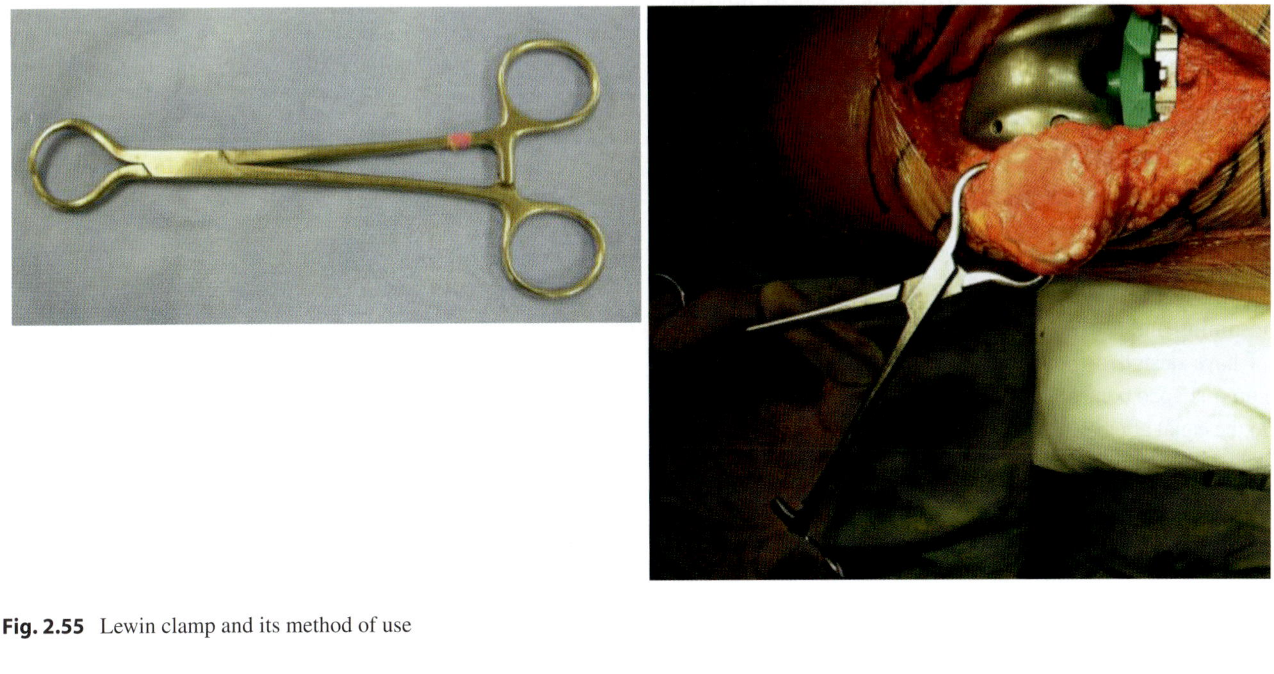

Fig. 2.55 Lewin clamp and its method of use

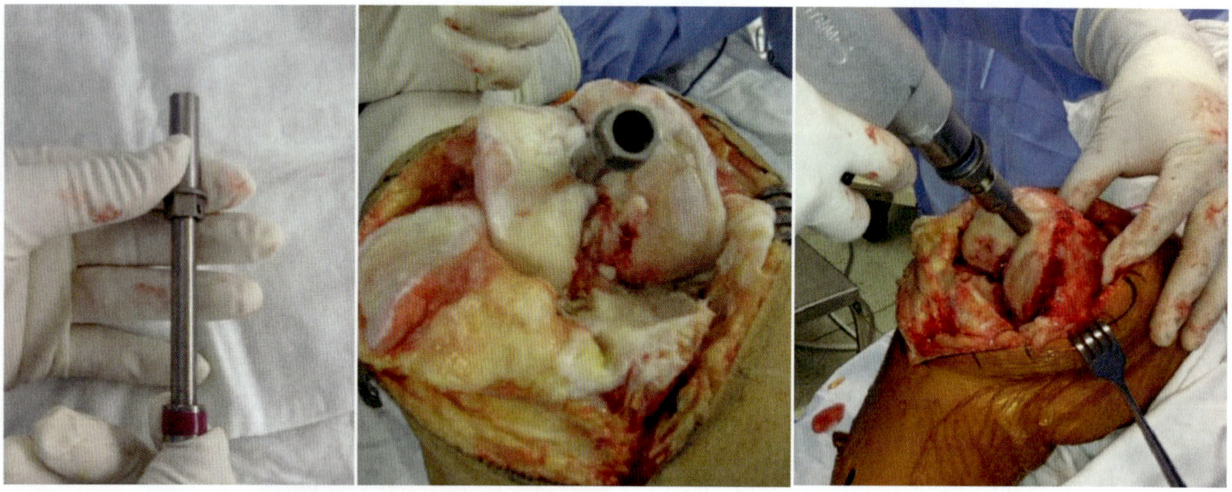

Fig. 2.56 Bone harvester and its method of use

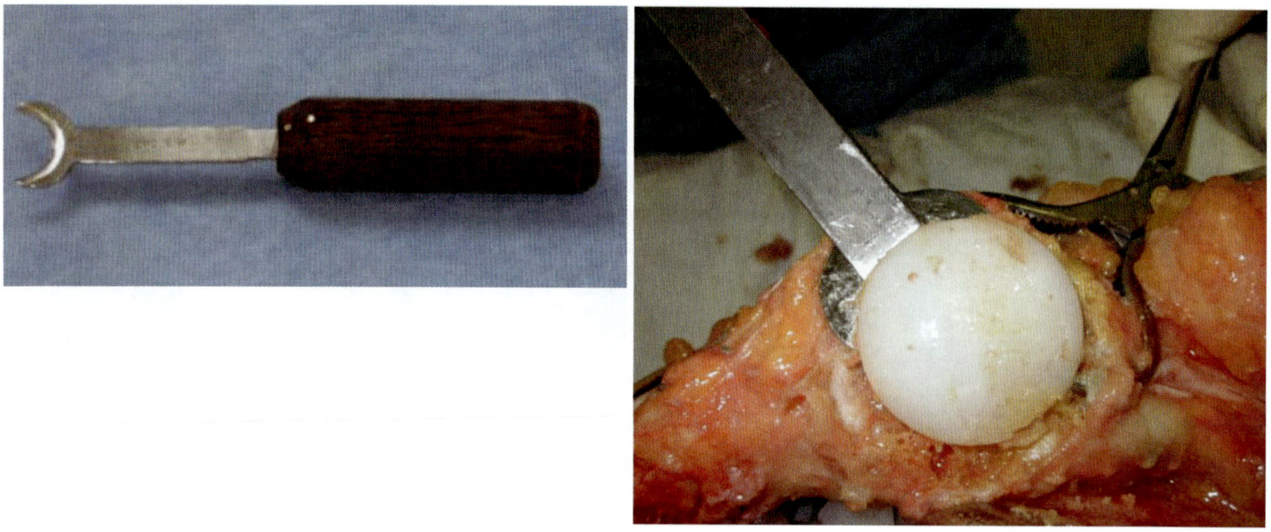

Fig. 2.57 Patella remover and its method of use

The Lewin clamp (Fig. 2.55) can be used to hold the patella firmly with only one hand and this makes it easier to perform the osteotomy.

2.4.1.10 Bone Harvester

In order to reduce bleeding from the femoral medullary canal postoperatively, sealing the canal with cement or bone fragment is needed. Cementing is easy, but it causes bone loss and interferes with screw fixation in the treatment of periprosthetic fracture. Bone impaction method is time-consuming and is often incomplete.

I have designed the bone harvester, which can take out a column-shaped bone plug before reaming, that can be reinserted into the canal after being enveloped with SURGICEL (Ethicon; Acclarent, Menlo Park, CA) or together with bone fragments.

It is just like the bone harvester that is used for bone biopsy. A serrated harvester with a 10 mm diameter is attached to the drill and the bone is harvested, and then the medullary cavity is enlarged with a medullary trocar.

This method has several advantages. The first is that the intramedullary pressure does not increase significantly and hence the risk of embolism may be decreased. The second advantage is that bleeding from the medullary cavity is almost completely blocked. Lastly, more bone is preserved, which can be beneficial in revision TKA or in periprosthetic fracture treatment (Fig. 2.56).

2.4.1.11 Patella Remover

I have designed an instrument that protects the patella from fracture while removing the patellar component during revision surgery (Fig. 2.57).

It is a crescent-shaped, thin instrument that can be inserted beneath the patellar component. After separating the marginal portion of the patellar component from the bone with a saw, a patella remover is inserted beneath the patella and the patella is lifted with an osteotome so that it can be removed easily with less risk of a patellar fracture.

2.4.2 Implant-Specific Surgical Instruments

Specific surgical instruments are needed for each implant. These are the femoral, tibial, and patellar osteotomy instruments together with a tensioning device or gapper for balancing the soft tissues. *Implant-specific surgical instruments used in TKA should be designed according to the characteristics of each implant, no matter who uses these instruments.*

These instruments should not cause any damage to the surrounding tissues, should be accurate, and should be designed so as to fit each implant, and *there should be supplemental devices available for correction when osteotomy goes wrong.*

With the introduction of minimally invasive surgery (MIS), new surgical instruments have been designed. The earlier forms of the MIS instruments were much different from the conventional instruments since the sequence and method of operation were different. But most of the MIS instruments used currently are slightly modified and smaller in size compared to the conventional instruments, because most of the surgical procedures are performed in a manner similar to the conventional method. Some of the instruments are designed to be compatible for computer-assisted surgery.

2.4.2.1 Femur

An intramedullary guide is required for the femoral alignment. *The intramedullary guide* should have two options, one long guide and one short guide. And an extramedullary guide should also be ready for use. The short guide and the extramedullary guide are needed for patients who have a severe deformity or have undergone THA. *The intramedullary guide should have a certain diameter with a groove or hole to evacuate blood so as to reduce the intramedullary pressure.*

When performing anterior and posterior osteotomy, there are two referencing systems, *the anterior referencing system and the posterior referencing system*. They are different according to which part, anterior or posterior of the femoral condyle, is set as a baseline for the osteotomy. So the instruments for osteotomy are a little different from each other depending on the system used. The chamfer cutting also varies from implant to implant and it is usually performed simultaneously with the anterior and posterior osteotomy. All procedures of femoral osteotomy can be done in one step by the use of one instrument. This can save time, but it may not provide a tight fit of the implant and correction is difficult when osteotomy is not done properly.

2.4.2.2 Tibia

Tibial instruments include guide for alignment, cutting jig, and instruments for preparation of stem fixation. For alignment, *an extramedullary guide is used more commonly*, but an intramedullary guide is necessary in case of revision or in other special situations. Hence, it is necessary to keep both the extramedullary and intramedullary guides ready.

The guide rod at the bottom of the extramedullary guide is designed to adjust the coronal and sagittal axes. The fitting can get loose while sawing or drilling resulting in alteration of axis. Some designs have a locking system in order to prevent this occurrence.

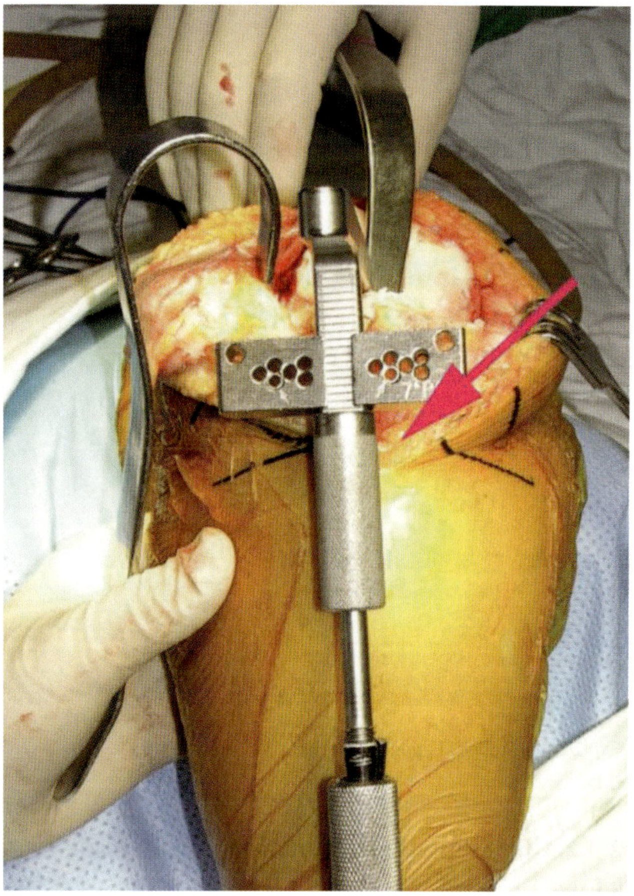

Fig. 2.58 Tibial cutting guide. With a fine adjuster (*arrow*), it is easier to control the amount of the osteotomy (Depuy, Warsaw, IN)

In some designs, the amount of osteotomy to be performed can be finely adjusted, and there are cutting jigs that can perform a step-cut osteotomy for metal augmentation (Fig. 2.58).

In order to verify whether the tibia has been accurately osteotomized, it is desirable to have an easily detachable test rod.

To fix the tibial plate, instruments are designed to ream or punch according to the shape of the stem. Punching can save more bones, but it can cause a fracture. Reaming can prevent a fracture, but it causes more bone loss.

2.4.2.3 Patella

For patellar osteotomy, a clamp type of instrument with a slot is used. However, it is difficult to determine the amount of osteotomy with this instrument, and it tends to slip during osteotomy causing an inaccurate osteotomy.

Therefore, many surgeons perform osteotomy manually by holding the patella with towel clips or the Lewin clamp. There is a holder or a clamp to hold the patella in place for cement fixation. The gripping power of the holding clamp should be strong enough to prevent slipping of the holding clamp.

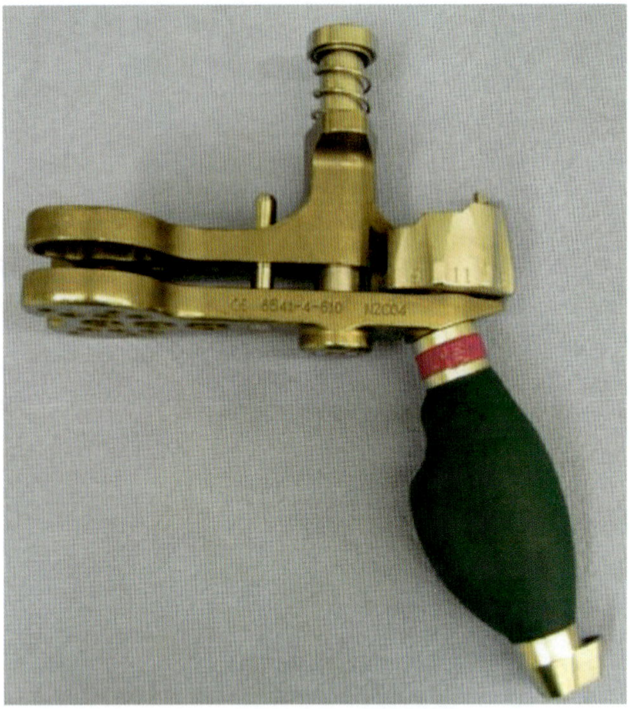

Fig. 2.59 Gapper (Triathlon; Stryker, Mahwah, NJ)

2.4.2.4 Equipment for Balancing

Flexion and extension gap balancing is closely related to the prognosis. The mobile-bearing type and most of the current implants provide a *gapper or tensioner* so as to be able to check the gap balance (Fig. 2.59).

2.4.2.5 Miscellaneous Instruments

Different impactors should be used to insert the implants into the femur and the tibia. It would be useful to have a femoral and tibial holder that can easily extract the trial implants. This holder is also useful for guiding the correct positioning of the implant while cementing is being performed.

Each company offers a different method for inserting the PE. Lesser damage to the PE is expected with the use of PE inserter than with the use of an impactor or hammer.

Bibliography

Abdel MP, Morrey ME, Jensen MR, et al. Increased long-term survival of posterior cruciate-retaining versus posterior cruciate-stabilizing total knee replacements. J Bone Joint Surg Am. 2011; 93-A:2072–8.

Aebli N, Krebs J, Schwenke D, et al. Progression of radiolucent lines in cementless twin-bearing low contact-stress knee prostheses: a retrospective study. J Arthroplasty. 2004;19:783–9.

Aglietti P, Baldini A, Buzzi R, et al. Comparison of mobile-bearing and fixed-bearing total knee arthroplasty: a prospective randomized study. J Arthroplasty. 2005;20:145–53.

Ahmed A, Tissakht M, Shrivastava S, Chan K. Dynamic stress response of the implant/cement interface: an axisymmetric analysis of a knee. J Orthop Res. 1990;8:435–47.

Akizuki S, Takizawa T, Horiuchi H. Fixation of a hydroxyapatite-tricalcium phosphate-coated cementless knee prosthesis. Clinical and radiographic evaluation seven years after surgery. J Bone Joint Surg Br. 2003;85-B:1123–7.

Akasaki Y, Matsuda S, Shimoto T, et al. Contact stress analysis of the conforming post-cam mechanism in posterior-stabilized total knee arthroplasty. J Arthroplasty. 2008;23:736–43.

Anand A, McGlynn F, Jiranek W. Metal hypersensitivity: can it mimic infection? J Arthroplasty. 2009;24:825–8.

Argenson JN, Komistek RD, Mahfouz M, et al. A high flexion total knee arthroplasty design replicates healthy knee motion. Clin Orthop. 2004;428:174–9.

Arola D, Toffel KA, Yang DT. Fatigue of the cement/bone interface: the surface texture of bone and loosening. J Biomed Mater Res. 2005; 76:287–97.

Banks SA. Understanding knee arthroplasty kinematics: news you can use. In: Scott WN, editor. Surgery of the knee. 4th ed. Philadelphia: Churchill Livingstone; 2006. p. 258–64.

Banks SA, Markovich GD, Hodge WA. In vivo kinematics of cruciate-retaining and substituting knee arthroplasties. J Arthroplasty. 1997; 12:297–304.

Barrack R. Factors influencing polyethylene wear in total joint arthroplasty. Orthopedics. 1998;21:937–40.

Bartel DL, Bicknell VL, Wright TM. The effect of conformity, thickness, and material on stresses in ultra-high molecular weight components for total joint replacement. J Bone Joint Surg Am. 1986;68-A:1041–51.

Bassett RW. Results of 1,000 performance knees: cementless versus cemented fixation. J Arthroplasty. 1998;13:409–13.

Becker MW, Insall JN, Faris PM. Bilateral total knee arthroplasty. One cruciate retaining and one cruciate substituting. Clin Orthop. 1991;271:122–4.

Bellemans J, Carpentier K, Vandenneucker H, et al. The John Insall Award: both morphotype and gender influence the shape of the knee in patients undergoing TKA. Clin Orthop. 2010;468:29–36.

Berend ME, Davis PJ, Ritter MA, et al. "Thicker" polyethylene bearings are associated with higher failure rates in primary total knee arthroplasty. J Arthroplasty. 2010;25:17–20.

Berend ME, Small SR, Ritter MA, et al. Effects of femoral component size on proximal tibial strain with anatomic graduated components total knee arthroplasty. J Arthroplasty. 2010;25:58–63.

Berger RA, Lyon JH, Jacobs JJ, et al. Problems with cementless total knee arthroplasty at 11 years follow up. Clin Orthop. 2001;392: 196–207.

Berry DJ, Currier JH, Mayor MB, et al. Knee wear measured in retrievals: a polished tray reduces insert wear. Clin Orthop. 2012;470: 1860–8.

Bert JM. Dislocation/subluxation of meniscal bearing elements after New Jersey low-contact stress total knee arthroplasty. Clin Orthop. 1990;254:211–5.

Bert JM, McShane M. Is it necessary to cement the tibial stem in cemented total knee arthroplasty? Clin Orthop. 1998;356:73–8.

Bettinson KA, Pinder IM, Morgan CG, et al. All-polyethylene compared with metal-backed tibial components in total knee arthroplasty at ten years. A prospective, randomized controlled trial. J Bone Joint Surg Am. 2009;91-A:1587–94.

Bhan S, Malhotra R, Kiran EK, et al. A comparison of fixed-bearing and mobile-bearing total knee arthroplasty at a minimum follow-up of 4.5 years. J Bone Joint Surg Am. 2005;87-A:2290–6.

Black J. Biomaterials overview. In: Callaghan JJ, editor. The adult hip. 1st ed. Philadelphia: Lippincott-Raven Publishers; 1998. p. 87–96.

Blaha JD. The rationale for a total knee implant that confers anteroposterior stability throughout range of motion. J Arthroplasty. 2004;19 Suppl 1:22–6.

Blaha JD, Wojty E. Motion and stability of the normal knee. In: Scott WN, editor. Surgery of the knee. 4th ed. Philadelphia: Churchill Livingstone; 2006. p. 227–39.

Bloebaum RD, Bachus KN, Jensen JW, et al. Postmortem analysis of consecutively retrieved asymmetric porous-coated tibial components. J Arthroplasty. 1997;12:920–9.

Bloebaum RD, Nelson K, Dorr LD, et al. Investigation of early surface delamination observed in retrieved heat-pressed tibial inserts. Clin Orthop. 1991;269:120–7.

Bobyn JD, Pilliar RM, Cameron HU, et al. The optimum pore size for the fixation of porous surfaced metal implants by the ingrowth of bone. Clin Orthop. 1980;150:263–70.

Bobyn JK, Jacobs JJ, Tanzer M, et al. The susceptibility of smooth implant surfaces to peri-implant fibrosis and migration of polyethylene wear debris. Clin Orthop. 1995;311:21–39.

Bonutti PM, Zywiel MG, Rudert LA, et al. Femoral notch stenosis caused by soft tissue impingement in semi- or open-box posterior-stabilized total knee arthroplasty. J Arthroplasty. 2010;25:1061–5.

Booth RE. Millenium arthroplasty: materials, methods & mechanisms. Orthopedics. 1998;21:929–31.

Brassard MF, Insall JN, Scuderi GR, et al. Does modularity affect clinical success? A comparison with a minimum 10 year follow up. Clin Orthop. 2001;388:26–32.

Buechel Sr FF, Buechel Jr FF, Pappas MJ, et al. Twenty-year evaluation of the New Jersey LCS rotating platform knee replacement. J Knee Surg. 2002;15:84–9.

Callaghan JJ, Lin SS. Posterior cruciate ligament-substituting total knee arthroplasty. In: Scott WN, editor. Surgery of the knee. 4th ed. Philadelphia: Churchill Livingstone; 2006. p. 1531–57.

Callaghan JJ, O'Rourke MR. Implant options in primary total knee joint replacement. In: Callaghan JJ, editor. The adult knee. 1st ed. Philadelphia: Lippincot Williams & Wilkins; 2003. p. 1059–66.

Cameron HU, Hu C, Vyamont D. Hinge total knee replacement revisited. Can J Surg. 1997;40:278–83.

Cameron HU, Mills RH, Jackson RW, et al. The structure of polymethylmethacrylate cement. Clin Orthop. 1974;100:287–91.

Carothers JT, Kim RH, Dennis DA, et al. Mobile-bearing total knee arthroplasty: a meta-analysis. J Arthroplasty. 2011;26:537–42.

Catani F, Leardini A, Ensini A, et al. The stability of the cemented tibial component of total knee arthroplasty: posterior cruciate-retaining versus posterior-stabilized design. J Arthroplasty. 2004; 19:775–82.

Cho WS, Moon HS, Park SS, et al. The shape and size discrepancy between bone and prosthesis in total knee arthroplasty. J Korean Orthop Assoc. 1998;33:1045–55.

Cho WS, Youm YS. Migration of polyethylene fixation screw after total knee arthroplasty. J Arthroplasty. 2009;24:825–9.

Cho WS, Youm YS, Ahn SC, et al. What have we learned from LCS mobile-bearing knee system? Knee Surg Sports Traumatol Arthrosc. 2010;18:1345–51.

Clarke HD, Fuchs R, Scuderi GR, et al. The influence of femoral component design in the elimination of patellar clunk in posterior-stabilized total knee arthroplasty. J Arthroplasty. 2006;21:167–71.

Clarke HD, Hentz JG. Restoration of femoral anatomy in TKA with unisex and gender-specific components. Clin Orthop. 2008; 466:2711–6.

Collier JP, Williams IR, Mayor MB. Retrieval analysis of mobile bearing prosthetic knee devices. In: Hamelynck KJ, editor. LCS mobile bearing knee arthroplasty. 1st ed. Heidelberg: Springer Verlag; 2002. p. 74–80.

Collier MB, Engh Jr CA, McAuley JP, et al. Osteolysis after total knee arthroplasty: influence of tibial baseplate surface finish and sterilization of polyethylene insert. Findings at five to ten years postoperatively. J Bone Joint Surg Am. 2005;87-A:2702–8.

Conditt MA, Ismaily SK, Alexander JW, et al. Backside wear of modular ultra-high molecular weight polyethylene tibial inserts. J Bone Joint Surg Am. 2004;86-A:1031–7.

Conditt MA, Noble PC, Bertolusso R, et al. The PCL significantly affects the functional outcome of total knee arthroplasty. J Arthroplasty. 2004;19:107–12.

Conditt MA, Thompson MT, Usrey MM, et al. Backside wear of polyethylene tibial inserts: mechanism and magnitude of material loss. J Bone Joint Surg Am. 2005;87-A:326–31.

Cooke C, Walter WK, Zicat B. Tibial fixation without screws in cementless total knee arthroplasty. J Arthroplasty. 2006;21: 237–41.

Dalury DF, Pomeroy DL, Gonzales RA, et al. Midterm results of all-polyethylene tibial components in primary total knee arthroplasty. J Arthroplasty. 2009;24:620–4.

Davis JP, Harris WH. Tensile bonding strength of the cement-prosthesis interface. Orthopedics. 1994;17:171–4.

Dargel J, Michael JW, Feiser J, et al. Human knee joint anatomy revisited: morphometry in the light of sex-specific total knee arthroplasty. J Arthroplasty. 2011;26:346–53.

Dennis DA, Komistek RD, Hoff WA, et al. In vivo knee kinematics derived using an inverse perspective technique. Clin Orthop. 1996;331:107.

Dennis DA, Komistek RD, Mahfouz MR, et al. Mobile-bearing total knee arthroplasty: do the polyethylene bearings rotate? Clin Orthop. 2005;440:88–95.

D'Lima DD, Chen PC, Colwell CW. Polyethylene contact stresses, articular congruity, and knee alignment. Clin Orthop. 2001; 392:232–8.

Dodd CAF, Hungerford DS, Krackow KA. Total knee arthroplasty fixation: comparison of the early results of paired cemented versus uncemented porous coated anatomic knee prostheses. Clin Orthop. 1990;260:66–70.

Dorr LD, Ochesner JL, Gronly J, et al. Functional comparison of posterior cruciate-retained versus cruciate-sacrificed total knee arthroplasty. Clin Orthop. 1988;236:36–43.

Duffy GP, Berry DJ, Rand JA. Cement versus cementless fixation in total knee arthroplasty. Clin Orthop. 1998;356:66–72.

Engh CA, Hooten Jr JP, Zettl-Schaffer KF, et al. Evaluation of bone ingrowth in proximally and extensively porous-coated anatomic medullary locking prostheses retrieved at autopsy. J Bone Joint Surg Am. 1995;77-A:903–10.

Engh GA, Parks NL, Ammeen DJ. Tibial osteolysis in cementless total knee arthroplasty. A review of 25 cases treated with and without tibial component revision. Clin Orthop. 1994;309:33–43.

Evans MC, Parsons EM, Scott RD, Thornhill TS, Zurakowski D. Comparative flexion after rotating platform vs Fixed-bearing total knee arthroplasty. J Arthroplasty. 2006;21:985–91.

Ezzet KA, Hershey AL, D'Lima DD, et al. Patellar tracking in total knee arthroplasty: inset versus onset design. J Arthroplasty. 2001; 16:838–43.

Ezzet KA, Hermiad JC, Steklov N, et al. Wear of polyethylene against oxidized zirconium femoral componentseffect of aggressive kinematic conditions and malalignment in total knee arthroplasty. J Arthroplasty. 2012;27:116–21.

Fan CY, Hsieh JT, Hsieh MS, et al. Primitive results after medial-pivot knee arthroplasties: a minimum 5-year follow-up study. J Arthroplasty. 2010;25:492–6.

Faris PM, Ritter MA, Keating EM, Meding JB, Harty LD. The AGC all-polyethylene tibial component: a ten-year clinical evaluation. J Bone Joint Surg Am. 2003;85-A:489–93.

Fehring TK, Berend KR, Hofmann S, et al. Advanced technologies in performing total knee arthroplasty: roundtable discussion. In:

Scott WN, editor. Surgery of the knee. 5th ed. Philadelphia: Churchill Livingstone; 2011. p. 1283–92.
Fehring TK, Mason JB. Cemented total knee replacement: the gold standard. In: Scott WN, editor. Surgery of the knee. 4th ed. Philadelphia: Churchill Livingstone; 2006. p. 1626–30.
Fornasier VL, Cameron HU. The femorall stem/cement interface in total hip replacement. Clin Orthop. 1976;116:248–52.
Freeman MA, Swanson SA, Todd RC. Total replacement of the knee using the Freeman-Swanson knee prosthesis. Clin Orthop. 1973;94:153.
Freeman MA, Tennant R. The scientific basis of cement versus cementless fixation. Clin Orthop. 1992;276:19–25.
Frye BM, Floyd MW, Pham DC, et al. Effect of femoral component design on patellofemoral crepitance and patella clunk syndrome after posterior-stabilized total knee arthroplasty. J Arthroplasty. 2012;27:1166–70.
Furman BD, Lipman J, Kligman M, et al. Tibial post wear in posterior-stabilized knee replacements is design-dependent. Clin Orthop. 2008;466:2650–5.
Gilbert JL. Metals. In: Callaghan JJ, editor. The adult hip. 1st ed. Philadelphia: Lippincott-Raven Publishers; 1998. p. 123–34.
Greene KA. Gender-specific design in total knee arthroplasty. J Arthroplasty. 2007;22:27–31.
Haas SS, Brauer GM, Dickson G. A characterization of polymethylmethacrylate bone cement. J Bone Joint Surg Am. 1975; 57-A:380–91.
Haider H, Weisenberger JN, Kurtz SM, et al. Does vitamin E-stabilized ultrahigh-molecular-weight polyethyelne address concerns cross-linked polyethylene in total knee arhtroplasty? J Arthroplasty. 2012;27:461–9.
Hamai S, Miura H, Matsuda S, et al. Contact stress at the anterior aspect of the tibial post in posterior-stabilized total knee replacement. J Bone Joint Surg Am. 2010;92-A:1765–73.
Han HS, Kang SB, Yoon KS. High incidence of loosening of the femoral component in legacy posterior stabilised-flex total knee replacement. J Bone Joint Surg Br. 2007;89-B:1457–61.
Harper EJ, Bonfield W. Tensile characteristics of ten commercial acrylic bone cements. J Biomed Mater Res. 2000;53: 605–16.
Hartford JM, Harned ME, Kaufer H, et al. Primary meniscal-bearing knee replacements: 8- to 15-year followup. Clin Orthop. 2007;465:227–31.
Heck DA, Robinson RL, Partridge CM, et al. Patient outcome after knee replacement. Clin Orthop. 1998;356:93–110.
Heimke G, Legen S, Willman G. Knee arthroplasty: recently developed ceramics offer new solution. Biomaterials. 2002;23: 1539–51.
Helm AT, Kerin C, Ghalayini SR, et al. Preliminary results of an uncemented trabecular metal tibial component in total knee arthroplasty. J Arthroplasty. 2009;24:941–4.
Hirsch HS, Lotke PA, Morrison LD. The posterior cruciate ligament in total knee surgery: save, sacrifice, or substitute? Clin Orthop. 1994;309:64–8.
Hodrick JT, Severson EP, McAlister DS, et al. Highly crosslinked polyethylene is safe for use in total knee arthroplasty. Clin Orthop. 2008;466:2806–12.
Hofmann AA, Evanich JD, Ferguson R, et al. Ten-to 14-year clinical follow-up of the cementless Natural Knee System. Clin Orthop. 2001;388:85–94.
Hofmann AA, McCandless J. Posterior cruciate sacrificing total knee arthroplasty. In: Scott WN, editor. Surgery of the knee. 5th ed. Philadelphia: Churchill Livingstone; 2011. p. 1132–4.
Ho FY, Ma HM, Liau JJ, et al. Mobile-bearing knees reduce rotational asymmetric wear. Clin Orthop. 2007;462:143–9.
Hsu HP, Walker PS. Wear and deformation of patellar components in total knee arthroplasty. Clin Orthop. 1989;246:260–5.
Huddleston JI, Wiley JW, Scott RD. Zone 4 femoral radiolucent lines in hybrid versus cemented total knee arthroplasties: are they clinically significant? Clin Orthop. 2005;441:334–9.
Hui C, Salmon L, Maeno S, et al. Five-year comparison of oxidized zirconium and cobalt-chromium femoral components in total knee arthroplasty: a randomized controlled trial. J Bone Joint Surg Am. 2011;93-A:624–30.
Hungerford DS, Kenna RV. Preliminary experience with a total knee prosthesis with porous coating used without cement. Clin Orthop. 1983;176:96–107.
Illgen R, Tueting J, Enright T, et al. Hybrid total knee arthroplasty: a retrospective analysis of clinical and radiographic outcomes at average 10 years follow-up. J Arthroplasty. 2004;19 Suppl 2: 95–100.
Incavo SJ, Mullins ER, Coughlin KM, et al. Tibiofemoral kinematic analysis of kneeling after total knee arthroplasty. J Arthroplasty. 2004;19:906–10.
Insall JN, Clarke HD. Historic development, classification, and characteristics of knee prosthesis. In: Insall JN, editor. Surgery of the knee. 3rd ed. Philadelphia: Churchill Livingstone; 2001. p. 1516–51.
Insall JN, Clarke HD. Historic development, classification, and characteristics of knee prosthesis. In: Scott WN, editor. Surgery of the knee. 5th ed. Philadelphia: Churchill Livingstone; 2011. p. 952–87.
Insall JN, Clarke HD. Total knee arthroplasty with posterior cruciate ligament substitution designs. In: Insall JN, editor. Surgery of the knee. 3rd ed. Philadelphia: Churchill Livingstone; 2001. p. 1660–93.
Ishii Y, Noguchi H, Takeda M, et al. Changes in the medial and lateral posterior condylar offset in total knee arthroplasty. J Arthroplasty. 2011;26:255–9.
Jacobs JJ, Gilbert JL, Urban RH. Current concepts review. Corrosion of metal orthopedic implants. J Bone Joint Surg Am. 1998;80-A: 268–82.
Johnson AJ, Costa CR, Mont MA. Do we need gender-specific total joint arthroplasty. Clin Orthop. 2011;469:1852–8.
Jones LC, Hungerford DS. Cement disease. Clin Orthop. 1987;225:192–206.
Kamath AF, Lee GC, Sheth NP, et al. Prospective results of uncemented tantalum monoblock tibia in total knee arthroplasty: minimum 5-year follow-up in patients younger than 55 years. J Arthroplasty. 2011;26:1390–5.
Kaper BP, Smith PN, Bourne RB, et al. Medium term results of a mobile bearing total knee replacement. Clin Orthop. 1999;367: 201–9.
Keating EM, Meding JB. Implant fixation-cement. In: Callaghan JJ, editor. The adult knee. 1st ed. Philadelphia: Lippincot Williams & Wilkins; 2003. p. 1067–70.
Kelly NH, Fu RH, Wright TM, et al. Wear damage in mobile-bearing TKA is as severe as that in fixed-bearing TKA. Clin Orthop. 2011;469:123–30.
Kim RH, Dennis DA. Mobile-bearing total knee arthroplasty. In: Scott WN, editor. Surgery of the knee. 5th ed. Philadelphia: Churchill Livingstone; 2011. p. 1152–60.
Kim YH, Choi Y, Kim JS. Comparison of standard and gender-specific posterior-cruciate-retaining high-flexion total knee replacements: a prospective, randomised study. J Bone Joint Surg Br. 2010;92-B:639–45.
Kim YH, Choi Y, Kim JS. Range of motion of standard and high-flexion posterior cruciate-retaining total knee prostheses a prospective randomized study. J Bone Joint Surg Am. 2009;91-A: 1874–81.
Kim YH, Choi Y, Kwon OR, et al. Functional outcome and range of motion of high-flexion posterior cruciate-retaining and high-flexion posterior cruciate-substituting total knee prostheses.

A prospective, randomized study. J Bone Joint Surg Am. 2009;91-A:753–60.

Kim YH, Yoon SH, Kim JS. The long-term results of simultaneous fixed-bearing and mobile- bearing total knee replacements performed in the same patient. J Bone Joint Surg Br. 2007;89-B: 1317–23.

Klein GR, Parvizi J, Rapuri VR, et al. The effect of tibial polyethylene insert design on range of motion: evaluation of in vivo knee kinematics by a computerized navigation system during total knee arthroplasty. J Arthroplasty. 2004;19:986–91.

Kocmond JH, Delp SL, Stern SH. Stability and range of motion of Insall-Burstein condylar prostheses: a computer simulation study. J Arthroplasty. 1995;10:383.

Komistek RD, Dennis DA, Mahfouz MR. Fluoroscopic analysis of total knee replacement. In: Scott WN, editor. Surgery of the knee. 4th ed. Philadelphia: Churchill Livingstone; 2006. p. 1592–612.

Krause WR, Krug W, Eng B, et al. Strength of the cement-bone interface. Clin Orthop. 1982;163:290–9.

Kumar PJ, Doir LD. Posterior cruciate-sacrificing total knee arthroplasty. In: Scuderi GR, editor. Surgical techniques in total knee arthroplasty. 1st ed. New York: Springer; 2002. p. 61–74.

Lachiewicz PF, Bolognesi MP, Henderson RA, et al. Can tantalum cones provide fization in complex revision knee arthroplasty? Clin Orthop. 2012;470:199–204.

Larson CM, McDowell CM, Lachiewicz PF. One-peg versus three peg patella component fixation in total knee arthroplasty. Clin Orthop. 2001;392:94–100.

Laskin RS. The Insall Award. Total knee replacement with posterior cruciate ligament retention in patients with a fixed varus deformity. Clin Orthop. 1996;331:29–34.

Laskin RS. An oxidized Zr ceramic surfaced femoral component for total knee arthroplasty. Clin Orthop. 2003;416:191–6.

Laskin RS. Improving flexion in TKA. In: Callaghan JJ, editor. The adult knee. 1st ed. Philadelphia: Lippincott Williams & Wilkins; 2003. p. 1233–44.

Laskin RS. Total knee arthroplasty using an uncemented, polyethylene tibial implant. A seven-year follow-up study. Clin Orthop. 1993;288:270–6.

Lee GC, Cushner FD, Vigoritta V, et al. Evaluation of the anterior cruciate ligament integrity and degenerative arthritic patterns in patients undergoing total knee arthroplasty. J Arthroplasty. 2005;20: 59–65.

Lee R, Volz R, Sheridan D. The role of fixation and bone quality on the mechanical stability of tibial knee components. Clin Orthop. 1991;273:177–83.

Lemns JE. Ceramics. In: Callaghan JJ, editor. The adult hip. 1st ed. Philadelphia: Lippincott-Raven Publishers; 1998. p. 97–104.

Li G, Most E, Sultan PG, et al. Knee kinematics with a high-flexion posterior stabilized total knee prosthesis: an in vitro robotic experimental investigation. J Bone Joint Surg Br. 2004; 86-A:1721–9.

Linden U. Porosity in manually mixed bone cement. Clin Orthop Relat Res. 1988;231:110–2.

Lombardi AV, Mallory TH, Fada RA, et al. An algorithm for the posterior cruciate ligament in total knee arthroplasty. Clin Orthop. 2001;392:75–87.

Lombardi Jr AV, Ellison BS, Berend KR. Polyethylene wear is influenced by manufacturing technique in modular TKA. Clin Orthop. 2008;466:2798–805.

Lu YC, Huang CH, Chang TK, et al. Wear-pattern analysis in retrieved tibial inserts of mobile-bearing and fixed-bearing total knee prostheses. J Bone Joint Surg Br. 2010;92-B:500–7.

MacDonald D, Hanzlik J, Sharkey P, et al. In vivo oxidation and surface damage in retrieved ehtylene oxide-sterilized total knee arthroplasties. Clin Orthop. 2012;470:1826–33.

Maistrelli GL, Antonelli L, Fornasier V, et al. Cement penetration with pulsed lavage versus syringe irrigation in total knee arthroplasty. Clin Orthop. 1995;312:261–5.

Mahoney OM, Kinsey TL, D'Errico TJ, et al. No functional advantage of a mobile bearing posterior stabilized TKA. Clin Orthop. 2012;470:33–44.

Maloney W. Enhanced cross-linked polymers: the promise in the affirmative. Orthopedics. 2002;25:936–7.

Mann KA, Ayers DC, Werner FW, et al. Tensile strength of the cement-bone interface depends on the amount of bone interdigitated with PMMA cement. J Biomech. 1997;30:339–46.

Mann KA, Werner FW, Ayers DC. Mechanical strength of the cement-bone interface is greater in shear than in tension. J Biomech. 1999;32:1251–4.

Maruyama S, Yoshiya S, Matsui N, et al. Functional comparison of posterior cruciate-retaining versus posterior stabilized total knee arthroplasty. J Arthroplasty. 2004;19:349–53.

Massin P, Gournay A. Optimization of the posterior condylar offset, tibial slope, and condylar rollback in total knee arthroplasty. J Arthroplasty. 2006;21:889–96.

Matsuda S, Ishinishi T, Whiteside LA. Contact stresses with an unresurfaced patella in total knee arthroplasty. The effect of femoral component design. Orthopedics. 2000;23:213–8.

McAuley J, Eikmann T. Choosing your implant. In: Scott WN, editor. Surgery of the knee. 4th ed. Philadelphia: Churchill Livingstone; 2006. p. 284–9.

McAuley JP, Engh GA. Constraint in total knee arthroplasty: when and what? J Arthroplasty. 2003;18(3 Suppl 1):51–4.

McCalden RW, MacDonald SJ, Bourne RB, et al. A randomized controlled trial comparing "high-flex" vs "standard" posterior cruciate substituting polyethylene tibial inserts in total knee arthroplasty. J Arthroplasty. 2009;24(6 Suppl):33–8.

McCaskie AW, Deehan DJ, Green TP, et al. Randomised, prospective study comparing cemented and cementless total knee replacement at five years. J Bone Joint Surg Br. 1998;80-B:971–5.

McEwan HMJ, McNulty DE, Auger DD, et al. Wear analysis of mobile bearing knee. In: Hamelynck KJ, editor. LCS mobile bearing knee arthroplasty. 1st ed. Heidelberg: Springer Verlag; 2002. p. 67–73.

McNulty DE, Liao YS, Haas BD. The influence of sterilization method on wear performance of the low contact stress total knee system. Orthopedics. 2002;25:243–6.

Medel FJ, Kurtz SM, Hozack WJ, et al. Gamma insert sterilization: a solution to polyethyelne oxidation? J Bone Joint Surg Am. 2012;91-A:839–49.

Mehin R, Burnett RS, Brasher PM. Does the new generation of high-flex knee prostheses improve the postoperative range of movement? A meta-analysis. J Bone Joint Surg Br. 2010;92-B: 1429–34.

Merchant AC, Arendt EA, Dye SF, et al. The female knee: anatomic variations and the female-specific total knee design. Clin Orthop. 2008;466:3059–65.

Menchetti PP, Walker PS. Mechanical evaluation of mobile bearing knees. Am J Knee Surg. 1997;10:73–81.

Meneghini RM, Hanssen AD. Management of bone defects in revision total knee arthroplasty: augments, structural and impaction grafts, and cones. In: Scott WN, editor. Surgery of the knee. 5th ed. Philadelphia: Churchill Livingstone; 2011. p. 1367–74.

Mihalko WM, Creek AT, Mary MN, et al. Mechanoreceptors found in a posterior cruciate ligament from a well-functioning total knee arthroplasty retrieval. J Arthroplasty. 2011;26:504.e9–e12.

Mihalko WM, Miller C, Krackow KA. Total knee arthroplasty ligament balancing and gap kinematics with posterior cruciate ligament retention and sacrifice. Am J Orthop. 2000;29: 610–6.

Miller MA, Race A, Gupta S, et al. The role of cement viscosity on cement-bone apposition and strength: an in vitro model with medullary bleeding. J Arthroplasty. 2007;22:109–16.

Miura H, Whiteside LA, Easley JC, et al. Effects of screws and a sleeve on initial fixation in uncemented total knee tibial components. Clin Orthop. 1990;259:160–8.

Moran CG, Pinder IM, Lees TA, et al. Survivorship analysis for the uncemented porous coated anatomic knee replacement. J Bone Joint Surg Am. 1991;73-A:848–57.

Morgan H, Battista V, Leopold SS. Constraint in primary total knee arthroplasty. J Am Acad Orthop Surg. 2005;13:515–24.

Morra EA, Greenwald AS. Polymer insert stress in total knee designs during high-flexion activities: a finite element study. J Bone Joint Surg Am. 2005;87-A:120–4.

Nakayama K, Matsuda S, Miura H, et al. Contact stress at the post-cam mechanism in posterior stabilised total knee arthroplasty. J Bone Joint Surg Br. 2005;87-B:483–8.

Nett MP, Roehrig GJ, Scuderi GR, et al. Posterior cruciate ligament substituting total knee arthroplasty. In: Scott WN, editor. Surgery of the knee. 5th ed. Philadelphia: Churchill Livingstone; 2011. p. 1135–51.

Nilsson KG, Karrholm J, Linder L. Femoral component migration in total knee arthroplasty: randomized study comparing cemented and uncemented fixation of the Miller-Galante I design. J Orthop Res. 1995;12:347–56.

Nusbaum HJ, Rose RM. The effects of radiation sterilization on the properties of ultra high molecular weight polyethylene. J Biomed Mater Res. 1979;13:557–76.

O'Keefe TJ, Winter S, Lewallen DG, et al. Clinical and radiographic evaluation of a monoblock tibial component. J Arthroplasty. 2010;25:785–92.

Oh KJ, Pandher DS, Lee SH, et al. Meta-analysis comparing outcomes of fixed-bearing and mobile-bearing prostheses in total knee arthroplasty. J Arthroplasty. 2009;24:873–84.

Onishi M. Surgical use of ceramic apatites. Nippon Shika Ishikai Zasshi. 1983;36:803–10.

Oral E, Malhi AS, Wannomae KK, et al. Highly cross-linked ultrahigh molecular weight polyethylene with improved fatigue resistance for total joint arthroplasty: recipient of the 2006 Hap Paul Award. J Arthroplasty. 2008;23:1037–44.

Parks NL, Engh GA, Topoleski LD, et al. Modular tibial insert micromotion: a concern with contemporary knee implants. Clin Orthop. 1998;356:10–5.

Park JW, Kim YH. Simultaneous cemented and cementless total knee replacement in the same patients. J Bone Joint Surg Br. 2011;93-B:1479–86.

Pilliar RM, Lee JM, Maniatopoulos C. Observations on the effect of movement on boneingrowth into porous-surfaced implants. Clin Orthop. 1986;208:108–13.

Pittman GT, Peters CL, Hines JL, Bachus KN. Mechanical bond strength of the cement-tibial component Interface in total knee arthroplasty. J Arthroplasty. 2006;21:883–8.

Pritchett JW. Patients prefer a bicruciate-retaining or the medial pivot total knee prosthesis. J Arthroplasty. 2011;26:224–8.

Ranawat AS, Mohanty SS, Goldsmith SE, et al. Experience with an all-polyethylene total knee arthroplasty in younger, active patients with follow-up from 2 to 11 years. J Arthroplasty. 2005;20 Suppl 3:7–11.

Rand JA. Cement or cementless fixation in total knee arthroplasty? Clin Orthop. 1991;273:52–62.

Reckling FW, Dillon WL. The bone-cement interface temperature during total joint replacement. J Bone Joint Surg Am. 1977; 59-A:80–2.

Ries MD, Cabalo A, Bozic KJ, et al. Porous tantalum patellar augmentation: the importance of residual bone stock. Clin Orthop. 2006;452:166–70.

Ries MD, Salehi A, Widding K, et al. Polyethylene wear performance of oxidized zirconium and cobalt-chromium knee components under abrasive wear. J Bone Joint Surg Am. 2002;84-A:129–35.

Rimnac CM, Klein RW, Betts F, et al. Post irradiation aging of ultra-high molecular weight polyethylene. J Bone Joint Surg Am. 1994;76-A:1052–6.

Ritter MA. Enhanced cross-linked polymers: the promise-in opposition. Orthopedics. 2002;25:938.

Ritter MA. High-flexion knee designs: more hype than hope? In the affirmative. J Arthroplasty. 2006;21 Suppl 1:40–1.

Ritter MA, Herbst SA, Keating EM, et al. Radiolucency at the bone cement interface in total knee replacement. J Bone Joint Surg Am. 1994;76-A:60–5.

Ritter MA, Wing JT, Berend ME, et al. The clinical effect of gender on outcome of total knee arthroplasty. J Arthroplasty. 2008; 23:331–6.

Rosenberg AG. Posterior cruciate ligament retention in total knee arthroplasty. In: Scott WN, editor. Surgery of the knee. 5th ed. Philadelphia: Churchill Livingstone; 2011. p. 1125–31.

Sawaguchi N, Majima T, Ishigaki T, et al. Mobile-bearing total knee arthroplasty improves patellar tracking and patellofemoral contact stress: in vivo measurements in the same patients. J Arthroplasty. 2010;25:920–5.

Schindler OS. Patellar resurfacing in total knee arthroplasty. In: Scott WN, editor. Surgery of the knee. 5th ed. Philadelphia: Churchill Livingstone; 2011. p. 1161–90.

Scott RD. A brief history of three decades of evolution of total knee arthroplasty in Boston. In: Scott RD, editor. Total knee arthroplasty. 1st ed. Philadelphia: Saunders; 2006. p. 1–7.

Scott RD, Volatile TB. Twelve years experience with posterior cruciate-retaining total knee arthroplasty. Clin Orthop. 1986;205:100–7.

Sculco TP. The role of constraint in total knee arthroplasty. J Arthroplasty. 2006;21(4 Suppl 1):54–6.

Seon JK, Park SJ, Lee KB, et al. Range of motion in total knee arthroplasty: a prospective comparison of high-flexion and standard cruciate-retaining designs. J Bone Joint Surg Am. 2009;91-A: 672–9.

Shannon FJ, Cronin JJ, Cleary MS, et al. The posterior cruciate ligament-preserving total knee replacement: do we 'preserve' it? A radiological study. J Bone Joint Surg Br. 2007;89-B: 766–71.

Sharma A, Komistek RD, Ranawat CS, Dennis DA, Mahfouz MR. In vivo contact pressures in total knee arthroplasty. J Arthroplasty. 2007;22:404–16.

Shimizu N, Tomita T, Yamazaki T, et al. The effect of weight-bearing condition on kinematics of a high-flexion, posterior-stabilized knee prosthesis. J Arthroplasty. 2011;26:1031–7.

Simmons S, Lephart S, Rubash H, et al. Proprioception following total knee arthroplasty with and without the posterior cruciate ligament. J Arthroplasty. 1996;11:763–8.

Small SR, Berend ME, Ritter MA, et al. A comparison in proximal tibial strain between metal-backed and all-polyethylene anatomic graduated component total knee arthroplasty tibial components. J Arthroplasty. 2010;25:820–5.

Sorrels RB, Stiehl JB. Long-term outcomes of a rotating platform mobile bearing prosthesis after total knee arthroplasty. J Arthroplasty. 2004;19:255.

Springer BD, Mason JB. Cemented total knee arthroplasty: the gold standard. In: Scott WN, editor. Surgery of the knee. 5th ed. Philadelphia: Churchill Livingstone; 2011. p. 1108–11.

Stern SH, Sills RD, Gilbert JL. The effect of tibial stem design on component micromotion in knee arthroplasty. Clin Orthop. 1997;345:44–52.

Stiehl JB. Mobile bearings in total knee arthroplasty. In: Scott WN, editor. Surgery of the knee. 4th ed. Philadelphia: Churchill Livingstone; 2006. p. 1558–73.

Stiehl JB, Komistek RD, Dennis DA, et al. Fluoroscopic analysis of kinematics after posterior cruciate-retaining knee arthroplasty. J Bone Joint Surg Br. 1995;77-B:884–9.

Vail TP, Lang JE, Sikes III CV. Surgical techniques and instrumentation in total knee arthroplasty. In: Scott WN, editor. Surgery of the knee. 5th ed. Philadelphia: Churchill Livingstone; 2011. p. 1042–99.

Van Citters PW, Collier JP. The retrieval laboratory: making sense of knee implant revision. In: Scott WN, editor. Surgery of the knee. 4th ed. Philadelphia: Churchill Livingstone; 2006. p. 290–303.

Victor J, Banks S, Bellemans J. Kinematics of posterior cruciate ligament-retaining and -substituting total knee arthroplasty: a prospective randomised outcome study. J Bone Joint Surg Br. 2005; 87-B:646–55.

Victor J, Mueller JK, Komistek RD, et al. In vivo kinematics after a cruciate-substituting TKA. Clin Orthop. 2010;468:807–14.

Vince KG, Malo M, Thadan PJ. Posterior stabilization in total knee arthroplasty. In: Callaghan JJ, editor. The adult knee. 1st ed. Philadelphia: Lippincot Williams & Wilkins; 2003. p. 1145–61.

Voigt J, Mosier M. Cemented all-polyethylene and metal-backed polyethylene tibial components used for primary total knee arthroplasty: a systematic review of the literature and meta-analysis of randomized controlled trials involving 1798 primary total knee implants. J Bone Joint Surg Am. 2011;93-A:1790–8.

Wang A, Yau SS, Essner A, et al. A highly crosslinked UHMWPE for CR and PS total knee arthroplasties. J Arthroplasty. 2008; 23:559–66.

Wasielewski RC, Komistek RD, Zingde SM, et al. Lack of axial rotation in mobile-bearing knee designs. Clin Orthop. 2008; 466:2662–8.

Whiteside LA. Cementless total knee design. In: Scott WN, editor. Surgery of the knee. 4th ed. Philadelphia: Churchill Livingstone; 2006. p. 1613–25.

Whiteside LA. Cementless total knee design. In: Scott WN, editor. Surgery of the knee. 5th ed. Philadelphia: Churchill Livingstone; 2011. p. 1112–24.

Whiteside LA, Nagamine R. Biomechanical aspects of knee replacement design. In: Scott WN, editor. The knee. 1st ed. St. Louis: Mosby; 1994. p. 1079–96.

Wilson DA, Astephen JL, Hennigar AW, et al. Inducible displacement of a trabecular metal tibial monoblock component. J Arthroplasty. 2010;25:893–900.

Wixson RL, Lautenschlager EP. Methylmethacrylate. In: Callaghan JJ, editor. The adult hip. 1st ed. Philadelphia: Lippincott-Raven Publishers; 1998. p. 135–57.

Yoshii I, Whiteside LA, Anouch YS. The effect of patellar button placement and femoral component design on patellar tracking in total knee arthroplasty. Clin Orthop. 1992;275:211–9.

Yoshiya S, Matsui N, Komistek RD, et al. In vivo kinematic comparison of posterior cruciate retaining and posterior stabilized total knee arthroplasties under passive and weight-bearing conditions. J Arthroplasty. 2005;20:777–83.

Zhang K, Mihalko WM. Posterior cruciate mechnoreceptors in osteoarthritic and cruciate-retaining TKA retrievals: a pilot study. Clin Orthop. 2012;470:1855–9.

3 Preparation for the Operation

Once the patient is admitted for the operation, it is necessary to carefully review again whether TKA is really needed and whether the patient's condition is suitable for undergoing the surgery. The knee joint and general condition must be carefully reassessed through history taking and physical examination on preoperative checkup. If no specific problems are noted during the preoperative checkup, the patients should be educated regarding postoperative care, progress, prognosis, and complications of TKA, and meticulous preparation should be carried out for the operation in order to prevent the occurrence of any incidents or complications perioperatively.

3.1 Admission Checkup

3.1.1 History Taking

On admission, *it is necessary to carefully assess whether arthroplasty is the only method to relieve the pain and to improve the function*, because many items for operation may be missed during the outpatient assessment. Since the intensity of pain is not always the same, the current severity of pain may be different from that at the time when it was decided to perform the TKA. In terms of function, it is necessary to assess the current level of function. Two questions that may help the surgeon to assess the current level of function are, "how much discomfort is the patient feeling due to the loss of function?" and "how much is the motivation to improve the function?"

It is inappropriate to perform TKA not only in those patients who have less pain and functional disturbance but also in those patients whose general condition is very poor. Lavernia et al. reported that the patients with a *preoperative WOMAC score more than 51 showed a higher postoperative WOMAC score*.

The patient's past history and current condition of the knee joint should be enquired in detail. In particular, the history of previous knee surgery including the timing and the type of operation performed should be known as it might have altered the anatomy of the knee joint.

It is also very important to assess *the condition of spine and hip joints and the vascular status of the lower limb*. Elderly patients often experience radiating pain and/or muscle weakness due to spinal problems. In such cases, pain and/or functional disturbance may persist even after arthroplasty, and the patient satisfaction may decrease despite of functional improvement after TKA. *Vascular claudication is often masked in the patients with arthritis because of restriction of activity*, and hence careful history taking is required. If the vascular status of the lower limb is not normal, it can cause a vague pain, increase the risk of swelling or thrombosis postoperatively, or aggravate arteriosclerosis to cause postoperative circulatory disturbance.

Past medical history should include the history of cardiopulmonary diseases, diabetes mellitus, endocrine diseases, gastrointestinal diseases, and renal diseases. Medical checkup should be done in order to know the patients' current general condition in case they have a history of any of the above diseases.

The risk of cardiopulmonary complications during the perioperative period of TKA is so high that in case of any doubt, a detailed study should be performed. Since many elderly patients have diabetes mellitus, the surgeon should be aware of the type and method used to control the ailment as well as how it is being controlled currently.

The possibility of iatrogenic Cushing's syndrome should be excluded if the patient displays features of moon face or generalized body edema. Some patients may have functional disturbance of the thyroid, which they may inform in advance most of the times.

Since infection is the most serious complication of TKA, it is essential to check for the possibility of activation of infection if they had recently undergone tooth extraction, received acupuncture or moxibustion, or suffered from genitourinary infections.

If the patients had undergone any other operation, enquire regarding the name and timing of the operation. If necessary, the surgeon who had performed the operation should be contacted, or a specialist for that particular operation should be

W. Cho, *Knee Joint Arthroplasty*,
DOI 10.1007/978-3-642-39389-1_3,

consulted in order to determine whether the patient can undergo arthroplasty.

If these procedures are ignored, there may be an unacceptably high risk of morbidity or mortality after TKA which is just an elective surgery to reduce the pain and to improve function.

3.1.2 Physical Examination

First of all, the *skin condition should be checked.* The yielding behavior or the elasticity of skin are very important for the wound healing and postoperative rehabilitation. If there is a preexisting surgical scar on the knee joint, its location and adhesions with the subcutaneous tissues should be examined by palpation. Information regarding recent skin problems and whether or not acupuncture or moxibustion has been performed is helpful in eliminating the sources of an occult infection.

Also, the presence of a tender point, heat sensation, joint swelling should be checked, and an effusion should be differentiated from a synovial hypertrophy. Patellar compression test is helpful in order to decide whether or not to resurface the patella in selective patellar replacement.

The type and the degree of deformity will affect the selection of implants as well as the operative procedures. Hence, the deformity should be examined carefully. *Flexion contracture* is well observed when the knee is rested on a flat surface. Flexion contracture should be differentiated from the extension lag in which the knee can be extended passively but cannot be extended actively, since the surgical procedures for flexion contracture and extension lag may be different.

Preoperative evaluation of *the knee instability* is also important. Mediolateral knee instability as well as A–P knee instability should be assessed preoperatively by physical examination and stress X-ray.

Active and passive ROM should be checked with the use of a goniometer. Lavernia et al. stated that when the ROM is checked by the naked eye, it is overestimated than the real ROM.

One of the most important points to be checked, although it is often skipped, is examining the power of the quadriceps and hamstrings. In particular, *the power of the quadriceps* is closely related to the prognosis.

The examination of the knee joint is followed by the *examination of the spine and hip joints*. Although it is obviously important, examination of the *vascular system* is often overlooked during the physical examination. However, it is critical to examine the vascular system to prevent circulatory compromise postoperatively. When there is a weak pulse, skin ulcers, or toe necrosis, the possibility of vascular disease is very high.

3.1.3 Preoperative Evaluation

Preoperative evaluation can be divided into two sections, general routine checkup and checkup of the knee joint. The routine checkup is a basic examination, and the past medical history or abnormalities found during the routine checkup need to be studied in more detail.

Echocardiogram or thallium scan is necessary when abnormal findings are noted on the EKG. In case of hypertension, diabetes mellitus, endocrine diseases, or disorders of brain or central nervous system, it is recommended to consult a specialist of the respective field so as to perform an appropriate examination, control the ailment, and make a decision regarding the operative risk. In case of osteoporosis, bone densitometry is performed, and treatment can be started postoperatively, if needed.

In cases the patients who have a history of thrombosis or who are at a high risk for DVT, duplex sonography or RI venography may also be performed. If the pulse is weak or calcification along the vessels is seen on the plain X-ray, a Doppler test should be performed, and this can be followed by an angiography if required.

For back pain, radiating pain, or muscle weakness in the lower limb, a plain X-ray as well as MRI or CT of the spine are helpful.

For examining the knee joint, a *simple X-ray* is the routine, and additional images may be taken according to the knee joint condition. The *standing true A–P, lateral X-rays*, the axial views, and a *scanogram* for choosing the appropriate size of the implant are fundamental.

In order to evaluate the tibiofemoral angle in the coronal plane, *the A–P X-rays of the whole lower limb* must be taken with the patella facing anteriorly. Otherwise, the limb can undergo rotation and an inaccurate angle of the axis may be measured. *In case of rotational deformity of the knee, the X-rays must be taken one after another separately to measure the correct angle of axis.* Even in the patients without knee instability, taking the *valgus and varus stress X-rays is very useful* (Fig. 3.1).

The MRI of the knee is only necessary to determine the causes of knee pain other than osteoarthritis. Hence, it is not needed in patients in whom the decision of performing an arthroplasty has already been made.

If inflammatory disease is suspected on routine checkup, joint aspiration or WBC bone scan may be helpful.

3.2 Final Decision

After a thorough preoperative checkup, the final decision regarding whether or not to perform the operation should be made. If TKA is not really needed at the moment or there are significant risks associated with TKA operation, it must be either cancelled or postponed.

Once the decision is made to perform TKA, it must be decided whether to perform TKA simultaneously on both the knees (one-stage TKA), or perform TKA on one knee followed by the other knee after a certain time interval (two-stage TKA). This decision is usually made before

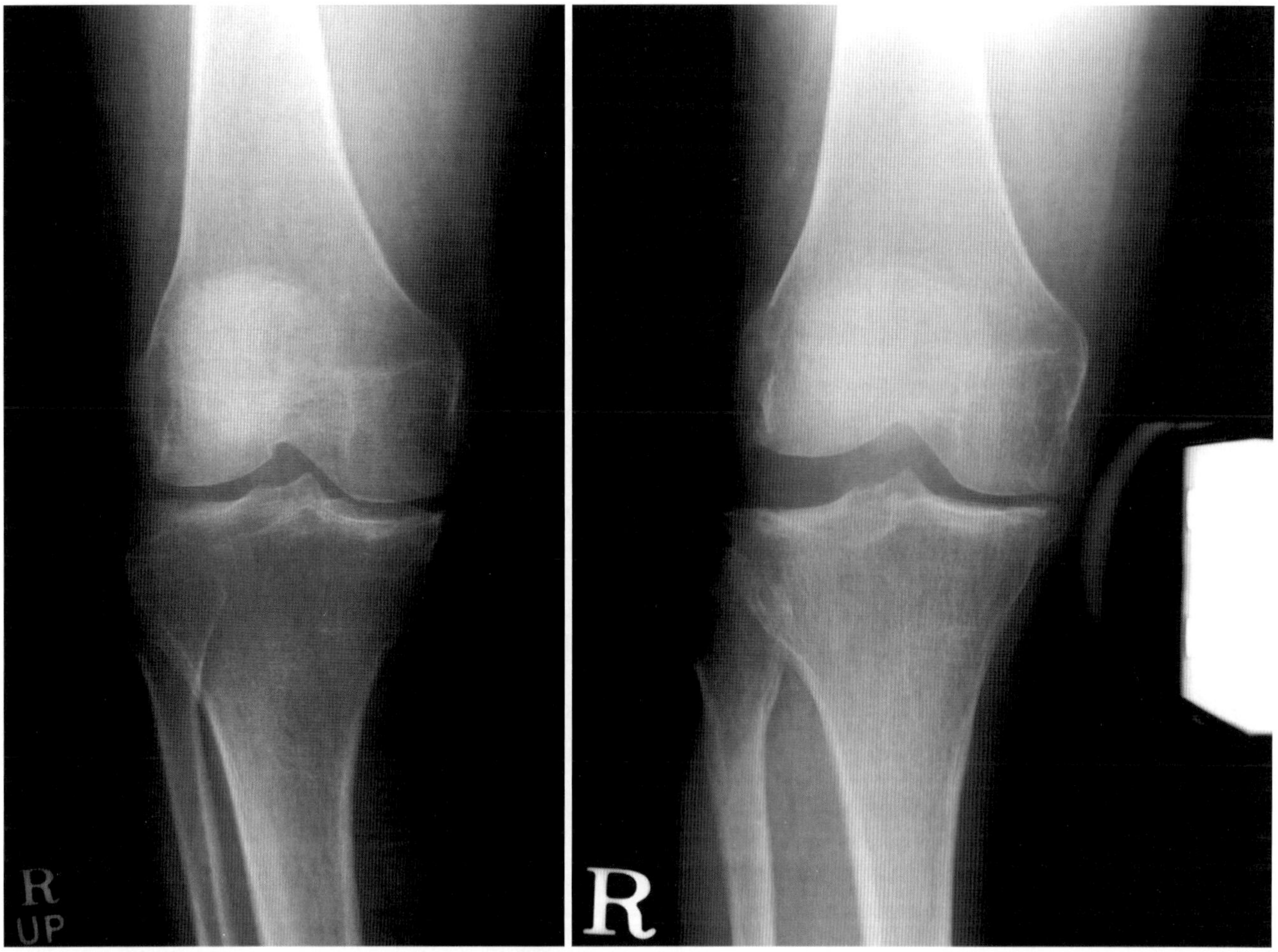

Fig. 3.1 The *left image* shows a weight-bearing standing view, and the *right image* shows a stress X-ray of the same knee joint. The *right image* appears more lax on the lateral side than the *left image*

admission, but the results of preoperative checkup can change the decision.

In case of the *one-stage operation, it can save costs and shorten the rehabilitation period.* However, the one-stage operation *can increase the risks associated with TKA. Hence the age of the patient, general condition, and condition of the knee joint should be taken into account.* On the other hand, the *two-stage operation* prolongs the duration of hospital stay which is a *great burden to both the patients and their families.*

As for the terminology, concomitant or simultaneous operation indicates that two teams of surgeons perform the operation on one leg each at the same time. In such a case, the duration of anesthesia can be reduced, but it can lead to overburdening of the heart hemodynamically, thereby increasing the risks. Also, it may be inconvenient for the two teams of surgeons to work simultaneously and the risk of infection is elevated. Hence, this operation is only undertaken in exceptional cases at specialized centers. In general, a simultaneous operation means one-stage operation or sequential bilateral operation under one anesthesia. Performing the operation on one knee followed by the other knee after some time interval is called the two-stage or sequential operation under two anesthesias.

It is generally agreed that the *results of TKA are not different whether it is done simultaneously on both knees or on one knee followed by the other.* The biggest controversial issue is the incidence of complications; the *one-stage surgery* is generally *thought to have greater risks* because the operation time is longer, the need for transfusion is increased due to more bleeding, the incidence of congestive heart failure is raised due to a hemodynamic shift, and the incidence of acute delirium is increased due to fat embolism. Restrepo et al. reviewed 27,807 patients through a meta-analysis of 18 literatures and reported that a significantly higher incidence of pulmonary embolism, cardiovascular complications, and mortality was seen in the patients who underwent one-stage operation than that in the patients who underwent two-stage operation. Lynch et al. reported that the patients above 80 years of age showed a higher rate of complications after simultaneous operation compared to that after two-stage operation. They also reported that *these complications were related to the preoperative cardiac conditions and the duration of operation.*

On the other hand, Kollettis et al., Lewallen, and Hooper et al. reported that *the chances of complications were not increased after the simultaneous operation in ordinary patients*. Vince et al. reported that it may be true that the simultaneous operation was associated with a higher rate of complications, but this complication rate was still lower than that after the second operation of the two-stage operation. Kim et al. reported that there were no differences in the complications and mortality between one-stage and two-stage operation even in the high-risk patients. Morrey et al. also reported the following rates of complications: 7 % for the two-stage operation performed during the same admission period, 9 % for the simultaneous operation, and 12 % for the two-stage operation performed during two separate admissions. Soudry et al. stated that the incidence of thrombosis rather increases with the two-stage operation. Ritter and Hardy found a higher mortality rate after the simultaneous operation, but the incidence of wound infection was decreased to almost half.

With regard to the time interval between the two operations in the two-stage operation, Foster et al. reported that the bleeding was reduced when the two operations were performed 1 week apart, and Sliva et al. recommended that the two operations should be performed 4–7 days apart during the same admission period. On the other hand, Ritter and Hardy recommended that the two operations should be performed 3–6 months apart since it is the safest and least expensive and is associated with lowest mortality.

Recommended indications for simultaneous operation are when anesthesia is difficult due to rheumatoid arthritis or ankylosing spondylitis in which several operations are required to be performed for other lesions besides the knee joints and the socioeconomic conditions are not favorable. In case of severe deformity (varus–valgus deformity and flexion contracture) of both knee joints, the one-stage operation is recommended as the nonoperated knee may have a negative impact on the operated knee postoperatively. Harato et al. stated that the loading was increased on the operated knee when the opposite limb had a flexion contracture. If the subsequent TKA is done within a shorter interval, it does not cause any problems. But there is always a possibility of delay in the operation on the other knee joint for a long time due to unexpected reasons.

Scott preferred the one-stage operation, and I would like to introduce his method here because it could be a realistic and helpful method. If patients have medical problems or are not willing to undergo the one-stage operation, the two-stage operation is performed. If one knee is less severely affected than the other knee, the patients should be asked whether they want to undergo an operation on the less painful knee assuming that the more severely affected side would be pain-free. If they want to undergo the operation on the less painful knee, the simultaneous operation is performed.

Regional anesthesia, especially epidural anesthesia, is preferred, and warfarin is used as an antithrombotic agent from the night before the operation. *Antibiotics are administered thrice: twice before each operation and once after the operation.*

The operation should start on the more severely affected knee joint, because it is possible that the operation can be cancelled due to the patient's condition. Operation on the second knee joint is started after skin closure of the first operated knee joint. New set of surgical instruments should be used, and everyone involved in the first operation should change their gloves. An attempt is made to make a skin incision of the same length.

Postoperative pain control is achieved with patient-controlled analgesia (PCA), and warfarin is administered for 4–6 weeks. Rehabilitation program would be the same as that for the one-stage operation.

In case skin incisions of different lengths are made on the two knee joints and if the patients ask about it, they are told that more things were needed to be done in one knee joint. If the progress of the TKA is different between the two knee joints, the patients are explained that the less affected knee joint is showing much better results than usual.

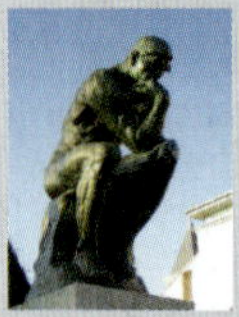

Author's Opinion

I think that the one-stage operation has many benefits as it saves costs, shortens the rehabilitation period, and increases the patient satisfaction. In case of the two-stage operation, there is a possibility of cancellation of the operation on the second knee. The nonoperated knee joint can have an adverse effect on the operated knee joint in case there is a deformity, severe instability, or ankylosis. So, the one-stage operation is performed in these cases unless there are special reasons for not doing so.

However, the two-stage operation should be performed if the patients are older than 80 years of age, patient's general condition is poor, there is a history of cardiac problem, or other risk factors were detected in the preoperative checkup.

I have performed more than 6,000 TKAs based on this principle, and I have not found any significant difference in the complications.

3.3 Outcome Study

Although the evaluation of TKA is done after the operation, its outcome should be compared with the preoperative status of the knee joint. Therefore, the outcome study should start from the preoperative period. This is not only important for the development of arthroplasty, but it is also essential for the surgeon to check the patient's preoperative condition and the feedback after surgery.

To accomplish this purpose, *a long-term follow-up should be done with the most widely used evaluation methods*. If this is not done, it is difficult to evaluate the commonly accepted results by the researchers because of the bias arising from the differences in patient selection or regional differences.

No matter which evaluation method is used, *it should be applicable to all patients and provide reproducibility and accuracy*. In order to achieve these, a well-trained examiner or interviewer is needed, and *the patients should be able to understand the survey correctly*.

As knee surgeries, especially arthroplasty, have become popular, several evaluation methods have been introduced until now. There are about 40 evaluation methods available currently. *There are basically two methods, one is evaluation by the medical personnel or interviewer and the other is evaluation according to the survey or through the recordings by the patients themselves.*

The most widely used methods by the medical staff are the Hospital for Special Surgery Knee score (HSS score) and Knee Society score (KSS) which was basically derived from the HSS score. These scores are calculated from the interview or from the examination by a physician or a trained medical staff. There is also a patellar scoring system for evaluating the patellofemoral conditions. These methods are based on the evaluation of pain and function in the knee joints. Hence, the socioeconomic factors, such as income and family relations as well as the psychological factors are excluded.

However, subjective evaluation by the patient is as equally important as the objective evaluation. The results of surgery may be affected by the nonphysical factors such as those mentioned above and the patients' expectations. The WOMAC score (Western Ontario and McMaster Universities Osteoarthritis Index score) evaluates the patient's pain and function, and the SF-36 (short form 36) evaluates the patient's quality of life through the patient survey or recordings by the patients themselves. However, Hamilton et al. suggested that patients' reporting of functional outcome after TKA is influenced more by their pain level than their ability to accomplish tasks.

The Knee Society Total Knee Arthroplasty Roentgenographic Evaluation System is a radiological method of evaluation.

3.3.1 HSS Score

The HSS Knee Score (Table 3.1) was introduced by the Hospital for Special Surgery (HSS) in the 1970s *to evaluate the results of hip and knee joint surgery*. It is also used to evaluate the results of other hip and knee surgeries besides arthroplasty and offers different versions for the hip and knee joints. The evaluation is accomplished *through the interview and physical examination by the medical personnel or by a well-trained specialist* appointed for performing the evaluation.

The HSS scoring system comprises of seven basic categories—pain, function, range of motion, muscular strength, flexion deformity, instability, and subtractions—with a total of 100 points. Pain has the largest impact for the score (30 points), followed by function (22 points), range of motion (18 points), muscular strength, flexion deformity, and instability (10 points each). *Fifty out of the 100 points are assigned by an interview and the remaining 50 points by the physical examination. Higher scores mean better results.*

For a better understanding, the background of the HSS score needs more explanation. Although distance of a block is ambiguous, originally one block means a block in the streets of Manhattan, which is about 1/20 miles (approx. 80–100 m). The walking distance refers to the distance which the patients can walk without taking rest.

In the climbing up and down the stairs item, 5 points are given if the patients can do so without any aid, 2 points if they need some aid such as holding the handrails, and 0 point if they need a lot of help. Transfer receives 5 points if the patients can rise from a chair without any aid, 2 points if they need to grab the armrest, and 0 point if they need a lot of help.

For the range of motion, the maximum range of motion is set at 144° and the angle of motion is divided by 8 and is rounded to the nearest integer (e.g., 0–95° = 11 points).

For muscular strength, the patients are asked to sit and extend the knees. Break refers to bending the legs with the use of the examiner's force. Therefore, "cannot break quadriceps" means that the examiner cannot bend the patient's knees with examiner's applied force.

Instability is measured by the instability found on varus and valgus stress test in full extension or flexion at 90°. If there is instability in flexion or extension, it should be measured.

For subtraction, normal alignment is set at 7° of valgus tibiofemoral angle in full extension, and any angle that exceeds 7° or is less than 7°, either a valgus or varus, 1 point is subtracted per every 5°.

For the overall evaluation, the knee is rated as excellent if the HSS score is between 85 and 100, good if the HSS score is between 70 and 84, fair if the HSS score is between 60 and 69, and poor if the HSS score is below 60.

Table 3.1 The Hospital for Special Surgery scoring system

THE HOSPITAL FOR SPECIAL SURGERY

KNEE SERVICE
Knee Rating Sheet

Name__________ HSS# __________ Preoperative date __________

	Score	LEFT						RIGHT					
PAIN (30 points)		pre	6mo	1yr	2yr	3yr	4yr	pre	6mo	1yr	2yr	3yr	4yr
Walking: None	15												
Mild	10												
Moderate	5												
Severe	0												
At rest: None	15												
Mild	10												
Moderate	5												
Severe	0												
FUNCTION (22 points)													
Walk: Walking and standing unlimited	12												
5–10 blocks. standing > 30 min	10												
1–5 blocks. standing 15–30 min	8												
Walk < 1 block	4												
Cannot walk	0												
Stairs: Normal	5												
With support	2												
Transfer: Normal	5												
With support	2												
ROM (18 points) Each 8*= 1 point													
MUSCLE STRENGTH (10 points)													
Cannot break quadriceps	10												
Can break quadriceps	8												
Can move through arc of motion	4												
Cannot move through arc of motion	0												
FLEXION DEFORMITY (10 points)													
None	10												
5–10°	8												
10–20°	5												
>20°	0												
INSTABLILITY (10 points)													
None	10												
5–10°	8												
10–20°	5												
>20°	0												
TOTAL													
SUBTRACTIONS:													
One cane	1												
One crutch	2												
Two crutches	3												
Extension lag of 5°	2												
10°	3												
15°	5												
Deformity (5° = 1 point)													
varus													
vaigus													
TOTAL SUBTRACTIONS													
KNEE SCORE													

The advantage of this evaluation method is that it is used worldwide, and hence a comparison can be done between the researchers as well as between the implants according to the time sequence. The drawback of this evaluation method is that examiner's bias can influence the score, and the score may change according to the patient's physical condition or age even though the condition of the knee joints is the same. Cho et al. reported that the score could change according to single and bilateral TKA, or other physical and medical conditions. Also, there is a probability of an interobserver and intraobserver bias.

In spite of these drawbacks, the HSS score can provide an objective evaluation of the patient's physical condition including pain and function of the knee joint. Regarding the interpretation of the HSS score, for example, if the KSS is good and the HSS score is low, it means that the condition of the knee joint is good, but the patient's physical condition is poor.

3.3.2 Knee Society Score

The Knee Society was organized in 1983 by the surgeons who were interested in knee joint surgery. In 1989, *the KSS (Table 3.2) was designed to overcome the drawbacks of the HSS score*. The KSS added the A–P and mediolateral instability to the HSS, and the patients were divided into three groups based on the associated medical conditions which could affect the evaluation score.

The KSS has a different scoring system as compared to the HSS, and *it consists of three sections: knee score (100 points), knee function score (100 points), and a patient classification system. This evaluation, like the HSS score, is accomplished through an interview and examination by a surgeon or a trained medical staff.*

The knee score is divided into pain, range of motion, and mediolateral and A–P instability with subtractions for flexion contracture, extension lag, and malalignment. The *maximum 50 points are assigned to pain*. Twenty-five points are given to ROM and stability, respectively. For the evaluation of range of motion, 1 point is added for every 5° to get a full 25 points if it is more than 125°. For the evaluation of stability, 15 points are given for mediolateral stability and 10 points for A–P stability.

In terms of alignment, 5–10° of valgus is considered normal, and any angle exceeding 10° or less than 5° is subtracted from 5 to 10°, and the remainder is multiplied by 3, and then these points are subtracted. For example, if there is 3° of valgus, 3 is subtracted from 5 (as 5–10° of valgus is normal), and the remainder 2 (5–3) is multiplied by 3, and thus 6 (2×3) points are subtracted.

The knee function score consists of walking and going up and down the stairs; each item has 50 points. Fifty points are given if there are no limitations on walking, 40 points are given if one can walk more than 10 blocks, 30 points if one can walk 5–10 blocks, 20 points if one can walk less than 5 blocks, 10 points if one can only ambulate within the home, and 0 point if one cannot walk at all. Here, one block refers to 1/20 miles (approx. 80–100 m). For walking the stairs, 50 points are given if there is no problem going up and down the stairs, 40 points when no problem is noted on going up the stairs but one needs to hold the handrails when going down the stairs, 30 points if one needs to hold the handrails when going up and down the stairs, 15 points if one cannot go down the stairs, and 0 point if one cannot go up and down the stairs.

There are also subtractions for the knee function score: 5 points are subtracted if one cane is used for walking, 10 points are subtracted if two canes are used for walking, and 20 points are subtracted if clutches or walkers are needed.

The overall evaluation, like the HSS score, is rated excellent if the score is higher than 85 points, good if the score is higher than 70 points, fair if the score is higher than 60 points, and poor if the score is lower than 60 points.

The purpose of the patient classification system is to classify the factors that affect the results of surgery. It is classified into three categories: *Category A* comprises of the patients who underwent arthroplasty on one or both the knees or hip joint, but this has no effect on the knee being evaluated (*not affecting the knee being evaluated*); *Category B* comprises of the patients who underwent operation of one or both the sides of the knees or hip joint, and this affects the results of the operated limb (*the knee being evaluated is affected by the problems of other parts of the limbs*); and *Category C* comprises of *the patients whose physical activities are affected by polyarthralgia or other causes. This classification standardizes the knee function score* by establishing the foundation for comparing them *under the same conditions*.

The benefits of the KSS are that, although it shares similar items with the HSS scoring system, it is simpler, more accurate, more objective, and more realistic. For example, the fact that one uses a cane or clutches means there is a serious functional disturbance. However, in the HSS score, only 1–2 points are subtracted. Another advantage of the KSS is that the patients whose activities are influenced by general factors that affect arthroplasty can be identified, and a more clear comparison can be made with the other patients with similar condition. In case of the HSS score, for example, the walking distance may be decreased due to the general condition which may lower the score although the condition of the operated knee is the same. *In the KSS system, the score remains constant if the condition of the knee is unchanged, even though the patients get older or the general conditions change*. In other words, if the operation is successful, the KSS score is good regardless of the patient's general condition.

The drawback of the KSS, like the HSS, is that there can be an examiner bias, and it overlaps with the HSS score in various items, and the evaluation of function score is too simple.

Table 3.2 The Knee Society scoring system

The Knee Society Score

Name ____________ Operative date ________

	Score	LEFT						RIGHT					
		pre	1yr	2yr	3yr	4yr	5yr	pre	1yr	2yr	3yr	4yr	5yr
PAIN None	50												
Mild or Occ	45												
Stairs only	40												
Walking and stairs	30												
Moderate Occ	20												
Cont	10												
Severe	0												
ROM: (5°= 1 point)	25												
STABILITY (max mov any pos)													
A/P < 5	10												
5–10mm	5												
10mm	0												
M/L < 5°	15												
6–9°	10												
10–14°	5												
15°	0												
TOTAL													
Deductions (minus)													
FLEXION CONTRACTURE													
None	0												
5–10°	2												
11–15°	5												
16–20°	10												
>20°	15												
EXTENSION LAG													
None	0												
<10°	5												
10–20°	10												
>20°	15												
ALIGNMENT													
5–10° (None	0												
0–4° (3pt each deg)													
11–15° (3pt each deg)													
Other	20												
Total Deductions													
KNEE SCORE													
(If total is a minus, score is zero)													
FUNCTION													
WALKING: Unlimited	50												
>10 blocks	40												
5 to 10 blocks	30												
<5 blocks	20												
Housebound	10												
Unable	0												
STAIRS: Norm up and down	50												
Norm up: down rail	40												
Up and: down rail	30												
Up rail: unable down	15												
Unable	0												
TOTAL													
Deductions (minus)													
Cane	5												
Two canes	10												
Crutches/Walker	20												
Total Dedcutions													
FUNCTION SCROE													

Patient category: A. Unilateral or bilateral (opposite knee successfully replaced)
B. Unilateral - other knee symptomatic
C. Multiple anthritis or medical infirmity

3.3.3 Knee Society Total Knee Arthroplasty Roentgenographic Evaluation System

Knee Society Total Knee Arthroplasty Roentgenographic Evaluation System was developed to evaluate the radiological results after TKA (Fig. 3.2). Using this system, it is possible to make a radiological comparison of the results between different hospitals or institutions and between different implants.

The advantage of this method is that it is easy to use and fast, and the results are recorded in one sheet of paper. The

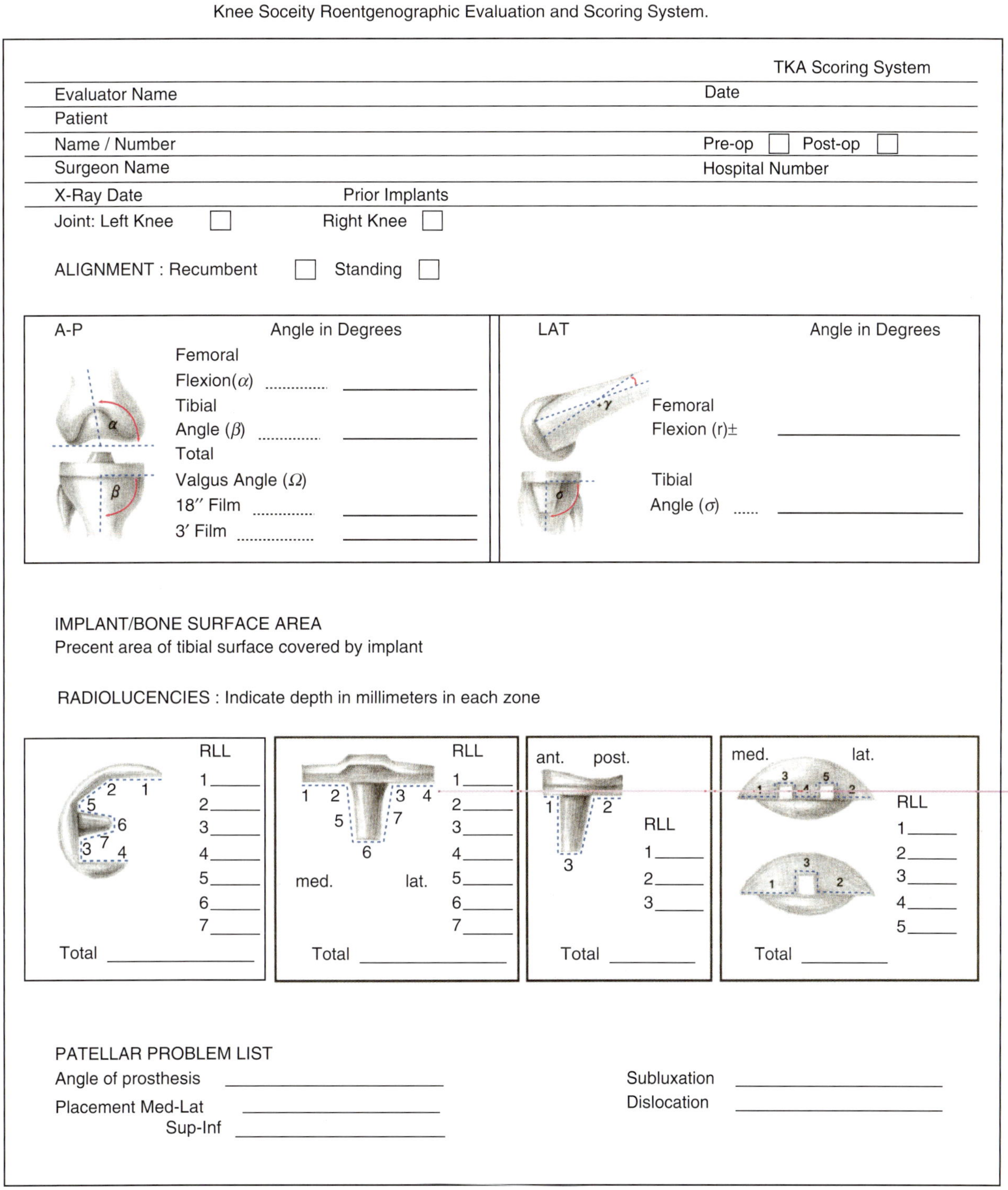

Knee Soceity Roentgenographic Evaluation and Scoring System.

TKA Scoring System

Evaluator Name — Date

Patient

Name / Number — Pre-op ☐ Post-op ☐

Surgeon Name — Hospital Number

X-Ray Date — Prior Implants

Joint: Left Knee ☐ Right Knee ☐

ALIGNMENT : Recumbent ☐ Standing ☐

A-P — Angle in Degrees

Femoral Flexion(α) .... ________

Tibial Angle (β) .... ________

Total Valgus Angle (Ω)

18″ Film .... ________

3′ Film .... ________

LAT — Angle in Degrees

Femoral Flexion (r)± ________

Tibial Angle (σ) ...... ________

IMPLANT/BONE SURFACE AREA

Precent area of tibial surface covered by implant

RADIOLUCENCIES : Indicate depth in millimeters in each zone

RLL 1___ 2___ 3___ 4___ 5___ 6___ 7___ Total ________

med. lat. RLL 1___ 2___ 3___ 4___ 5___ 6___ 7___ Total ________

ant. post. RLL 1___ 2___ 3___ Total ________

med. lat. RLL 1___ 2___ 3___ 4___ 5___ Total ________

PATELLAR PROBLEM LIST

Angle of prosthesis ________ Subluxation ________

Placement Med-Lat ________ Dislocation ________

Sup-Inf ________

Fig. 3.2 Knee Society roentgenographic evaluation and scoring system

drawbacks of this method are that the criteria for loosening zone are set up too arbitrary and some radiolucencies cannot be recorded correctly. This method not only calculates the angles and positions of the prosthesis, but it also introduces a scoring system that assesses the fixation state between the implants and the bones. The radiological results can be stored in a database.

In order to apply this method, it is necessary to standardize the method for checking the X-rays. To minimize the errors, several X-rays are taken and the most representative films are chosen, or fluoroscopic-aided X-ray can be used.

3.3.3.1 Method

The distance between the tube and film is fixed at 101.6 cm, and a 91.44 cm cassette is used to evaluate the alignment if possible. The distance of 101.6 cm is the distance between the tube and film of the C-arm.

With respect to the position of the knee joint, patella should face the ceiling while the patient is lying down, and for the A–P view, the beam is projected perpendicular to the center of the joint line. For the lateral view, the X-ray beam is directed at 90° to the A–P view. For patellar evaluation, the skyline or Merchant view is taken.

3.3.3.2 Recording

The alignment of prostheses is measured for precision by measuring the angle of implants on the A–P and lateral X-rays. *On the A–P X-ray, the α-angle is the obtuse angle where the anatomical axis meets the femoral prosthesis, and the β-angle is the angle between the tibial prosthesis and the anatomical axis of the tibia. The Ω-angle is the valgus angle between the femur and the tibia. On the lateral view, the γ-angle is the angle between the femoral prosthesis and the anatomical axis of the femur, and the δ-angle is the posterior slope of the tibial prosthesis.* The stability of prosthesis is expressed as the sum of radiolucency scores. The tibia is divided into seven zones on the A–P view: zones 1 and 2 represent the medial condyle; zones 3 and 4 the lateral condyle; and zones 5, 6, and 7 the area around the stem. If the prosthesis does not have a stem, zones 5, 6, and 7 are assigned from the medial to lateral side at the site of the imaginary stem. On the lateral view, the tibia is divided into three zones: zone 1 represents the anterior side, zone 2 the posterior side, and zone 3 the area around the stem. The lateral view of the femur is also divided into seven zones: zones 1 and 2 represent the anterior side; zones 3 and 4 the posterior side; and zones 5, 6, and 7 the area around the stem. If there is no stem, zones 5, 6, and 7 are assigned from the anterior to the posterior side of the site of the imaginary stem. Patella is divided into three zones: zone 1 represents the medial side, zone 2 the lateral side, and zone 3 the lug site if there is one lug. If there are two or more lugs, the patella is divided into five zones, of which zones 3, 4, and 5 are assigned around the lug sites.

If there are any problems with the patellofemoral joint, then additional measurements such as patellofemoral angle, height of the patellar prosthesis (skyline view or lateral view), severity of subluxation, and presence of dislocation should be included in the recordings.

Radiolucency of each numbered zone around the three prostheses is measured in millimeters (mm), and the total sum is expressed as points. *If the score is less than 4 points, it is not a sign of loosening and no observation is necessary. Whereas if the score is between 5 and 9, it requires observation, and if the score is higher than 10, there is a high probability of loosening. However, if the prosthesis has migrated or shifted, loosening of the prosthesis is thought to have occurred regardless of the score.*

3.3.4 WOMAC Score (The Western Ontario and McMaster Universities Osteoarthritis Index Score)

WOMAC score was first developed *to evaluate the efficacy of treatment according to the treatment method.* However, this method became a good tool to evaluate the results of TKA. *The WOMAC questionnaire is filled out by surveying the patients and consists of 24 questions grouped into three categories of pain, stiffness, and function with a total of 96 points* (Table 3.3). Each question is given 0 points in case there is no problem, 1 point for mild problems, 2 points for moderate problems, 3 points for severe problems, and 4 points for extreme problems. Therefore, *a higher WOMAC score indicates poor results, and the score is judged as excellent if it is below 14, good if it is between 15 and 28, fair if it is between 29 and 38, and poor if it is above 38 points.*

The advantage of the WOMAC system is that it is a patient-oriented survey that eliminates the examiner's bias, it is easy to calculate the score as the questions are simplified, it reflects the patients' satisfaction better, and it can be

Table 3.3 WOMAC questionnaire

WOMAC questionnaire
Section A (Pain)
How much pain do you have?
1. Walking on a flat surface
2. Going up or down stairs
3. At night while in bed
4. Sitting or lying
5. Standing upright
Section B (Stiffness)
6. How severe is your stiffness after first awakening in the morning?
7. How severe is your stiffness after sitting, lying down, or resting later in the day?
Section C (Function)
What degree of difficulty do you have while:
8. Descending stairs?
9. Ascending stairs?
10. Rising from sitting?
11. Standing?
12. Bending to the floor?
13. Walking on a flat surface?
14. Getting in/out of car?
15. Going shopping?
16. Putting on socks/stocking?
17. Rising from bed?
18. Taking off socks/stocking?
19. Lying in bed?
20. Getting in/out of bath?
21. Sitting?
22. Getting on/off toilet?
23. Heavy domestic duties?
24. Light domestic duties?

used to evaluate the results of operation or conservative treatments for arthritis.

The drawback of the WOMAC system may be that the pain score is assigned to a greater extent from the surgeon's viewpoint. If there is only a minor pain and when the responses are filled out by the patient, the score is not very different from that when interviewed by the medical staff. However, if there is moderate to severe pain, the scores turn out to be very different between the surgeons and patients. This is because the surgeons mostly focus on joint motion, alignment, and stability, which are directly related with operation, whereas the patients tend to express all the functions in relation to the pain. Also, there is an overlap between the questions for pain and physical function, and the score is likely to be higher if there are problems associated with either the pain or limited motion. For example, the score is considerably different when the knee flexion is above 95° or below 95°

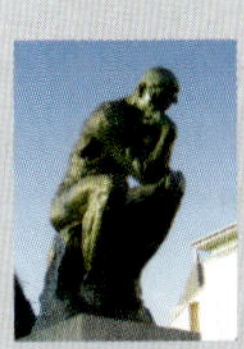

Author's Opinion

I think it would have been easier to understand and compare the results if there was one more question to make a total score of 100 points and if the rating system is reversed so that patients would have a higher score when they are in a good physical condition.

3.3.5 SF-36 (36-Item Short-Form Health Survey) or MOS (Medical Outcomes Study)

SF-36 (Table 3.4) was developed to know the effects of treatment methods according to the medical expenses and to establish public health policies. But it is also used to evaluate the clinical results and work-up to compare the effects of treatment methods for various diseases.

This method evaluates the *health-related quality of life* (HRQOL) by examining which treatment methods give better satisfaction for a certain disease when the cost of treatment was the same and how the results progress over time. For example, the treatment results can be compared between osteoarthritis and rheumatoid arthritis, mild osteoarthritis and severe osteoarthritis, and unicompartmental knee arthroplasty and total knee replacement in relation to the cost of treatment.

This method includes the effects of treatment according to the physical, psychological, and socioeconomic conditions.

Table 3.4 SF-36 survey form

Item groupings and abbreviated item content for the MOS SF-36 survey

Health scale	Item	Abbreviated item content
Physical functioning (PF)	PF1	Vigorous activities, such as running, lifting heavy objects, strenuous sports
	PF2	Moderate activities, such as moving a table, vacuuming, bowling
	PF3	Lifting or carrying groceries
	PF4	Climbing several flights of stairs
	PF5	Climbing one flight of stairs
	PF6	Bending, kneeling, or stooping
	PF7	Walking more than a mile
	PF8	Walking several blocks
	PF9	Walking one block
	PF10	Bathing or dressing yourself (yes, limited a lot, yes, limited a little, no, not limited at all)
Role physical (RP)	PF1	Limited in the kind of work or other activities
	PF2	Cut down the amount of time spent on work or other activities
	PF3	Accomplished less than would like
	PF4	Difficulty performing the work or other activities (yes or no)
Bodily pain (BP)	BP1	Intensity of bodily pain (none, very mild, mild, moderate severe, very severe)
	BP2	Extent pain interfered with normal work (not at all, a little bit, moderately, quite a bit, extremely)
General health perceptions (GH)	GH1	Is your health (excellent, very good, good, fair, poor)?
	GH2	My health is excellent
	GH3	I am as healthy as anybody I know
	GH4	I seem to get sick a little easier than other people
	GH5	I expect my health to get worse (yes or no)
Vitality (VT)	VT1	Feel full of pep[a]
	VT2	Have a lot of energy
	VT3	Feel a lot of energy
	VT4	Feel tired (all the time, most of the time, a good bit of time, some of the time, none of the time)
Social functioning (SF)	SF1	Frequency health problems interfered with social activities
	SF2	Extent health problems interfered with normal social activities (yes or no)
Role emotional (RE)	RE1	Cut down the amount of time spent on work or other activities
	RE2	Accomplished less than would like
	RE3	Didn't do work or other activities as carefully as usual (yes or no)
Mental health (MH)	MH1	Been a very nervous person
	MH2	Felt downhearted and blue
	MH3	Felt so down in the dumps nothing could cheer you up
	MH4	Been a happy person
	MH5	Felt calm and peaceful (all of the time, most of the time, a good bit of time, some of the time, a little of the time, none of the time)
Reported change	TRAN	Rating of health as of now compared to 1 year ago (much better, somewhat better, same, somewhat worse, much worse)

[a]pep: energy or vitality

It is basically *a survey form filled out by the patients*, but it can also be filled out *through an interview or a phone call.*

SF-36 consists of 36 questions divided into nine domains: eight basic concepts and one domain that asks about the differences compared to 1 year ago.

The scores are usually not summed together but are calculated separately for each question, except for the last item which asks about any changes compared to 1 year ago. The score calculation is complicated and performed through a special program. It is based on the Likert method in which the scores are given in relation to the emotional factors. It can be computed more easily and converted to a total of 100 points. *Higher scores are indicative of better health conditions, better function, and less pain.*

Kiebzk et al. reported that the SF-36 physical functioning score is similar to the knee function score for TKA evaluation, and that the score was higher in males than in females. It rapidly increased during the first 3 months after the operation to reach the highest point after a year and gradually decreased thereafter due to other medical diseases or the death of the spouse.

When THA and TKA were compared, the preoperative scores were the same, but the postoperative scores were higher for THA, and the pain was particularly more severe and long lasting after TKA.

The advantages of this method are that it can rate the differences in the effects of treatment methods between the diseases in relation to the cost, *reflects the patient satisfaction well,* and helps in establishing public health policies and treatment methods. Its drawbacks are that it can give a very high score in the physical role part, but a very low score in the emotional role part. Also, it is very complex, there are some ambiguous questions which the patients cannot answer correctly, it is costly, and it is difficult to calculate the score.

Because SF-36 contains too many questixons, SF-12 consisting of only 12 questions was recently developed. SF-12 is thought to achieve the purpose of SF-36.

3.3.6 Patellofemoral Scoring System

The HSS score and the knee score are most widely used to evaluate the results of TKA, but these scoring systems are not enough to evaluate the *results associated with the patellofemoral joints.* However, the need for a patellofemoral scoring system increased so as to be able to detect the problems associated with the patellofemoral joints before and after the operation in order to suggest treatment methods and evaluate the results of the operation of the patellofemoral joint.

These include the Bristol patellar score, Bartlett patellar score, Fulkerson patellofemoral joint evaluation score, HSS patellofemoral scoring system, and Lonner patellofemoral score. These methods focus on the functions represented by anterior knee pain and climbing up and down the stairs, and physical examination has been added in some of the methods.

3.3.7 Miscellaneous Methods

3.3.7.1 Oxford Knee Score (OKS)

The Oxford Knee Score was developed to evaluate the clinical results of hip and knee surgery in 1996 and has been revised several times thereafter. It is most commonly used in the United Kingdom.

The score is designed such that *the answers are filled up by the patients*, which can be replaced by a letter. *It has an advantage in the cohort study, but it has a drawback since it consists of some questions which cannot be answered correctly.*

This system has 12 basic questions which are related to the function and how the function affects the quality of life. Each question is given 1–5 points; 1 point is the best result and 5 points is the worst result. Therefore, a score of 12 points indicates a normal function and a score of 60 points indicates the worst result. If the score is more than 24 points, it means that the patient needs close observation.

3.3.7.2 High-Activity Arthroplasty Score

It is designed *to evaluate the function of arthroplasty in physically active patients.* It may be inappropriate to use the same evaluation method for the physically active and relatively less active patients. For example, activity may be restricted in the physically active patients even though they have a good HSS score.

The High-Activity Arthroplasty Score (HAAS) consists of four items: walking (5 points), running (4 points), stair walking (3 points), and general activities (6 points). For example, five points are given if the patient can walk on an uneven road for more than 1 h. Four points are given when the patient can run for more than 5 km; 3 points are given when he or she can go two stairs up in one step; and 6 points are given when the patient can play singles tennis, perform 10 km of running, or more than 80 km of bicycling. Scores between 0 and 18 points can be given and the best score is 18 points.

However, this method is too extreme for evaluating the results of arthroplasty.

3.3.7.3 Survival Rate

The survival rate cannot be evaluated preoperatively, but I would like to describe it here as this is a very important method for evaluating the clinical results. *Survival is defined as the time elapsed till the end point.*

In arthroplasty, survival rate is the index of how long the patient can use the arthroplasty, and it is expressed as the non-revision rate in a certain period of time. The 10-year and 15-year survival rate is commonly used in TKA, and it is very helpful for evaluating the surgical techniques and implant properties. Hence, revision due to an infection is sometimes excluded because it does not have a significant relationship with the surgical technique and implant used.

The most commonly used method is the *Kaplan–Meier method*, which is calculated in relation to the follow-up period, revision rate, and life expectancy. Some surgeons state that the results of the Kaplan–Meier method are overestimated due to the calculation method in correlation with the patient's mortality.

3.3.7.4 Satisfaction Rate

This is the method to evaluate the patient's satisfaction with the operation. The operation may not be successful if the patients are not satisfied with the operation, no matter how well the operation has been done. Satisfaction rate is related to the preoperative knee condition, patient's expectations, clinical results, patient's psychological condition, age, sex, and socioeconomic status. However, *the clinical result with respect to resolution of pain is the most decisive factor*. It is known that the WOMAC score reflects the patient satisfaction quite well.

3.4 Patient Education

Patient education increases the patient satisfaction and helps to reduce perioperative anxiety and to avoid litigation through a better understanding of arthroplasty. Patient education is needed during the whole admission period. However, it is more effective when it is done preoperatively. Immediately after surgery, the patients are not fully conscious and may not pay attention to the instructions. If proper education is not imparted, the patient may feel anxious that something went wrong during the operation, even though postoperative course is not deviated.

Preoperatively, the patients should have information regarding the following: the goal of arthroplasty, postoperative progress, perioperative rehabilitation, and the possible early complications. The other informations which the patients need to know are the duration of hospitalization and the amount of transfusion needed, etc.

The patient satisfaction may decrease postoperatively due to unrealistic expectations. It must be emphasized that normal knee function may not be achieved after arthroplasty and TKA has a survival time. The goal of TKA is to enable the patient to walk without pain, go up and down the stairs, and engage in light sports or low impact sports.

To inform the postoperative progress is helpful to enhance postoperative rehabilitation. The important education of rehabilitation is the breathing exercise. Deep breathing

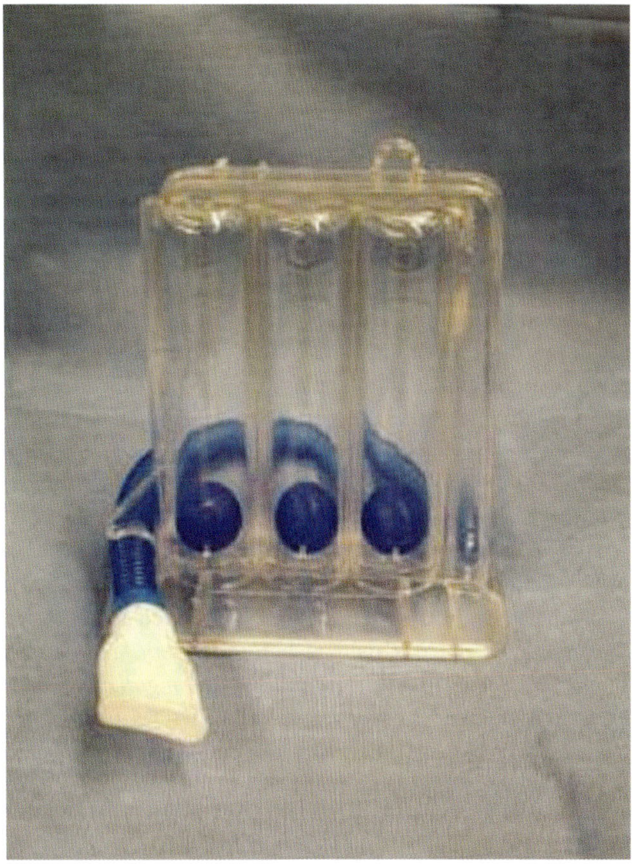

Fig. 3.3 Inspirometer

exercise can be performed using a simple device (inspirometer: Fig. 3.3). It is desirable to instruct the patients preoperatively regarding the isometric and isotonic exercises for the knee joint; lifting the legs and other exercises for increasing the quadriceps and hamstring power as well as the ROM exercises of the knee joint.

3.5 Final Checkup for the Operation

Final checkup for the operation includes seeking patients or their families consent for the operation, medical preparation, premedication for anesthesia, and surgical preparation. All the prerequisites for the operation should be fulfilled so as to ensure smooth progression of the operation.

3.5.1 Consent Form

It is mandatory to obtain consent from the patients or their families preoperatively for the purpose of legal protection. When an electronic medical record is used, it is recommended to prepare a separate written sheet. It is necessary to make a note or drawings of the risks and complications associated with the operation. It is recommended that the patients should write their name and should sign on the consent form. If necessary, a camcorder or video recording can be used for the preservation of testimony.

3.5.2 Medical Preparation

General conditions such as hypertension and diabetes mellitus should be optimized as per the instructions of the anesthesiologist. If the patients have hypertension, it is recommended that the blood pressure is controlled such that the diastolic pressure is less than 95 mmHg and a systolic pressure is less than 160 mmHg, and *the blood pressure should not be more than 180/110 mmHg at best. However, too drastic reduction in the blood pressure in a short time period can be risky for the cardiovascular and cerebrovascular system.*

Diabetes mellitus (DM) should be controlled according to the modified Alberti's method before surgery, and *fasting blood sugar level should be less than 200 mg/dl.* Marchant et al. and Bolognesi et al. reported that if DM is not controlled, the incidence of urinary infection, pneumonia, and stroke increases, and the amount of transfusion needed also increases. Hence, *"how well the blood sugar level has been controlled" is more important than "how much is the blood sugar level as of now."*

Physician consultation is desirable for appropriate perioperative management of patients with Cushing's syndrome or other endocrine disorders such as thyroid dysfunction.

Antithrombotic agents can be administered with the amount of recommended dosage according to the risk level. The cases of patients who are at a high risk of thrombotic complications should be discussed with the physicians in order to plan the preventive measures. This is further described in Chap. 8.

Sometimes, the patients show symptoms of common cold preoperatively, and it is advisable to *postpone the surgery if they have too much secretion or have high-grade fever.*

There are some controversies about *discontinuation of nonsteroidal anti-inflammatory drugs (NSAIDs) preoperatively.* The NSAIDs prolong the bleeding time by inhibition of platelet aggregation which is reversible. In general, the basic principle is to *stop the NSAIDs at least 1 week prior to the operation.* However, there were some reports suggesting that the platelet function did not decrease with continuous medication. The current trend is to give analgesics or anti-inflammatory drugs with the concept of preemptive pain control.

The general concept is to discontinue warfarin, but Rhodes et al. reported that no difference was seen in the amount of transfusion needed, incidence of wound problem, and revision rate in the cases in which warfarin administration was continued.

3.5.3 Preparation for Anesthesia

Although the type of anesthesia is finally decided by the anesthesiologist, it is recommended that, if possible, the patient should be given the opportunity to choose the method among the various anesthetic modalities. The types of anesthesia include general anesthesia, spinal anesthesia, epidural anesthesia, and peripheral nerve block. More than one type of anesthesia is used in combination sometimes to relieve the pain postoperatively.

If the patients have rheumatoid arthritis or ankylosis of multiple joints, X-rays of the cervical spine should be taken in order to check the condition of the cervical spine before intubation. Also, X-rays of the lumbar spine can be of help if spinal anesthesia is planned.

General anesthesia has a high success rate and it is also a time-saving technique, but there may be accompanying pain and nausea or vomiting postoperatively. Spinal or epidural anesthesia is associated with reduced morbidity rate, incidence of thrombosis, and pain postoperatively, but complications including hypotension due to sympathetic block, bradycardia, urinary retention, postural headache due to dural puncture, spinal hematoma, and epidural abscess have been reported.

Peripheral nerve block is a type of regional anesthesia and provides high patient satisfaction and early ambulation postoperatively. For achieving a satisfactory level of anesthesia during TKA, it is necessary to block the femoral nerve, obturator nerve, lateral femoral cutaneous nerve, and sciatic nerve, and the first three nerves can be blocked simultaneously. However, peripheral nerve block is rarely used in both the legs since there is a probability of overuse of the drugs, and it is often replaced by general anesthesia due to inadequate anesthetic effect. Sharma et al. experienced 12 cases of fall followed by 3 cases of revisions, 5 cases of femoral neuritis, and one new case of atrial fibrillation after femoral nerve block among 709 knees. They concluded that femoral nerve block is not a safe method as expected. On the other hand, Macfarlane et al. reviewed the meta-analysis of 1,538 patients from 28 literatures, and they reported no difference in the mortality and cardiovascular morbidity, and that the regional block enhances the postoperative rehabilitation compared to the general anesthesia.

It is essential to establish an IV route and insert a Foley catheter and keep at least 2 pints of blood ready preoperatively although there is not much bleeding during TKA. The anesthesiologist usually chooses the type of blood, whole blood or packed cells, to be transfused. In most of the cases, the packed cells are preferred.

Antibiotics are administered before the operation to prevent postoperative infections, and 1.0 g IV injection of the *first-generation cephalosporin 1–2 h preoperatively is recommended.*

Other preparations such as fasting or giving sedatives are the same as in the other operations.

3.5.4 Knee Joint Preparation

If the patients have a flexion contracture, it should be released preoperatively by stretching or traction as much as possible. It is recommended that the residual flexion contracture to be less than 45°. If the residual flexion contracture is greater than 45°, the patients may need to undergo a special surgical procedure or a two-stage operation.

As different implants may be needed according to the degree of deformity, instability, or bone defect, it is necessary to decide upon which prosthesis to use based on these conditions.

The angle between the anatomical and mechanical axes should be calculated on the plain A–P X-ray and the size of implants should be chosen by the scanogram, which is the X-ray with a metal ruler reflecting the magnification ratios. The templates that fit the implants are used for determination of the implant size. *Of course, the implant size measured in this manner is not always the same as the actual size of implants that need to be used, but the errors can be reduced by checking the size again during operation if there are any discrepancies.*

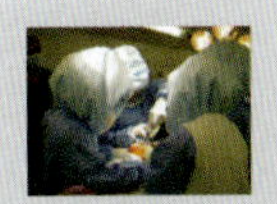

Author's Method

Mechanical and anatomical axes are generally measured on the femoral A–P X-ray preoperatively. However, I also draw a line from the end of the medial condyle to the lateral condyle, which is perpendicular to the mechanical axis of the tibia, to determine how much the lateral condyle should be resected during osteotomy. By doing so, I can prepare metal augment or allogeneic graft, and I can verify the accuracy of tibial osteotomy by comparing between an imaginary lateral resection and a real resection.

For preparation of the operation site, clean the limb thoroughly. Hair removal may be done by shaving or by using depilatory ointment. It is controversial as to whether or not shaving is beneficial. Shaving does not affect the infection rate to a great extent, and it may even increase the risk of infection if the skin is injured while shaving.

In case of a large bone defect, metal augment or allograft is prepared, and allograft tendon should be available in cases of ankylosed knee or extension lag. It is recommended to keep the antibiotics available in the operating room all the time

The knee preparation must be done consistently and uniformly. Since the surgeon cannot check everything personally regardless of the size of hospital, and it is likely that a few items may be missed out or may not be prepared properly due to the changes in the medical staff, it is desirable to prepare a preoperative checklist so as not to miss out any item and for being uniformly prepared.

Bibliography

Alicea J. Scoring systems and their validation for the arthritic knee. In: Insall JN, editor. Surgery of the knee. 3rd ed. New York, NY: Churchill Livingstone; 2001. p. 1507–15.

Alicea J. Knee scores in total knee arthroplasty. In: Scuderi GR, editor. Surgical techniques in total knee arthroplasty. 1st ed. New York, NY: Springer; 2002. p. 31–8.

Baldini A, Anderson JA, Zampetti P, et al. A new patellofemoral scoring system for total knee arthroplasty. Clin Orthop. 2006;452:150–4.

Benjamin JB. Safety and efficacy of bilateral total knee arthroplasty. J Arthroplasty. 1997;12:497–502.

Bolognesi MP, Marchant Jr MH, Viens NA, et al. The impact of diabetes on perioperative patient outcomes after total hip and total knee arthroplasty in the United States. J Arthroplasty. 2008;23:92–8.

Bould M, Freeman BJ, Pullyblank A, et al. Blood loss in sequential bilateral total knee arthroplasty. J Arthroplasty. 1998;13:77–9.

Brull R, Sharrock NE. Anesthesia for knee surgery. In: Scott WN, editor. Surgery of the knee. 4th ed. Philadelphia, PA: Churchill Livingstone; 2006. p. 1064–73.

Cho WS, Park SS, Kim DH, et al. The reliability of HSS knee rating system. J Korean Knee Society. 2000;12:43–1248.

Cohen RG, Forrest CJ, Benjamin JB. Safety and efficacy of bilateral total knee arthroplasty. J Arthroplasty. 1997;12:497–502.

Fennema P, Lubsen J. Survival analysis in total joint replacement: an alternative method of accounting for the presence of competing risk. J Bone Joint Surg Br. 2010;92-B:701–6.

Forster MC, Bauze AJ, Bailie AG, et al. A retrospective comparative study of bilateral total knee replacement staged at a one-week interval. J Bone Joint Surg Br. 2006;88-B:1006–10.

Hamilton DF, Gaston P, Simpson AH. Is patients reporting of physical function accurate. Following total knee replacement ? J Bone Joint Surg Br. 2012;94-B:1506–10.

Harato K, Nagura T, Matsumoto H, et al. Extension limitation in standing affects weight-bearing asymmetry after unilateral total knee arthroplasty. J Arthroplasty. 2010;25:225–9.

Hooper GJ, Hooper NM, Rothwell AG, et al. Bilateral total joint arthroplasty: the early results from the New Zealand National Joint Registry. J Arthroplasty. 2009;24:1174–7.

Insall JN, Dorr LD, Scott RD, et al. Rationale of the Knee Society clinical rating system. Clin Orthop. 1989;248:13–4.

Kevin JM, Todd CV, Thomas EB, et al. Scoring systems and their validation for the arthritic knee. In: Scott WN, editor. Surgery of the knee. 4th ed. Philadelphia, PA: Churchill Livingstone; 2006. p. 1295–300.

Kiebzak GM, Campbell BS, Maurerhan DR. The SF-36 general health status survey documents the burden of osteoarthritis and the benefits of total joint arthroplasty: but why should we use it ? Am J Manag Care. 2002;8:463–74.

Kim TK, Kwon SK, Kang YG, et al. Functional disabilities and satisfaction after total knee arthroplasty in female Asian patients. J Arthroplasty. 2010;25:458–64. e451-452.

Kim YH, Choi YW, Kim JS. Simultaneous bilateral sequential total knee replacement is as safe as unilateral total knee replacement. J Bone Joint Surg Br. 2009;91-B:64–8.

Kolettis GT, Wixson RL, Peruzzi WT, et al. Safety of one-stage bilateral total knee arthroplasty. Clin Orthop. 1987;309:102–9.

Kwon SK, Kang YG, Kim SJ, et al. Correlations between commonly used clinical outcome scales and patient satisfaction after total knee arthroplasty. J Arthroplasty. 2010;25:1125–30.

Lavernia C, D'Apuzzo M, Rossi MD, et al. Accuracy of knee range of motion assessment after total knee arthroplasty. J Arthroplasty. 2008;23:85–91.

Lavernia C, D'Apuzzo M, Rossi MD, et al. Is postoperative function after hip or knee arthroplasty influenced by preoperative functional levels? J Arthroplasty. 2009;24:1033–43.

Lewallen DG. Bilateral total knee arthroplasty. In: Callaghan JJ, editor. The adult knee. 1st ed. Philadelphia, PA: Lippincott Williams & Wilkins; 2003. p. 1285–9.

Likert R. A technique for the measurement of attitudes. Arch Psychol. 1932;140:1–55.

Lonner JH. Patellofemoral arthroplasty. In: Scott WN, editor. Surgery of the knee. 4th ed. Philadelphia, PA: Churchill Livingstone; 2006. p. 1440–54.

Lynch NM, Trousdale RT, Ilstrup DM. Complications after concomitant bilateral total knee arthroplasty in elderly patients. Mayo Clin Proc. 1997;72:799–805.

Macfarlane AJ, Prasad GA, Chan VW, et al. Does regional anesthesia improve outcome after total knee arthroplasty? Clin Orthop. 2009;467:2379–402.

Marchant Jr MH, Viens NA, Cook C, et al. The impact of glycemic control and diabetes mellitus on perioperative outcomes after total joint arthroplasty. J Bone Joint Surg Am. 2009;91-A:1621–9.

Morrey BF, Adams RA, Ilstrup DM, et al. Complications and mortality associated with bilateral or unilateral total knee arthroplasty. J Bone Joint Surg Am. 1987;69-A:484–8.

Murray DW, Fitzpatrick R, Rogers K, et al. The use of the Oxford hip and knee scores. J Bone Joint Surg Br. 2007;89-B:1010–4.

Ng KF, Lawmin JC, Li CC, et al. Comprehensive preoperative evaluation of platelet function in total knee arthroplasty patients taking diclofenac. J Arthroplasty. 2008;23:424–30.

Noble PC, Gordon MJ, Weiss JM, et al. Does total knee replacement restore normal knee function? Clin Orthop. 2005;431:157–65.

North American Knee Arthroplasty Revision (N.A.K.A.R.) Study Group. Predictive validity of the Knee Society Index of Severity: a prospective, multicenter cohort study. J Arthroplasty. 2004;19:322–8.

Pavone V, Johnson T, Saulog PS, et al. Perioperative morbidity in bilateral one-stage total knee replacements. Clin Orthop. 2004; 421:155–61.

Restrepo C, Parvizi J, Dietrich T, et al. Safety of simultaneous bilateral total knee arthroplasty. A meta-analysis. J Bone Joint Surg Am. 2007;89-A:1220–6.

Rhodes DA, Severson EP, Hodrick JT, et al. Discontinuation of warfarin is unnecessary in total knee arthroplasty. Clin Orthop. 2010;468:120–6.

Ritter MA, Harty LD. Debate: simultaneous bilateral knee replacements: the outcomes justify its use. Clin Orthop. 2004;428:84–6.

Rothwell AG, Hooper GJ, Hobbs A, et al. An analysis of the Oxford hip and knee scores and their relationship to early joint revision in the New Zealand Joint Registry. J Bone Joint Surg Br. 2010; 92-B:413–8.

Scott RD. Bilateral simultaneous total knee arthroplasty. In: Scott RD, editor. Total knee arthroplasty. 1st ed. Philadelphia, PA: Saunders; 2006. p. 100–2.

Sharma S, Iorio R, Specht LM, et al. Complications of femoral nerve block for total knee arthroplasty. Clin Orthop. 2010;468: 135–40.

Sliva CD, Callaghan JJ, Goetz DD, et al. Staged bilateral total knee arthroplasty performed four to seven days apart during a single hospitalization. J Bone Joint Surg Am. 2005;87-A:508–13.

Soudry MA, Binazzi R, Insall JN, et al. Successive bilateral total knee replacement. J Bone Joint Surg Am. 1985;67-A:573–6.

Talbot S, Hooper G, Stokes A, et al. Use of a new high-activity arthroplasty score to assess function of young patients with total hip or knee arthroplasty. J Arthroplasty. 2010;25:268–73.

Yoon HS, Han CD, Yang IH. Comparison of simultaneous bilateral and staged bilateral total knee arthroplasty in terms of perioperative complications. J Arthroplasty. 2010;25:179–85.

Vince KG. Bilateral total knee arthroplasty under one anesthesia: a safe protocol. Mayo Clin Proc. 1997;72:883–5.

Ware JE, Sherbourne CD. The MOS 36-item short form health survey (SF-36). I. Conceptual framework and item selection. Med Care. 1992;30:473–83.

4 Surgical Techniques

The surgical techniques of TKA demand probably the highest degree of precision. Achieving the primary purpose of TKA, which is pain relief and restoration of function with minimal complications, depends on whether or not the operation has been performed properly, and these surgical factors also affect the long-term survival of TKA.

For a successful operation, the surgeon should be able to perform the surgical techniques appropriately based on the knowledge of anatomy and biomechanics of the knee joint. The surgeon should be experienced and he/she is also required to have an understanding of the implants to be used. Also, there should be good teamwork among the attending medical staff and the surgical environment should also be favorable.

Since the operation comprises of successive steps which are interrelated, it cannot be divided into separate procedures. But I would like to describe the successive steps here by dividing them into: drape, surgical approach, soft tissue procedure, osteotomy and bone preparation, balancing, fixation, closure, and miscellaneous techniques.

4.1 Drape

Drape is the first step to preventing surgical infection. Tourniquet should be applied as proximal as possible so that it does not slip down and the limb should be cleaned up to the toes with Betadine and alcohol. After drying, the ankle and toes are wrapped lightly with rubber gloves twice so as to allow the detection of landmarks around the ankle joint easily (Fig. 4.1). The drape should not interfere with the knee joint motion, and the topographical landmark on the hip joint should be detectable easily in case of a special situation. A sufficient amount of adhesive surgidrape is used so that the skin is not exposed at all. Alternatively, a commercially available surgical drape can be used. The operation table should be covered with a waterproof sheet. C-arm compatible operation table should be available for revision cases.

Since the knee has a tendency to rotate externally, the operation table is tilted so that the knee to be operated faces towards the ceiling.

Everyone who attends the operation should wear *double gloves* to prevent contamination and to protect themselves. Also, protective goggles or body exhaust suit is necessary when operating on the patients who have infectious disease.

The Esmarch bandage or elastic bandage is used to exsanguinate the limb to be operated upon, and a tourniquet pressure of up to 300–350 mmHg is applied. Theoretically, a tourniquet pressure which is either 100 mmHg greater than the systolic pressure or twice that of the systolic pressure is enough. But, *in patients with obesity and bigger skeleton, a lot of bleeding from the cancellous bones and the medullary canal can occur with a tourniquet pressure that is less than 300 mmHg*.

It is safe to release and reinflate the tourniquet if the operation lasts more than 90 min. The use of tourniquet contributes to provide a better operation field which enables the surgeon to perform the operation more accurately, to reduce the operation time and bleeding, and to achieve better durable cement fixation. However, Wakankar et al. reported that the operation time was not prolonged, the bleeding did not increase, and the incidences of postoperative pain, superficial infection, and deep vein thrombosis were reduced in cases in which a tourniquet was not used.

The drawbacks of tourniquet inflation are that it increases the cardiovascular blood flow to cause cardiovascular overloading with transient increase in blood pressure and may cause pulmonary edema or cardiac failure when the tourniquet is released. Other drawback is that it may provoke ischemic condition in the limb to be operated. Therefore, *caution should be paid when using a tourniquet in the patients who have cardiovascular diseases or peripheral vascular problems*.

4.2 Surgical Approach

The surgical approach is the first step to an operation, and it is very important as an inappropriate surgical approach makes the subsequent procedures inaccurate and difficult to

W. Cho, *Knee Joint Arthroplasty*,
DOI 10.1007/978-3-642-39389-1_4,

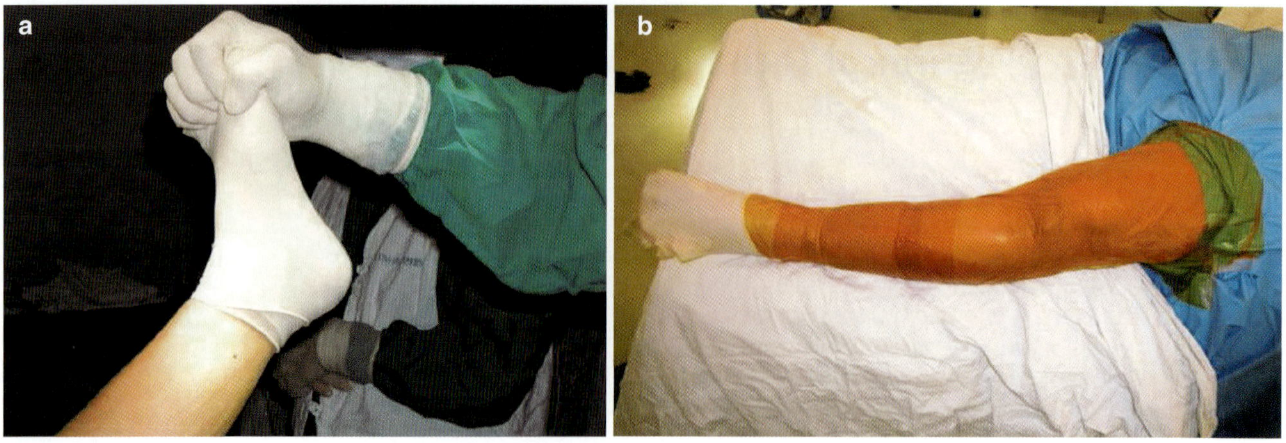

Fig. 4.1 (a) Drape on the foot and ankle, (b) after full drape

perform, and a longer operation time is required, which influences the results of the operation significantly.

A poor surgical approach can cause skin and deep tissue necrosis in patients with a severe deformity, history of previous knee operation, or poor skin conditions. If any skin and soft tissue problem develops, the recovery is delayed and the prognosis becomes poor. *A good surgical approach should provide adequate exposure, protect the important tissues such as vessels and nerves, preserve the function of TKA as much as possible, and provide convenience and reproducibility.*

Minimally invasive surgery reduces the length of the skin incision and arthrotomy. This is further described in Chap. 10.

The anterior approach is adopted in TKA because all the important nerves and vessels are located posteriorly. In practice, the skin incision, arthrotomy, and other ancillary procedures such as the treatment of the extensor mechanism are performed independently to each other. However, most of the literature suggest as if one skin incision belongs to one arthrotomy. I would like to describe these approaches in three separate categories: skin incision, arthrotomy, and ancillary procedures to the extensor mechanism.

4.2.1 Skin Incision

Skin incision should be determined based on the subsequent exposure, extensibility, cosmesis, and wound healing.

4.2.1.1 Neurovascular Anatomy

Blood Supply

Skin incision for TKA should be done precisely to achieve good wound healing. In order to do so, it is important to know the vascular supply. *The blood supply comprises of the extrinsic arteries from the outside of the knee joint and the intrinsic arteries that form a ring around the patella.* The extrinsic arteries exist in the subcutaneous layer and include

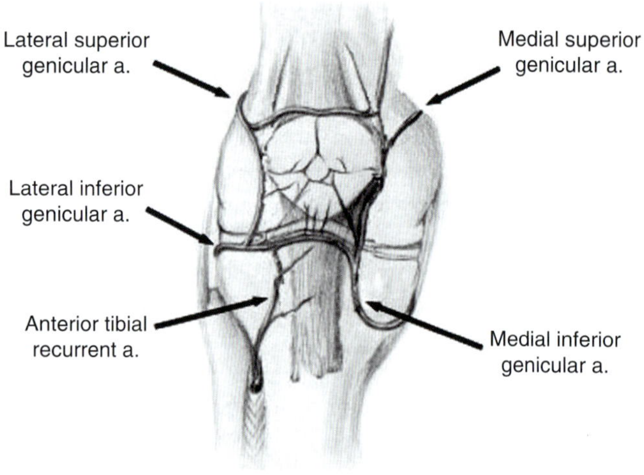

Fig. 4.2 Intrinsic arteries around the knee joint

the saphenous artery, the descending genicular artery, and the muscular branches coming from the medial side. The intrinsic arteries exist in the subfascial layer and comprise of the medial superior genicular, the medial inferior genicular, the lateral superior genicular, the lateral inferior genicular, and the anterior tibial recurrent arteries, which together form a ring around the patella (Fig. 4.2). The extrinsic arteries mostly impact the wound healing. *The vessels in the superficial layer anastomose with the deep-seated intrinsic arteries through the perforating arteries, rather than anastomosing with each other.*

Due to this pattern of the vascular supply, when the skin incision is made more medially, more vascular disruption occurs on the lateral side. Too much dissection of the deep fascia compromises the perforating arteries to cause a wound healing problem (Fig. 4.3). Therefore, *making the skin incision too far medially and too much subcutaneous dissection on the lateral side of the incision should be avoided* (Fig. 4.3).

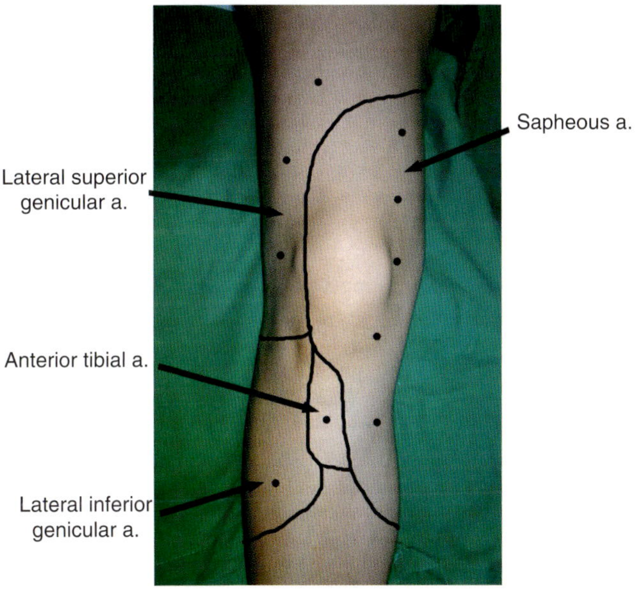

Fig. 4.3 Schematic drawing of the point where perforating arteries appear to the superficial layer from deep arteries

Nerve Innervation

In the anterior part of the thigh, the medial and intermediate cutaneous nerve of the thigh runs from the medial to the lateral side and innervates the anterior area of the thigh. On the tibial side, the infrapatellar branch of the saphenous nerve runs from the medial to the lateral side. If the skin incision is extended too proximally, the nerves of the thigh that are mentioned above are most likely to get injured. The injury to the branch of the saphenous nerve is inevitable.

4.2.1.2 Principles of Skin Incision

If a wound healing problem develops during the postoperative period of TKA, it increases the risk of deep infection as the knee joint is close to the skin and it affects the rehabilitation program resulting in a poor prognosis. Hence it is necessary to keep certain principles of skin incision.

The method of skin incision differs between the ordinary patients, patients with history of knee surgeries, and patients with a severe deformity. The skin incision in the elderly patients should be long enough so as to reduce the skin tension during retraction. *The end of the incision should not be U-shaped but V-shaped on retraction.* The recently introduced minimally invasive surgery should be applied to patients with no major skin problems.

The skin incision is made vertically in TKA. In the patients with history of previous knee operation, the arthroscopy portal scar may be ignored, and a transverse incision scar may not cause problems if the new incision is made perpendicular to the old scar. If the scar is small, it is recommended that the new incision should meet the old scar at an obtuse angle. If the scar is long, it is recommended to follow the existing scar as far as possible. If making an incision along the previous scar seems to compromise the operative field, *a new incision can be made lateral to the existing scar. However, the distance between the new incision and the existing scar should be at least 7 cm apart.* If the wound healing is doubtful with the above methods, sham incision can be considered.

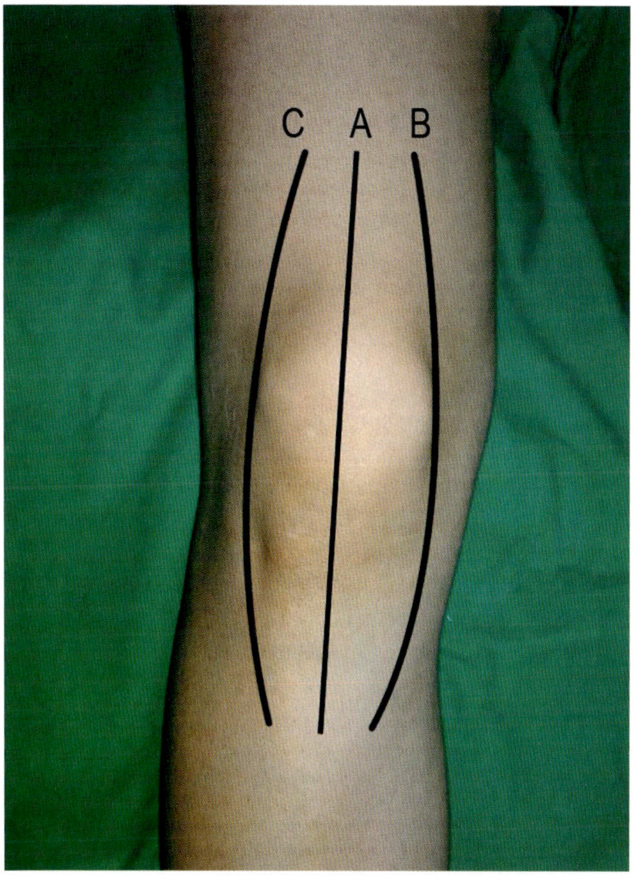

Fig. 4.4 Skin incision. A: midline, B: paramedial, C: lateral

If the skin has poor elasticity due to the previous surgery, it is also possible to expand the skin using a tissue expander.

4.2.1.3 Methods of Skin Incision

There are three methods of making a skin incision, and the infrapatellar branch of the saphenous nerve is cut in every method (Fig. 4.4).

Midline Incision

In this method, a straight incision about 12–14 cm long is made at the center of the knee joint. The proximal incision starts from 4 to 5 cm proximal to the patella and the distal incision ends at about 1 cm medial to the tibial tuberosity. A too short distal incision is to be avoided as the skin is thin and vascularity is poor in this area. When the incision is made directly over the tibial tuberosity, it can cause problems related to wound healing and pain. If the incision ends lateral to the tibial tuberosity, Yacoubian and Scott stated that it has an advantage of reducing tension on the incision scar when the tibia is internally rotated or during kneeling.

This is the most widely used incision because it can ensure a better blood supply than that provided by the paramedial incision, it is possible to perform any arthrotomy through this skin incision, it can be easily extended proximally and distally, and it can be used in revision cases.

Paramedial Incision

This is a curved incision with its center located on the medial side of the patella and its proximal and distal ends are just the same as or a little medial to those of the midline incision. It has been widely used in the past, but it often causes skin problems on the lateral side due to excessive subcutaneous dissection over the patella when the curve is too acute. Also, this incision may be difficult to use in revision TKA. Therefore, it is only used in exceptional cases.

Lateral Incision

In this type of incision, the center of the incision is located on the lateral side of the patella. This incision preserves more blood supply, but it provides poor exposure because arthrotomy also needs to be performed on the lateral side. Besides, this incision can cause orientation problems to the surgeons who are accustomed to the usual midline incision. Hence, this *incision is used exceptionally for TKA in the patients with valgus deformity*.

4.2.2 Arthrotomy

While performing an arthrotomy, it is important to know the distribution of blood supply around the patella. This is because various arthrotomy methods differ according to the blood supply. An anastomosis of six intrinsic arteries forms a ring around the patella. The relationship between each type of arthrotomy and arterial supply is shown in Fig. 4.5.

The arthrotomy methods include the paramedial, subvastus, midvastus, and medial trivector-retaining arthrotomy for the medial side and lateral arthrotomy for the lateral side (Fig. 4.6).

4.2.2.1 Paramedial Arthrotomy (Fig. 4.7a)

As it provides good exposure and allows for proximal extension, the paramedial arthrotomy is the most commonly used arthrotomy.

The quadriceps tendon can be incised longitudinally in the center, at the medial one-third or at the medial musculocutaneous junction. However, the quadriceps tendon is usually incised at the medial one-third because it is associated with less bleeding, less fibrosis, and less difficulty in suturing

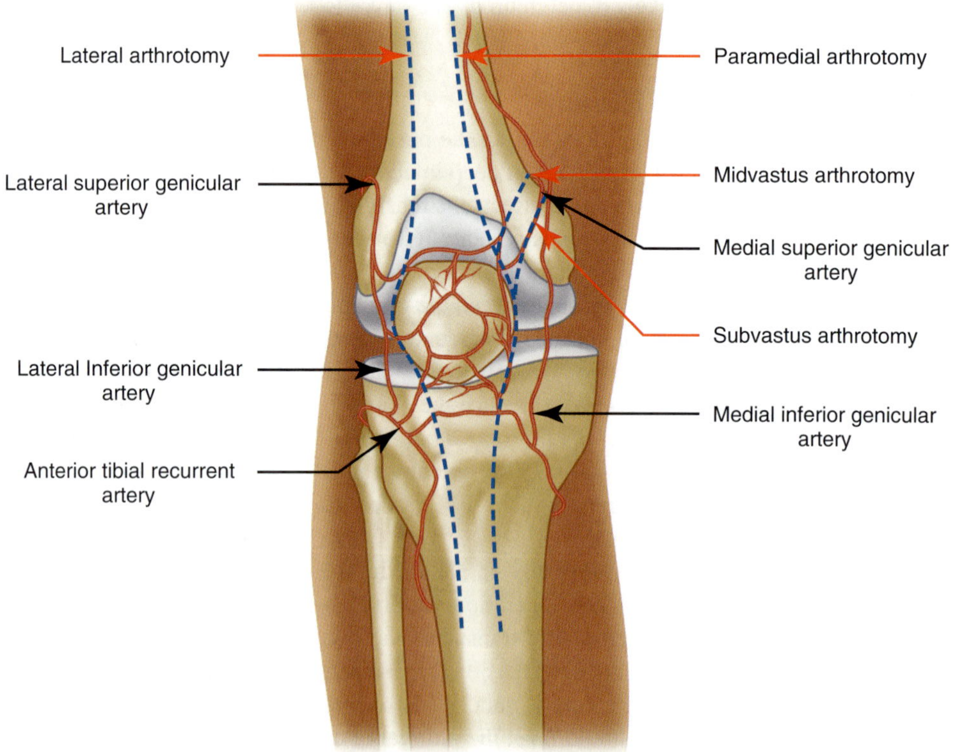

Fig. 4.5 Relationship between the arteries around the patella and arthrotomy

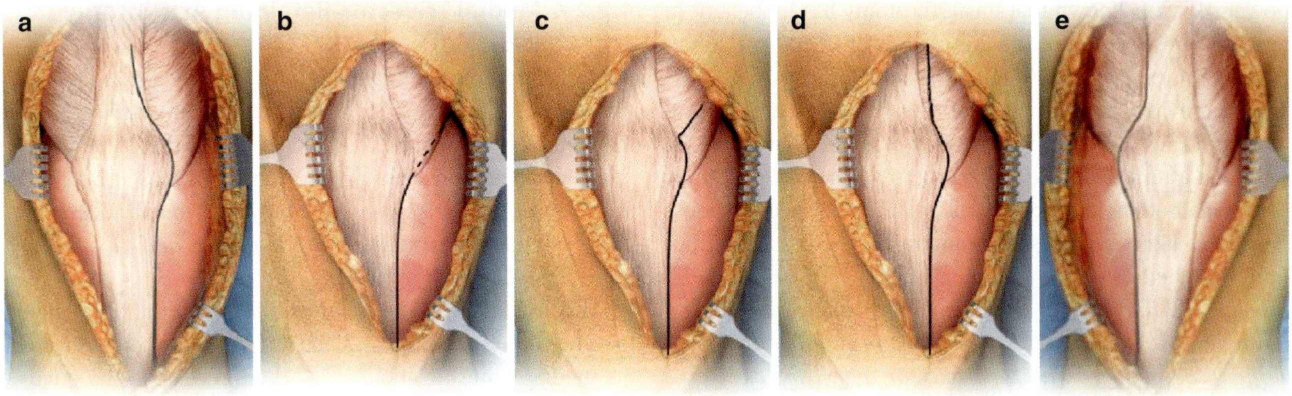

Fig. 4.6 Various arthrotomies. (**a**) Paramedial, (**b**) subvastus, (**c**) midvastus, (**d**) medial trivector, (**e**) lateral

Fig. 4.7 Paramedial arthrotomy, (**a**) Insall method, (**b**) standard method

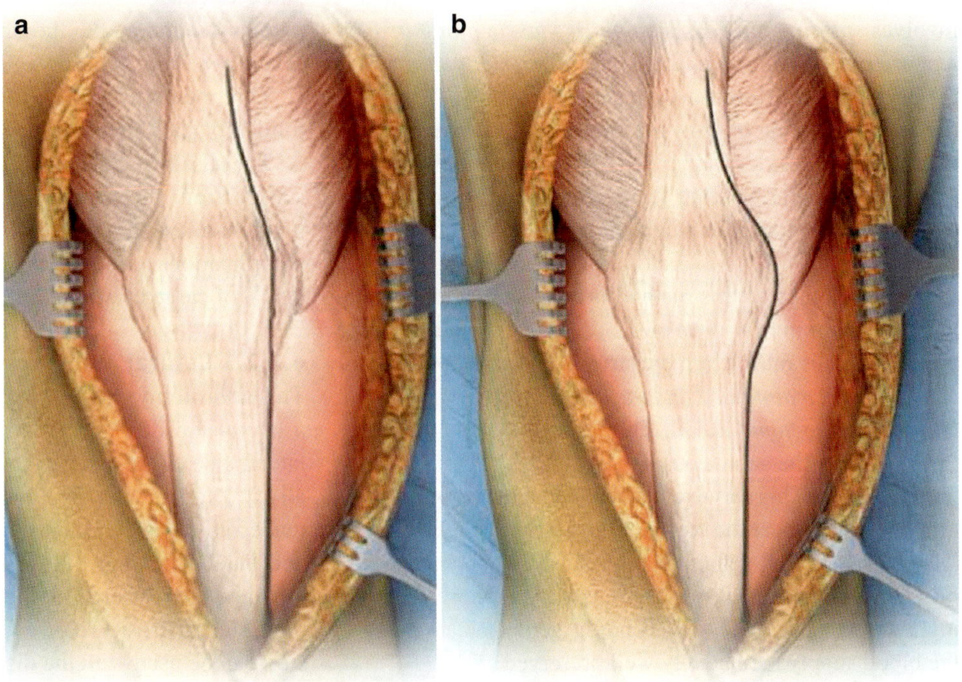

compared to that with the incision through the muscle. In fact, the width of the quadriceps tendon differs in each patient and the incision can be placed at the center or on the sides during arthrotomy according to the width of the tendon.

In the patellar area, Insall recommended peeling off a part of the anterior longitudinal fiber in order to prevent cutting of the longitudinal fibers of the extensor mechanism. But many surgeons prefer cutting at 5 mm medial to the patella because it takes less time and is easier to suture (Fig. 4.7). In the tibial portion, incision should be placed far medial to the tibial tuberosity in order to protect the patellar tendon.

The drawbacks of this arthrotomy are that when the quadriceps tendon is incised, it can cause weakening of the extensor mechanism postoperatively and it disrupts all the blood vessels on the medial side.

4.2.2.2 Subvastus Arthrotomy (Fig. 4.6b)

Subvastus arthrotomy involves *blunt oblique dissection beneath the vastus medialis muscle starting from the superomedial part of the patella extending proximally up to the intermuscular septum* which is located at about 10 cm proximal to the adductor tubercle, and the medial joint capsule is incised distally to form an L shape. Mostly the patella is not everted but is retracted laterally.

The advantages of this method are that the extensor mechanism is not incised, and the supreme genicular artery on the medial side of the patella is preserved. The arthrotomy method in which the quadriceps tendon is cut causes weakening of the muscle strength and increases the incidence of lateral subluxation of the patella. When the patella is not everted, it is also helpful for early restoration of muscle power. But it is known that this arthrotomy has no benefit in terms of preservation of the muscle power in comparison to the other arthrotomies at the long-term follow-up.

The drawbacks of this arthrotomy are inadequate surgical exposure and increased postoperative pain in comparison with that after the midvastus arthrotomy. The complications of this method include hematoma in the vastus medialis muscle and weakness of muscle strength when excessive retraction is applied.

This arthrotomy is not recommended in obese patients, muscular patients, patients with a history of previous knee surgery, or patients with deformity or ankylosis, as it provides poor surgical exposure in these cases.

4.2.2.3 Midvastus Arthrotomy (Fig. 4.6c)

This arthrotomy has been developed by Engh, and it involves *splitting the vastus medialis muscle along its center starting 4–5 cm proximal to the superomedial portion of the patella*. The arthrotomy is extended distally by incising the insertion area of this muscle to the patella and the medial joint capsule. Distal incision is located either on the medial side of the patellar tendon or on the medial 1/4 of the patellar tendon. The patella can be everted or retracted laterally.

The advantage of this method is that the quadriceps tendon in the proximal portion of the patella and one-half of the vastus medialis muscle are preserved. Thereby, *the extensor mechanism is maintained and the blood supply to the patella is preserved to some extent*. The vastus medialis muscle is innervated by the saphenous nerve which is a branch of the femoral nerve. This nerve remains undamaged in this arthrotomy as it enters near the origin of the vastus medialis muscle. Also, the superior genicular artery has two branches and proximal one of them is preserved as it anastomoses with the highest genicular artery (descending genicular artery). So, the blood supply is relatively well preserved.

This arthrotomy allows for full retraction or eversion of the patella and can be extended to a rectus snip. Engh states that *this arthrotomy can be utilized in obese patients, patients with severe deformity, or in revision cases in which this arthrotomy had been done previously*, provided the knee can be bent more than 90°.

However, there are reports that this approach has problems of poor orientation of surgical field, bleeding, and decrease of muscle power. White et al. reported that the incidence of lateral retinacular release was lower with this arthrotomy than the paramedial arthrotomy, and benefits of this arthrotomy were seen for the first postoperative 6 months in terms of postoperative pain and leg elevation, which became similar to those with the paramedial arthrotomy thereafter. Meanwhile, Keating et al. reported that there was no difference in the prognosis between the midvastus arthrotomy and the paramedial arthrotomy.

4.2.2.4 Medial Trivector-Retaining Arthrotomy (Fig. 4.6d)

The most common complication of TKA is abnormal patellar tracking. The theoretical background of this arthrotomy is that most of the maltracking occurs due to the imbalance of the quadriceps muscles. *If the incision passes through the center of the quadriceps vector, the forces that naturally stabilize the quadriceps tendon are balanced and this helps to normalize the patellar tracking.*

This method was designed by Bramlett et al. who stated that the center of the quadriceps muscle vector is on the vastus medialis muscle about 1.5–2.0 cm medial to the quadriceps tendon.

In this arthrotomy, the *vastus medialis muscle is vertically incised about 1.5–2.0 cm medial to the quadriceps tendon*, and the incision is extended distally to 1 cm medial to the patellar tendon and to the tibial tuberosity in order to *maintain the intrinsic stability of the vastus medialis muscle*.

This method resembles the paramedial arthrotomy anatomically and the midvastus arthrotomy biomechanically.

The disadvantages of this arthrotomy are that the blood supply from the medial side is interrupted and the vastus medialis muscle is incised. Bramlett et al. reported that the complications of the extensor mechanism were found only in 0.5 % of cases in which this arthrotomy was used.

4.2.2.5 Lateral Arthrotomy (Fig. 4.6e)

This arthrotomy was first introduced by Keblish and involves a lateral incision on the skin and opening the joint on the lateral side of the patella. This arthrotomy is used exceptionally in patients with a valgus deformity. The skin incision is made on the lateral side of the quadriceps tendon, patella, and patellar tendon following the *Q* angle and ends at the medial edge of Gerdy's tubercle, which is 1–2 cm lateral to the tibial tuberosity. However, a standard midline skin incision can be used with the distal incision ending at the lateral side of the tibial tuberosity.

Keblish's lateral approach comprises of six steps from making a skin incision to the closure including soft tissue balancing according to the degree of deformity. This is because the knee joint cannot be visualized only with the lateral arthrotomy in patients with a valgus deformity, and tissue necrosis can be reduced when soft tissue management is performed in conjunction with the arthrotomy. When the paramedial arthrotomy is done in patients with a valgus deformity, it may aggravate the existing external rotation deformity of the tibia, cause problems in patellar tracking, and increase the risk of peroneal nerve injury or infection. Approaching the lateral structures in valgus deformity is difficult with the use of paramedial arthrotomy and requires an additional release of the lateral retinacular ligament, which increases the risk of circulatory disturbance from both the medial and lateral sides during the operation. *The first step is to release the iliotibial band (ITB)*, because ITB is the main structure that causes the valgus and external rotation deformity of the tibia. *The second step is arthrotomy with Z-plasty of the lateral retinacular ligament in the coronal plane.* In patients with a valgus deformity, it is possible to perform coronal Z-plasty due to hypertrophy of the lateral retinacular ligament. *The third step is to dislocate the patella. The fourth step is to release the soft tissues on the lateral side of the tibia from Gerdy's tubercle. The fifth step is to release the lateral collateral ligament, popliteus tendon, and posterolateral capsule. The sixth step is to close the wound.*

The advantages of this arthrotomy are that it allows the deformed site to be approached directly, it helps in better preservation of the blood supply, and it allows for natural release of the lateral retinacular ligament during arthrotomy. Its other advantages are that it reduces skin dissection which results in lesser skin problems and *allows for gradual release of the soft tissues.*

Its drawbacks are that it does not provide a good operation field on the medial side, makes eversion of the patella difficult, and is associated with the problem of disorientation for the surgeons who are accustomed to the medial approach, and the soft tissue defects on the lateral side cannot be repaired. In other words, it is a *good method for correcting a valgus deformity* and for releasing the contracture of soft tissues on the lateral side naturally, but *it may cause more problems when performed by the inexperienced surgeons.*

Buechel proposed three steps of lateral arthrotomy according to the degree of valgus deformity. This is described in Sect. 5.2.1.2.

4.2.3 Ancillary Procedures

Ancillary procedures are performed when sufficient surgical exposure is not possible due to severe deformity or ankylosis in primary TKA, and when the desired range of motion (ROM) cannot be achieved due to quadriceps contracture, or sufficient surgical exposure is difficult in cases of revision TKA.

When eversion or retraction of the patella is not possible, the first step is to extend the incision proximally followed by cutting the lateral patellofemoral ligament (Fig. 4.8) and the lateral joint capsule, or releasing the lateral retinacular ligament in advance.

If the patella cannot be everted or adequately retracted laterally despite of the above methods or injury to any portion of the extensor mechanism is likely, ancillary measures to the extensor mechanism are needed. Alternatively, ancillary procedures may be performed right from the beginning in difficult cases.

The methods of managing the extensor mechanism include rectus snip, multiple puncture, Z-plasty or V–Y quadricepsplasty, and tibial tubercle osteotomy. Comparing the three ancillary methods to the extensor mechanism, the rectus snip is the modest technique with good results and lower morbidity, and hence it is recommended in most of the cases. While comparing between tibial tubercle osteotomy and quadriceps turndown, Barrack et al. reported that quadriceps turndown offers a better range of motion and has a higher patient satisfaction. Whereas with *tibial tubercle osteotomy*, although the muscle power is preserved, *it makes kneeling difficult and is followed by pain which makes many of the patients feel that the operation has failed.*

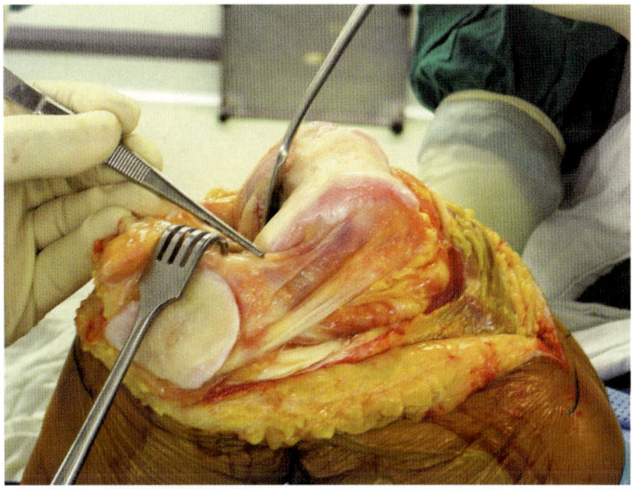

Fig. 4.8 Release of the patellofemoral ligament

Subperiosteal peel is a method of extensive medial release in case severe medial contracture is noted.

4.2.3.1 Rectus Snip (Fig. 4.9)

Rectus snip includes cutting (snipping) the rectus femoris muscle at the musculotendinous junction. This method was developed by Coonse and Adams and was modified by Insall.

The benefit of this method is that it is *simple, the integrity of the vastus medialis muscle is maintained, and the superolateral genicular artery is preserved.* So, extension lag rarely occurs postoperatively. *This is the modest and the most conservative ancillary method to manage the extensor mechanism in revision and ankylosed knee.*

The quadriceps tendon is cut superolaterally at an angle of 45° from the proximal end of the medial arthrotomy (Fig. 4.10). But it may be extended inferolaterally according to the level of the medial incision or may be extended superomedially from the lateral side in the lateral arthrotomy.

If a rectus snip is not enough for adequate exposure, the cut can be extended distally to the lateral side, and this makes the arthrotomy similar to the quadriceps turndown technique except for the shape and level of proximal apex. Lateral retinacular release is sometimes performed along with a rectus snip to preserve the superolateral genicular artery.

After rectus snip, immobilization in the extended position is required for 3 weeks postoperatively.

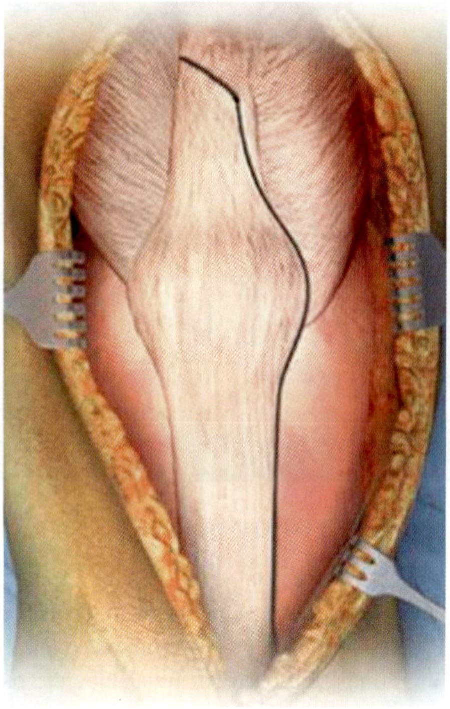

Fig. 4.9 Rectus snip

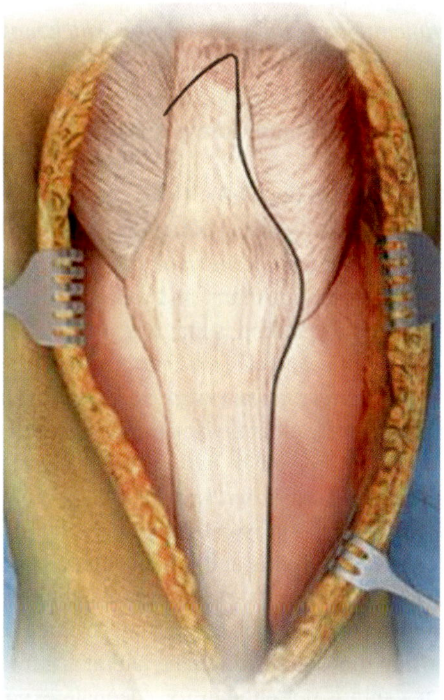

Fig. 4.10 Modified rectus snip

4.2.3.2 V–Y Quadricepsplasty (Quadriceps Turndown; Fig. 4.11) and Z-Plasty

V–Y quadricepsplasty was developed by Coonse and Adams and it also allows for elongation of the extensor mechanism. This method can be modified into various types based on the shape of the incision over the quadriceps tendon. The Z-plasty is another form of quadriceps turndown which is performed to lengthen the quadriceps tendon. The patella can be turned down after Z-plasty. Both the V–Y and Z-plasty ensure good exposure, but the V–Y is more recommended because it elongates the tendon more gradually.

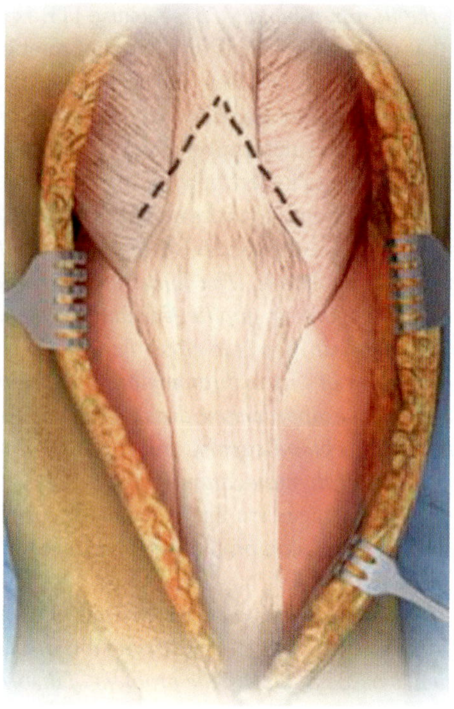

Fig. 4.11 V–Y quadricepsplasty

V–Y quadricepsplasty has been used when eversion of the patella is not possible after a rectus snip, the range of flexion is less than 60°, or the overall arc of motion is only 30–40°.

The drawbacks of V–Y quadricepsplasty are that the blood supply to the patella is disrupted, thereby increasing the incidence of avascular necrosis of the patella, and the strength of quadriceps muscle is inevitably weakened or an extension lag develops.

Therefore, too much elongation of the extensor mechanism is not recommended, and meticulous suturing together with allograft augmentation may be needed.

During postoperative care, ROM exercises should be restricted for about 6–8 weeks.

4.2.3.3 Tibial Tubercle Osteotomy (Fig. 4.12)

This method was originally developed by Dolin, but the method that is being used as of now has been modified by Whiteside.

It is useful for patients with severe contracture of the quadriceps tendon or fibrotic ankylosis. *The benefits of this method are that it can provide a good exposure, the position of the tibial tubercle can be adjusted, and it can be used to remove the tibial component during revision surgery*. Also, it allows for early rehabilitation and maintains the strength of the quadriceps muscle as a result of bone-to-bone healing.

The *drawbacks* of this method are *the possible complications, such as postoperative pain, nonunion of the osteotomy site, fragment fracture, patellar tendon rupture, infection*, and it is a time-consuming method.

The bony fragment should be about 3 in. in length, 2 cm in width, and 1 cm in thickness on the thicker side. The distal part may be gradually beveled to reduce the incidence of tibial fracture.

During osteotomy, it is important to preserve the blood supply by not detaching the periosteum from the bone on the lateral side. If screws are used for fixation, fracture of bony fragments may develop, so it is recommended to use wires. Three wires are used most of the times and wire holes may be drilled for fixation before performing the osteotomy. The topmost wire may pass through the bony fragment to prevent slipping, and the two lower wires are fastened from the outer side for application of a compressive force. Postoperative care is not different from that after the usual TKA.

4.2.3.4 Subperiosteal Peel (Fig. 4.13)

The soft tissue envelope is peeled off from the distal femur in the form of continuous sleeve along with the origin of medial collateral ligaments and is retracted posteriorly, allowing the distal femur to be buttonholed.

This exposure was first described by Windor and Insall. Combined with the medial subperiosteal dissection of the proximal tibia, this method allows the knee to be flexed

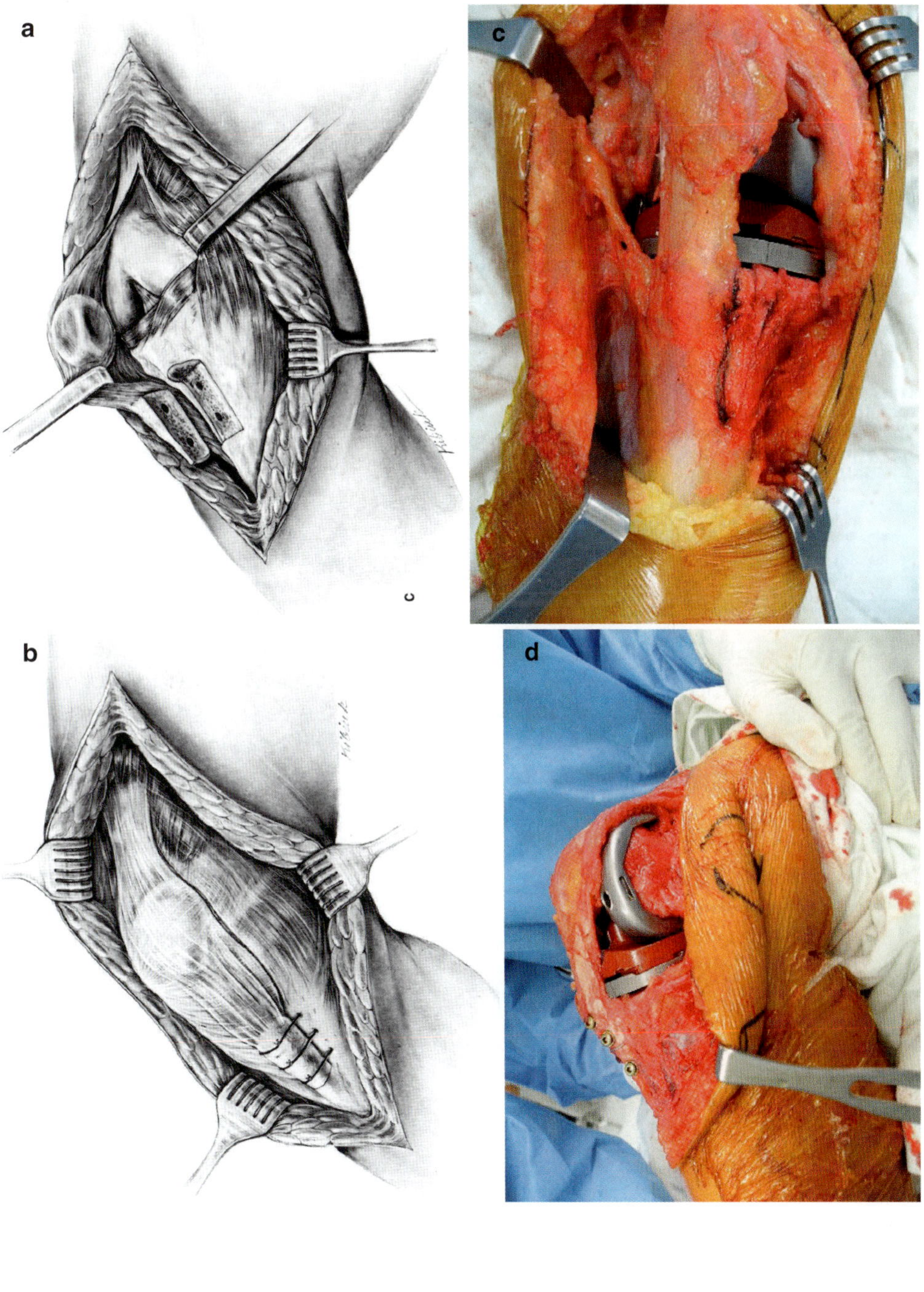

Fig. 4.12 Frontal and lateral views of tibial tubercle osteotomy. *Left schematic drawings* of wiring method (**a**, **b**) and *right photographs* show screw fixation method. (**c**) Osteotomy, (**d**) after fixation, (**e**) postoperative X-ray

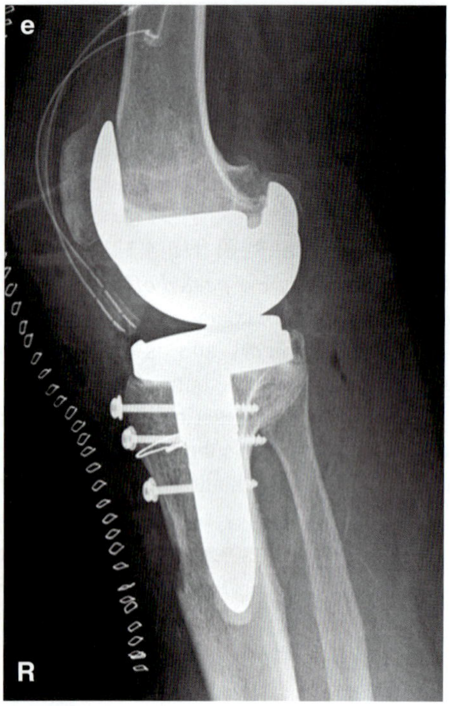

Fig. 4.12 (continued)

without the danger of damage or injury to the important soft tissue structures. The technique is useful for long-standing ankylosis of the knee joint, for reimplantation after infection, and in other difficult cases. *The risk associated with extensive subperiosteal peel is devascularization with subsequent osteonecrosis* of the condyle. As such, *extensive subperiosteal release should be reserved for only the most extreme cases.*

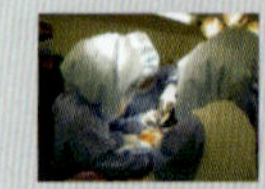

Author's Method

With respect to the surgical approach, I usually use the midline skin incision and paramedial arthrotomy. They are simple to perform, provide a good exposure, have reproducibility, and do not cause serious problems even with lateral retinacular release. Therefore, they are suitable for most of the TKAs. I do not hesitate to extend the distal skin incision to minimize skin tension during the operation.

Paramedial arthrotomy is performed not by using the straight Insall's arthrotomy, but by using a curved incision which is located 5 mm away from the medial border of the patella. The lateral patellofemoral ligament is incised when it is too tight during patellar eversion. If the patella cannot be everted, I perform lateral retraction of the patella or release of the lateral retinacular ligament in advance.

Forceful eversion of the patella may cause the patellar tendon to be stripped off from the tibial tubercle, or rupture of the patellar, or quadriceps tendon, or fracture of the patella may develop. This tends to happen more often in patients with advanced rheumatoid arthritis or severe osteopenia. I use pins, miniplate, or special instruments in these patients to prevent stripping off of the patellar tendon.

I have experienced some inconveniences while performing subvastus arthrotomy.

In patients with a valgus deformity, I have tried the lateral approach, but have experienced difficulties because I was not familiar with this approach. I perform the ordinary paramedial arthrotomy even in severe valgus deformity.

Among the ancillary methods, I believe that the rectus snip is the most recommended method. In case of V–Y turndown, the quadriceps tendon was weakened to a great extent. Even in cases when I reinforced the tendon with a tendon allograft, an extension lag or extensor weakness developed. When I did tibial tubercle osteotomy, the operation became more complicated and more time consuming, and the patients were not very satisfied.

4.3 Soft Tissue Procedure

4.3.1 Cruciate Ligament Treatment

Even though the posterior cruciate-retaining (CR) type is intended to be used initially, the posterior-substituting (PS) type should be used when the posterior cruciate ligament (PCL) shows severe degenerative changes or looks abnormally thin. If the PCL is tight, a recession can be considered after the insertion of trial implants.

If the PS type is used, the *posterior cruciate ligament may be removed at any time*, but it is generally removed during tibial osteotomy or before femoral notch cutting. However *with the use of a mobile-bearing joint, the PCL should be removed after tibial osteotomy and before starting femoral osteotomy for proper gap balancing*. Since the middle genicular artery is cut during resection of the posterior cruciate ligament, it is recommended to coagulate the bleeding focus immediately.

4.3.2 Meniscectomy

The medial meniscus is so firmly attached to the deep medial collateral ligament that the boundary between the two is not clear to the naked eye. Excessive resection of the medial meniscus can weaken the deep medial

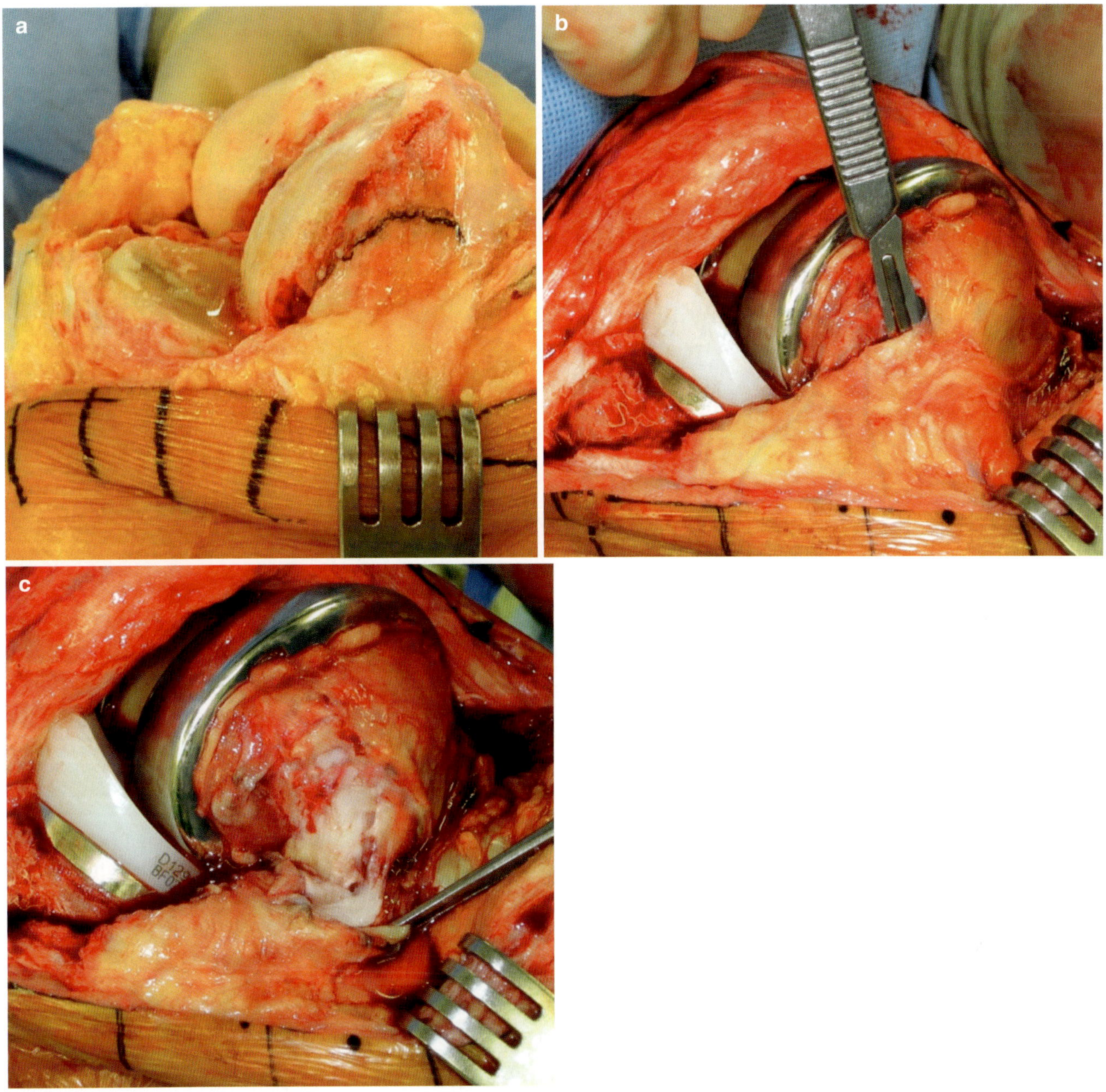

Fig. 4.13 Subperiosteal peel. (**a**) Planning, (**b**) subperiosteal peel, (**c**) after peel

collateral ligament and too little resection hinders the performance of the surgical procedure and causes impingement.

The lateral meniscus can cause impingement when it is resected to a lesser extent, and the *lateral inferior genicular artery* can be injured thereby increasing the bleeding when more amount of lateral meniscus is resected. Since *this artery runs around the boundary of the lateral meniscus, it can be cut longitudinally. Hence, cauterization of every bleeding point should be done immediately after the lateral meniscectomy* (Fig. 4.14).

If the joint space is too narrow for performing lateral meniscectomy, preliminary medial release can be performed in advance in order to make performance of the lateral meniscectomy a little easier.

4.3.3 Soft Tissue Release

Mediolateral balance should be achieved through *soft tissue release on the tibial side if there is a varus deformity or on the femoral side if there is a valgus deformity.* The reason for

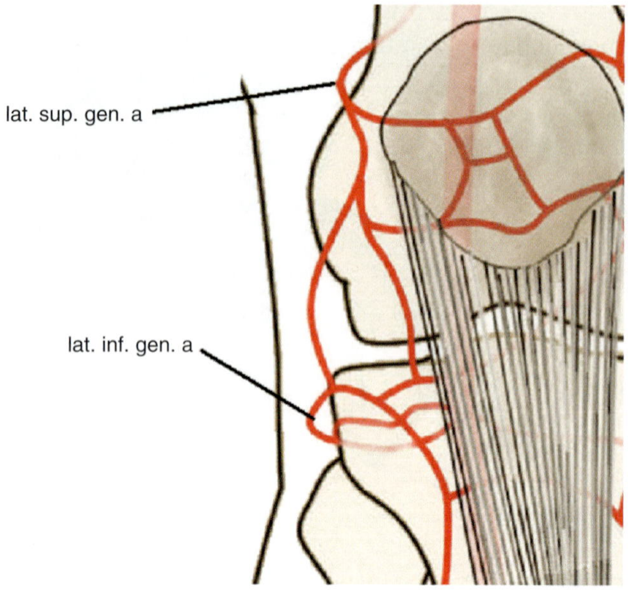

Fig. 4.14 Course of the lateral inferior genicular arteries (*arrow*)

the soft tissue release on the femoral side in case of a valgus deformity is to reduce the risk of peroneal nerve injury.

The ligaments should be released vertically and left in the form of a sleeve instead of cutting them transversely. First, all or part of the deep medial collateral ligament (MCL) should be released in most of varus deformities so that the tibia can be translated anteriorly and externally rotated. *After the preliminary release of the superficial MCL, final balancing is performed during checking the balance or after insertion of the trial implants.*

4.3.4 Fat Pad Removal

The fat pad is supplied by the superior genicular artery. The amount of fat pad to be retained in order to preserve the blood flow may be a controversial issue. If the fat pad can be retained too much in order to preserve the blood flow, but this may interfere with the surgical procedure and cause pain due to impingement and scar formation. Hence, removal of a certain amount of fat pad is inevitable for a better exposure and to prevent impingement postoperatively. Lemon et al. reported *the occurrence of patella baja when a large amount of fat pad has been removed*. However, in patients with a valgus deformity, it is necessary to preserve the lateral fat pad to cover the lateral portion of the joint.

4.3.5 Removal of Posterior Soft Tissues

Soft tissues in the posterior joint space not only restrict the joint motion but also cause pain due to impingement. The posterior space should be clean for achieving better ROM (Fig. 4.15). It is easier to remove these tissues after osteotomy. There can be remaining menisci, loose synovial tissue, and some fibrotic tissue in the posterior space.

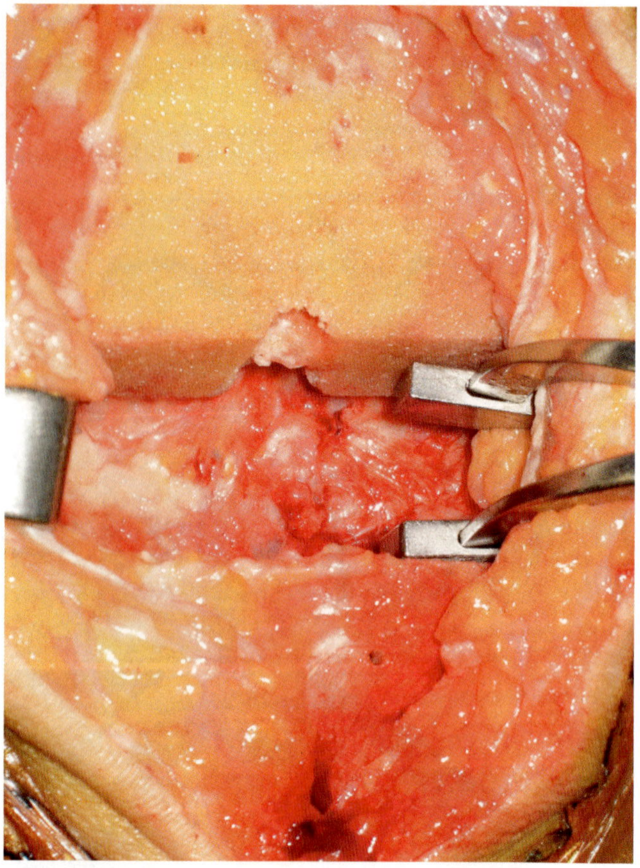

Fig. 4.15 A clean posterior space after the removal of soft tissues

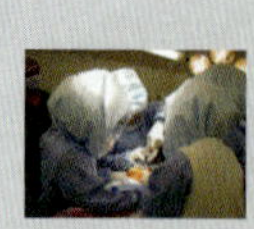

Author's Method

After resection of the ACL, I perform a medial meniscectomy. The medial meniscectomy starts from the mid-portion, 1–2 mm away from the peripheral border. On the anterior part, the incision should not extend along the shape of the meniscus but should extend straight anteriorly and distally so that all the anteromedial soft tissues can be removed at this time. This is because these tissues not only interfere with the operative procedure but also cause anterior impingement postoperatively.

The posterior portion of medial meniscus cannot be removed at this time and the remaining meniscus is removed after osteotomy (Fig. 4.16).

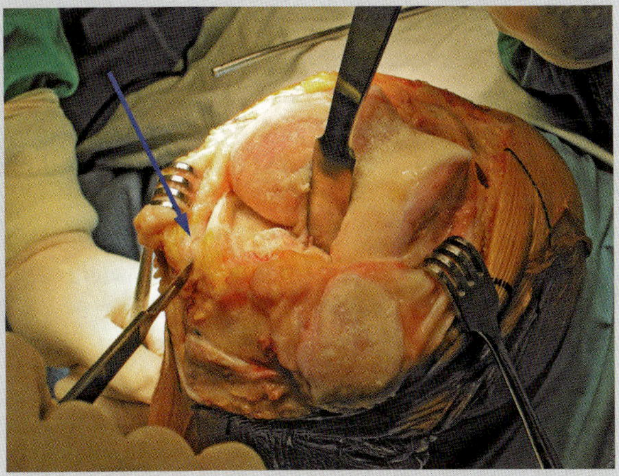

Fig. 4.16 Adequate amount of medial meniscal resection

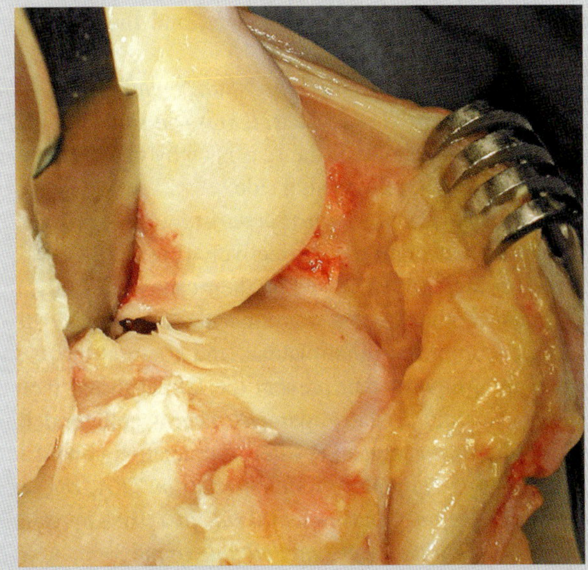

Fig. 4.17 Operation field after appropriate fat pad removal

After this, preliminary release of the MCL is performed for better visualization of the lateral side. I perform medial release by pushing down a periosteal elevator into the posteromedial corner and turning its handle anteriorly to 90°. After this, further medial release is performed by palpating the tight ligamentous structure.

The lateral meniscectomy is performed starting from the hiatus. The anterior portion of the hiatus is resected along the shape of the meniscus and the anterior horn is detached. A complete meniscectomy is performed by pulling the detached anterior horn anteriorly.

This is followed by removal of the fat pad. When the patella is everted, a groove is found between the fat pad and the patellar tendon. The scissors are inserted into the groove and then opened. The fat pad located above the scissors is removed. By doing this, the fat pad can be safely removed without damaging the patellar tendon.

After forceful eversion of the patella, any remaining fat pad over the lateral plateau is removed (Fig. 4.17).

If bleeding is noted at the lateral meniscectomy site during this procedure, every bleeding point is coagulated.

PCL resection can be done at any time of surgery. Generally, I perform PCL resection after femoral osteotomy for fixed-bearing joint and after tibial osteotomy and before femoral osteotomy for mobile-bearing joint.

When the CR type is used, particular attention is paid to protect the PCL. Sometimes, I create a bony island at the point of PCL attachment site. *I do not recess the PCL because PCL recession has critical drawback: the tension is unreliable and the ligament markedly weakens even with minor recession.*

I perform soft tissue removal in the posterior joint space meticulously after osteotomy of the femur and tibia.

4.4 Osteotomy and Bone Preparation

Osteotomy and bone preparation is the *most critical step for alignment of implant, balancing of the joint, and secure fixation of prosthesis in arthroplasty, which starts from choosing the right size of the implant.*

Osteotomy should be highly reproducible, but it is prone to errors not only due to incorrect alignment but also due to the technical problems during installation of instruments or during osteotomy. In soft bones, the instrument can displace during sawing and drilling. In hard bones, the instrument may be positioned incorrectly during fixation or less amount of bone cutting may occur during osteotomy due to deviation of the saw blade.

Use of the navigation system increases the reproducibility by reducing errors caused due to incorrect alignment, but malalignment cannot be prevented if osteotomy is not done properly.

4.4.1 Osteotomy

4.4.1.1 Differences in Technique According to the Resection Method

The method of osteotomy is largely divided into the measured technique and the tension technique (gap technique).

The *measured technique* was the traditional method of osteotomy for the CR type. The basic concept is to *resect the bone of the same thickness as that of the implant thickness* in order to maintain the anatomical joint line. For example, if the thickness of tibial plate plus PE is 10 mm, the amount of tibial resection plus meniscal thickness should also be 10 mm. The amount of femoral condylar osteotomy is approximately the same as the thickness of the femoral prosthesis.

This method was designed based on the assumption that the ligament is balanced if the amount of osteotomy performed is the same as the thickness of the prosthesis. Hence the size of the implant is important. Theoretically, the posterior cruciate ligament (PCL) should be intact and soft tissue balancing should be done after osteotomy. Currently, however, various shapes and sizes of implants are available and new surgical techniques have been developed. So, the measured technique is used regardless of the PCL retention and soft tissue balancing is sometimes done before osteotomy.

The benefit of this method is that it is easy and convenient to perform osteotomy, whereas its drawback is that osteotomy of each bone is done independently causing soft tissue imbalance.

The *tension technique* was used when there were limited sizes and shapes of femoral implants available in the early stage of the PS type. This technique prevents over-resection of the posterior condyle of the femur and the flexion gap is adjusted through appropriate tibial resection.

In this technique, all spurs are removed from the beginning, *the ligament is balanced before osteotomy, and osteotomy is performed according to the flexion and extension gap balance.* Thus, osteotomy of the femur and tibia is correlated sequentially. Although the procedure may differ from surgeon to surgeon or from implant to implant, most of the times, the procedure starts with a tibial osteotomy. *The external rotation of the femur is automatically determined* by the tension technique. This method *makes ligament balancing easy*, but often *inadequate-sized implants are used for ligament balancing. The joint line is elevated* as the distal femur has to be resected more in order to widen the extension gap in a flexion contracture. And *there may be instability in mid-flexion if the posterior joint capsule is tight* as the ligament balancing test is done in 90° flexion and full extension state.

In brief conceptually, in the measured technique, the amount of osteotomy is determined according to the size of implant and ligament balancing is independent of the osteotomy. In the tension technique, the amount of osteotomy varies according to the ligament balance and no further ligament balancing is needed after osteotomy. Both these techniques have their advantages and drawbacks, and the current osteotomy technique is done in combination of both the techniques (Fig. 4.18).

4.4.1.2 Concept of Alignment

Mechanical Alignment

Alignment is critical for long-term survival of the implant regardless of the osteotomy method. Alignment includes coronal, sagittal, and rotational alignment. For ensuring correct alignment, it is necessary to consider the mechanical aspect based on the anatomy.

In the coronal plane, *the line from the center of the femoral head to the center of the talus is called the mechanical axis.* In TKA, most of the surgical techniques focus on this mechanical axis with the aim so as this axis to pass through the center of the knee joint.

The axis extending along the femoral and the tibial shaft is called the anatomical axis. In the femur, the angle between the mechanical and anatomical axes is about 6° (4–7°), whereas the two axes are coincident in the tibia.

However in an upright position, the center of weight transmission is actually on the medial side of the femoral head and the angle between the gravity line and the mechanical axis is about 3°. Therefore, the angle between the gravity line and the anatomical axis is 7–10° in the femur. The point where the gravity line falls upon the knee joint depends on the pelvic width, femoral neck offset, and the length and shape of the femur and tibia.

If the gravity line falls at more than 5 mm to the medial side, more than 40–70 % of the weight is transmitted onto the medial side. This is one of the reasons why osteoarthritis is found more often on the medial side.

The tibial plateau is inclined in varus by 3°, in order to be able to bear the weight more effectively (Fig. 4.19).

Green et al. reported, based on their cadaveric study, that in a varus osteotomy, stress was concentrated on the posteromedial portion of the tibial plateau, and a lateral thrust was noted. The structures that prevent the lateral thrust include the joint capsule, arcuate ligament, lateral collateral ligament, popliteus muscle, and posterior cruciate ligament.

If the limb is aligned physiologically in TKA, the wear may progress rapidly on the medial side just like osteoarthritis occurs more often on the medial side of the joint. Also, if the structures that resist lateral thrust are weakened by arthritis or operation, the lateral thrust cannot be prevented, thereby causing instability and accelerating the wear.

In summary, osteotomy is designed such that the mechanical axis falls upon the center of the knee joint so as to reduce the PE wear and loosening. This is not physiological, but it is the mechanics of TKA.

A mild varus alignment is acceptable since it is physiological. Also, in patients who have had medial compartmental arthritis due to a varus deformity since their young age, the axis may have got adjusted according to their lifestyle, and hence it is questionable whether it is desirable to align the limb according to the mechanical axis in these patients. Bellemans et al. reported 32 % of men and 17 % of women have constitutional varus which had varus alignment since they reached skeletal maturity, and restoring neutral alignment in these cases may be abnormal and undesirable.

On the contrary, *valgus alignment should best be avoided.* Valgus alignment may cause walking disturbance along with

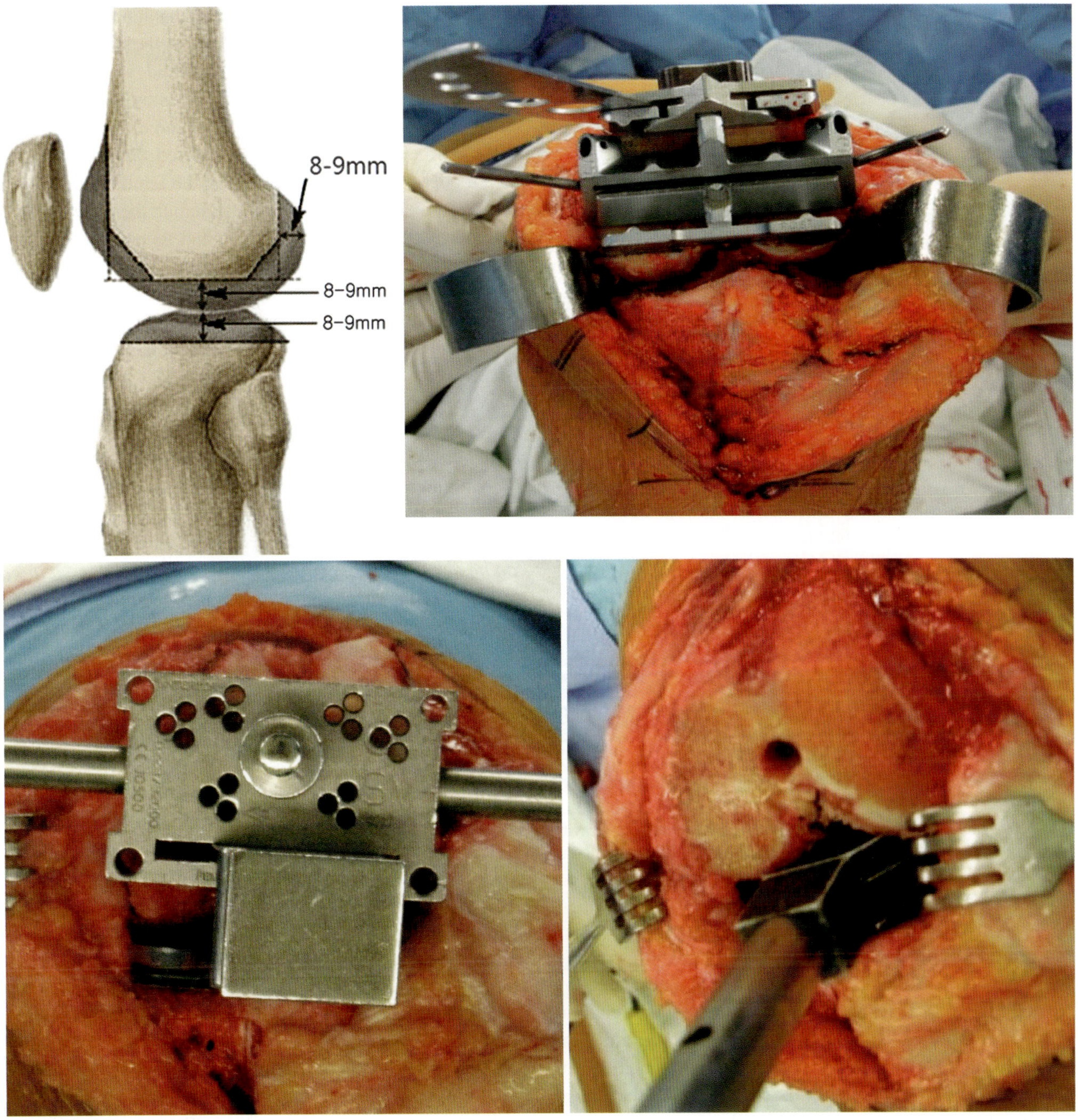

Fig. 4.18 Comparison between the measured technique and the tension technique. The *top images* show the measured technique. The thickness of osteotomy is nearly the same as the thickness of prosthesis. The *bottom images* show tension technique. Osteotomy is done according to ligament tension

cosmetic problems. In obese patients, it is important to limit the amount of valgus to 5° so as to avoid contact of the medial soft tissues of the both thighs.

Interestingly, Mullaji et al. suggested the importance of *hindfoot alignment and that hindfoot alignment should be reflected in the overall alignment.* They emphasized that limb alignment after TKA should reflect the ground mechanical axis. In hindfoot valgus deformity, the axis passes lateral to the center of the knee joint even though tibiofemoral alignment is correct, and this could have implications on the long-term survival of the implant.

In the sagittal plane, the mechanical axis is a line from the center of the hip to the center of the ankle. However, since weight shift is so marked by the knee and ankle motion, *there is no fixed theory about the sagittal axis.*

Axial alignment affects extensor mechanism and ROM, and femoral rotation is closely related with mediolateral gap in flexion state.

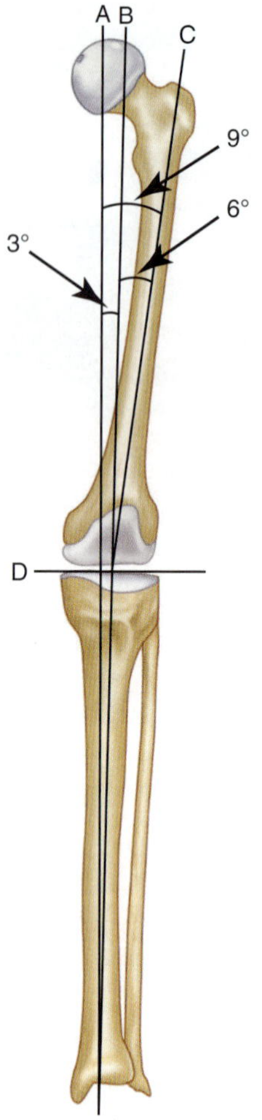

Fig. 4.19 Anatomical and mechanical axis of the limbs. A: Gravity line, B: mechanical axis, C: anatomical axis of femur, D: tibial articular surface. A – B = 3°, B – C = 4 – 7°, B – D = 93°, A – D = 90°

Kinematic Alignment

The concept of kinematic alignment was introduced by Howell and Hull. Kinematics refers to the relative relationship of the femur, patella, and tibia at any flexion angle without application of force to the knee joint. About 20 % of patients are not satisfied with the conventional mechanical alignment method because of continued pain and poor functioning in activities of daily living. They emphasized that kinematic alignment can reduce the loss of flexion and extension motion, stiffness, instability, pain, and prolonged recovery associated with mechanical alignment.

For the kinematics of a TKA to be the same as that of a normal knee joint, the three-dimensional placement of the femoral and tibial components have to be chosen so that the orientation of the three kinematic axes is unchanged from the normal knee joint.

After acquisition of MRI scans, three-dimensional arthritic knee model and normal knee model are generated. Shape matched patient-specific cutting guides are made on the basis of the transverse axis around which the femur flexes and extends, the transverse axis around which the tibia flexes and extends, and the longitudinal axis around which the tibia rotates internally and externally. The osteotomy planes corresponding to the positions of the femoral and tibial components in the normal knee model are transferred onto the arthritic knee model. After shape matching of the femoral component to the restored articular surface of the femur, there are just four subsequent steps to restore motion and to balance the knee joints: osteophyte removal, adjusting the tibial cutting plane, releasing the posterior capsule off the femur, and medialization or lateralization of the tibial component. For this purpose, single radius femoral component is an optimal design.

However, *there are some controversies regarding this concept. First, this method cannot be used without the patient-specific template system. Second, kinematic alignment is used despite of the fact that normal kinematics is altered due to the sacrifice of the ACL and both the menisci. Third, the kinematics without weight bearing is different from that with weight bearing. Fourth, ligament balancing can be achieved by sacrificing the alignment, although there are reports that the mechanical axis in kinematically aligned TKA is similar to that in conventional and computer-assisted TKA. Finally, there are no reports of clinically established long-term results.*

Resection Technique for Ensuring Mechanical Alignment

Based on the mechanical alignment, there are two osteotomy methods for ensuring mechanical alignment in the coronal plane: the classic method and the anatomical method.

The classic method was introduced by Lotke and Ecker in which *distal osteotomy of the femur and proximal osteotomy of the tibia are performed perpendicular to the mechanical axis*, and then the soft tissues of the knee joint are balanced thereafter. In this method, the line from the center of the hip joint to the center of the ankle joint passes through the center of the knee joint. In other words, *since the discrepancy between the mechanical axis and anatomical axis is a 4–7° of valgus in the femur, a 4–7° valgus osteotomy is performed perpendicular to the mechanical axis*. Even though the articular surface of the tibia has a 3° varus, *osteotomy perpendicular to the tibial axis makes the mechanical axis to pass through the center of the knee joint* (Fig. 4.20a).

As the human eyes are accustomed to the perpendicular or parallel angle, perpendicular cutting can be done almost similarly on every occasion. This is the *most commonly used method as it ensures high reproducibility*.

On the other hand, the *anatomical method* was developed by Hungerford et al. and is used mostly for the CR type (Fig. 4.20b). *As the tibial plateau has a 3° varus, this method consists of varus cutting of the tibial plateau at 3° and an additional valgus cutting at 3° from the mechanical axis of*

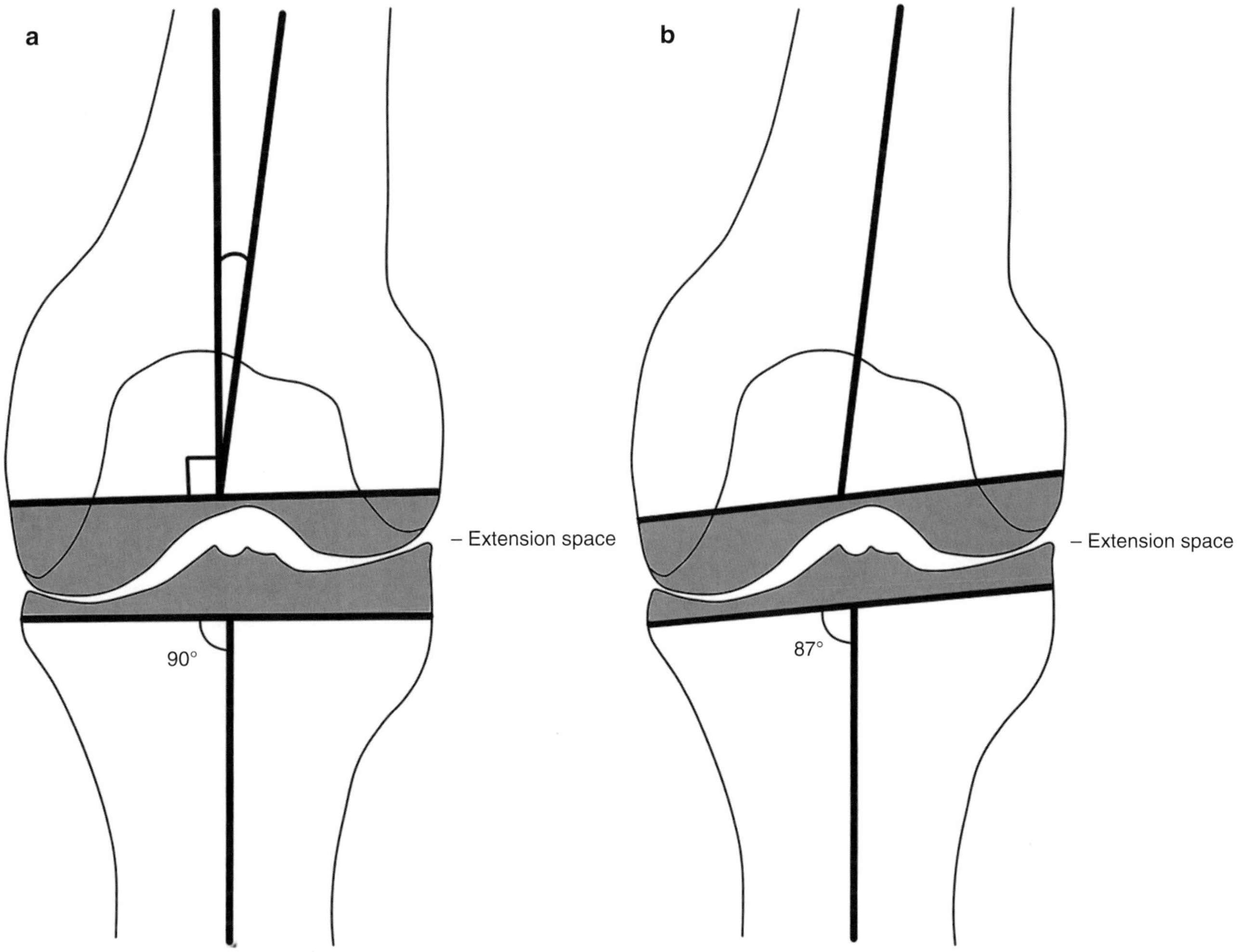

Fig. 4.20 Classic and anatomical method of osteotomy. (**a**) Classic method, (**b**) anatomical method

the femur, resulting in a total valgus cutting of femur at 7–10°. This method reflects the ground force more biomechanically. But as mentioned before, *it lowers reproducibility* to result in more than 3° of varus tibial osteotomy and may damage the lateral collateral ligament and/or popliteus tendon due to excessive valgus osteotomy on the femoral side.

In any method, the mechanical axis passes through the center of the knee joint and the tibiofemoral angle is 6° ± 1–2° valgus.

On the other hand, some surgeons recommend 5–6° of femoral valgus osteotomy routinely, since in most of the cases the difference between the anatomical and mechanical axis is 5–6°.

In the sagittal plane, *there is no definite theory* and the angle of osteotomy varies slightly according to the implants. Usually femoral osteotomy is performed according to the anatomical axis of the distal femur. The mechanical axis can also be considered in the sagittal plane, but it is very difficult to perform the osteotomy along the mechanical axis as most of the instruments are designed to fit the anatomical axis. Furthermore, the center of gravity shifts markedly according to the motion of the knee and ankle joints during walking, and the knee tends to be hyperextended due to anterior bowing of the femur. In navigation surgery, anterior notching develops frequently when the osteotomy is performed according to the mechanical axis, since the implant and the instrument are adjusted according to the anatomical axis of the distal femur.

The posterior slope of the tibial articular surface is known to be 10° in the sagittal plane, but some surgeons state that the posterior slope of the lateral condyle is less than 10° (Fig. 4.21). *Others state that even though the posterior slope is 10°, it is actually less than 10° considering the menisci. They emphasize that there is no posterior slope as the posterior horn of the meniscus is thicker than the anterior horn.*

The posterior slope affects the range of motion to a great extent. Bellemans et al. reported the result of a cadaveric study which suggested that an average increase of 1.7° knee flexion was noted for every degree increase in the posterior slope. According to the Bellemans' report, the knee joint can get 17–20° more flexion by increasing the posterior slope by 10°.

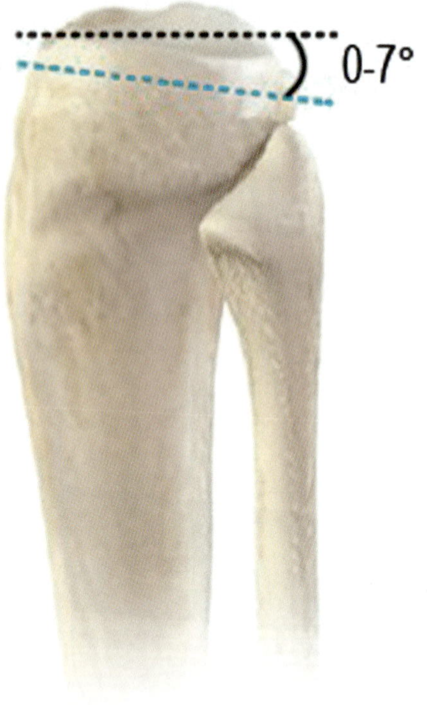

Fig. 4.21 Posterior slope of tibial resection

If the anterior and posterior thickness of the PE is almost the same, the posterior slope of 10° is too great. *In particular with the PS type, posterior slope of 7° or more imposes too much stress on the post to cause an early post wear. The recommended degree of posterior slope varies from implant to implant, and it is mostly between 3 and 7°*. However, it is often set at 0° when using extension stem.

The fibula is known to be parallel to the tibial axis in the sagittal plane, and it is believed that cutting perpendicular to the fibular axis in the sagittal plane is similar to cutting perpendicular to the tibial axis.

Rotational alignment greatly affects patellar tracking and femoral rotation is closely related to the flexion gap. Hence, these two factors should be considered in rotational alignment. This has been described in more details under "External Rotation" in this chapter.

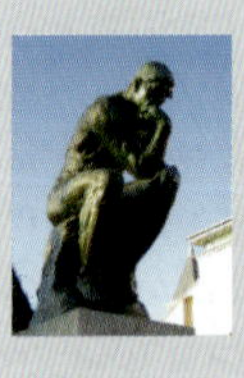

Author's Opinion

I think femoral valgus osteotomy of more than 9° in the coronal plane is to be avoided even when the angle between the anatomical and mechanical axes is more than 9°. This is because the LCL and popliteus tendon is likely to be injured and the mechanics of flexion and extension can be altered by too much valgus osteotomy of the distal femur.

Also, I am not in favor of performing an osteotomy according to the mechanical axis in the sagittal plane, since the weight shifts markedly according to the knee and ankle motion on walking in the sagittal plane. So the mechanical axis is less meaningful in the sagittal plane than in the coronal plane.

In the sagittal plane, the extensor mechanism and flexion–extension motion of the knee joint are more important. Hence, osteotomy in the sagittal plane should be performed according to the anatomical axis of the distal femur and the design of each prosthesis.

Another opinion is that the center of flexion–extension motion is different from the mechanical center, since the posterior part of the femur and the tibia plays a major role not for the weight transmission, but for the joint motion. In other words, the point of weight transmission falls anterior to the center of flexion–extension motion. Thus, the center of the knee joint in navigation system is not the center of the mechanical axis in the sagittal plane. This is the reason why anterior notching develops more often after navigation surgery.

4.4.2 Osteotomy of Each Bone and Preparation for Fixation

Osteotomy and preparation for fixation can be started from any bone. Most of the surgeons start the osteotomy from the femur except in the case of a mobile-bearing joint.

4.4.2.1 Femur

Removal of Spurs

It is necessary to remove the spurs before osteotomy. *By removing the spurs, it becomes possible to select the correct implant size, balance the ligament accurately, remove the source of pain, and achieve a better ROM*. In particular, spurs buried under the superficial MCL should be completely removed for correct ligament balancing.

Also, the spurs on the articular surface of the medial condyle of femur project too far distally in severe osteoarthritis, and these spurs keep the cutting guide away from the articular surface during distal cutting, which results in less distal osteotomy. Hence, they need to be removed so as to be able to perform distal osteotomy accurately (Fig. 4.22).

The *spurs on the posterior condyle* impinge on the PE and hence *reduce the ROM*. These spurs should also be removed after femoral and tibial osteotomy for achievement of a better

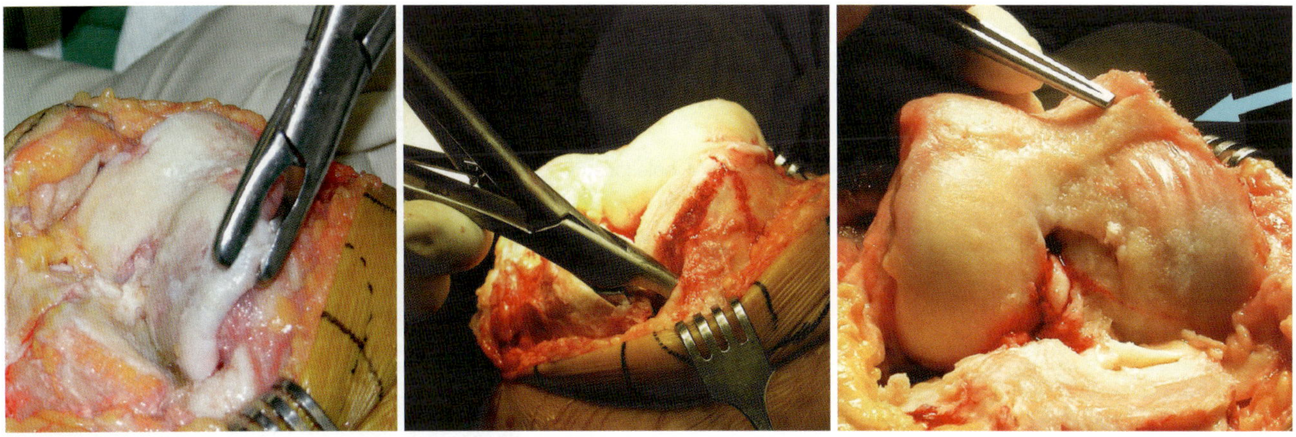

Fig. 4.22 Spur removal before femoral osteotomy. The *left image* shows removal of the peripheral spur. The *middle image* shows removal of the spurs hidden beneath the medial collateral ligament. The *right image* shows spurs in the tidemark in the articular surface of the medial femoral condyle. These spurs should be removed before osteotomy for correct implant size, ligament balancing, more ROM, and accurate distal osteotomy

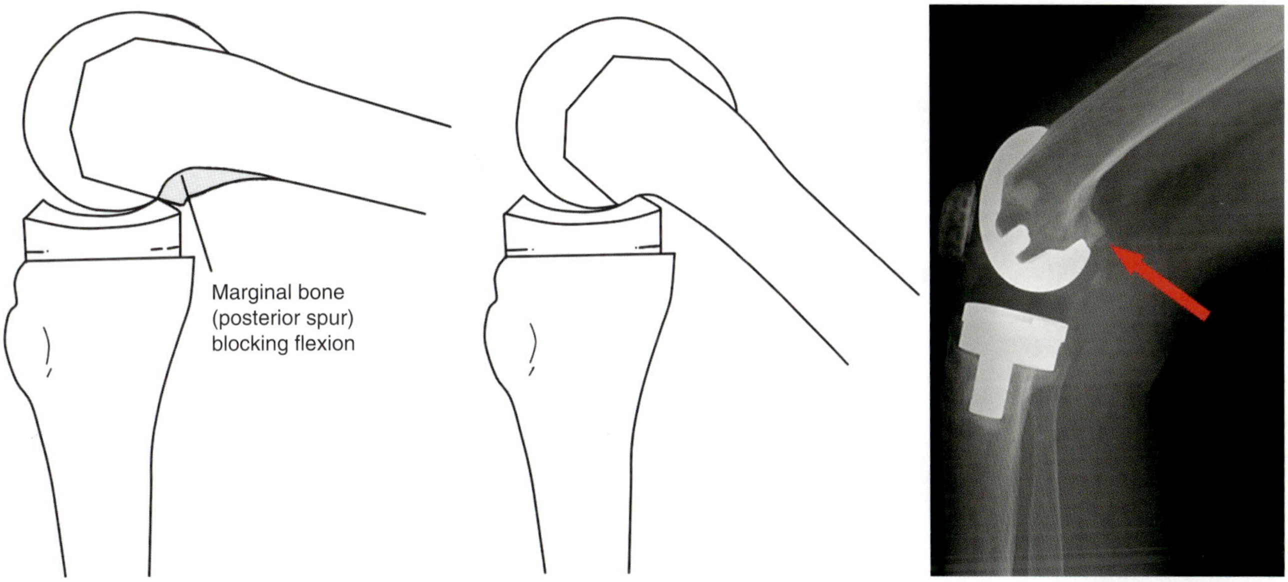

Fig. 4.23 The reason why the posterior spurs (*arrow*) interfere with flexion and its X-ray

ROM. In the PS type, *the composite of trial implant of the tibial plate and the PE should be inserted smoothly into the posterior side (Fig.* 4.23*) in a flexed position.*

Axial Alignment

An intramedullary guide or an extramedullary guide may be used for coronal alignment, but it is difficult to point out the landmark of the hip joint with an extramedullary guide and hence its accuracy is decreased. It is only used when an intramedullary guide cannot enter into the medullary canal such as THA on the ipsilateral side, the presence of IM nailing, severe deformity of femoral shaft, or patients with an extremely small skeleton.

The pilot point of the intramedullary guide is 5–10 mm anterior to the notch on the A–P and at the center or slightly medial to the center mediolaterally (Fig. 4.24). This is because the anatomical axis of the femoral shaft falls at this point. Even though the pilot point is located at the center, a slightly lateral placement of the prosthesis is recommended for better patellar tracking. The more posterior is the entry portal, the greater is the anterior angulation of the prosthesis. Mihalko et al. suggested inserting the intramedullary guide as posteriorly as possible. By doing so, osteotomy is performed more anatomically, notching is prevented as the prosthesis is angulated anteriorly, and flexion motion is increased.

Reaming

It is desirable to use a reamer that minimizes the risk of fat embolism, especially when performing a simultaneous

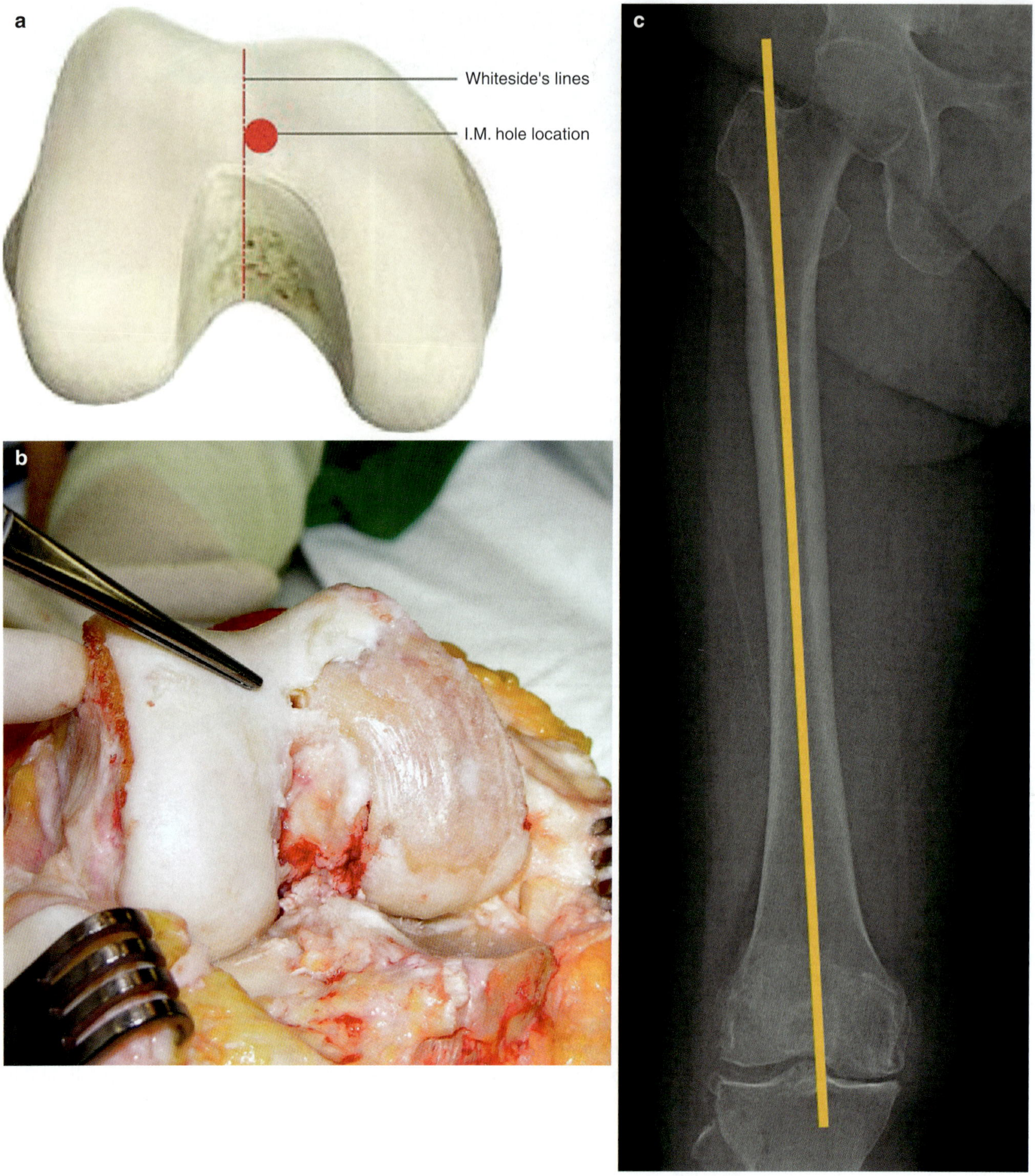

Fig. 4.24 Point of insertion of an intramedullary guide in the femur. The point is a little medial to the center. (**a**) Schematic drawing, (**b**) operation findings, (**c**) the reason why the point is a little medial to the center

bilateral operation or when using an intramedullary guide in the femur and the tibia concomitantly. Ries et al. reported that larger flute-shaped reamers would reduce the risk of fat embolism. Adequate reaming should be performed so as to be able to insert the alignment guide smoothly. It is *desirable to insert the guide gently* and to suction out the contents of the medullary canal when inserting the guide rod after reaming.

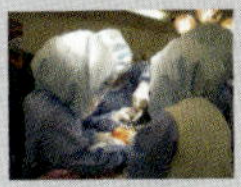

Author's Method

When reaming, I recommend not to apply excessive force and I allow the reamer to follow naturally the path of the medullary canal. In order to do so, it is recommended to hold the reamer with just the thumb and the index finger.

I do not perform reaming currently, but I take out a bone plug using the bone harvester which I have designed and then I widen the medullary canal with a trocar which is used in IM nailing (Fig. 4.25). Before insertion of the medullary guide, I perform suction routinely.

This method has certain benefits especially in reducing the intramedullary pressure and reduce the incidence of fat embolism. The bone plug is reinserted with the bone fragment or is wrapped with Surgicel® (Johnson and Johnson Medical, Arlington, TX) for a tight fit into the canal just before cement fixation in order to block bleeding from the medullary canal.

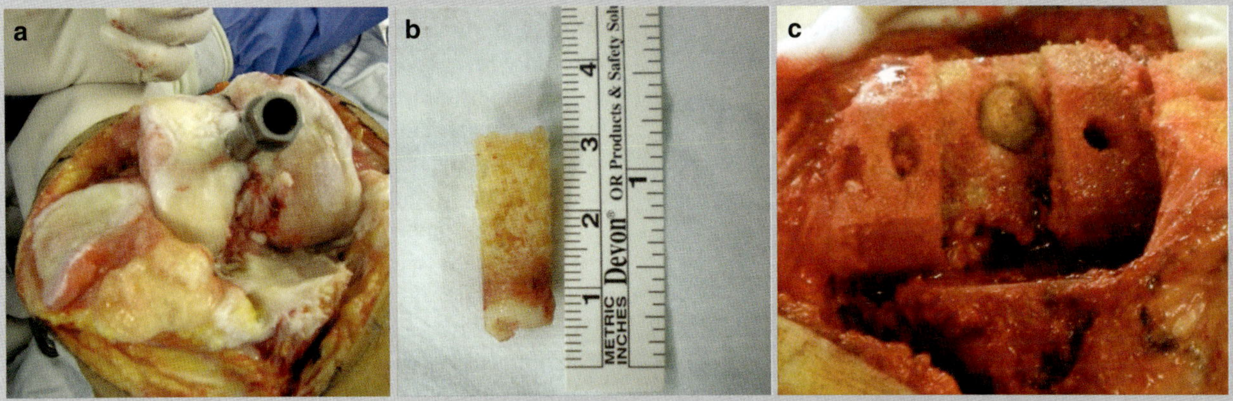

Fig. 4.25 Harvesting the bone plug (**a**), harvested bone plug (**b**), reinserted bone plug (**c**)

External Rotation

The amount of external rotation of the femur is related to patellar tracking, mediolateral balancing in flexion, and the axis of flexion–extension motion. *If femoral rotation is inaccurate, patellar tracking is adversely affected causing patellar subluxation/dislocation and anterior knee pain. Flexion instability and changes in the axis of flexion–extension motion due to poor rotational alignment may cause eccentric wear and loosening of the prosthesis.*

As the landmarks are not clear and each patient has a unique bony anatomy, it is not so easy to determine the amount of external rotation. Anyhow, *the femur should not be internally rotated* and the amount of external rotation *should be determined specific to each patient.* However, Scott stated that external rotation of the femur does not affect patellar tracking as much as expected, and he accepted internal rotation of the femur for mediolateral balancing in flexion in case of a valgus deformity, and he recommended adjustment of patellar tracking by adjusting the position of prosthesis or by other techniques.

The methods for determining external rotation include the transepicondylar method, transcondylar method, Whiteside's line, and transtibial or ligament tension method.

In the transepicondylar method, both the epicondyles are the references, while in the *transcondylar method both the posterior condyles are the reference. In Whiteside's method, a line perpendicular to the patellar groove is used. The transtibial method implies cutting perpendicular to the tibial axis, and the ligament tension method uses ligament tension after tibial osteotomy*. The transtibial method and the ligament tension method are often regarded as one and the same (Fig. 4.26).

These methods are used differently according to the gap technique and the measured technique. In the anterior reference system (ARS) of the measured technique, the external rotation is usually determined by the use of the transepicondylar or transcondylar method and the anterior osteotomy is done first. Whereas in the posterior reference system (PRS), generally distal osteotomy is performed first and external rotation is mostly predetermined at 3° by the instrument. In the gap technique, external rotation is determined by the ligament tension after tibial osteotomy.

The transepicondylar method is the most ideal method since both the epicondyles are the attachment sites of the collateral ligaments and they accurately reflect the axis of flexion and extension motion. It is often used when there is a valgus deformity or the shape of the condyle is abnormal, i.e., in revision. However, it is not very easy to locate the epicondyles and this is time-consuming. The lateral epicondyle is easier to locate since it is pointed, but the medial epicondyle is blunt. Berger et al. divided the medial epicondyle into two: one is the clinical epicondyle to which the superficial medial collateral ligament (MCL) attaches and the other is the surgical epicondyle where the sulcus between the deep MCL and the superficial MCL is located. They reported that the discrepancy in the transepicondylar axis between the two points was an average 4.7° in men and 5.2° in women. The average discrepancy between the surgical transepicondylar axis and the transcondylar axis was 3.5° in men and 0.3° in women.

Generally, the condylar vessel passes through the ridge to which the superficial MCL is attached anteriorly and proximally. Hence, the condylar vessel helps in identifying the accurate location of the clinical medial epicondyle. To locate the clinical medial epicondyle, the synovial tissues should be peeled off around the medial epicondylar area so as to identify the condylar vessel (Fig. 4.27).

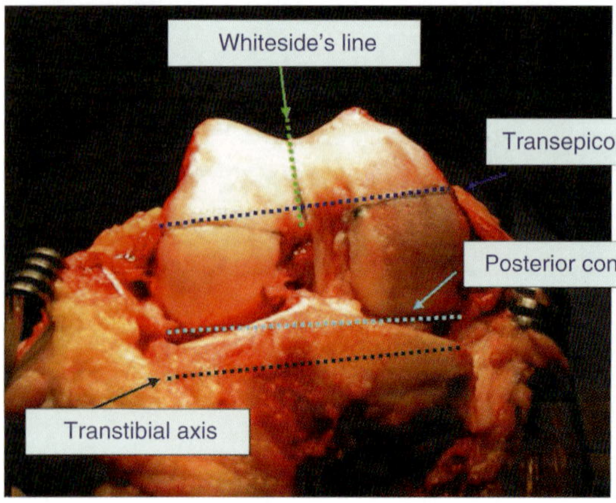

Fig. 4.26 Different guidelines for external rotation

Stoeckl et al. reported the results of a cadaveric study by four surgeons, which suggested that *the position of the medial epicondyle varied from surgeon to surgeon*. Wai Hung et al. also reported the results of comparison between ten cadavers and CT findings which suggested that there was an average difference of 2.6° between the examiners.

Most of the surgeons *prefer the transcondylar method as it is convenient*. Three degrees of external rotation is preferred by most of the surgeons or 3° of external rotation is fixed by the instrument. However, the use of this method may lead to errors due to wear of the articular cartilage in severe osteoarthritis, and *it is difficult to use this method if there is a severe deformity or a bone defect*. If the articular cartilage in the posterior portion of the medial condyle is worn out, more amount of external rotation is achieved by this method. The posterior condylar axis and the transepicondylar axis are known to have a difference of 4–7°, although it varies from surgeon to surgeon. So, many surgeons state that *it is not enough to set the angle of external rotation at 3° in all patients*. Berger et al. reported that the difference is about 3.5° in a cadaveric study, while Cho et al. reported a difference of about 4.8° by measuring the axes through computerized tomography (Fig. 4.28). Assuming that the cartilage of the medial condyle is worn out in severe medial osteoarthritis, 3° external rotation by the transepicondylar method may correctly reflect the true transepicondylar axis.

Whiteside's line defines a line connecting the deepest part of the trochlea and the center of the intercondylar notch, and a line perpendicular to it is *generally aligned with the transepicondylar axis*. However, there is significant variability in

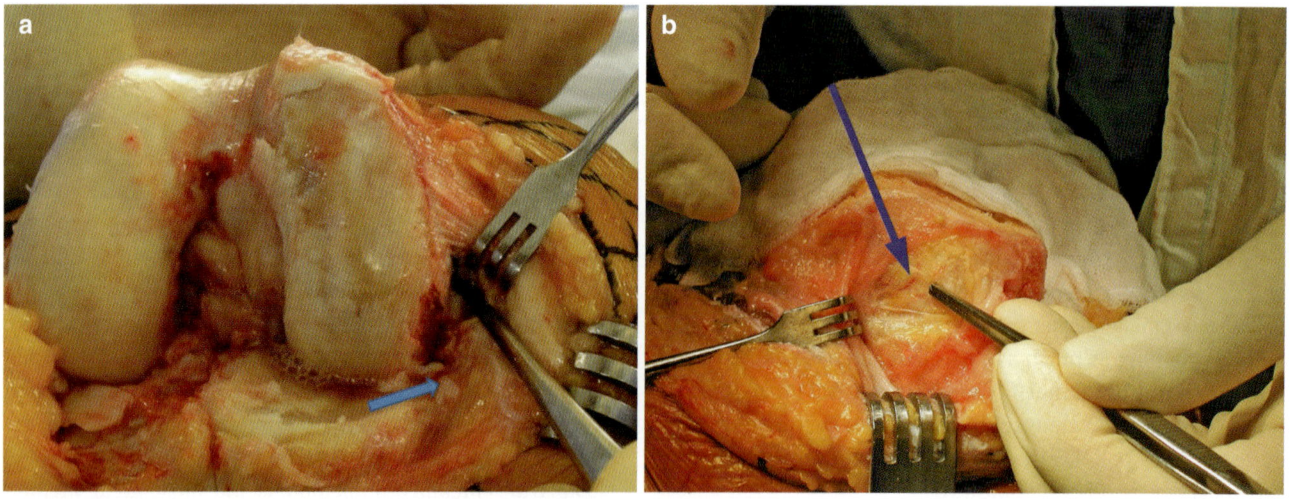

Fig. 4.27 The location of the medial epicondyle. (**a**) Superficial MCL is retracted and the *arrow* indicates deep MCL. The *blue line* (forceps) is sulcus line which is indicative of surgical medial epicondyle (*left*). (**b**) The line beneath the blue arrow is the condylar vessel and the forceps indicates the clinical medial epicondyle (*right*)

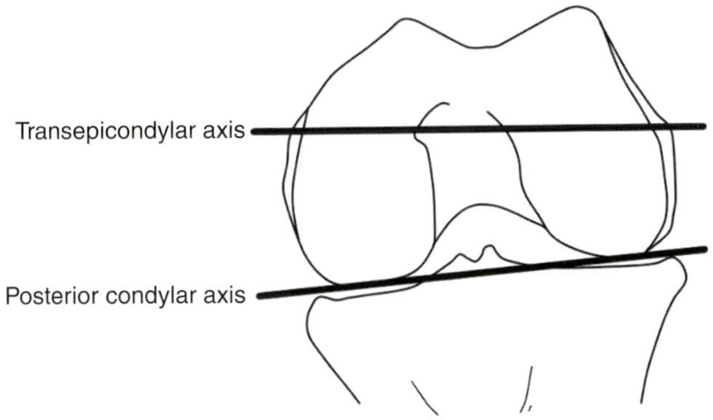

Fig. 4.28 The angle between the transepicondylar axis and the posterior condylar axis

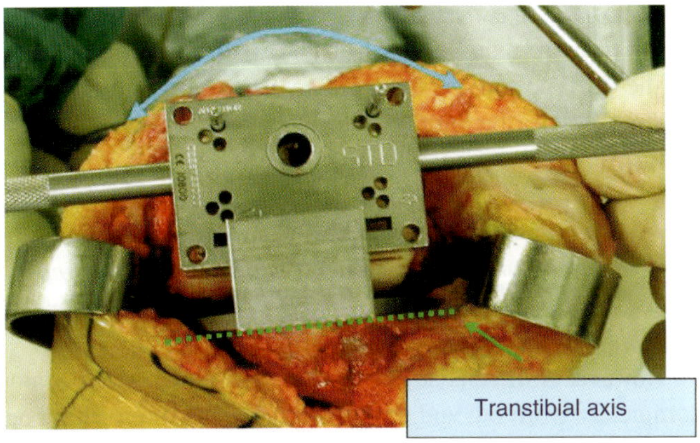

Fig. 4.29 Determining external rotation in the ligament tension technique. The concept of transtibial method is similar to that of the ligament tension technique

the anatomy of the trochlear groove, and this method *may be inaccurate if there are excessive spurs in the notch area or when there is condylar dysplasia.*

The transtibial method with cutting perpendicular to the tibial axis is similar to the ligament tension technique (gap technique), if the ligaments are balanced. The *ligament tension technique* is often used in a mobile-bearing joint in which the soft tissue balancing is utmost important. Osteotomy is generally started from the tibia followed by anterior and posterior cutting of the femur. Therefore, *the amount of external rotation is automatically determined according to the osteotomy of the tibia and tension in both the collateral ligaments* (Fig. 4.29). When mediolateral balance is established by the ligament tension technique, it results in less than 3° of external rotation in some cases, but good patellar tracking can be achieved most of the times.

Seon et al. stated that the transepicondylar method is the most ideal, but the ligament tension technique is more convincing as there are anatomical variances among the patients. Katz et al. reported that the axis of flexion and extension was maintained most reliably in the ligament tension method and there was a tendency for excessive external rotation with the transepicondylar axis compared to the ligament tension method. Fehring et al. reported that 45 % of cases showed at least 3° malrotation with the methods other than the ligament tension method. With respect to ligament balancing, Dennis et al. reported that the condylar lift-off is less common in the external rotation determined by the ligament tension technique than in the external rotation determined by the anatomical landmark. In this aspect, *the ligament tension technique is gradually becoming the standard method for determining the external rotation.*

However Hanada et al. stated that patellar tracking became worse by the ligament tension method due to shifting of the patellar groove to the lateral side, and a varus deformity was seen in 90° flexion with the external rotation determined by the ligament tension technique.

In order to achieve good patella tracking and mediolateral balance in flexion state, the surgeons' experience based on one or two of the aforementioned methods is the best way to determine the external rotation, while keeping in mind that the ultimate goal is to secure patellofemoral alignment, mediolateral balance in flexion and flexion motion.

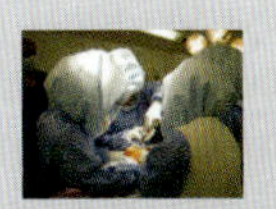

Author's Method

I use the ligament tension technique for a mobile-bearing joint and 3° of external rotation according to the transcondylar method for a fixed-bearing joint.

Although the transepicondylar axis is the basis, I have experienced cases in which much more time is taken to draw the index line due to unclear landmarks, and the amount of rotation was inaccurate.

I use the transcondylar axis because it is easy and convenient to use. I have some principles and tips for using the transcondylar axis. First, I do not use this method in a severe deformity including a valgus deformity and in revision cases. In these cases, I usually use the ligament tension method. Second, a little less amount of external rotation is preferred in severe osteoarthritis as the cartilage of the medial condyle has been worn out.

I am in favor of the theory of the ligament tension technique because of inaccuracy of the transcondylar method when there is a severe deformity and atrophy of the bone. Particularly, in a valgus deformity, the tibia is cut more on the medial side and the posterior condyle of the femur is also cut more on the medial side, causing an imbalance in flexion due to a wider medial gap by the use of the transcondylar method.

Sometimes, the lateral femoral condyle is cut more than the medial femoral condyle with the ligament tension technique, which indicates internal rotation. In such a case, I check the tibial resection and ligament tension again and continue with the osteotomy according to the ligament tension technique if there are no problems of tibial osteotomy and ligament tension. I have seen the "grand-piano sign" in the anterior cutting surface and good patellar tracking in many cases even when the posterior portion of the lateral condyle was cut more than the medial condyle.

In conclusion, I use the ligament tension technique with reference to the transepicondylar axis concomitantly when the anatomical structures have been altered.

Osteotomy

The method and sequence of osteotomy depends on the type of reference system used: anterior reference system (ARS) or posterior reference system (PRS).

Osteotomy According to the ARS

In the ARS, anterior osteotomy is performed after determination of external rotation. Since the *anterior osteotomy is the basis of all femoral osteotomies*, an accurate anterior osteotomy is the first step to a successful osteotomy of the femur. In ARS, the amount of posterior osteotomy differed according to size (Fig. 4.30).

The position of the stylus must be located accurately before anterior cutting. If resection has been done accurately, *the resected surface should be flush with the anterior cortex of the femur; should it neither be projecting (tenting) nor should it be notched. The "grand-piano sign" is the sign of good external rotation* (Fig. 4.31). If the shape of the cut surface resembles that of a boot (boot sign), it indicates that more external rotation has been achieved. And if the shape is round, it means that less external rotation has been done.

Anterior notching not only predisposes to periprosthetic fracture but also reduces posterior cutting which *decreases the flexion gap*. On the other hand, *too little anterior cutting causes anterior overstuffing to aggravate patellar maltracking and imposes much stress on the patella*, which may be the cause of pain and early failure, and can increase the amount of posterior cutting which *increases the flexion gap*.

After *anterior osteotomy*, the distal, posterior, and chamfer cutting are performed. Before distal cutting, the cutting guide should be adjusted according to the difference in the angle between the anatomical and mechanical axis, which is measured preoperatively. Anteroposterior inclination of distal osteotomy in the sagittal plane differs from prosthesis to prosthesis. During distal cutting, it is important to protect the collateral ligaments on both sides. First, the distal cutting guide should be fixed and it should be confirmed whether the distal cutting guide makes contact with the condyle. Due to the difference in the size of the condyles, valgus setting of the instrument, and the cartilage erosion, the distal cutting guide will not make contact with both the condyles. If the cutting guide does not contact with any of the condyles, the amount of distal cutting is reduced and the extension gap is narrowed. If the extension gap is narrowed due to less distal cutting, it causes a flexion contracture. Bengs and Scott reported that a flexion contracture of about 9° occurs with every 2 mm decrease in the extension gap.

If there is a *flexion contracture of more than 15° or if osteonecrosis exists, it is sometimes necessary to move the distal cutting jig proximally by one click to increase the amount of distal osteotomy so as to widen the extension gap.*

When more than 2 mm of distal osteotomy is performed for the CR type and 4–5 mm of distal osteotomy is performed for the PS type, the joint line elevation affects the knee kinematics seriously. *Changes in the joint line have various effects such as mid-flexion instability, an increase in PCL strain, alteration in the quadriceps function, and impingement of patella and patellar tendon on the tibial component. Hence, it is recommended not to perform distal osteotomy of more than 4–5 mm for the PS type.*

However if there is severe osteoarthritis, the cartilages are completely worn out and the distal condyle is often cut more than intended. There are some signs of excessive distal cutting in the operation field: the articular portion of the posterior condyles is not seen in the frontal view, fibers of the PCL and popliteus tendon are fluttering, and the popliteus tendon has a tendency to subluxate during flexion and extension motion. The cutting surface should be flat, and if it is not so, the femoral implant loses its stability and the coronal axis alters (Fig. 4.32).

Then, the appropriate size of the implant is selected and performs posterior osteotomy and chamfer cutting. *The A–P size is more important than the width; however it is not desirable that the implant overhangs.* As external rotation is achieved, the posterior portion of medial condyle is resected more than the lateral condyle. *If the amount of medial posterior osteotomy is more than 1 cm, it means the implant is small, and if it is less than 5–6 mm, it means that the implant is large. Using a smaller size of the implant in the ARS leads to more posterior resection causing instability in flexion. When a larger size of the implant is used, the flexion gap is decreased resulting in limitation of the flexion motion and increase stress on the PE.*

If the size of the implant is an in-between size, a smaller implant is recommended for the CR type, which increases the flexion gap as well as the flexion motion without causing serious problems. A larger implant is recommended for the PS type, because the flexion gap becomes wider than the extension gap when the posterior cruciate ligament is removed.

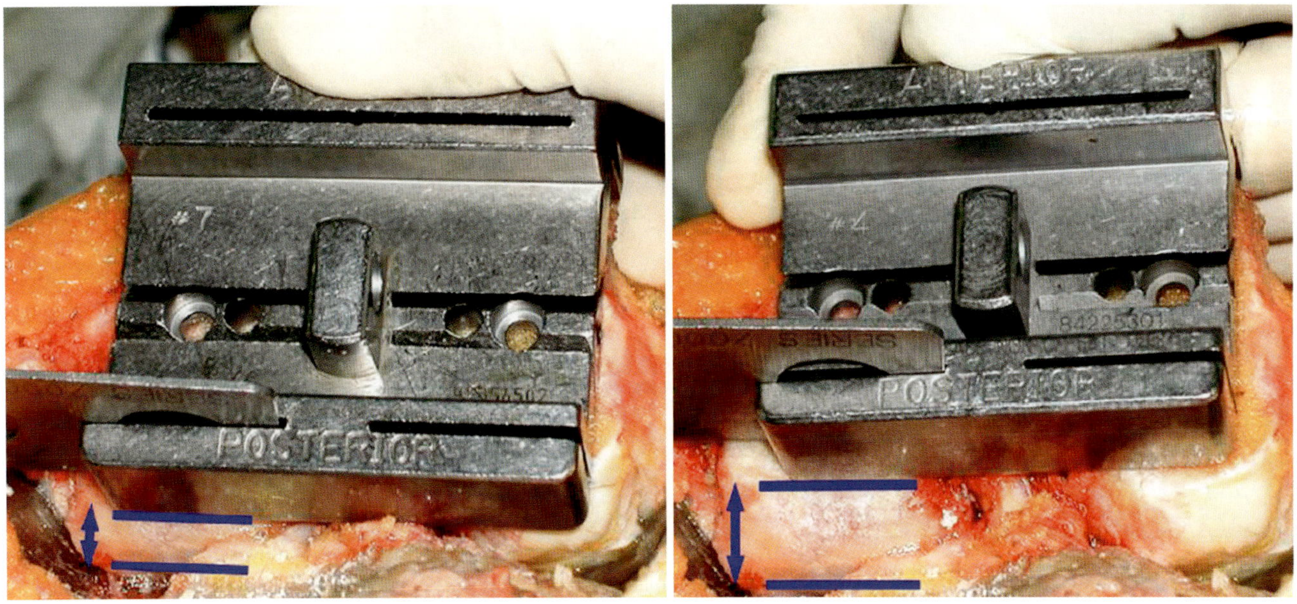

Fig. 4.30 Anterior reference system. The amount of posterior osteotomy is differed according to size of implant

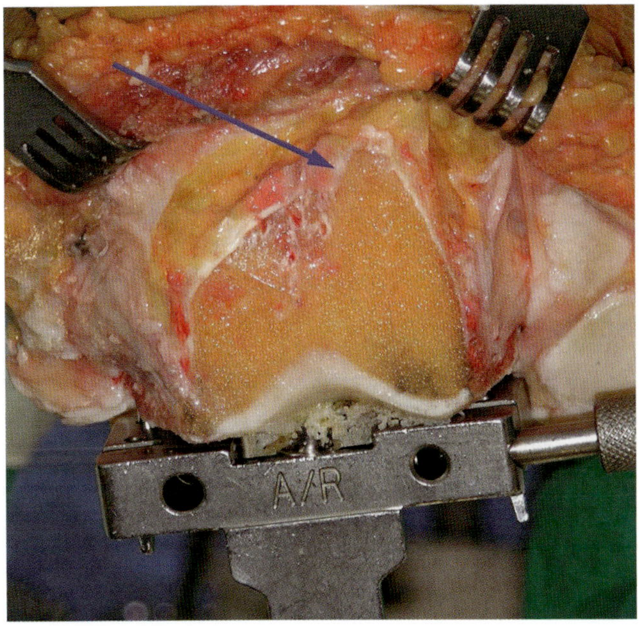

Fig. 4.31 The grand-piano sign (*arrow*). The lateral portion is cut more than the medial portion

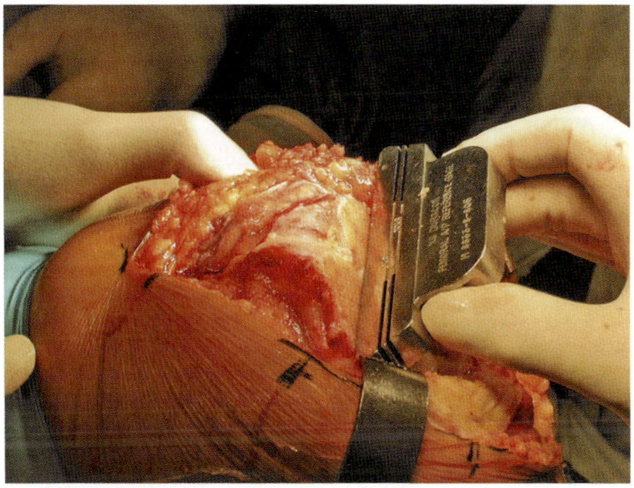

Fig. 4.32 Checking the flatness of the resected surface after distal osteotomy

Some implants need final anterior osteotomy since the anterior flange portion of the femoral component has a 3–5° of inclination. If notching develops during final anterior osteotomy, it indicates that distal osteotomy has not been performed correctly resulting in posterior angulation of the femoral component.

Osteotomy According to the PRS

In the PRS, the amount of posterior cutting is fixed regardless of the size of prosthesis and anterior cutting level is differed according to the implant size (Fig. 4.33).

PRS generally starts with distal cutting of the femur, followed by determination of the size of the implant, anterior, posterior, and chamfer cutting in that order. *Generally, external rotation is fixed at an angle of 3° to the transcondylar axis by an instrument. PRS helps maintain a consistent flexion gap. But if the size of the implant is too large, it reduces anterior cutting to cause overstuffing that imposes more stress on the patella and worsens patellar tracking. Even a slightly smaller prosthesis causes notching*; hence controlled osteotomy may have to be performed to allow the prosthesis to be inserted in flexion position within 3° in order to prevent notching.

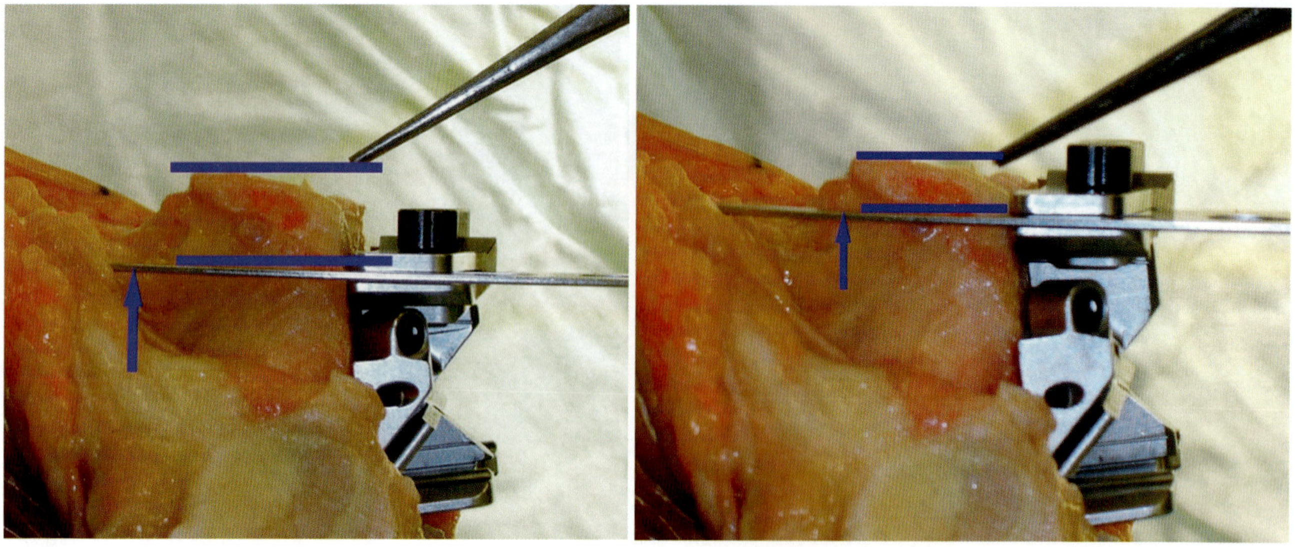

Fig. 4.33 Anterior cutting level is different according to the size of implant in PRS. *Left* is smaller in size and *right* is larger in size

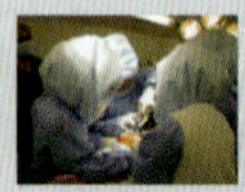

Author's Method

I perform femoral osteotomy according to the implant-specific manual. In mobile-bearing joint, I perform tibial osteotomy first and external rotation is determined by the gap technique. In fixed-bearing joint, I use either ARS or PRS according to the implant, and 3° of external rotation is given by the transcondylar axis.

In ARS, I perform anterior osteotomy first. I try to ensure that the surface of osteotomy is flushed with anterior femoral cortex. I usually use a drill to fix the osteotomy jig as the position of the jig may be altered when inserting the pins with a hammer. Resection is done from the periphery of the bone to reduce the occurrence of marginal fracture.

After anterior osteotomy, I determine the implant size. While choosing the implant size, I think the A–P length is more important than the width unless the implant overhangs. When the implant is of an in-between size, I choose a smaller size for the CR type and ARS, and a larger size for the PS type and PRS.

When doing distal cutting, I always trim the notch area routinely. As the bone in this portion is hard, it is likely to be cut less, which causes a seesaw effect resulting in instability and malalignment. In the patient who has a flexion contracture of more than 15°, I perform more amount of distal osteotomy from the beginning.

After distal osteotomy, I check the position of chamfer and posterior cutting jig. I use my thumb and index finger to check that the mediolateral position of the cutting jig is at the center of the bone. If the cutting guide is not at the center, it takes more time to make new lug holes later. I accept that it is better to place the jig slightly to the lateral side for better patellar tracking.

When fixing the cutting jig, I fix the pins first partly on both the sides to prevent slipping off of the cutting jig, which can be developed when firm fixation is done one after another. After this, final fixation is done.

Chamfer cutting is performed after posterior cutting and I perform chamfer cutting deeply for a tight fit of the implant.

In PRS, the osteotomy is performed according to the manual of each implant. If anterior notching is expected, I perform final anterior cutting manually so as to prevent notching.

4.4.2.2 Tibia

Removal of Spurs

The spurs on the medial side should be removed not only for pain relief but also to achieve ligament balance. If the bone is uncovered to a great extent on the medial side after insertion of the trial implant or fixation of the final implant, it is also desirable to remove this uncovered bone.

Axial Alignment

Tibial osteotomy can be done either with an extramedullary guide or with an intramedullary guide. As the landmarks are easily detectable topographically, the *extramedullary method*

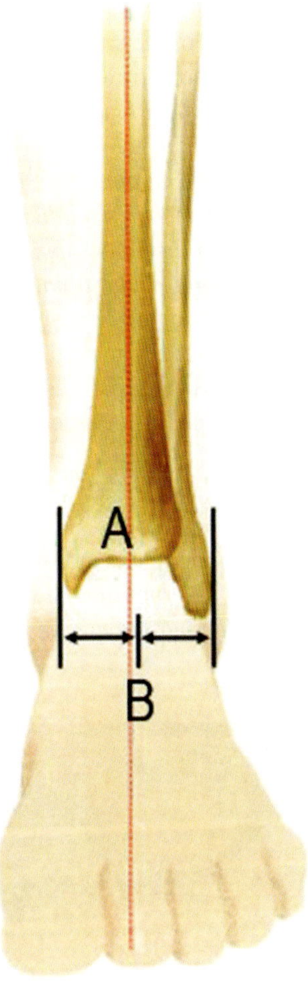

Fig. 4.34 The center of the tibial axis and the center of the ankle joint. A: axis center, B: ankle center. A is slightly medial to B

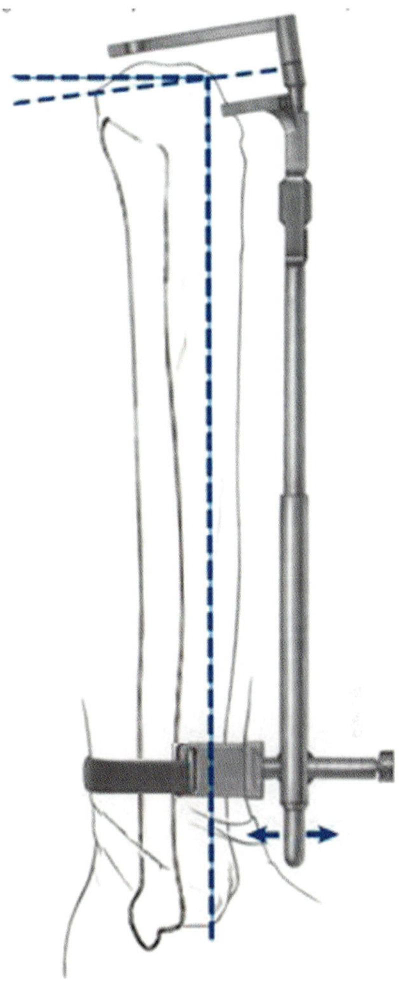

Fig. 4.35 Tibial axis in the sagittal plane

is commonly used for tibial alignment. The advantage of the extramedullary method is that it can be used when there is a deformity, it reduces the risk of fat embolism and the axis can be adjusted to any plane such as the posterior slope. However, alignment can be altered in obese patients. On the contrary, the intramedullary method allows for a relatively accurate osteotomy, but it cannot be used if there is a deformity of tibial shaft and it is associated with an increased incidence of fat embolism. Comparing the accuracy of the two methods, some surgeons state that the intramedullary method is better, but Dennis et al. reported that there is no significant difference in the accuracy between the two methods.

When the extramedullary method is used, *the proximal pilot point of axial alignment is not the center of the tibial plateau, but the point where the mechanical axis meets the tibial plateau on the coronal plane.* If this principle is followed, the osteotomy can be performed at a right angle to the mechanical axis. Hence, in a severe varus deformity, the mediolateral pilot point moves laterally. Therefore, it is recommended to draw a line along the mechanical axis on the preoperative X-ray and use the point where the mechanical axis meets the tibial plateau as a proximal pilot point of coronal axial alignment. *The distal pilot point is at the tibial crest, 2 in. above the ankle joint.* This point reflects the mechanical axis correctly. *This distal pilot point is slightly medial to the center of the ankle joint because the lateral malleolus of the ankle joint is larger than the medial malleolus; hence the center of the ankle joint is not coincident with the center of the tibial axis* (Fig. 4.34). In the past, *the second toe* was used as the distal pilot point, but *it was not accurate because the position of the second toe changes* according to the position of the foot.

In the sagittal plane, the fibular axis is nearly parallel to the tibial axis, and so the line that connects the fibular head to the lateral malleolus of the ankle joint is the index of sagittal axis. *The posterior slope should be adjusted according to the recommended angle for each implant* (Fig. 4.35).

However, *it is advisable to reduce the posterior slope if there is a flexion contracture, when the posterior slope has been reversed due to high tibial osteotomy or when the PS type is used.*

In a severe varus deformity, there is always an accompanying rotational deformity of the proximal tibia. If the rotational deformity is not taken into account, the desired posterior slope cannot be obtained accurately and the alignment on the coronal plane can be changed. So, it is not easy to obtain the correct angle in patient with both the rotational and varus deformity.

Osteotomy

The angle of osteotomy is perpendicular to the tibial axis in the classic method and corresponds to a 3° varus cut or parallel to the articular surface in the anatomical method. However, even if the cutting is done perpendicularly using the classic method, it often becomes a varus cut due to the shape of the articular surface. So, beginners should recheck the osteotomy with the aid of test rod in order to prevent a varus cut.

Tibial osteotomy may widen or narrow the flexion and extension gaps concomitantly according to the amount of resection; hence the difference between the two gaps does not change.

If the amount of resection is too small, alignment can be altered due to less cutting of the sclerotic bone on the medial side, the space becomes too narrow making it difficult to perform the operation, and the *PE is thinned to increase the incidence of wear dramatically*.

On the other hand, *if the amount of resection is too large, the tibial component size becomes smaller due to the funnel-shaped bony anatomy, and its bony support becomes weaker due to internal architecture of the tibial plateau*. Goldstein et al. suggested that resection of 20 mm or more would lead to structural changes causing a marked decrease in the supporting force. If more than 10 mm of resection is done on the thicker side in the CR type, it is needed to protect the PCL insertion site with special care.

Size and Rotation

The size of the tibial component is closely related to its rotational alignment. *When determining the size, good coverage is preferred theoretically, but good coverage may constrain*

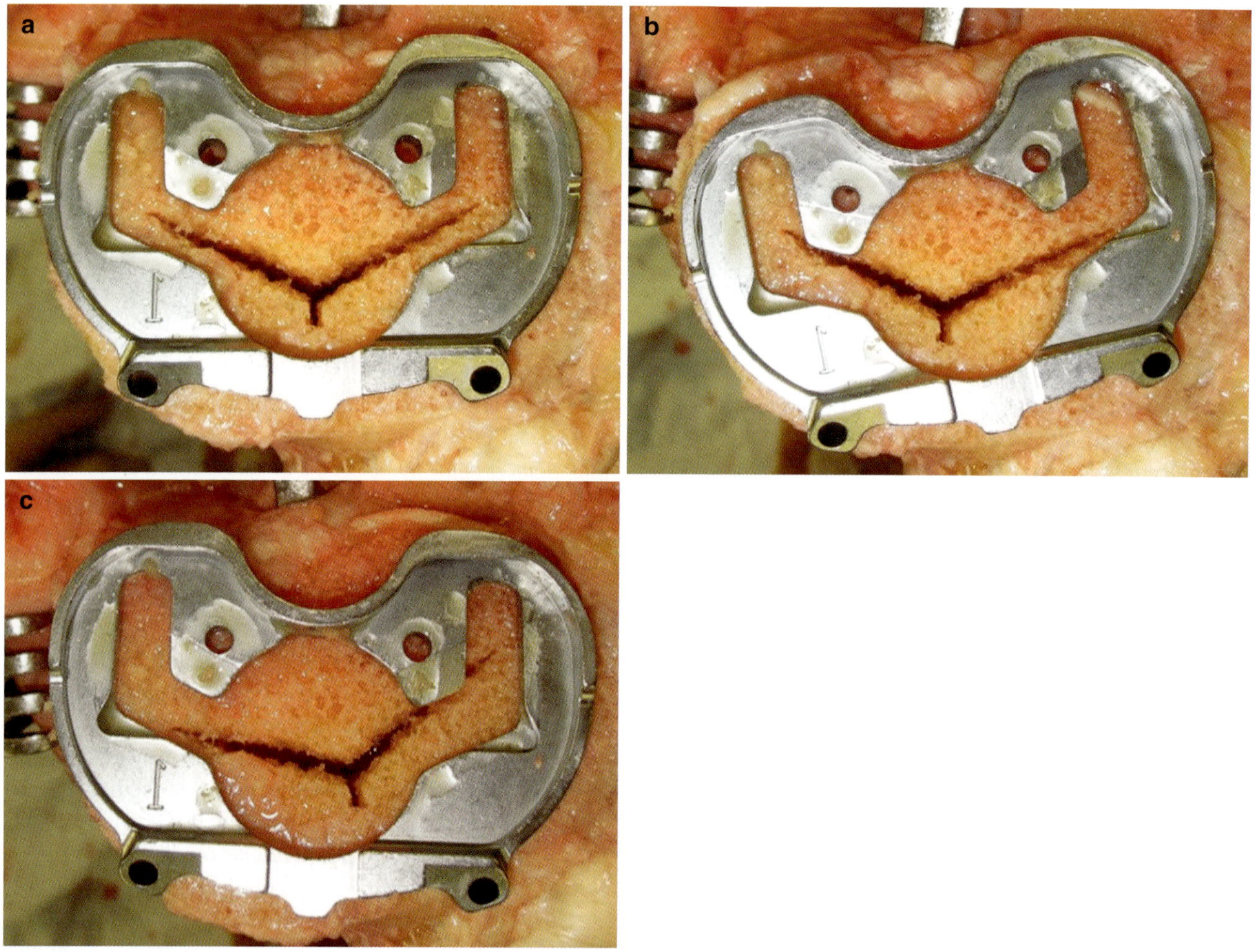

Fig. 4.36 Appropriate size and position of the tibial implant. (**a**) Neutral rotation. (**b**) External rotation. Excessive external rotation leads to posterolateral overhang of tibial prosthesis. (**c**) Internal rotation

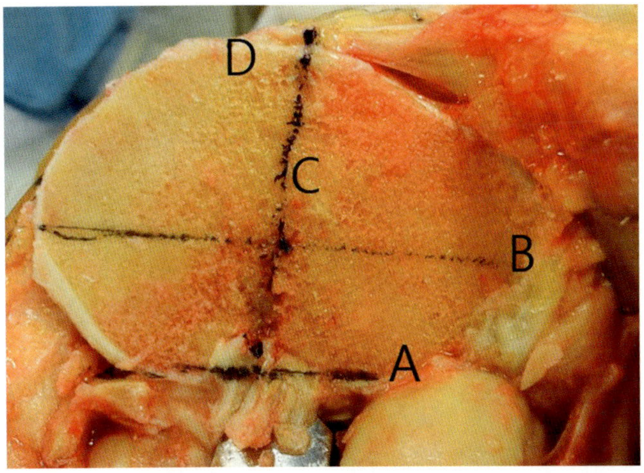

Fig. 4.37 Various rotational guideline of the tibial implant. A: posterior condylar axis, B: line along the largest distance between medial and lateral plateau, C: a line drawn from PCL insertion site to the center of plateau, D: medial 1/3 of tibial tubercle

the tibial external rotation as the medial condyle is 2–3 mm larger than the lateral condyle. If the size of the implant is fitted to the medial condyle, lateral overhang occurs. Therefore, a little smaller implant can be a better choice.

If the implant overhangs on the medial side, it irritates the MCL to cause pain and limited motion, and hence the implant should not overhang especially on the medial side. In case of a symmetric design, it is recommended to leave about 2 mm of bone on the medial side. The posterolateral portion allows for some overhang only to prevent internal rotation of the tibial implant as the LCL is a little away from the joint (Fig. 4.36).

There are several *methods for determining the tibial rotation*. Methods based on *anatomical landmarks* include using the axis of the most medial and lateral portion of the tibial plateau and using the axis of both the posterior condyles of the tibial plateau, aligning to the line drawn from insertion point of the PCL to the center of the plateau, a line connecting the midpoint of PCL to the medial border of patella tendon (Akagi line), medial one-third of the tibial tuberosity, and transepicondylar axis of femur. The aim of the rotational alignment is that the center of anterior portion of the tibial baseplate should be aligned with the tibial crest, which is equivalent to the medial one-third of the tibial tubercle (Fig. 4.37). Rotation can also be determined by *flexion and extension motion* (dynamic method). But this type of component positioning is subject to error if the leg is held with rotational force, the tourniquet is applied on the thigh, and the flexion gap is tight.

Many surgeons have reported quite different results and the navigation system is still not reliable for determining rotational alignment. Most of the surgeons prefer to use the method with the medial one-third of the tibial tuberosity as an anterior landmark. However Bonnin et al. reported that the use of the anterior tibial tubercle as a rotational landmark might cause several problems. First, orientation of the anterior tibial tuberosity may vary considerably with respect to the transepicondylar axis, which could induce excessive external rotation. Second, asymmetry between the medial plateau and the lateral plateau was more pronounced, which could compromise bone coverage of the tibial plateau. Finally, variations in morphology were greater. Khan et al. reported that reference axis based on posterior tibial condyles was most accurate and least variable for tibial component alignment among these methods. The fact that there are many methods to determine tibial rotation indicates that there is no established theory for the axis of rotation.

In conclusion, the shape of the plateau and the dynamic method can be used in combination with the transverse axis of the proximal tibia. However, internal rotation should be avoided. Nicoll and Rowley and Barrack et al. reported that *internal rotation of the tibia is closely related to patellar maltracking and postoperative pain*. Conversely, excessive external tibial component rotation may also result in abnormal patellar tracking as well as kinematic conflict in the tibiofemoral articulation such as notch–cam impingement in the PS type of prosthesis.

Preparation for Fixation

Once the size and rotation have been determined, preparation for fixation is done according to the manual of each implant. It is recommended to place the implant posteriorly if possible. If the prosthesis is located on the posterior side, it has a benefit in the ROM due to more rollback, it reduces stress on the patella, and it improves the lever action of the quadriceps muscle.

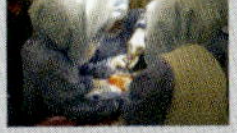

Author's Method

When performing tibial osteotomy, I always draw mechanical axis line to decide the proximal pilot point and a line perpendicular to the mechanical axis at the imaginary osteotomy level on preoperative X-ray to verify the alignment and the amount of osteotomy to be performed on the lateral plateau (Fig. 4.38).

I use the extramedullary method during tibial osteotomy. The proximal pilot point for coronal alignment is the point where the mechanical axis meets the tibia plateau on X-ray and the distal pilot point is the anterior tibial crest 2 in. above the ankle joint. The posterior slope

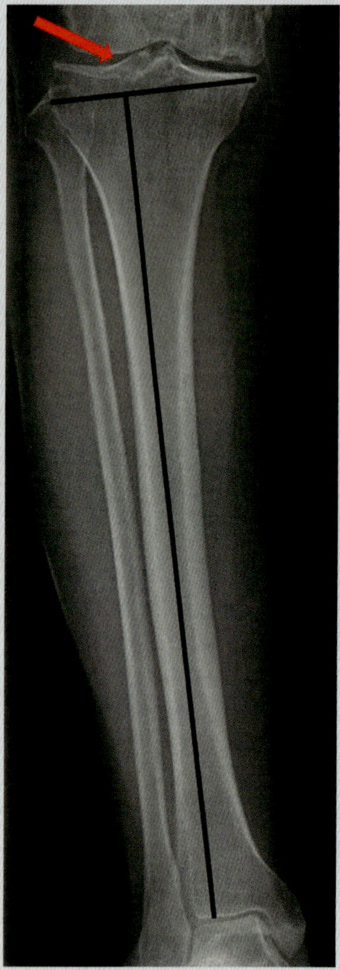

Fig. 4.38 Proximal tibial point (*arrow*) is moved to the lateral side in a severe varus deformity

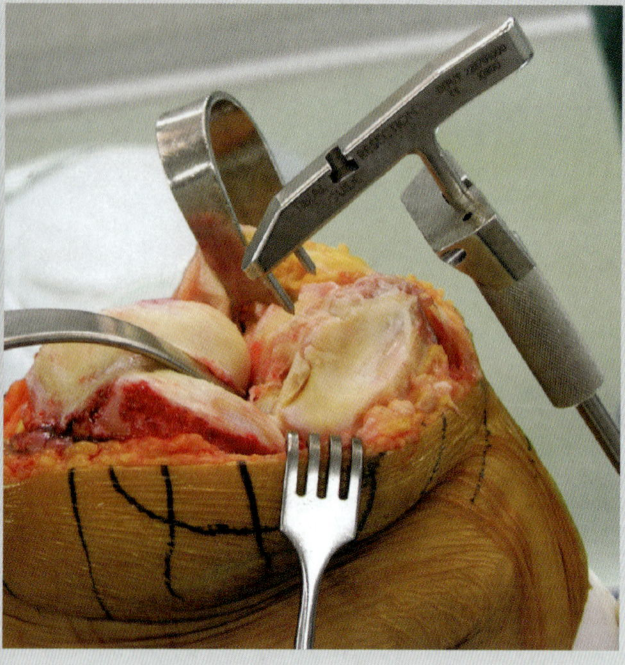

is determined according to the recommended angle for each implant. I try to perform about 1 mm of osteotomy on the thinner side (medial side in varus deformity) so as to expose some of the sclerotic bone, and I try not to exceed 10 mm of osteotomy on the thicker side (lateral side in varus deformity).

Once the cutting level is determined, pins are used for fixation of cutting jig. Fixation starts from the lateral side first because the bone on the medial side is harder and the pins may slip which can result in a change in the position of the cutting jig. I always use a drill for fixation of pin on the medial side.

For tibial cutting, cutting of the medial side is performed first and the cutting level is reassessed in order to verify the level of osteotomy. During the lateral osteotomy, I keep the saw blade within the bone to protect the patellar tendon. Also, every precaution is taken not to insert the saw blade too deep so as not to injure the iliotibial band.

In case of the CR type, I make every effort to preserve the PCL. Anatomically, the PCL is attached at the point 1 cm below the plateau. It is very hard to preserve the PCL when more than 1 cm of osteotomy is performed. In order to preserve the PCL when more than 1 cm of bone is resected, I make a bony island at the site where the PCL is attached, but extreme care is taken since avulsion fracture of the PCL may occur.

Since the subchondral bone can be pressed down when an osteotome is used as a lever to remove the resected bones, I lift up the osteotomized bone for removal.

After osteotomy, any bone remaining in the periphery of the lateral plateau is removed completely using the rongeur or saw, as this remaining bone can affect the size, location, and rotation of the prosthesis.

For the rotational alignment, I use the point of the medial one-third of the tibial tubercle and finally readjust by the dynamic method after insertion of trial implant. The size of tibial component is determined in relation to the femoral component. But I do not choose the implant which overhangs in the rotation-adjusted state. I prefer to use the plate size such that 2 mm of the medial plateau remains uncovered.

Before keeling of the sclerotic bones, I prefer to do sawing at the keel area before punching so as to prevent a fracture and migration of the prosthesis. If sclerotic bone is seen on the tibial surface, this area is drilled to allow decompression and for rigid cement fixation.

4.4.2.3 Patella

Restoration/reestablishment of physiological leg alignment, maintenance of Q angle and joint line, adequate component rotation, and balancing of the extensor mechanism are the key ingredients of a successful patellar surgery.

Resurfacing vs. Non-resurfacing

Before describing the patellar preparation, I would like to discuss as to whether to resurface the patella or not. In the early era of TKA, TKA was performed mainly in the patients with rheumatoid arthritis and patellar resurfacing was not done at that time. But resurfacing of the patella was introduced in 1974 with the Total Condylar system since patellofemoral pain was often reported postoperatively.

The purpose of patellar resurfacing is to reduce anterior knee pain and improve patellofemoral function. However, since the incidence of complications due to patellar resurfacing increased, the number of surgeons who did not prefer to resurface the patella also increased.

The controversy between patellar resurfacing and patellar non-resurfacing is due to the difference in the opinion regarding the *complications of patellar resurfacing*. The incidence of complications *of patellar resurfacing* varies greatly from 5 to 60 % according to the inclusion criteria of the complications.

There are surgeons who do routine patellar resurfacing and selective patellar resurfacing and who don't do resurfacing at all. Those who *prefer patellar resurfacing state that patella replacement reduces anterior knee pain, results in higher patient satisfaction and better overall function, and the incidence of complications caused due to patellar resurfacing is not very high* if the operation is successful. They particularly believe that *without patellar resurfacing, degenerative changes in the patella would worsen with time*. The articulation between the cartilage and the metal is considered nonphysiological, and *prolonged exposure to high compressive forces rapidly aggravates cartilage erosion*, even when cartilage erosion is not severe at the time of primary TKA. Soudry et al. reported that better clinical results were achieved after resurfacing, and Cameron and Fedorkow reported that it becomes easier to go up and down the stairs after patella resurfacing. Smith et al. stated that about 30 % of patients without resurfacing had anterior knee pain and about 40 % of patients gradually developed patellofemoral alignment problems. Wood et al. also stated that there was no difference in the revision rate between the patients with resurfacing and those without resurfacing, but the anterior knee pain was more severe in patients without resurfacing. Pavlou et al. reported the results of a comparative study through a meta-analysis of 7,075 cases which suggested that there was no significant difference between the resurfacing and non-resurfacing groups in terms of the incidence of anterior knee pain, but a higher reoperation rate was observed in the non-resurfacing group. They speculated that if the surgeon is not entirely satisfied with the overall soft tissue balance, it is preferable to perform patellar resurfacing so as to reduce the chances of reoperation. Shih et al. reported that about 40 % of patients developed patellofemoral arthritis and malalignment as a result of non-resurfacing at the 8.5-year follow-up, and these were closely related to the preoperative patellofemoral alignment. Pagnano et al. reported that about 50 % of revision was related to the problems with patellofemoral articulation due to non-resurfacing.

On the other hand, those surgeons who are *not in favor of patellar resurfacing* emphasize that *non-resurfacing can save time and cost, and reduce the patellar complications*. The values for the patellofemoral peak contact stress and contact area remain almost at the same level of those in the native knee if the patella was left unresurfaced. Following patellar resurfacing, patellofemoral contact stress increased beyond the yield strength of PE. They state that the *function of the patella is not that of a joint but that of a lever action which transmits the quadriceps power effectively*, and hence patella replacement is not needed. They suggested that the anterior knee pain in patients without resurfacing is not very different compared to that in patients with resurfacing and *anterior knee pain is not caused due to non-resurfacing in all cases. Also, fibrous tissue formation occurs between the articular surface of the patella and the femoral implant* after TKA, which *minimize the problems between the metal and the cartilage*. Enis et al. experienced *a lower incidence of lateral retinacular release in patients with non-resurfacing,* and Ranawat et al. reported that asymmetric resection occurred in about 7 % of operations in patients with patellar resurfacing. Sneppen et al. reported a subluxation rate of 14 % and a patellar tilt rate of 12 % in patients with resurfacing. Brick and Scott compared the revision rate between the patients with resurfacing and those without resurfacing, and no difference was noted; 2.5 % of patients with resurfacing and 2.4 % of patients without resurfacing underwent revision. Burnett et al. concluded through a 10-year follow-up study that patellar resurfacing is not required as there was no significant difference between the patients with resurfacing and those without resurfacing. But, they reported a higher complication rate in the non-resurfacing group in an article published at a later date.

Some surgeons who are not in favor of routine patellar resurfacing do *selective patellar resurfacing in cases of severe arthritis of the patellofemoral joint, rheumatoid arthritis* or any similar inflammatory arthritis or crystalline disease, *poor patellofemoral alignment, non-anatomical patella, or preoperative anterior knee pain*. Due to the difference in the modulus of elasticity, the articular surface of the patella adapts to the geometry of the opposing prosthetic surface by bedding-in. This process of remodeling which has been termed as "stress contouring" results in gradual adaptation of the retropatellar articular surface and subchondral bone to the shape of the trochlea. Keblish et al. have noted that *minimal remodeling is required if the patella is exposed to an anatomical design of the femoral component*, whereas excessive remodeling is observed in non-anatomical designs. Many surgeons believe that patellar resurfacing should be considered in patients with preoperative symptoms of patellofemoral arthritis. Rodriguez et al. reported that in Outerbridge grade IV patellofemoral arthritis, the revision rate was increased in patients without resurfacing. However, Bhan et al. reported that they achieved good results in patients with rheumatoid arthritis without patella replacement.

Also, those surgeons who prefer patella replacement do not resurface the patella if the patients are obese, young, and active with a relatively well-preserved articular cartilage or have severely eburnated patella with a poor bone stock of less than 15 mm in thickness. However, there is a difference in opinion regarding the obese patients. Bourne and Burnett suggested non-resurfacing when a patella-friendly femoral component is used in a young patient with mild patellofemoral arthritis and good patellofemoral alignment. In addition to these conditions, the patella should not be resurfaced when the patella is too small.

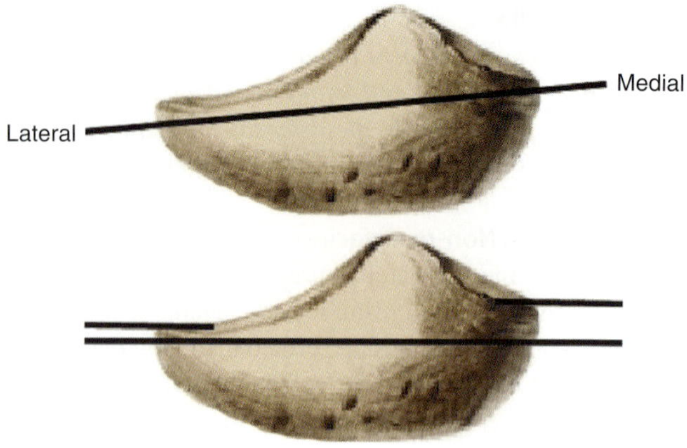

Fig. 4.39 The amount of medial and lateral resection of the patella. If the patella is cut parallel to the articular surface as shown in the *top image*, bone cut is made asymmetrically. The medial side should be cut more as shown in the *bottom image* to equalize the thickness of the remaining medial and lateral sides

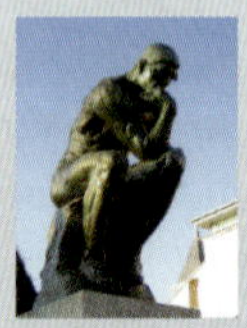

Author's Opinion

I perform patellar resurfacing in nearly every TKA case. The reason I prefer to perform patellar resurfacing is that it is a relative inexpensive procedure and does not take much time. I have experienced a few complications among more than 6,000 cases of patellar resurfacing, and revision arthroplasty due to development of anterior knee pain in patients without resurfacing has been reported quite frequently in the literature.

Rationale of patellar non-resurfacing seems reasonable, but non-resurfacing of the patella even in patients with severe osteoarthritis or rheumatoid arthritis may lead to problems. Hence, selective patellar resurfacing is recommended in such patients, even when the surgeon does not favor patella resurfacing.

Osteotomy

The goal of patellar osteotomy is to maintain the patellar thickness and improve patellofemoral alignment. The amount of resection depends on the pre-resurfacing patellar thickness so that the *post-resurfacing patellar thickness (composite thickness; total height of patellar shell plus patella implant) is equal or slightly lesser than the pre-resurfacing patellar thickness. If there is an increase in the patella composite thickness, it causes an increase in patellar pressure resulting in anterior knee pain, leads to early wear and/or loosening, or reduces joint motion due to poor patellofemoral tracking*. Greenfield et al. reported that the incidence of lateral retinacular release decreased from 55 % to 12 % by decreasing the composite thickness. Cho et al. and Yoshii et al. also reported that the incidence of patellar tilt decreased when the composite was not thicker than the native patella.

On the other hand, *if the patella is too thin, it weakens the quadriceps power* and perforation occurs when drilling the lug holes since the lug holes are located on the periphery, *thereby causing a patellar fracture*. Hence, many surgeons consider 12 mm to be the cutoff thickness for patellar osteotomy.

Patellar osteotomy can be done using an instrument or manually. *Cutting the same amount of bone on the medial and lateral sides will result in an asymmetric osteotomy because the lateral side is thinner than the medial side.* Therefore, *the medial side should be cut more than the lateral side* (Fig. 4.39). However, Chan and Gill observed that patellar tracking is improved when the patella is cut obliquely according to its natural shape; the medial side remaining thicker than the lateral side. After osteotomy, spurs on the periphery should be removed so that they do not cause irritation.

Position and Size

The position of the patellar component should be located on the medial side, as the anatomical position of the vertical ridge is located on the medial side. With regard to the position of the patella, Hofmann et al. reported that the ridge is about 3 mm medial to the center in normal anatomy, and Miller et al. recommended that it should be located at about 3.75 mm medially in the dome-shaped patellar component. While Anglin et al. recommended medialization of the patella by a maximum of 2.5 mm and

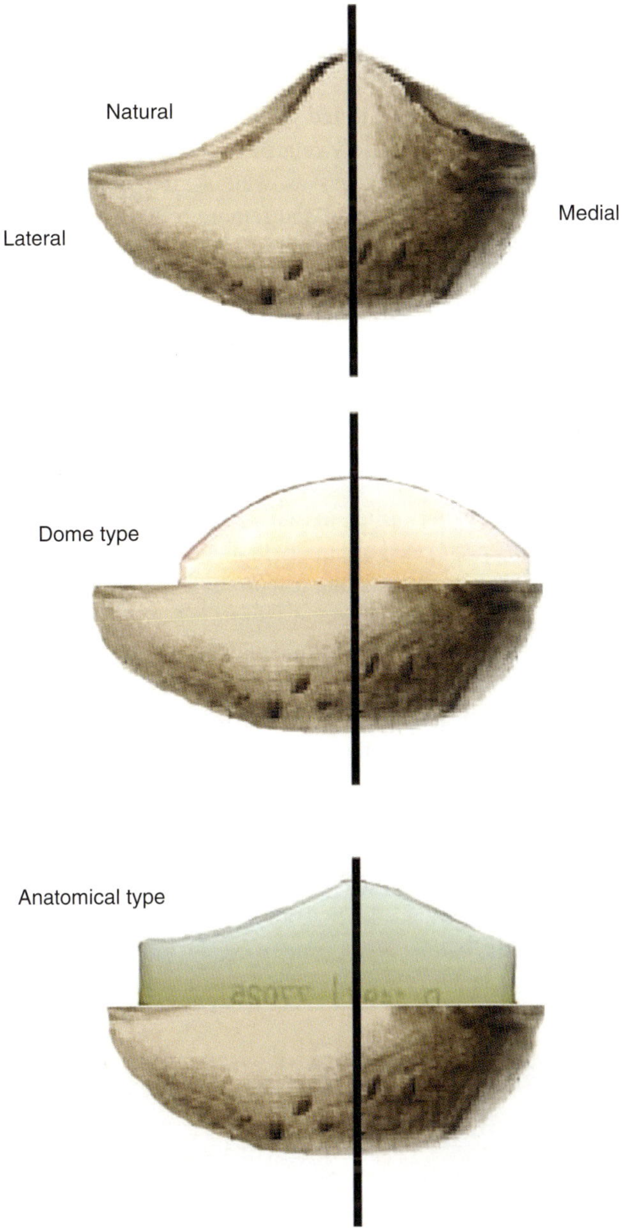

Fig. 4.40 The position of implant in patella replacement

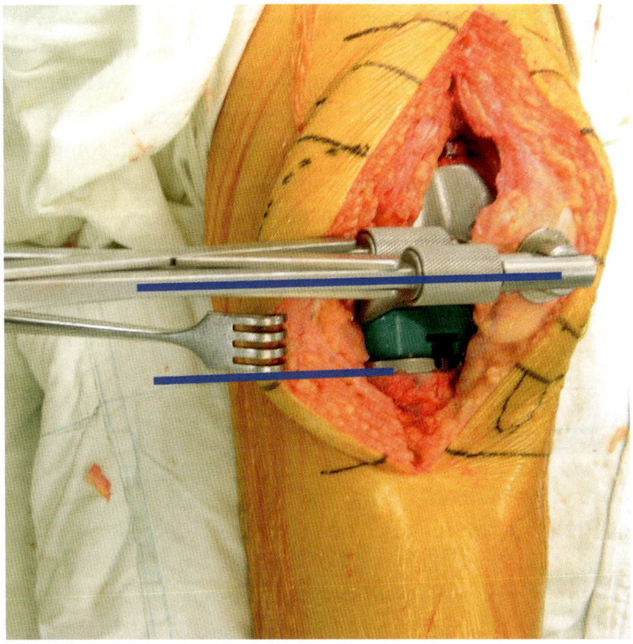

Fig. 4.41 Checking the rotational alignment of the patellar prosthesis of the anatomical type. The patellar axis should be parallel to the tibial prosthesis in extension

overzealous medialization leaves excessive bone exposed on the lateral patellar facet causing pain on contact with the femoral condyle.

Since an asymmetric patellar component is designed in the anatomical type, the ridge will be placed anatomically even if the implant is positioned in the center (Fig. 4.40).

In terms of patellar height, the height is reduced in about 50 % of TKAs, which makes it uncomfortable for the patients to go up and down the stairs. Hence, it is recommended to position the patella in the center or slightly proximal to the center. In case of patella baja, the patellofemoral compressive forces will be increased during early flexion and the overall range of motion is often compromised. On the other hand, patella alta is primarily associated with patellar instability and subluxation.

The size of the patellar component is to be determined considering the size of the patella and in correlation with the size of the femoral component. The size of the patellar component should neither be too small nor should the patella overhang. Most of the patellar sizes are compatible with the femoral sizes, but not all of them are compatible with each other.

When the patellar component design is oval or anatomical, it may worsen patellar tracking in case the axis is incorrect. Therefore, *it is necessary to align the patellar component along the flexion–extension axis, and it is regarded that the axis is aligned well when the patellar axis is parallel to the tibial component in extension* (Fig. 4.41). It is also recommended that the two lug holes should not be parallel to the joint line in order to reduce the risk of patellar fracture.

After preparing for resurfacing, it is important to remove all soft tissues surrounding the patella to prevent patellar clunk syndrome, to reduce pain, and to improve motion, especially when the PS type is used. During these procedures, the quadriceps tendon or patellar tendon should not be injured.

Almost all surgeons recommend patelloplasty when the patella is not resurfaced. The procedure is essentially aimed to re-create the shape and surface configuration of the patella similar to that of the natural patella. *Patelloplasty includes removal of spurs, smoothing of the articular surface, and drilling the sclerotic bone or resecting the articular surface on the lateral side of the patella, and/or cauterization along the peripheral margin of the patella* for a nerve block effect.

Zhang et al. reported that partial lateral facetectomy was an effective way to improve the function of patella-retaining TKA in patients with primary osteoarthritis. However, smoothing of the articular surface and drilling the sclerotic bone are controversial issues. Van Jonbergen et al. compared the effects of electrocautery with and without electrocautery. Electrocautery reduced the incidence of anterior knee pain, but the WOMAC score was similar to that in cases without electrocautery. However, Gupta et al. and Baliga et al. stated that the pain is not reduced with cauterization as was expected.

Patellar tracking is tested after insertion of the trial implants, and this is closely related to the implant size and patellar composite thickness as well as the position and external rotation of the tibial and femoral components. It is further described in this chapter under Sect. 4.5.

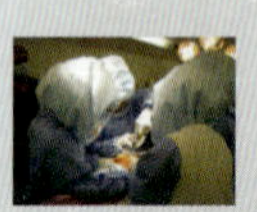

Author's Method

Before performing patella osteotomy, I measure the preoperative patellar thickness and then I perform the osteotomy while maintaining the thickness of the patella between 12 and 13 mm, because most of the Orientals have a smaller patella with an average thickness of 21 mm ranging from 20 to 23 mm.

Since the thickness of most of the patellar components is between 9 and 10 mm, the composite thickness ranges between 20 and 23 mm, which is the same or slightly lesser than the pre-resurfacing thickness. Some patients in whom the patellar thickness is less than 20 mm, I perform osteotomy as less as 11 mm (Fig. 4.42). If the preoperative patellar thickness is much lesser than 20 mm, I do not resurface the patella.

I usually perform osteotomy manually as most of patellar osteotomy instruments would slip off during the osteotomy. I personally stabilize the patella using one Lewin clamp which is larger than a towel clip (Fig. 2.56).

Osteotomy is performed in two steps. The medial side osteotomy is performed obliquely first and is followed by the finishing osteotomy. If the osteotomy is performed in one step, it results in a deeper osteotomy. Medial osteotomy is performed to a larger amount than lateral side and uniform thickness should be confirmed at every portion.

I place the patella on the medial side slightly mediolaterally and at the center or a little proximal supero-inferiorly.

The size of the patellar component is determined in relation to the femoral component and patella bone, and patellar overhang is avoided. The bone exposed to a large extent is removed and denervation with cauterization is done when the patella is not resurfaced.

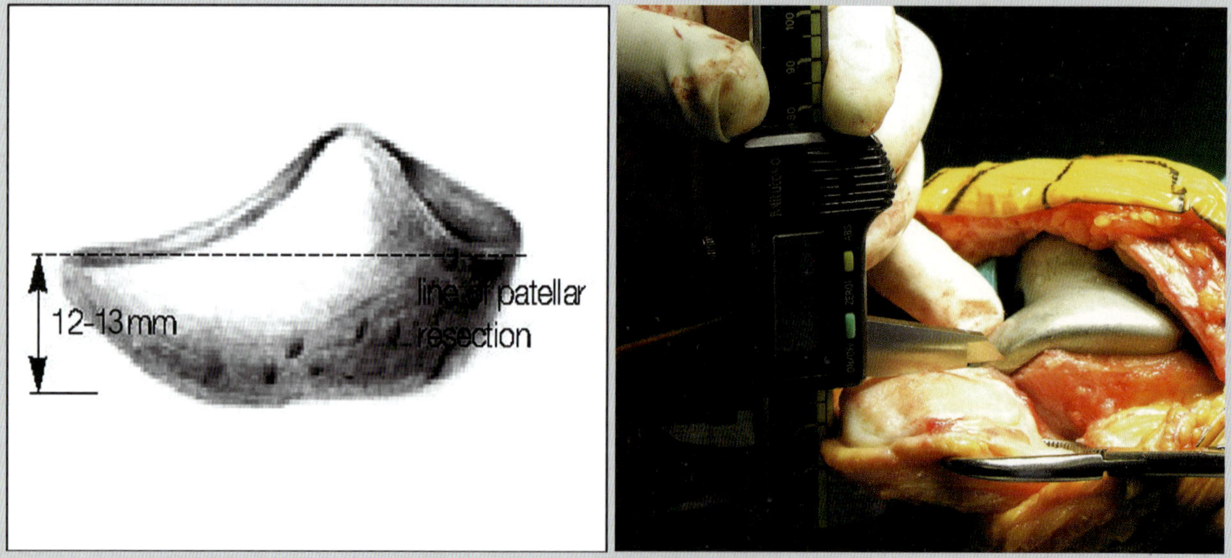

Fig. 4.42 Amount of patellar resection and measurement of the thickness of the patella

4.5 Balancing

If balancing is not performed properly during TKA, the patient experiences instability and pain from the early postoperative period, he/she suffers from walking difficulty due to giving way, and the incidence of early wear and loosening increases. Therefore, balancing is the most important procedure in TKA. Balancing includes flexion and extension gap balancing, mediolateral balancing, and patellofemoral balancing.

4.5.1 Flexion and Extension Gap Balancing

4.5.1.1 Causes of Imbalance

Gap imbalance can be caused as a result of an *incorrect osteotomy, improper size of the femoral prosthesis, and inadequate ligament balance*. Among these, more femoral distal cutting and improper size of the femoral prosthesis usually predispose to gap imbalance in most of cases. The posterior cruciate ligament also has a critical impact on gap balancing. Mihalko and Krackow reported that the flexion gap is widened on an average by more than 5.2 mm when the *posterior cruciate ligament is sacrificed,* and Cho et al. also reported that sacrificing the posterior cruciate ligament widens both the flexion and extension gaps, and the flexion gap is increased more than the extension gap by *an average of 2.8 mm.*

4.5.1.2 Checkup

Flexion and extension gap balance can be checked with the gapper or tensioner or by the flexion and extension motion after insertion of the trial implant. The *common method is to use the gapper or tensioner*. Lamina spreader may also be used, but the findings may be inaccurate when used by the inexperienced surgeons. Theoretically, *the gap should be same in flexion and extension without tightening or loosening when the same forces are applied. The method of using trial implants* involves checking the gap balance while flexing and extending the knee joint with insertion of trial implants after osteotomy. Scott uses the *POLO (pullout, lift-off) method* to check the flexion gap for the CR type. This method implies that *there is an adequate flexion gap if the selected thickness of composite (tibial plate + PE) cannot be pulled out easily by hands and is not lifted off when the knee is flexed by 80–100°* (Fig. 4.43).

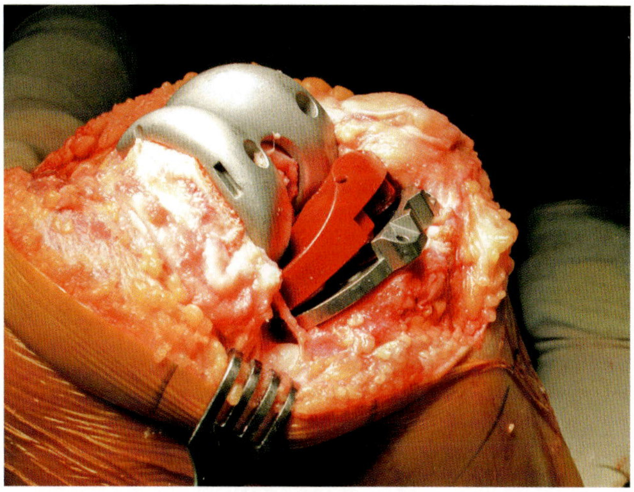

Fig. 4.43 If the flexion gap is narrow, the anterior portion of the PE spacer is lifted

There are other signs of a narrow flexion gap. *If the posterior cruciate ligament is too tight or excessive rollback occurs in the CR type, it indicates that the flexion gap is narrow*. In addition, when a crepitus sound is heard during flexion, when the flexion motion is limited, or when the femoral component or tibial composite translates forward during flexion, it also indicates that the flexion gap is narrow. On the other hand, the flexion gap is wide if the spacer can be inserted easily or shows instability in flexion state.

It is regarded that the *flexion and extension gap balance is good if the knee joint can be extended completely without hyperextension or flexion contracture when a composite of correct thickness for the flexion gap is inserted. If hyperextension of the knee develops, it indicates that the extension gap is wide and if a flexion contracture persists, it indicates that the extension gap is narrow.*

A wide extension gap and a narrow flexion gap both refer to similar conditions because the same phenomenon occurs with the change of the thickness of the PE. This is also applicable to a narrow extension gap and a wide flexion gap.

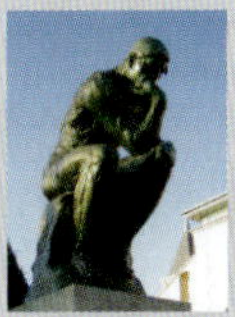

Author's Opinion

I use the gapper or tensioner whenever it is available and recheck the flexion and extension gap balance with the trial implant.

I use the PS type in almost all the cases. I select a thickness of the tibial composite that can be inserted with a little resistance and the composite should not be very loose in 90° flexion. Then, I check the condition of the knee in extension. I deduce that there is a good gap balance when there is neither a flexion contracture nor hyperextension.

However, the post of the PS type plays some role in preventing hyperextension, and hence hyperextension may not occur even though the extension gap is a little wider. For example, if a 15 mm PE is the correct thickness for the extension gap, hyperextension will not occur even when a 12 mm PE is tested with the PS type.

If hyperextension does not occur, it may be thought that it does not cause any clinical problem. But it is highly likely to increase stress on the post, thereby accelerating the wear of the post at the long-term follow-up. Therefore, when the PS type is used, use of the CR type of PE or gradually increasing the thickness of PS type of PE for testing is recommended (Fig. 4.44).

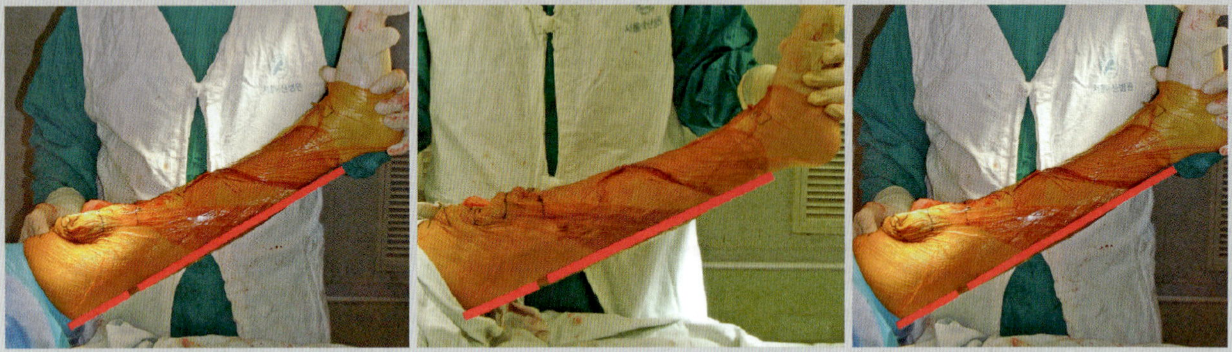

Fig. 4.44 Extension of the knee with a 12 mm CR type of PE (*left*), 15 mm CR type of PE (*middle*), and 12 mm PS type of PE implant (*right*). The knee in the *left image* shows hyperextension, but it will not be hyperextended if the same thickness of the PS type of PE is used like that in the *right image*

4.5.1.3 Correction of Gap Discrepancy

Narrow Flexion Gap (Wide Extension Gap)

If the flexion gap is narrow, it can be classified as a *narrow gap on both the anterior and posterior sides and a narrow gap on the posterior side only. If the flexion gap is narrow on the posterior side only, the tibial slope can be increased or PCL recession can be done.* However PCL recession is not recommended due to lack of reproducibility. If the flexion gap is narrow on both the sides, *a smaller femoral prosthesis can be used in the ARS for more posterior cutting or the PS type can be used to widen the flexion gap in case the CR type was planned for use* initially.

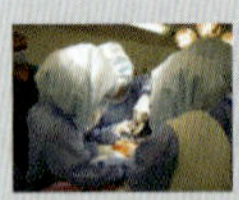

Author's Method

In case of a wide extension gap, I perform slice bone graft on the distal cut surface of femur to decrease the extension gap and use a thinner PE which is compatible with the flexion gap. By doing so, the extension gap is decreased and the chamfer portion is filled with cement. When it is intended to decrease the extension gap only with the use of cement, it is difficult to control the extension gap because the curing time from the dough stage of the cement is very short.

The slice bone is taken from the osteotomized autograft. What is important is that the thickness of the sliced bone should be greater than the intended extension gap restoration as the cancellous bone tends to get compressed (Fig. 4.45).

Recently, I use Choren pad which I designed to decrease the extension gap.

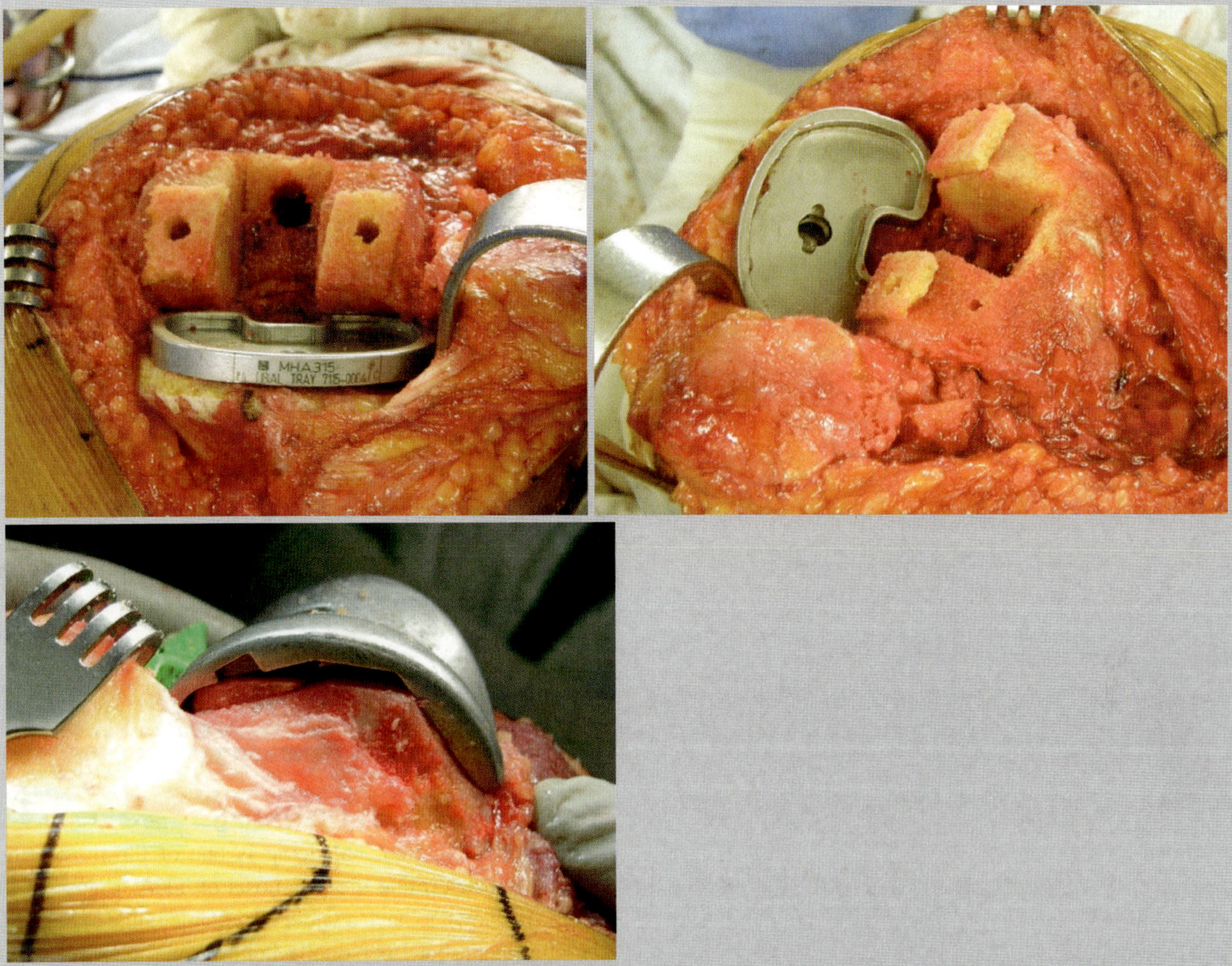

Fig. 4.45 A slice bone graft to decrease the extension gap

Wide Flexion Gap (Narrow Extension Gap)

If the extension gap is narrow, the easiest way to achieve gap balance is to perform more distal cutting. However, this elevates the joint line to alter the knee joint mechanics and weakens the quadriceps power. Therefore, distal cutting should not be more than 2 mm in the CR type and be 4–5 mm in the PS type. Using a femoral component that is one size larger and augmenting the posterior part is another option. This method is described under Sect. 5.2.1.3. *If a flexion contracture of 5 ~ 10° persists, posterior release is recommended.* By performing posterior release, the extension gap is increased more than the flexion gap.

It is acceptable if the flexion gap is a little wider in spite of the above procedures. This is because, the ROM increases as the flexion gap increases and the flexion gap can be decreased by relocation of the everted patella in situ and by flexion of the knee joint. Gejo et al. revealed that the flexion gap is decreased by about 1.9 mm at 90° flexion and by 5.5 mm at 135° flexion. There is no established theory regarding how much width of the flexion gap can be permitted. Some surgeons insist that the increase of the flexion gap can be up to 4–5 mm in the PS type. *If the flexion gap is too wide, thereby causing flexion instability, the use of a constrained type should be considered.*

More cutting of the tibia or changing the thickness of the PE does not balance the extension and flexion gap discrepancy, and this would only worsen the situation (Table 4.1).

Table 4.1 Factors affecting the extension and flexion gaps in TKA and the relevant changes

		Extension gap	Flexion gap
Femoral component (anterior reference system)	Upsizing	–	↓
	Downsizing	–	↑
Distal femur manipulation	Augmentation	↓	–
	Resection	↑	–
PE insert (spacer)	Thinner	↑	↑
	Thicker	↓	↓
Proximal tibia manipulation	Resection	↑	↑
	Posterior slope↑	–	↑
	Posterior slope↓	–	↓
Posterior capsule release		↑↑	↑
PCL resection		↑	↑↑

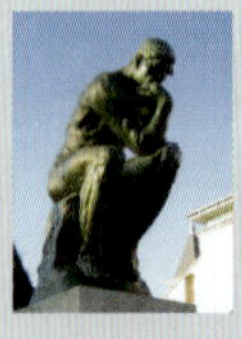

Author's Opinion

I agree that it is desirable to balance the flexion and extension gaps, but I have a strong doubt about whether it is essential.

I accept a little wider flexion gap because of the following reasons. First, when deciding the size of the femoral implant in the ARS, a smaller femoral implant is recommended when it is an in-between size. This means that a little wider flexion gap is permissible. Second, sacrificing the PCL widens the flexion gap by at least 2 mm more than the extension gap, but the CR type and the PS type of prosthesis have an equal A–P length even though *the PS type has an effect in increasing* the flexion gap. Third, a wider flexion gap is related to stability in flexion. As squatting is not allowed after TKA, the biggest problem of wide flexion gap is going up and down the stairs. If instability is not severe, the muscle strength can overcome the difficulties of stair walking. Fourth, the extension and flexion gap is tested with patellar eversion, but the flexion gap is actually decreased due to quadriceps tension when the patella is returned to its anatomical position and when the knee joint is flexed. Fifth, a wider flexion gap clearly increases the range of flexion and reduces stress on the PE in flexion.

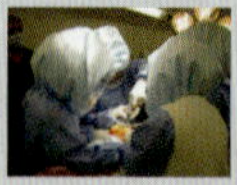

Author's Method

I try not to leave any flexion contracture uncorrected intraoperatively. I use different techniques according to the degree of flexion contracture that exists after the insertion of a PE of adequate thickness in a flexion state.

If the flexion contracture is more than 15° pre- and intra-operatively, I perform more distal osteotomy from the beginning. If the flexion contracture is less than 15°, I perform posterior release.

I allow a little wider flexion gap in patella everted state because the flexion gap decreases when the patella is brought back to its anatomical position and is held with a towel clip. If the flexion gap is wider than the acceptable range, thereby causing flexion instability with this method, I use the constrained type of implant.

4.5.2 Mediolateral Balancing

4.5.2.1 Importance of Balancing

Mediolateral ligament balancing is one of the most critical factors that determine the prognosis of TKA. Ligament balancing is known to have a wider acceptable range compared to the alignment, but I personally believe that balancing should be addressed more accurately than alignment, because instability causes difficulty in walking from the immediate postoperative period and it affects the long-term result more severely.

Accurate mediolateral balancing is particularly important in the PS type due to the absence of cruciate ligaments for stability of the knee joint and due to its relation with the range of motion. Matsuda et al. reported that the range of motion was decreased by about 11° when the mediolateral imbalance was more than 2°.

4.5.2.2 Definition of Imbalance

Although it is difficult to define imbalance, *the joint space should not be trapezoidal in shape, but it should be rectangular when the limb is distracted with an even force, and it should neither be tight nor loose on any side after insertion of the trial implant or the real implant in extension.*

The flexion gap should be rectangular. But, it is a generally accepted concept that the lateral side can be allowed to be wider than the medial side in flexion. However Matsumoto et al. emphasized that the soft tissue tension patterns differ between everted and reduced patellae state as well as between PS and CR TKA.

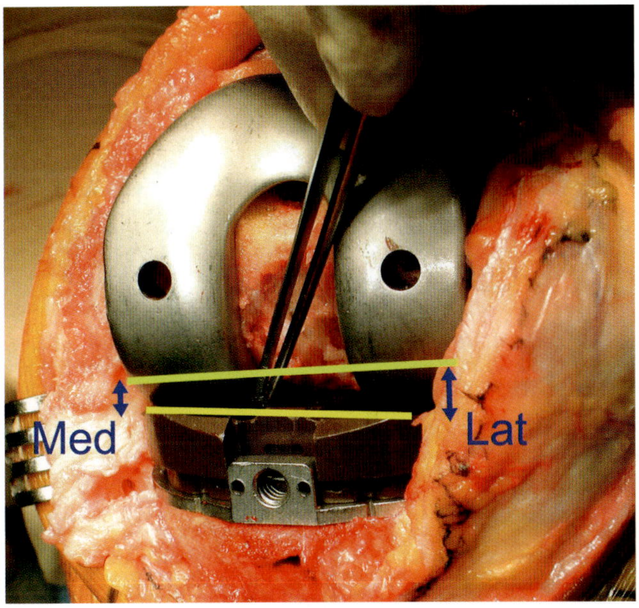

Fig. 4.46 If the medial portion is not released adequately, the medial portion is too tight and the lateral portion is opened

There are many intraoperative signs of imbalance. *When the PE can be inserted easily into one side but it is difficult to insert it into the other side*, when the ligament *shows bowstring pattern instead of a fan belt pattern* after insertion of the trial implant or fixation of the implant, *when one side is compressed while the other side is opened up after insertion of trial implant, and when the pivot phenomenon occurs along the axis of the compressed condyle* in flexion–extension motion, *they all indicate that there is a mediolateral imbalance* (Fig. 4.46).

Recently tibial trial liners with load-bearing and alignment sensors are introduced for ligament balancing. They can graphically show quantitative compartment load-bearing force and component track patterns.

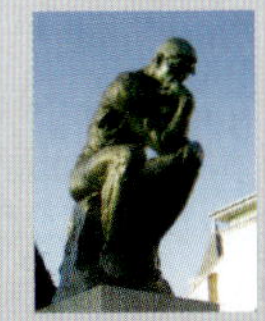

Author's Opinion

I have a different opinion regarding the theory that the medial and the lateral gap in flexion should be equal after osteotomy.

I think the goal of gap balancing is to have an even tension on both the sides after closure of the wound. But it is impossible to check the tension in this state, and it is considered that even distance has even tension regardless of whether or not the implant is inserted and whether or not the wound is closed. However, the tension can be altered according to the implant design, patella position and suture of the arthrotomy site, etc.

For example, multi-radius femoral component has asymmetric condyles. If both the sides are balanced after osteotomy, balance may be impaired after insertion of implant of this design. If the knee is flexed with the patella in an everted state, more tension is loaded on the lateral side, thereby opening up the medial side, particularly when the PCL is sacrificed. This is evident by opening up of the medial side when the PCL is resected, which was in neutral tension on both the sides before resection of the PCL (Fig. 4.47). So, it is not paradoxical but natural that the medial side is more widened in the PS type when the knee is flexed at 90° with the patella everted. And the tension before and after closure of the wound may vary.

A better method is to check the tension on both the sides with the patella returned to its natural position and the arthrotomy site held by a towel clip. With this method, the eccentric force due to patellar eversion will become neutral. However, it is also difficult to check practically in this state.

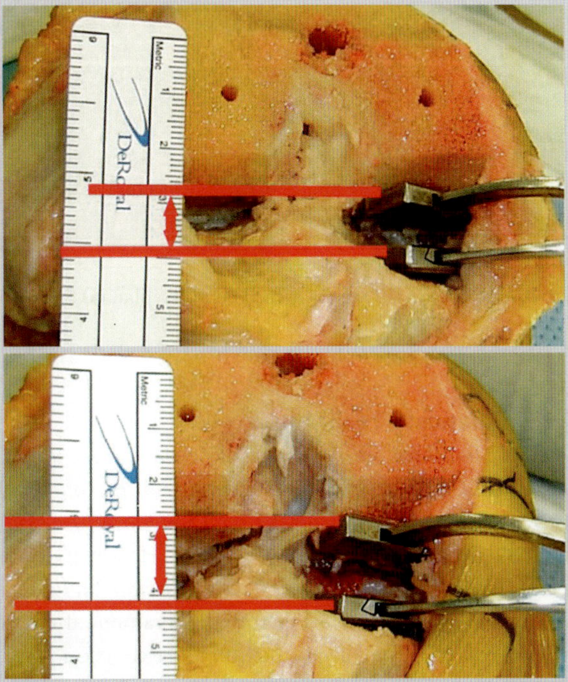

Fig. 4.47 Difference in the medial opening before/after sacrificing the PCL. *Left*: before sacrificing the PCL, *right*: after sacrificing the PCL

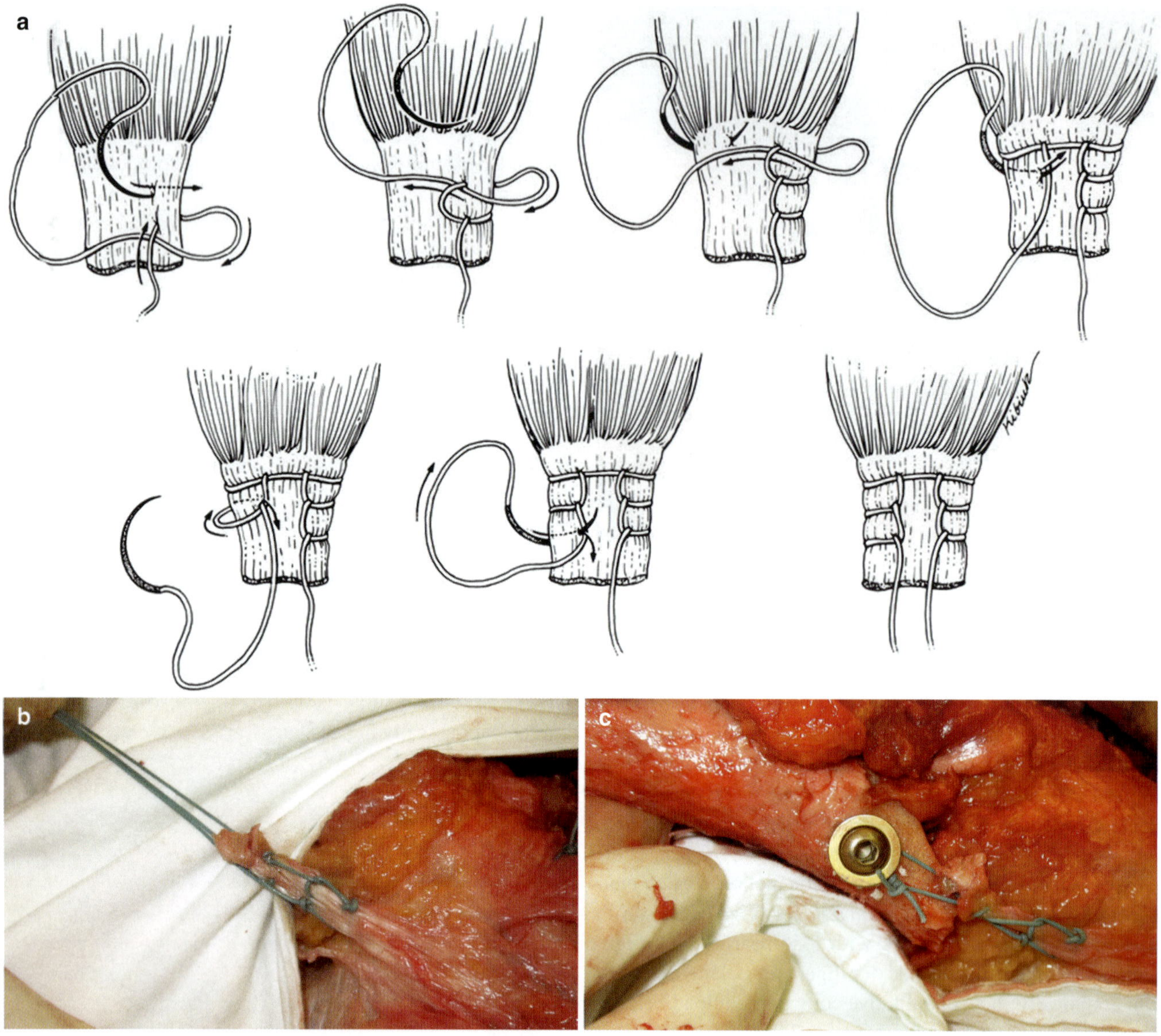

Fig. 4.48 Krackow's advancement method of fixation. (a) Schematic drawing (under the permission of Krackow KA), (**b**) after suture, (**c**) after advancement

4.5.2.3 Balancing Techniques

In general, ligament balancing is done thrice: after the ACL and meniscal resection in the early stage of the operation, when performing testing with the trial implant after osteotomy, and after fixation of the real implant. However, *in case of a mobile-bearing joint, it is desirable to establish ligament balance in the first step* as balancing the ligament after osteotomy can cause imbalance of flexion and extension gap.

It is recommended to release on the contracture side than to reef the relaxed ligament. This is because reefing is unreliable. Krackow stated that superolateral advancement of the LCL is better than using the constrained type of implant in exceptional cases when the deformity cannot be corrected by any of the methods. He stated that the cause of failed advancement is an insecure fixation method and poor rehabilitation and suggested a new advancement method (Fig. 4.48).

With regard to the PCL resection, Insall and Laskin emphasized that *ligament balancing cannot be achieved without PCL resection* if there is a severe varus deformity of more than 15°. However, Krackow and Matsueda disagree with the opinion of Insall and Laskin because PCL resection causes discrepancy between the extension and flexion gap.

If balancing cannot be achieved by any other method, using a constrained type is the last resort. If ligamentous tissues are elongated, it is recommended to detach the ligaments with the bone and fix it to the bone proximally with screws even though a constrained type of implant is used (Fig. 4.49).

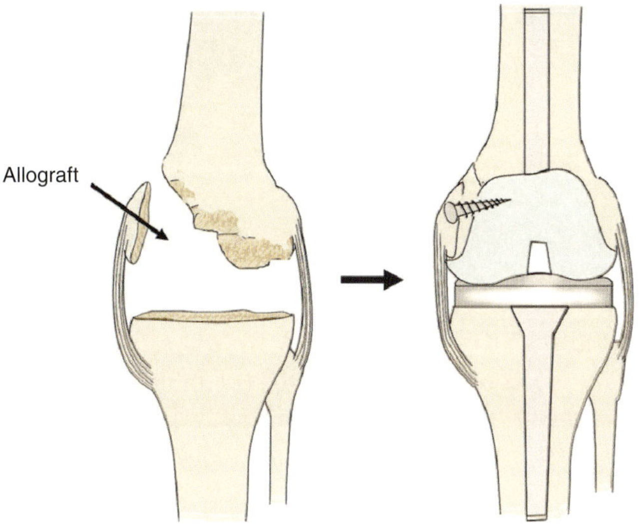

Fig. 4.49 Fixation of the bone–ligament composite

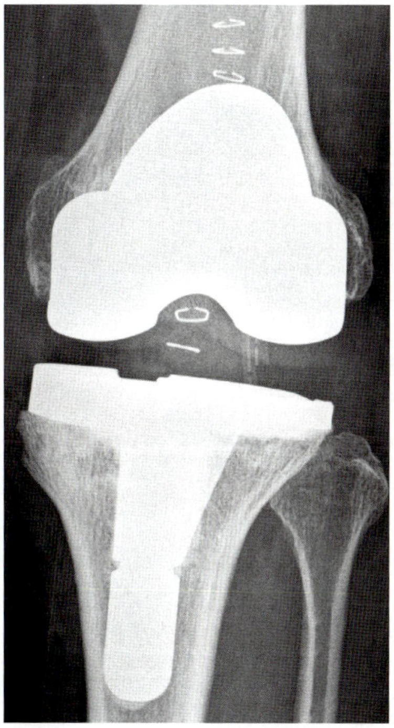

Fig. 4.50 Incomplete release of MCL. Medial side is tightened and lateral side is opened

Medial Release

Most patients with osteoarthritis show a certain degree of varus deformity regardless of the bone defect. When degenerative changes develop on the medial side, a contracture would occur at the medial capsule or the MCL and would be accompanied by relaxation of the LCL and a flexion contracture. The goal is to establish ligament balance while the femorotibial alignment is in a 5–10° valgus state.

In case of a varus deformity, release is generally performed on the tibial side. When release is performed in the form of a sleeve, ligament tissues will be scarred with thick fibrous connective tissues, and their functioning is not affected. But, if the MCL is cut transversely, it may cause functional loss; hence this should be avoided. Lee and Lotke experienced residual instability when an additional procedure was not performed in patients with intraoperative MCL injury which occurred due to transection of the MCL during osteotomy.

Most of the surgeons agree that *release of the MCL and pes anserinus is to be done step by step until balance is established.* If the deformity is not severe, the desired effect can be achieved simply by releasing the superficial MCL. *Clayton et al. recommended releasing the MCL up to 5–6 cm before the insertion site of pes anserinus.* Laskin classified the varus deformity into three types. He stated that the deformity should be tested under anesthesia as pain influences the balancing. The first type is a flexible deformity that gets corrected to normal alignment with a passive force, the second type is a fixed deformity that does not get corrected to normal alignment with a passive force, and the third type is a mixed deformity that is partially correctable. He recommended release only when the deformity is not correctable passively.

Alternatively, pie-crusting technique of the MCL can be performed with a 16 gauge needle by making multiple punctures. Whiteside introduced the *selective release technique depending on the MCL tightness in extension and flexion. In MCL tightness in extension, he recommended release of the posterior part of the MCL, and in MCL tightness in flexion, he recommended release of the anterior portion of the MCL.*

Some surgeons worry about the complete detachment, while the others believe that it is not a problem as instability does not occur, and this is just like the conservative treatment of the MCL tear. *Insall et al. emphasized that at least 7–8 cm of the MCL should be released to achieve the balancing in severe varus deformity*. In such a situation, the MCL is likely to be detached completely. Vince et al. stated that *the most common cause of imbalance is not excessive release, but incomplete release*. When balancing is not achieved and the MCL is partially detached, the MCL becomes tense due to incomplete release (Fig. 4.50). When weight bearing is started in this state, the MCL will be completely detached, thereby causing instability. When the signs of imbalance are noted during the operation, which have been described before, releasing the contracture on the tight side until the balance is established and using a thicker PE will solve the problem.

If balance cannot be achieved by releasing the superficial MCL, *release of the pes anserinus should be performed.* In such a situation, *the knee can be balanced in extension, but the medial portion will open up more when the knee is flexed*

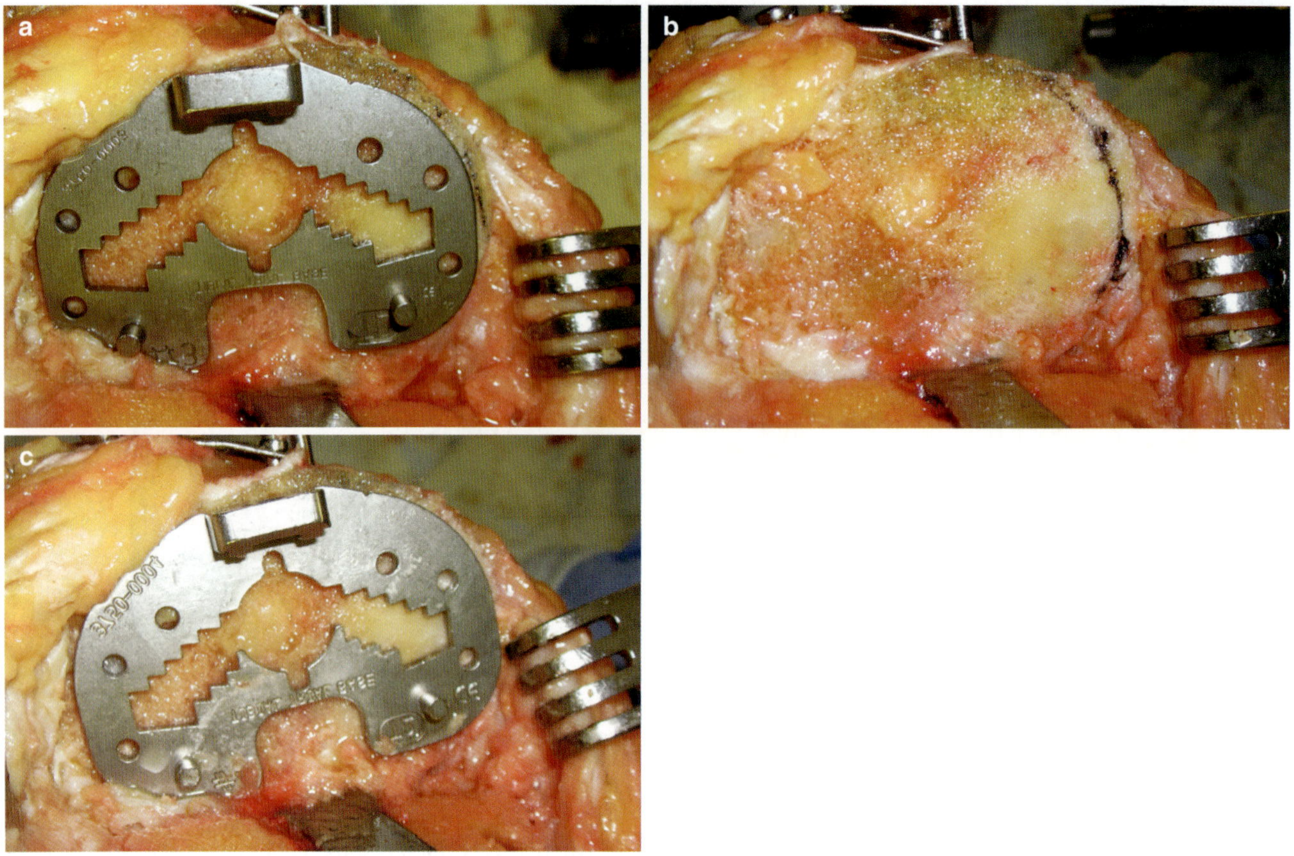

Fig. 4.51 Shift and resection method. (**a**) Correct size of implant is placed. Tight MCL is retracted. (**b**) Medial side of the tibia is to be resected. (**c**) Smaller tibial plate is used and shifted to the laterally

at 90°. This effect is even more prominent when the PCL is sacrificed. Some surgeons perform the release of the semimembranosus tendon from the beginning, while the others leave it until the end or perform partial release of the semimembranosus tendon.

When medial opening in flexion is noted, the surgeon should recheck for possible excessive external femoral rotation, a varus tibial resection, or full thickness damage to the superficial MCL. If there are no such errors as have been described above, mild medial opening of the flexion gap should be accepted. Insall insisted that a little larger than normal medial gap has no clinical consequences, but an excessive lateral gap can lead to posterolateral subluxation. In this case, the knee joint should be protected for a certain period of time until the development of scar adhesions, which includes the use of brace fitting and pursuance of postoperative rehabilitation in flexion less vigorously than usual.

As an alternative to medial release, *Dixon et al. suggested the "shift and resection" method*, which is partial resection of the medial tibial condyle along with the use of a smaller implant that is shifted to the lateral side to achieve the effect of MCL release (Fig. 4.51).

Engh et al. introduced medial epicondylar osteotomy as an alternative to medial soft tissue release (Fig. 4.52). It involves medial epicondylar osteotomy measuring 1 × 4 cm along with the MCL and leaving the osteotomized fragment unfixed. About 54 % of patients showed bony union postoperatively and the others showed fibrous union, which did not cause any serious functional disturbance.

Although this method does not cause damage to the soft tissues, it is not recommended in routine cases. It may be applied to revision TKA, allograft prosthetic component (APC), or ankylosed knee. Avulsion fracture of the medial epicondyle occurs occasionally while inserting the prosthesis when the medial side is tight. In such a situation, it is not necessary to fix the avulsed fragment, as it can be considered to be a natural medial epicondylar osteotomy.

If the LCL is too relaxed, one alternative to lateral collateral advancement is to release the MCL and reduce the amount of distal osteotomy of the femur.

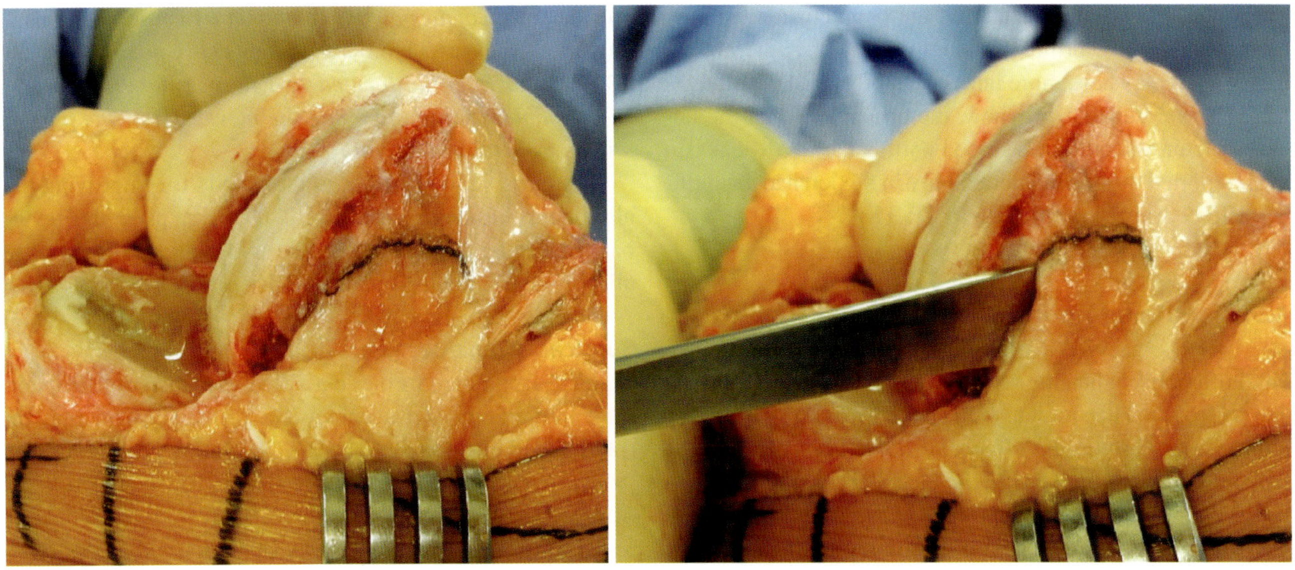

Fig. 4.52 Medial epicondylar osteotomy

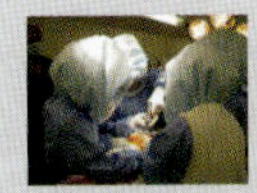

Author's Method

I use the periosteal elevator for release of the MCL from the anterior portion of the semimembranosus tendon and follow Claytons' suggestion to release the MCL up to 3–4 cm beneath the pes anserinus. I examine the balancing at this point and release the MCL more if needed.

However in many cases, I had to release the MCL up to 7–8 cm or detach the MCL completely as recommended by Insall. But, none of my patients complained of instability postoperatively. I try not to release the pes anserinus and the semimembranosus tendon as it can cause instability in flexion.

When performing complete release, I take special care so as not to create valgus alignment, to ensure that the lateral space is neither tight nor loose, and to place the detached MCL in situ. I believe that the lateral space is critical for instability when MCL is completely detached. If the lateral space is tight, the medial space is bound to open up, and if the lateral side is loose, both medial and lateral instability may occur.

As mentioned before, the optimal balance in flexion is tested by placing the patella in situ and holding it with a towel clip. If the knee is unstable or if the medial side still opens up in flexion intraoperatively, the ligament balance is readjusted and the PE thickness is changed, or the constrained type is used.

If the patient complains of instability when he/she starts walking, I perform the stress test. If the knee joint is unstable as per the stress test, I prescribe brace fitting for 6 weeks. If the knee joint is stable as per the stress test, I encourage performing muscle strengthening exercises.

Lateral Release

Valgus deformity of the knee joint is not as common as a varus deformity, and hence not many surgeons are familiar with it. It is difficult to correct valgus deformity because release of the contracture of the lateral compartment is very complicated.

The lateral approach suggested by Keblish or Buechel not only includes the skin incision but also lateral release of the soft tissues. The lateral release according to the principle of Keblish is partly described in this chapter under "Approach," and the method of lateral release in severe valgus deformity including iliotibial band and lateral structure is described in detail in Sect. 5.2.1.2.

The most controversial issue of the lateral release which can be found infrequently during checking the mediolateral balancing is whether to release the popliteus tendon when lateral side is tight. Kesman et al. evaluated the effect of resection of the popliteus tendon on knee ligament balancing in extension and flexion intraoperatively using posterior-stabilized TKA. They reported that resection of the popliteus tendon does not appear to change the static balance of the knee joint. They emphasized that the popliteus tendon may not have the same critical function in TKA, as the arthroplasty itself may have more inherent stability and the patients have a lower demand. Anyhow, the principle is that the lateral structures should be released until balanced. Kobayashi et al. reported that slack lateral laxity in flexion had a significant effect during knee flexion in CR TKA.

4.5.3 Patellofemoral Balancing

Patellofemoral balancing is closely related to the function and pain of the knee joint as well as the long-term survival of arthroplasty. *Patellar malalignment can cause anterior knee pain, motion limitation, instability*, patellar fracture, or quadriceps and patellar tendon rupture. Bindelglass et al. reported that the patella was in a neutral position on X-rays in only 54.7 % of the patients, while Laughlin et al. reported that the patella was in a neutral position in 62 % of patients. Laughlin et al. stated that poor patellar tracking leads to a higher risk of wear due to the cold flow. However despite these general concepts, Bindelglass et al. reported the results of the use of the all-poly patellar component, which suggested that maltracking was not related with the clinical results including pain, range of motion, and loosening.

Some surgeons state that patellar tracking does not change as time elapses, whereas Laughlin et al. reported that the lateral tilt aggravated with time due to the change of quadriceps mechanics and the scar contracture caused by lateral retinacular release.

4.5.3.1 Causes of Malalignment

Malalignment of the patellofemoral joint can be caused by three factors: patient-related factors, implant design, and surgical techniques.

Patient-Related Factors

Patient-related factors are those in which the causes of malalignment are already present in the knee joint preoperatively. Chan et al. found that preoperative patellofemoral malalignment is closely related to postoperative malalignment, and every 2° increase in preoperative tilt resulted in an increase in postoperative tilt by approximately 1°. Bindelglass et al. also stated that poor preoperative tracking led to poor postoperative tracking.

In case of a valgus deformity, rotational deformity due to condylar dysplasia or other causes, patellar tilting, subluxation or dislocation due to patellar atrophy, or abnormal height often leads to malalignment of the patellofemoral joint postoperatively. This can be anticipated on the basis of the preoperative X-rays.

Implant Design

In terms of the implant design, alignment may be affected by the depth and shape of the trochlea of the femoral component and the design of the patellar component. In order to improve alignment, the current femoral implants have *patella-friendly shapes with laterally located and deeper patellar groove, slightly oblique tracking along the movement of the patella and an accentuated lateral ridge.*

There are various shapes of the patella for improving the alignment. Although it is currently not being used, the metal-backed patella is known to cause more lateral tilt than the all-poly patellar component.

Surgical Techniques

Surgical factors are further classified into approach, implant size, the amount and accuracy of osteotomy, and implant rotation and position.

Approach

Subvastus and midvastus approaches that do not violate the quadriceps tendon are preferable for achieving good patellofemoral alignment and the medial trivector-retaining approach in which the vector of quadriceps muscle power is aligned in the center of axis is also preferred for achieving good patellofemoral alignment.

Resection of the lateral patellofemoral ligament (Fig. 4.12) improves patellar tracking; hence Pagnano et al. stated that they perform resection of the lateral patellofemoral ligament routinely.

Implant Size

The size of the femoral implant is important; *if the implant size is too large, the lateral retinacular ligament will become tense, thereby causing patellar maltracking* (Fig. 4.53), and if it is too small, there will be inadequate articulation between the femoral and the patellar components.

Osteotomy

Incorrect osteotomy of the patella can cause discrepancies in the thickness of the medial and the lateral side resulting in patellar maltracking. If the patellar composite is too thick, the lateral retinacular ligament becomes tight, thereby causing patellar maltracking. Cho et al. reported that if the *postoperative patellar thickness is more than the preoperative thickness, it could cause patellar maltracking.*

Rotation and Position of the Component

Most of the times, patellar maltracking is caused by rotational malalignment of the femur or the tibia. External rotation of both the femur and the tibia is desirable, but too much external rotation not only accelerates wear of the prosthesis but also results in an intoeing gait.

Implant position is also related to the alignment; if the femoral prosthesis is located medially, the lateral retinacular ligament becomes tight and interferes with good alignment, and hence *it is desirable to place the femoral*

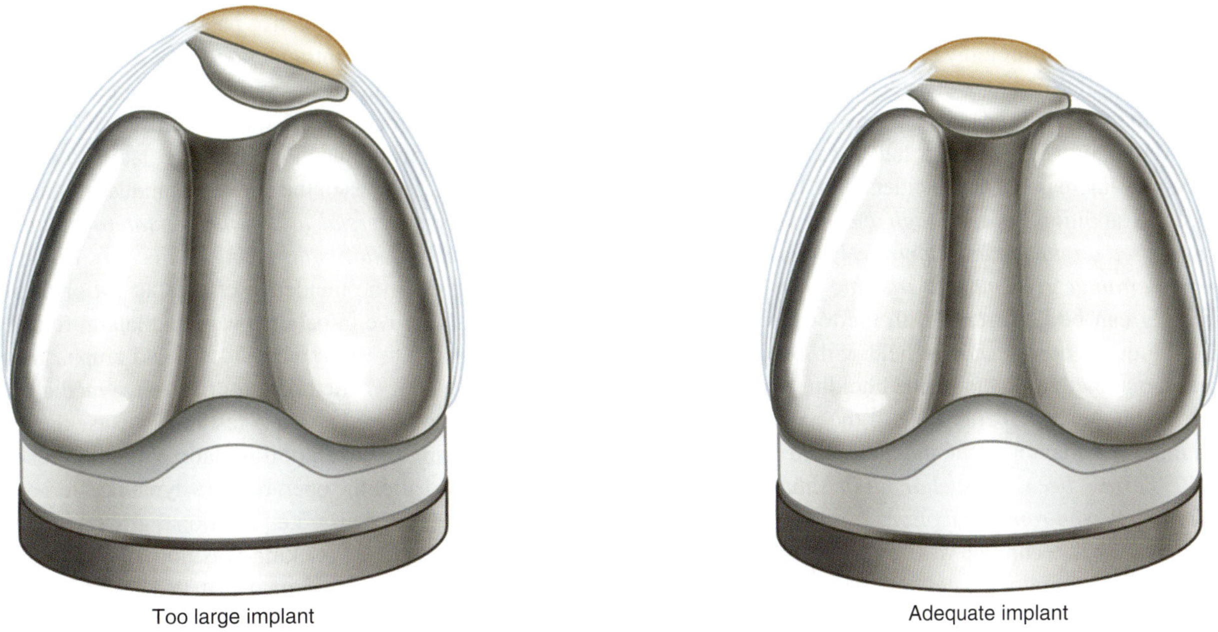

Fig. 4.53 Problems encountered when the femoral implant is too large

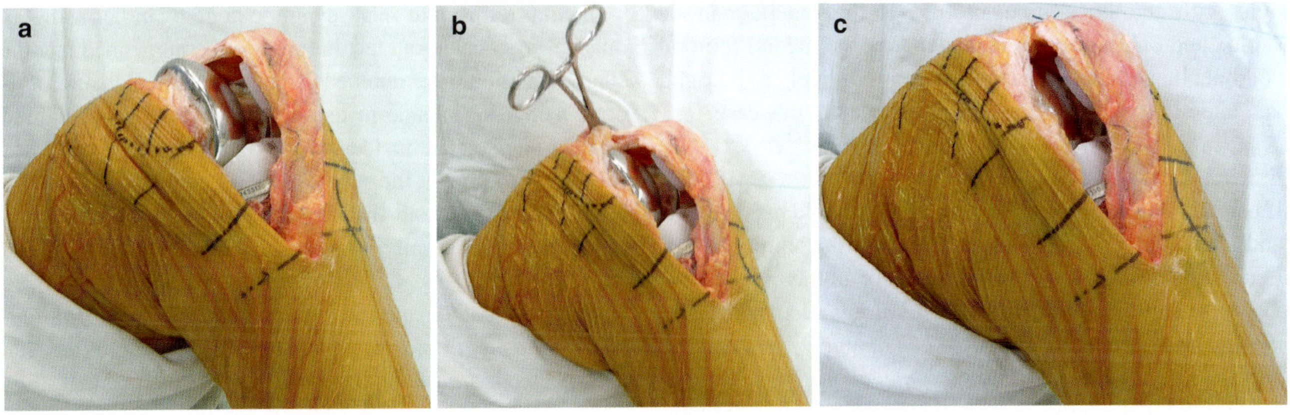

Fig. 4.54 The three methods of testing patellar tracking: (**a**) no-thumb technique, (**b**) towel clip technique, (**c**) one-stitch technique

prosthesis such that it is aligned with the lateral edge of the femur. However, if *the femoral prosthesis* is positioned beyond the lateral edge of the femur and overhangs, it causes tenting of the lateral retinacular ligament and the ligament becomes tight.

The tibial implant should also be positioned *on the lateral side to improve the alignment*. Since the lateral tibial plateau is smaller than the medial tibial plateau, fitting the implant size with the medial condyle causes the tibial implant to rotate internally. Therefore, it is desirable to select the implant size which fits to the lateral condyle and resect the remaining bones on the medial condyle.

If the patellar component is positioned on the lateral side, it also contributes to patellofemoral malalignment.

4.5.3.2 Checkup

Patellar tracking is checked after insertion of the implant, and if possible *it is done after tourniquet deflation in order to reduce the false-positive results caused due to the quadriceps grasping effect*. Husted et al. tested patellar tracking using the no-thumb technique after tourniquet deflation and reported that the incidence of lateral retinacular release was reduced by about 31 %.

Methods of testing patellar tracking include the no-thumb technique, towel clip technique, one-stitch technique, and patella medial subluxation test (Fig. 4.54). *The no-thumb technique* was introduced by Scott, and it tests patellar tracking without the use of any external forces while flexing the knee with an everted patella relocated back to its original position. This is known as *the most standard method of testing patellar tracking. But, it overestimates patellar maltracking, thereby increasing the incidence of lateral retinacular release.* When paramedial arthrotomy is performed, the tension of the medial retinacular ligament disappears. During knee flexion, the tension of vastus lateralis and rectus femoris muscles causes retraction of the patella laterally, which leads to an unnecessary increase in the incidence of lateral retinacular release. In addition, *even though the no-thumb technique shows a good alignment intraoperatively, it actually does not always guarantee good patellar tracking postoperatively.*

Testing can be performed with the towel clip technique while the quadriceps tendon is held with one or two towel clips. Pagnano et al. recommended holding the patellar tendon 8 cm above the superior pole of the patella and emphasized that the behavior of the *patella should be examined at 60 ~ 90° flexion, because patellar tilt or subluxation is common in this flexion range of motion.*

The one-stitch technique was developed by Rae et al., and it is considered that good patellar tracking is not achieved if the stitched synovial tissues around the patella are torn during flexion.

Another method of checking the lateral retinacular tightness is to subluxate the patella over the medial femoral condyle with the knee in extension. If the patella can be subluxated one-half of its diameter over the medial femoral condyle, then the lateral retinaculum is not likely to be tight, and lateral retinacular release is not needed in this case.

4.5.3.3 Correction

If patellar maltracking is noted, its causes should be identified and addressed. Lateral retinacular release is commonly carried out because it is simple, but it is not an inert procedure. *The problems associated with lateral retinacular release include persistent swelling due to hematoma, wound healing problems, and/or development of patellar necrosis.* Scuderi et al. noted that lateral retinacular release increases the incidence of circulatory disturbance from 15 to 50 % to cause patellar avascular necrosis, but Ritter and Campbell stated that patellar necrosis does not cause serious clinical problems and patellar revascularization was noted on bone scan within 1 year. However, careful assessment is required as it can also cause other complications such as patellar fracture. Therefore, if the alignment is poor intraoperatively, it is advisable to cut the lateral patellofemoral ligament, strip the lateral pillar of the patella, or perform lateral subfascial dissection first, and some surgeons recommend performing lateral retinacular release only in cases when the above techniques do not work.

It is also *controversial as to whether lateral retinacular release corrects patellar maltracking in all cases.* Bindelglass et al. reported that the incidence of patellar tilt or displacement did not improve in patients who had lateral retinacular release compared to those who did not and emphasized the need for performing meticulous suturing of the medial capsular incision. They stated that this result is because the testing performed during the operation is static, while the functions that are required after the operation are dynamic. Berger et al. emphasized that the cause, i.e., rotational alignment, should be examined if patellar tracking was normal preoperatively and also it should be confirmed that the lateral retinacular ligament is not tight. If none of these problems exist, lateral retinacular release would only be a temporary solution. In other words, they state that *lateral retinacular release can only be done when the lateral retinacular ligament is tense.*

Lateral retinacular release can be done by either using an outside-in or inside-out technique. It is recommended that the synovium should be retained if lateral retinacular release is done using the outside-in technique, so caution is required while doing so. The inside-out method should be performed cautiously to protect the superior lateral genicular artery. If it is necessary to extend the incision proximally, it should be directed superolaterally so as to protect the superior lateral genicular artery (Fig. 4.55). Release is done about 1.5–2.0 cm lateral to the patella and the *thick lateral patellofemoral ligament in the middle should be resected,* and a better effect can be expected by releasing the distal part of this ligament.

Wachtl et al. proposed a lateral patellar osteotomy as an alternative surgical procedure to the traditional lateral retinacular release. They insisted that the ligamentous structures on the lateral patella are thus decompressed, thereby relaxing the lateral retinacular ligament.

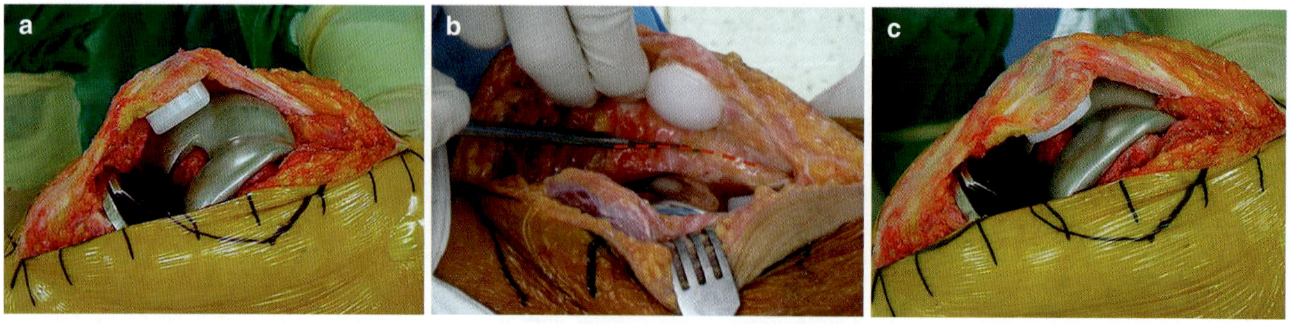

Fig. 4.55 The method and effect of lateral retinacular release. (**a**) before release, (**b**) during release, (**c**) after release

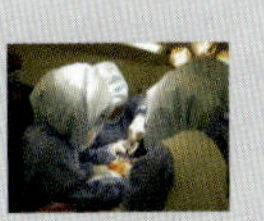

Author's Method

I basically use the "no-thumb technique" as a screening test and use the towel clip technique only when poor patellar tracking is noted with the no-thumb technique, because the incidence of lateral retinacular release is significantly increased with the no-thumb technique alone. If good patellar tracking is not seen with the no-thumb technique, I use the towel clip technique and observe the motion of the patella in a range of flexion from 60° to 90° for an accurate judgment.

I do lateral reticular release when poor patellar tracking still persists with the towel clip method. I was able to achieve good patellar tracking using this principle in most of the cases.

Postoperative poor patellar tracking was also experienced even when good patellar tracking was observed with the no-thumb technique during the surgery.

I cannot understand why most surgeons stick to the use of the "no-thumb technique" and why they insist to deflate the tourniquet in order to determine the need for the lateral retinacular release, while they test the patellar tracking with medial incision site open. I think holding the arthrotomy site with towel clips reflects the postoperative patellar tracking better than that using the no-thumb technique with tourniquet deflation.

4.6 Fixation

4.6.1 Fixation Methods

Fixation methods of TKA include all cement fixation and cementless mechanical (press fit) and biological (bony ingrowth) fixation. Hybrid fixation implies cementing on the tibial component and not on the femoral component. Due to many reports of an increased rate of loosening of cementless fixation in TKA, most surgeons now prefer cement fixation. *The advantage of cementing are as follows: the bleeding can be reduced, the surgical technique is easy to perform since the minor gap is filled with cement, early weight bearing is possible, and the incidence of osteolysis is reduced* as the cement prevents penetration of the polyethylene particles into the cancellous bone.

When the extension stem is used, cement can be applied only at the bottom of the tibial prosthesis, at the epiphyseal and metaphyseal portion, or along the whole length of the extension stem. *Partial cementation* refers to cementing of the tibial base plate or cementing on the metaphyseal area without cementing along the whole length of the stem. It is controversial as to which technique is better. *Generally, cement is used for the shorter stems or the long and slender stems.* Theoretically, *cement is not used when the extension stem is thought to be fixed by the press-fit method*; in such cases, reaming should be performed 1 mm less than the diameter of the stem. Fehring observed that partial cementation increases micromotion of the tibial prosthesis and may cause pain.

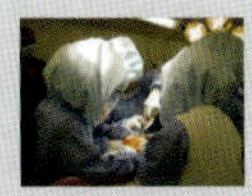

Author's Method

I use cement on the whole length of the prosthesis. Even though, the stem achieves a press-fit fixation, it is not reliable especially in patients with osteopenia. The purpose of using the extension stem is to achieve stable fixation, and cementing will further enhance the fixation.

Also, there may be an irregular bone defect in the medullary cavity in infected TKA which acts as a dead space, and hence I fill this dead space with antibiotic-loaded cement.

4.6.2 Cementing Techniques

The cementing techniques in hip arthroplasty have developed considerably. The knee joint is not identical to the hip joint, but there are many similarities in cementing technique between the two joints. First, vacuum mixing is ideally recommended. However, Insall believed that centrifugation is unnecessary in TKA because the cement layer is thin and air bubbles can escape easily. Second, *the cementing time is important.* If cementing is done while the cement is in the liquid stage, it may be contaminated with blood and/or fat and this weakens the cement strength. If cementing is done too late, the time required for penetration of the cement into the bone will be lost and the bonding strength will be decreased. Third, *use of pulsatile lavage is better for removal of blood and bone debris.* However, there are controversies concerning the use of pulsatile lavage in the knee joint. The ideal depth of cement penetration is about 2–3 mm below the subchondral bone. Walker et al. suggested that ideal cement penetration into the bone is 3–4 mm. When pulsatile lavage is used, cement penetrates more than 4–5 mm into the bone in osteoporotic patients, which causes *thermal necrosis of bone*, and the bone is weakened, thereby causing loosening. Fourth, *multiple drilling is required in the sclerotic bones for achieving more cement penetration. Lastly, a compressive force is applied to achieve stable fixation.*

The recommended thickness of cement is around 1 mm and if the cement thickness is more than 2 mm, the bonding strength is decreased.

4.6.2.1 Method According to Time Sequence

Cementing can be done in one stage or in two stages.

One-Stage Method

The one-stage method is less time-consuming and economical, but it is not recommended for the beginners since they need to hurry to perform the cementing or they would *miss the appropriate timing to perform cementing adequately*.

Another advantage is rigid cement fixation of both the femoral and tibial components by a compressive force. An added advantage of the one-stage method is that the implant is usually fixed in a balanced state in extension. Most of the times, the implant is inserted and the cement is compressed with the knee joint in extension before it cures. If the knee joint is not accurately balanced before cementing, the implant can be balanced after cementing, even though the alignment is slightly changed.

Two-Stage Method

The advantage of the two-stage method is that there is no need to hurry, and this makes it easier to remove the extruded cement. Its drawbacks are that it is more time consuming and costly, and fixation is jeopardized if the surgeon is in a hurry to perform the second stage of cementing before the first-stage cement is completely cured. For example, *if femoral cementing is started without waiting for a sufficient period of time after tibial cementing, the tibial prosthesis may move during curing, thereby causing suboptimal fixation.*

4.6.2.2 Procedure

Cementing starts when the cement is in the dough stage. The cement can be applied on the bone or on the implant. Some surgeons apply digital pressure on the cement after applying it onto the bone, but this may delay the contact time between the cement and the implant, which reduces the bonding strength between the cement and the prosthesis.

Some surgeons apply the cement on both bone and prosthesis with digital compression on the bony side. Vanlommel et al. demonstrated that applying cement to both the undersurface of the tibial baseplate and onto the tibial bone, either by spatula or finger packing technique, leads to an optimal cement penetration of 3–5 mm.

Care should be taken so as not to contaminate the articular surface of the prosthesis with the cement. If there is too much cement on the posterior femoral condyle, the excess cement will extrude out, and it takes time to remove this cement, especially when the one-stage method is used (Fig. 4.56). The extruded cement should be removed, otherwise it could restrict the joint motion or cause third body wear (Fig. 4.57).

Cement will take more time to cure if it is less in volume. In fact, a thin film of cement is needed in TKA, so it needs a longer time requiring compression to cure the cement until the film of cement is completely hardened.

If cement extrusion is noted after setting of the cement, it is recommended to leave the extruded cement as it is unless it irritates the soft tissues or constrains motion, because removing the hardened cement on the outside of the component may break up the cement which is located beneath the prosthesis.

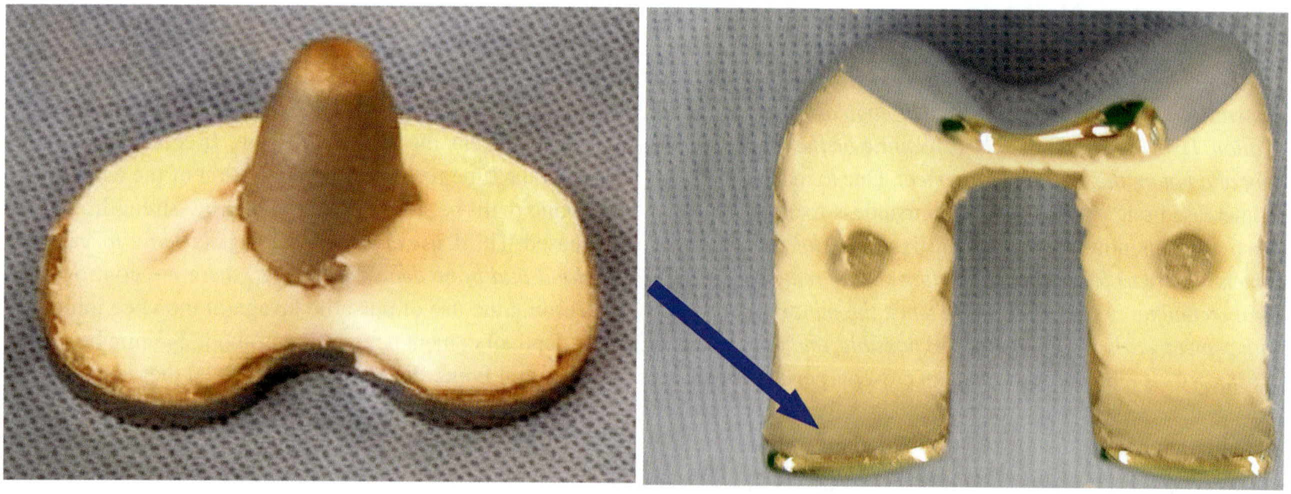

Fig. 4.56 Applying the cement onto the tibial and femoral prosthesis. It is not desirable to apply too much cement on the posterior condyle of the femur (*arrow*)

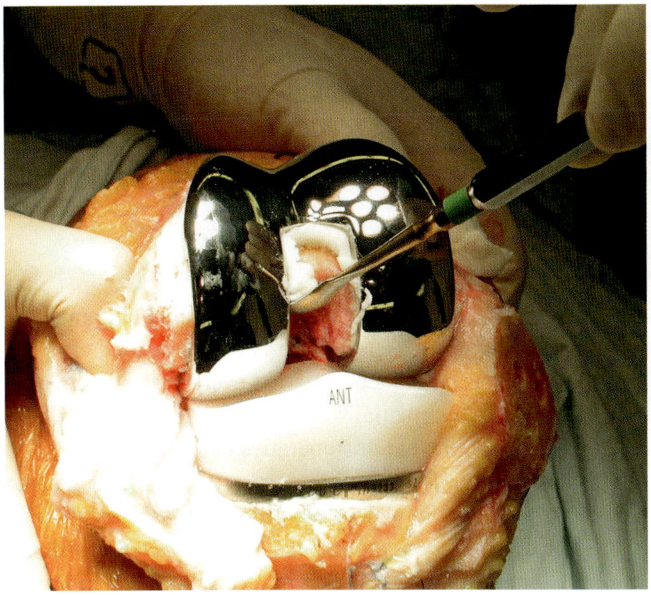

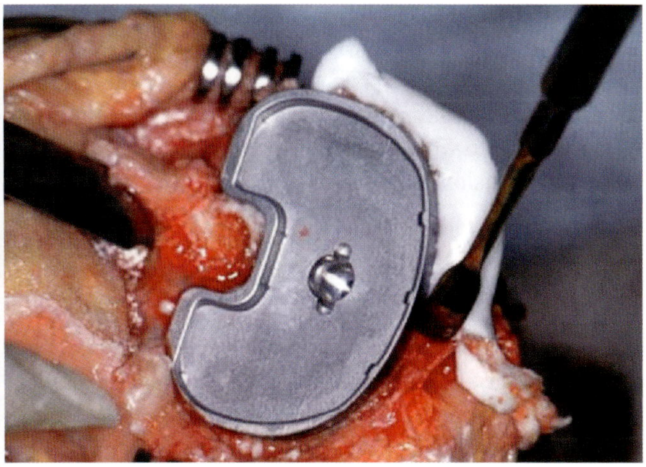

Fig. 4.57 Removing the extruded cement after inserting the prosthesis

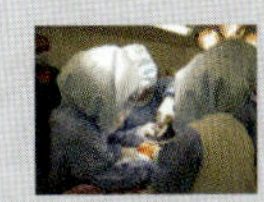

Author's Method

I do not use vacuum mixing or pulsatile lavage because a thin cement layer is used in TKA.

I mix antibiotics into the cement in the ratio of 1:1 (1 g of antibiotics in 1 pack of cement) in patients with high risk of infection in order to prevent the occurrence of infection.

I do cementing in one stage. I apply the cement onto the prosthesis first. The reason why I apply the cement onto the prosthesis first is that the contact between the cement and the prosthesis should not be delayed later than 5–6 min. If I apply cement onto the bone first, adequate time for contact between the cement and the femoral prosthesis would be passed by when I perform femoral fixation. If so, the bonding strength between the cement and the femoral prosthesis would be markedly decreased. The bonding strength between the cement and the bone is mainly achieved by penetration of the cement into the bone. It is not a problem even if 5–6 min has passed by, because the cement is still in the dough stage and a compression force would penetrate the cement into the bone adequately.

Fixation of the patella, tibia, and femur is done in that order. The reason why I perform fixation of the patella first is that it is convenient to do so, and I am afraid that late fixation of the patella would increase the incidence of loosening.

When fixing the tibial component, more force is applied on the posterior and lateral sides first to ensure even thickness of the cement. Otherwise, the thickness of the cement on the posterolateral side would often be more than that of the cement on the anterior side.

When lifting the femur to fix the femoral component, I press the tibial component down with my fingers; otherwise the tibial component may be lifted off during lifting of the femur.

When inserting the femoral prosthesis, I apply force in the direction of extension, since most of the implants tend to be inserted at an anterior angulation. At this time, I remove any extruded cement.

After insertion of the implant, I apply pressure with the knee in full extension and wait until complete curing of the cement occurs. To check the curing time, I make a thin film of cement from the remaining cement (Fig. 4.58).

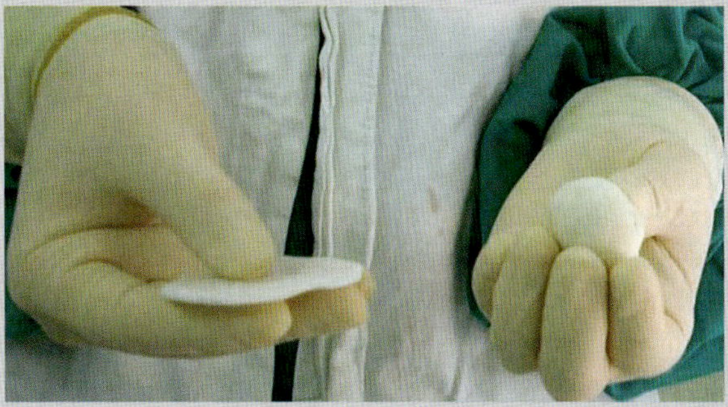

Fig. 4.58 A model to check the curing time of cement. The *left thin film* of the cement can reflect the actual time required for curing of cement used in TKA

4.7 Closure

There are some controversies with respect to the closure such as when to release the tourniquet, whether to insert a Hemovac, and to what extent the knee should be bent while closing the incision.

4.7.1 Hemostasis

Some surgeons state that the amount of bleeding does not differ to a great extent even when the tourniquet is released after skin closure, but releasing the tourniquet in advance and performing hemostasis before closure helps to reduce the amount of bleeding and prevent unexpected accidents. In particular, the lateral inferior genicular arteries have a tendency of being cut longitudinally while removing the lateral meniscus, and this may result in a considerable amount of bleeding.

Irrigation with norepinephrine before closure is known to be one of the methods to reduce the bleeding. Cho et al. reported that irrigation with norepinephrine diluted to 1:2,00,000 reduced the postoperative bleeding and consequently decreased the amount of transfusion required. An autogenous bone or cement can also be used to block the opening in femoral medullary canal to reduce the intramedullary bleeding. Using an autogenous bone is more physiological; however, it is more time consuming and incomplete. This is the opposite of using the cement.

4.7.2 Hemovac Insertion

Some surgeons state that Hemovac insertion is not recommended because it does not reduce the incidence of postoperative complications and it interferes with the rehabilitation process, and yet it increases the incidence of infection. Esler et al. reported that placing a Hemovac could not prevent hematoma formation, but it increased the bleeding. They observed that Hemovac constrains the rehabilitation process and interferes with the nursing care with no contribution to the clinical improvement in terms of infection or range of motion. Omonbude et al. reported that the *incidence of hematoma was increased when a Hemovac was not inserted, but there was no difference in the clinical course and complications*. Li et al. also reported that there was no clear advantage to the use of wound drains after unilateral TKA. However, Kim et al. reported that even though it does not contribute to the long-term clinical results, more number of patients without a Hemovac showed petechiae, swelling, and extravasation of blood more frequently and 2 of 69 cases showed deep infection, although this was not statistically significant.

In fact, Hemovac does not stay in place for more than 2 days, and because the amount of bleeding after Hemovac removal is more than the capacity of the knee joint, the amount of blood remaining in the joint space is the same with or without the use of a Hemovac.

Currently, the Hemovac is used in combination with cell saver to reduce the need for allogeneic transfusion.

4.7.3 Suturing Technique

Suturing should be done along the longitudinal alignment of soft tissues, and for this purpose it is recommended to make markings before the incision. However, Insall suggested suturing the vastus medialis obliquus muscle a little lower down distally to prevent postoperative extension lag.

To improve the joint motion postoperatively, it is recommended to suture the wound with the knee bent at 45–60°. The knee could be bent more, but by doing so, tension in the tissues increases and this makes suturing difficult. Emerson et al. stated that flexion motion improved for the first 6 months and the length of rehabilitation period was shortened when the wound was closed with the knee joint bent at 90–110°.

Careful compression dressing is needed after closure. If the wound is wrapped too tightly, it can cause peroneal nerve palsy and swelling of the lower limb accompanied by bullae.

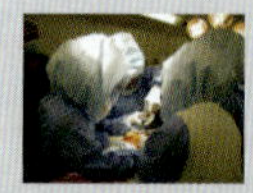

Author's Method

I deflate the tourniquet before closing the wound. When closing the wound, I bend the knee in about 40–50° flexed position. I believe that it is not necessary to bend the knee joint in 90–110° flexed position as better ROM could be achieved than that suggested by Emerson et al., even though the wound was sutured with the knee joint in about 40–50° flexed position.

Continuous suturing saves time but there are problems when wound revision is needed. Hence, I personally recommend using the interrupted suturing technique. In particular, subcutaneous suture should be done meticulously for clean wound healing without dimpling of the skin. I always use staples for skin closure to save the time.

I routinely insert a Hemovac before closure.

4.8 Miscellaneous Techniques

Various techniques have been described in Chap. 2 and in the other part of this chapter, but I think it is necessary to describe some of the techniques in brief. These techniques include methods for increasing the range of motion, techniques in mobile-bearing joint, and techniques in the PCL-substituting type.

4.8.1 Methods for Increasing the ROM

4.8.1.1 Importance of ROM

The range of motion has a great impact on improving function. *The knee joint must be able to flex at least 95° to go up and down the stairs, 120° to be able to squat, and 135° or flex completely to have no constraint during the activities of daily living*. In the HSS score, 18 of 100 points are assigned for the ROM, which is quite a lot, taking into account the impact of ROM on function. The fact that 25 of 100 points in the knee score are assigned for the ROM also emphasizes the importance of ROM. Ritter et al. stated that ROM plays the most important role in the HSS and KSS scoring systems, not only because of ROM itself but also because it affects walking and stair walking.

4.8.1.2 Anatomy and Biomechanics

In physiological conditions, the maximum range of flexion is up to the angle at which the thigh touches the calf, but this angle varies from person to person and flexion between 145° and 160° is regarded as maximal flexion. In order to achieve this flexion motion after TKA, the articular geometry and mechanics of the articular surface should be near normal. There should be no spurs, and ligaments and soft tissues should be balanced.

The articular geometry and biomechanics of the knee joint should fulfill a few conditions for achieving good flexion. First, the femoral condyle is not spherical, but it has the offset that is projected more posteriorly to ensure adequate room when the articular surface of the tibia meets the femur. *Second, the cruciate ligaments allow femoral rollback. Third, the distal radius of the lateral femoral condyle is larger than that of the medial femoral condyle, and the A–P dimension of the lateral tibial condyle is smaller than that of the medial tibial condyle*. This implies that the lateral femoral condyle rotates and rollback occurs when the knee joint flexes, and the lateral meniscus slips posteriorly concomitantly to increase the stability and range of motion in flexion. *Fourth, the tibial plateau should have a posterior slope* of 5–10° (Fig. 4.59).

The surgical techniques and implants should fulfill the above conditions in order to improve postoperative flexion.

4.8.1.3 Factors affecting ROM

Factors involved in postoperative ROM include patient's preoperative ROM, surgical techniques, prosthesis design, and rehabilitation method.

Preoperative Patient Conditions

The preoperative patient conditions include preoperative ROM, causative diseases, degree of the deformity, age, sex, and obesity. Cho et al. reported that *preoperative ROM is constant and the most important factor* among the other factors that govern the postoperative ROM. If the preoperative range of motion is normal, the ROM is often decreased a little postoperatively. If the preoperative range of motion is less than 75°, the range of motion is expected to increase more after TKA, although it is usually difficult to achieve an angle greater than 100°.

Intraoperative Factors

Intraoperative factors consist of the approach and surgical techniques.

Approach

It is thought that the midvastus or subvastus approach would improve flexion motion because the quadriceps tendon is not

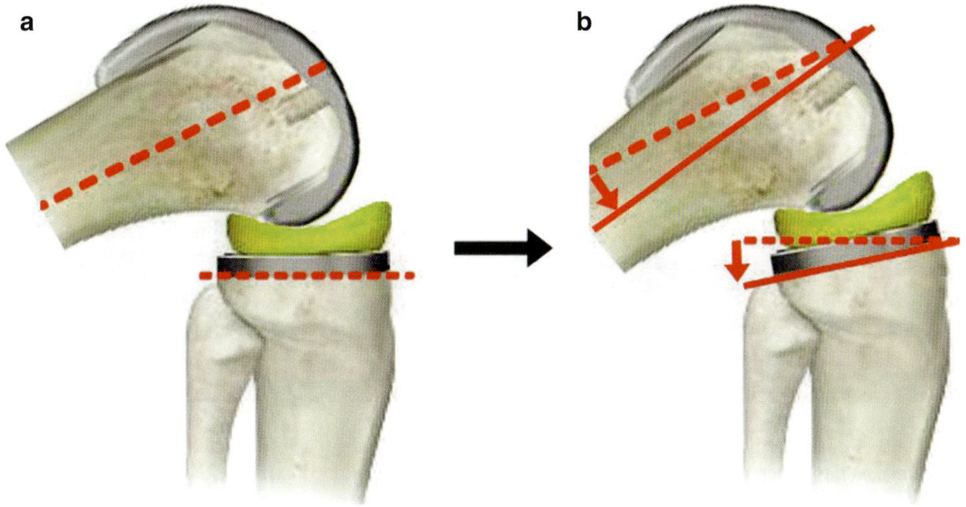

Fig. 4.59 The rationale of posterior tibial slope for achieving an increase in flexion motion. (**a**) less posterior slope, (**b**) more posterior slope

violated in these approaches. However, Keating et al. stated that neither of these approaches actually improve the flexion motion.

MIS (minimally invasive surgery) increases the ROM in the early postoperative period, but there is no difference in the ROM at the long-term follow-up.

Surgical Techniques

In terms of surgical techniques, *flexion motion as well as stability can be increased when the knee joint is balanced.* Other factors are impingement, selection of proper size of the implants, location of implants, accurate osteotomy, etc.

The key structure to achieve ligament balance and improve ROM is the PCL. The PCL contributes to rollback, thereby improving flexion motion. Walker et al. reported that rollback occurs when the tension in the PCL increases by about 15 %, but the rollback decreases when the tension is decreased. The impact of sacrificing the PCL on flexion motion is controversial; however it is generally accepted that the PCL sacrifice and substitution improves rollback and increases the flexion gap, thereby increasing flexion motion.

The spurs on the posterior condyle of the femur should be removed meticulously during the operation because flexion can be increased when the PE does not make any contact with the spurs during flexion. Soft tissues in the posterior space should either be resected for achieving more flexion or should be released in order to improve extension motion (Fig. 4.60).

The tibial slope is also very important; *when the posterior tibial slope is not incorporated in the osteotomy*, the flexion gap will be narrowed and tension in the PCL will decrease, thereby *reducing the femoral rollback and flexion motion.* On the other hand, too much posterior slope widens the flexion gap and causes instability in flexion.

Implant size also affects flexion motion. In particular, implant size is closely related to tension of the PCL in the CR type. *If the implant is too small, posterior condylar offset is reduced to cause impingement in flexion, and a wide flexion gap decreases tension of the PCL, thereby reducing rollback. If the implant is too large, it narrows the flexion gap causing overstuffing in flexion, which also results in decreased flexion motion.* In any case, implant size is important and a smaller implant is recommended for the ARS when the implant is of an in-between size.

Implant location also affects the ROM; *the tibial component should be placed on the posterior side so as to increase flexion motion.* Walker et al. reported the results of a computer-aided analysis which suggested that if the tibial component is located about 5 mm to the posterior side, flexion motion is increased by 5°, but if it is located too far posteriorly such that it overhangs, it causes impingement and may also cause an increase in the incidence of loosening (Fig. 4.61).

Femoral location is also related to flexion motion; if it is *located anteriorly, it has the effect of increasing the flexion gap* resulting in an increase in the flexion motion, if positioned on the posterior, the flexion motion is decreased. But, it should be considered in relation to the quadriceps function.

The rotational alignment also affects the flexion motion. Internal rotation of the femur will cause decrease in the flexion gap on the medial side during flexion and worsen patellofemoral alignment, thereby reducing flexion motion.

If the *patellar composite thickness* increases postoperatively, the patellofemoral joint is under more tension, and when the knee flexes by more than 70°, the flexion motion is restricted and incidence of wear is increased.

The location of the patella is also related to flexion motion. Joint line elevation or patella baja can lead to impingement between the patella and the PE resulting in reduced flexion. Proximal location of the patellar component or a beveled PE is required in these cases for more flexion. It is known that patellar resurfacing is not related to the joint motion.

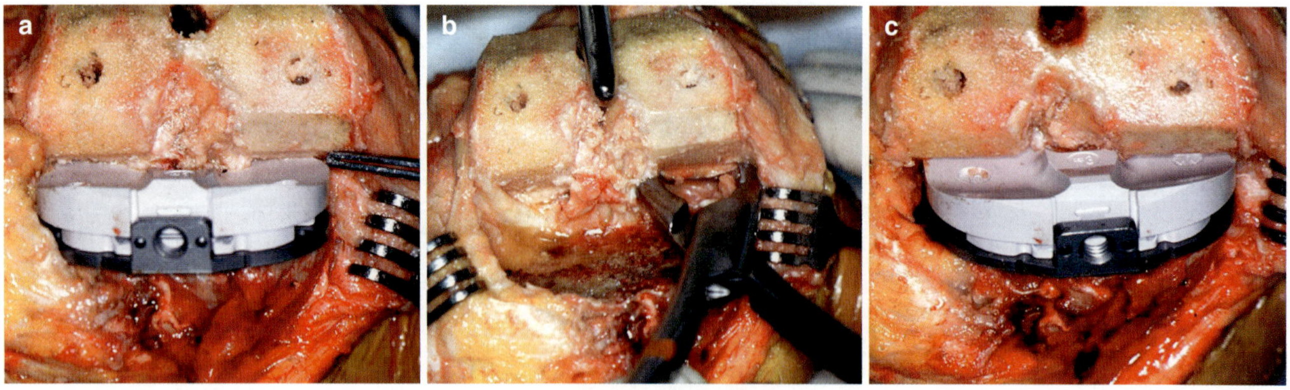

Fig. 4.60 Removing the posterior spurs. (**a**) The presence of posterior spurs makes the placement of the spacer to the posterior side difficult, thereby causing limited flexion. (**b**) Removing the spurs. (**c**) The spacer can be moved to the posterior side more easily, which increases the flexion motion

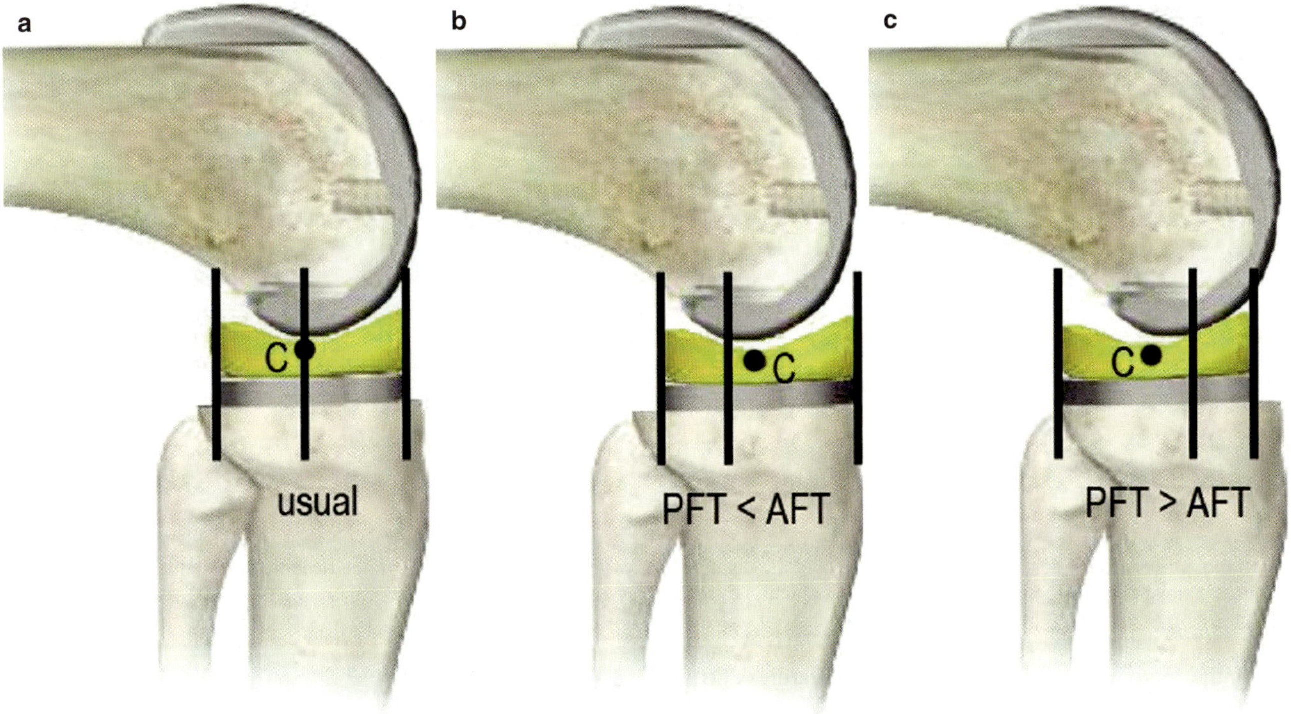

Fig. 4.61 Influence of tibial implant location on the flexion angle. (**a**) Normal location, (**b**) anterior location, (**c**) posterior location. If the tibial implant is pushed to the posterior as shown in (**c**), posterior femoral translation is increased, thereby increasing the flexion motion

In terms of *closure*, Emerson et al. emphasized that flexion motion increases when closure is done in 90–110° of flexion, but many surgeons disagree with their opinion.

Implants

In terms of implant design, conventional implants are designed to achieve flexion up to about 120°. Some surgeons have recently reported that the flexion motion is increased by using implants that are specifically designed to achieve more flexion. This is described in Chap. 2.

4.8.2 Techniques for the Mobile-Bearing Joint

The mobile-bearing joint offers several benefits, but its drawback is that it causes spinout due to instability when ligament balancing is not achieved. Therefore, *it is most important to balance the ligaments during the operation, and it is recommended to perform tibial osteotomy first since the gap technique is used for this purpose*.

Ligament balancing and tibial osteotomy are the first steps of a successful operation and *PCL resection should be done before femoral osteotomy in the PCS type so as not to cause flexion and extension gap discrepancy*.

There are many mobile-bearing prosthesis and the surgical procedures are also different. I would like to describe the surgical procedure of low-contact stress (LCS), as it is the most standard type of a mobile-bearing joint. In case of LCS, the tibial osteotomy is done with a posterior slope of about 7° after ligament balancing and it is designed to match the anterior inclination of the distal portion of the femoral prosthesis. The preparation and positioning of the tibial component is done with the same way as in routine arthroplasty. The gap technique is used to decide the external rotation of the femoral implant and followed by anterior and posterior femoral osteotomy. Then, distal osteotomy is performed perpendicular to the mechanical axis in the coronal plane. After anterior–posterior resection and distal osteotomy, a gapper is used to recheck the flexion and extension gap balance. Then, a cutting jig is used to perform chamfer cutting and to remove the spurs on the posterior condyle. Tibial malrotation is automatically corrected by the virtue of mobile PE, to provide a certain scope of error for tibial malrotation. Although the malrotation of the PE is automatically corrected in a mobile-bearing joint, it is recommended to align the rotational axis appropriately (Fig. 4.62).

The size of the PE and the patellar component follows the femoral size for providing better stability.

The surgical advantage of LCS is that the operation is performed very smoothly if accurate soft tissue balancing is achieved and tibial osteotomy is performed correctly. The mediolateral gap in flexion can be accurately balanced, and the external rotation of the femur is determined by the gap technique.

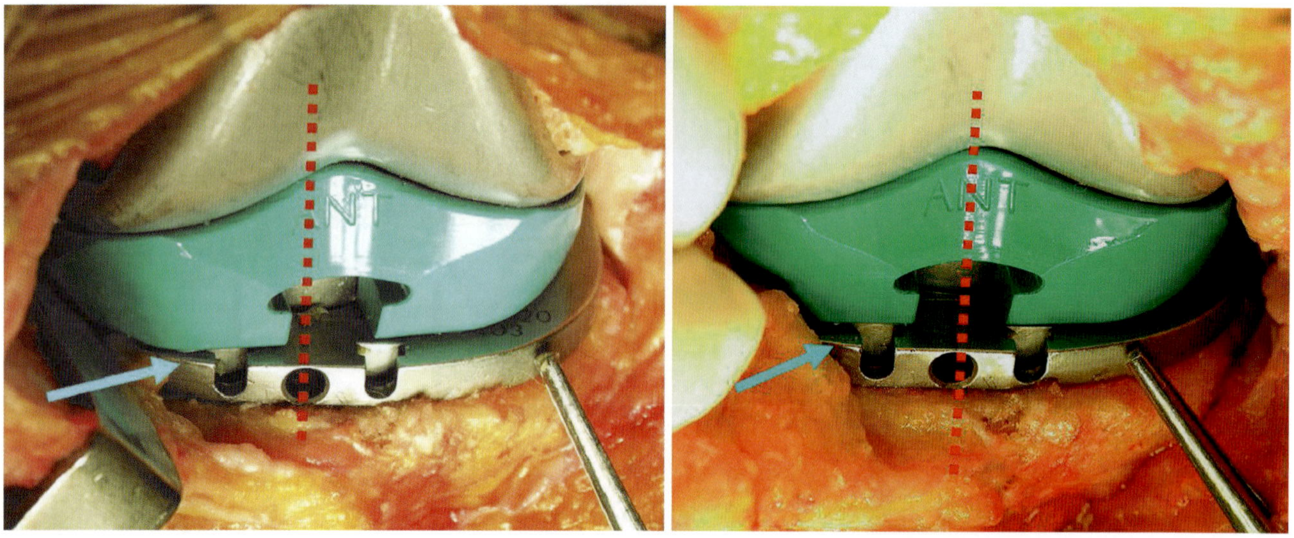

Fig. 4.62 Verification of correct rotational alignment of the tibial plate. *Left photograph* shows an asymmetric mediolateral distance between the PE and the tibial plate (*arrow*), which indicates malrotation of the tibial plate. *Right photograph* shows correct rotational alignment

As the femoral component is the same regardless of the PCL sacrifice or not, even if the PCL is injured or needs to be resected during the operation, no additional procedure is needed for the femur except for changing of the mobile-bearing PE.

Its surgical drawback is that it is a little difficult to perform the operation since the tibia is cut first and all the surgical procedures have to be readjusted if ligament balancing is not established or tibial osteotomy is inaccurate. In small bones, the stem, which is in the shape of a cone, comes in contact with the posterior cortex of the proximal tibia causing the tibial component to shift anteriorly (Fig. 4.63).

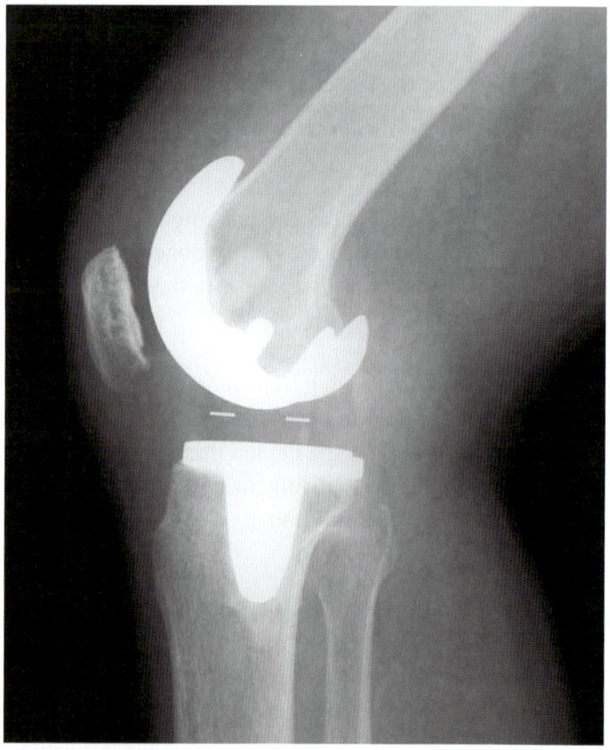

Fig. 4.63 Location of stem and relationship with tibial cortex in LCS. Stem is in contact with posterior cortex, which affects the location of tibial prosthesis

4.8.3 Techniques for the Posterior Cruciate-Substituting Type

Surgical techniques used for the PS type are basically not different from those applied for the CR type. However, it is necessary to consider some of the phenomena or incidents that are not seen with the CR type.

First, *the collateral ligament balancing should be accurate*. If there is a severe deformity, soft tissue release should be done accordingly and the gap may become wider than expected. Hence, a constrained type of prosthesis should be used to compensate for the marked flexion and extension gap discrepancy in patients with severe deformities. In other words, the constrained type of prosthesis may be used if the PCL is resected in case of severe deformity and instability. In order to determine whether or not to use the constrained type, the knee is bent in a figure of 4. If the post gets dislocated, the constrained type should be used.

Second, *sacrificing the PCL may increase the flexion gap more than the extension gap and cause gap imbalance*. Therefore, *an implant with a thicker PE than CR type should be used if the PCL has been sacrificed*. Also, a more distal osteotomy may be needed to balance the flexion and extension gaps as the flexion gap becomes wider than the extension gap, or a larger femoral component can be chosen in case of the ARS to decrease the flexion gap if the size of the implant is an in-between size. On the other hand, if the flexion gap turns out to be too narrow with CR types, the PCL may be sacrificed in order to balance the extension and flexion gaps.

Third, *since the cam and the post prevent hyperextension, it is recommended to either use a CR type of trial PE to test the extension and flexion gaps or increase the PE thickness of the PS type step by step until flexion contracture develops.*

Fourth, it requires care when *performing box cutting* of the femur. Accurate osteotomy is needed to prevent an intercondylar fracture. Too much amount of osteotomy weakens the bones and *causes a fracture*, but too little amount of osteotomy can also cause a bursting fracture while inserting a trial implant.

Fifth, it is *not necessary to remove too much bone during tibial osteotomy*. Since the extension and flexion gaps are widened by sacrificing the PCL, it is possible to maintain an appropriate gap even when minimal osteotomy of the tibia is performed. Hence, the bone supporting the tibial implant can be much more stronger.

Sixth, *the posterior slope should not be more than 7° so as to reduce the incidence of wear of the post.*

Seventh, *if the notch portion is of the open-box type, the bone cement should be removed meticulously so that it does not come in contact with the post.*

Lastly, it is *desirable to remove the soft tissues surrounding the patella meticulously in order to reduce the incidence of patellar clunk syndrome.*

Bibliography

Akagi M, Mori S, Nishimura S, et al. Variability of extraarticular tibial rotation references for total knee arthroplasty. Clin Orthop. 2005;436:172–6.

Akagi M, Oh M, Nonaka T, et al. An anteroposterior axis of the tibia for total knee arthroplasty. Clin Orthop. 2004;420:213–9.

Anglin C, Brimacombe JM, Wilson DR, et al. Biomechanical consequences of patellar component medialization in total knee arthroplasty. J Arthoplasty. 2010;25:793–802.

Anouchi YS, Whiteside LA, Kaiser AD. The effects of axial rotational alignment of the femoral component on knee stability and patellar tracking in total knee arthroplasty demonstrated on autopsy specimens. Clin Orthop. 1993;287:170–7.

Arima J, Whiteshide LA, McCarty DS, et al. Femoral rotational alignment, based on the anterior posterior axis, in total knee arthroplasty in a valgus knee. J Bone Joint Surg. 1995;77-A:1331–4.

Baliga S, McNair CJ, Barnett KJ, et al. Does circumpatellar electrocautery improve the outcome after total knee replacement?: a prospective, randomized, blinded controlled trial. J Bone Joint Surg. 2012;94-B:1228–33.

Babazadeh S, Dowsey MM, Swan JD, et al. Joint line position correlates with function after primary total knee replacement: a randomised controlled trial comparing conventional and computer-assisted surgery. J Bone Joint Surg. 2011;93-B:1223–31.

Barrack RL, Bertot AJ, Wolfe MW, et al. Patellar resurfacing in total knee arthroplasty. A prospective, randomized, double-blind study with five to seven years of follow-up. J Bone Joint Surg. 2001;83-A:1376–81.

Barrack RL, Schrader T, Bertot AJ, et al. Component rotation and anterior knee pain after total knee arthroplasty. Clin Orthop. 2001;392:46–55.

Barrack RL, Smith P, Munn B, et al. The Ranawat award. Comparison of surgical approaches in total knee arthroplasty. Clin Orthop. 1998;356:16–21.

Barrack RL, Wolfe MW, Waldman DA, et al. Resurfacing of the patella in total knee arthroplasty. A prospective, randomized, double-blind study. J Bone Joint Surg. 1997;79-A:1121–31.

Bellemans J, Robijns F, Duerincks J, et al. The influence of tibial slope on maximal flexionafter total knee arthroplasty. Knee Surg Sports Traumatol Arthrosc. 2005;13:193–6.

Bellemans J, Vandenneucker H, Van Lauwe J, et al. A new surgical technique for medial collateral ligament balancing: multiple needle puncturing. J Arthroplasty. 2010;25:1151–6.

Bellemans J, Colyn W, Vandenneucker H, et al. Is neutral mechanical alignment normal for all patients? The concept of constitutional varus. Clin Orthop. 2012;470:45–53.

Bengs BC, Scott RD. The effect of distal femoral resection on passive knee extension in posterior cruciate ligament-retaining total knee arthroplasty. J Arthroplasty. 2006;21:161–6.

Berger RA, Crossett LS, Jacobs JJ. Malrotation causing patellofemoral complications after total knee arthroplasty. Clin Orthop. 1998;356:144–53.

Berger RA, Lyon JH, Jacobs JJ, et al. Problems with cementless total knee arthroplasty at 11 years followup. Clin Orthop. 2001;392:196.

.Berger RA, Rubash HE, Seel MJ. Determining the rotational alignment of the femoral component in total knee arthroplasty using the epicondylar axis. Clin Orthop. 1993;286:40–7.

Berth A, Urbach D, Neumann W, et al. Strength and voluntary activation of quadriceps femoris muscle in total knee arthroplasty with midvastus and subvastus approaches. J Arthroplasty. 2007;22:83–8.

Bhan S, Malhotra R, Eachempati KK. Total knee arthroplasty without patellar resurfacing in patients with rheumatoid arthritis. Clin Orthop. 2006;450:157–63.

Bindelglass DF, Cohen JL, Dorr LD. Patellar tilt and subluxation in total knee arthroplasty. Relationship To pain, fixation, and design. Clin Orthop. 1993;286:103–9.

Bonnin MP, Saffarini M, Mercier PE, et al. Is the anterior tibial tuberosity a reliable rotational landmark for the tibial component in total knee arthroplasty? J Arthroplasty. 2011;26:260–7.

Bourne RB, Burnett RS. The consequences of not resurfacing the patella. Clin Orthop. 2004;428:166–9.

Boyd AD, Ewald FC, Thomas WH. Long term complications after total knee arthroplasty with or without resurfacing of the patella. J Bone Joint Surg. 1993;75-A:674–81.

Bramlett KW, Haller WN, Krauss WD. The trivector retaining approach. In: Scuderi GR, editor. Surgical techniques in total knee arthroplasty. 1st ed. New York: Springer; 2002. p. 131–6.

Brick GW, Scott RD. The patellofemoral component of total knee arthroplasty. Clin Orthop. 1988;231:163–78.

Buechel FF. A sequential three-step lateral release for correcting fixed valgus knee deformities during total knee arthroplasty. Clin Orthop. 1990;260:170–5.

Burnett RS, Boone JL, McCarthy KP, et al. A prospective randomized clinical trial of patellar resurfacing and nonresurfacing in bilateral TKA. Clin Orthop. 2007;464:65–72.

Burnett RS, Boone JL, Rosenzweig SD, et al. Patellar resurfacing compared with nonresurfacing in total knee arthroplasty. A concise follow-up of a randomized trial. J Bone Joint Surg. 2009;91-A:2562–7.

Callaghan JJ, Windsor RE. V-Y quadricepsplasty. In: Scuderi GR, editor. Surgical techniques in total knee arthroplasty. 1st ed. New York: Springer; 2002. p. 155–8.

Cameron HU, Fedorkow DM. The patella in total knee arthroplasty. Clin Orthop. 1982;165:197–9.

Chan KC, Gill GS. Postoperative patellar tilt in total knee arthroplasty. J Arthroplasty. 1999;14:300–4.

Cho WS, Kim JM, Ahn HS, et al. The effect of norepinephrine in primary total knee replacement arthroplasty. J Korean Orthop Assoc. 2004;39:247–51.

Cho WS, Kim JM, Kim MY, et al. Gap discrepancy in posterior cruciate ligament-sacrificing total knee joint arthroplasty. J Korean Knee Soc. 2004;16:8–14.

Cho WS, Park SS, Kim JJ, et al. The discrepancy between epicondylar and posterior axis of femur in total knee arthroplasty. J Korean Knee Soc. 1999;11:8–11.

Christensen CP, Jacobs CA, Jennings HR. Effect of periarticular corticosteroid injections during total knee arthroplasty. A double-blind randomized trial. J Bone Joint Surg. 2009;91-A:2550–5.

Clayton ML, Thompson TR, Mack RP. Correction of alignment deformities during total knee arthroplasties: staged soft-tissue releases. Clin Orthop. 1986;202:117–24.

Cobb JP, Dixon H, Dandachli W, et al. The anatomical tibial axis: reliable rotational orientation in knee replacement. J Bone Joint Surg. 2008;90-B:1032–8.

Cushner FD. The subvastus approach to the knee. J Knee Surg. 2003;16:52–4.

D'ambrosio F, Scott WN. Ligament releases in the arthritic knee. In: Scott WN, editor. The knee. 1st ed. St. Louis: Mosby; 1994. p. 1199–210.

Dennis DA, Channer M, Suman MH. Intramedullary versus extramedullary tibial alignment systems in total knee arthroplasty. J Arthroplasty. 1993;8:43–7.

Dennis DA, Komistek RD, Kim RH, et al. Gap balancing versus measured resection technique for total knee arthroplasty. Clin Orthop. 2010;468:102–7.

Didden K, Luyckx T, Bellemans J, et al. Anteroposterior positioning of the tibial component and its effect on the mechanics of patellofemoral contact. J Bone Joint Surg. 2010;92-B:1466–70.

Dixon MC, Parsch D, Brown RR, et al. The correction of severe varus deformity in total knee arthroplasty by tibial component downsizing and resection of uncapped proximal medial bone. J Arthroplasty. 2004;19:19–22.

Doerr TE, Eckhoff DG. Lateral patellar burnishing in total knee arthroplasty following medialization of the patellar button. J Arthroplasty. 1995;10:540–2.

Dolin MG. Osteotomy of the tibial tubercle in total knee replacement: a technical note. J Bone Joint Surg. 1983;65-A:704–6.

Dorr LD, Boiardo RA. Technical considerations in total knee arthroplasty. Clin Orthop. 1986;205:5–11.

Dossett GH. Total knee replacement study using standard cutting guide vs. Otismed MRI generated cutting guide. Phoenix, AZ: Department of Veterans Affairs; 2010.

Easley ME, Insall JN, Scuderi GR, et al. Primary constrained condylar knee arthroplasty for the arthritic valgus knee. Clin Orthop. 2000;380:58–64.

Emerson RJ, Ayers C, Head W, et al. Surgical closing in total knee arthroplasty: flexion versus extension. Clin Orthop. 1996;331: 74–80.

Engh GA. Medial epicondylar osteotomy: a technique used with primary and revision to improve surgical exposure and correct varus deformity. Instr Course Lect. 1999;48:153–6.

Engh GA. Midvastus approach. In: Scuderi GR, editor. Surgical techniques in total knee arthroplasty. 1st ed. New York: Springer; 2002. p. 127–30.

Engh GA. The difficult knee. Clin Orthop. 2003;416:58–63.

Engh GA, Holt BT, Parks NL. A midvastus muscle-splitting approach for total knee arthroplasty. J Arthroplasty. 1997;12:322–31.

Enis J, Gardner R, Robledo M, et al. Comparison of patellar resurfacing versus nonresurfacing in bilateral total knee arthroplasty. Clin Orthop. 1990;260:38–42.

Esler CN, Blakeway C, Fiddian NJ. The use of a closed-suction drain in total knee arthroplasty. A prospective, randomised study. J Bone Joint Surg. 2003;85-B:215–7.

Fehring TK. Rotational malalignment of the femoral component in total knee arthroplasty. Clin Orthop. 2000;380:72–9.

Garvin KL. Quadriceps snip. In: Scuderi GR, editor. Surgical techniques in total knee arthroplasty. 1st ed. New York: Springer; 2002. p. 149–54.

Gejo R, Morita Y, Matsushita I, et al. Joint gap changes with patellar tendon strain and patellar position during TKA. Clin Orthop. 2008;466:946–51.

Goldstein SA, Wilson DL, Sonstegard DA, et al. The mechanical properties of human tibial trabecular bone as a function of metaphyseal location. J Biomech. 1983;16:965–9.

Gomez S, Yasgur DJ, Scuder GR, et al. Draping technique for total knee anthroplasty. In: Scuderi GR, editor. Surgical techniques in total knee arthroplasty. 1st ed. New York: Springer; 2002. p. 168–73.

Gooding CR, Garbuz DS, Masri BA, et al. Extensile surgical exposures for revision total knee replacement. In: Scott WN, editor. Surgery of the knee. 5th ed. Philadelphia: Churchill Livingstone; 2011. p. 1320–6.

Green GV, Berend KR, Berend ME, et al. The effects of varus tibial alignment on proximal tibial surface strain in total knee arthroplasty: the posteromedial hot spot. J Arthroplasty. 2002;17:1033–9.

Greenfield MA, Insall JN, Case GC, et al. Instrumentation of the patellar osteotomy in total knee arthroplasty: the relationship of patellar thickness and lateral retinacular release. Am J Knee Surg. 1996;9:129–32.

Griffin FM, Scuderi GR, Insall JN. Lateral release for fixed-valgus deformity. In: Scuderi GR, editor. Surgical techniques in total knee arthroplasty. 1st ed. New York: Springer; 2002. p. 197–204.

Gustke K. Use of smart trials for soft-tissue balancing in total knee replacement surgery. J Bone Joint Surg. 2012;94(11 Suppl A):147–50.

Gupta S, Augustine A, Horey L, et al. Electrocautery of the patellar rim in primary total knee replacement: beneficial or unnecessary? J Bone Joint Surg. 2010;92-B:1259–61.

Haertsch PA. The blood supply to the skin of the leg: a post-mortem investigation. Br J Plast Surg. 1981;34:470–7.

Hanada H, Whiteside LA, Steiger J, et al. Bone landmarks are more reliable than tensioned gaps in TKA component alignment. Clin Orthop. 2007;462:137–42.

Harada Y, Wevers HW, Cooke TD. Distribution of bone strength in the proximal tibia. J Arthroplasty. 1988;3:167–75.

Heesterbeek PJ, Jacobs WC, Wymenga AB. Effects of the balanced gap technique on femoral component rotation in TKA. Clin Orthop. 2009;467:1015–22.

Helmy N, Anglin C, Greidanus NV. To resurface or not to resurface the patella in total knee arthroplasty. Clin Orthop. 2008;466:2775–83.

Hofmann AA, Goldberg TD, Tanner AM, et al. Surface cementation of stemmed tibial components in primary total knee arthroplasty: minimum 5-year follow-up. J Arthroplasty. 2006;21:353–7.

Hofmann AA, Plaster RL, Murdock LE. Subvastus (southern) approach for primary total knee arthroplasty. Clin Orthop. 1991;269:70–7.

Hooper GJ, Rothwell AG, Frampton C, et al. Does the use of laminar flow and space suits reduce early deep infection after total hip and knee replacement?: the ten-year results of the New Zealand Joint Registry. J Bone Joint Surg. 2011;93-B:85–90.

Howell SM, Hull M. Kinematic alignment in total knee arthroplasty. In: Scott WN, editor. Surgery of the knee. 5th ed. Philadelphia: Churchill Livingstone; 2011. p. 1255–68.

Hsu H-P, Walker PS. Wear and deformation of patellar components in total knee arthroplasty. Clin Orthop. 1989;246:260–5.

Hungerford DS, Krackow KA. Total joint arthroplasty of the knee. Clin Orthop. 1985;192:23–33.

Husted H, Toftgaard JT. Influence of the pneumatic tourniquet on patellar tracking in total knee arthroplasty: a prospective randomized study in 100 patients. J Arthroplasty. 2005;20:694–7.

Incado SJ, Ronchetti PJ. Tibial plateau coverage in total knee arthroplasty. Clin Orthop. 1994;299:81–5.

Insall JN. A midline approach to the knee. J Bone Joint Surg. 1971;53-A:1584–6.

Insall JN, Easley ME. Surgical techniques and instrumentation in total knee arthroplasty. In: Insall JN, editor. Surgery of the knee. 3rd ed. New York: Churchill Livingstone; 2001. p. 1553–620.

Johnson D, Eastwood D. Lateral patellar release in knee arthroplasty: effect on wound healing. J Arthroplasty. 1992;7:427–31.

Kaper BP, Bourne RB. Patellar replacement in total knee arthroplasty. In: Insall JN, editor. Surgery of the knee. 3rd ed. New York: Churchill Livingstone; 2001. p. 1739–49.

Katz MA, Beck TD, Silber JS, Seldes RM, Lotke PA. Determining femoral rotational alignment in total knee arthroplasty: reliability of techniques. J Arthroplasty. 2001;16:301–5.

Kayler D, Lyttle D. Surgical interruption of patellar blood supply by total knee arthroplasty. Clin Orthop. 1988;229:221–7.

Keating EM, Faris PM, Meding JB, et al. Comparison of the midvastus muscle-splitting approach with the median parapatellar approach in total knee arthroplasty. J Arthroplasty. 1999;14:29–32.

Keblish PA. The lateral approach. In: Scuderi GR, editor. Surgical techniques in total knee arthroplasty. 1st ed. New York: Springer; 2002. p. 137–48.

Keblish PA. The lateral approach for total knee arthroplasty. J Knee Surg. 2003;16:62–8.

Keblish PA, Varma AK, Greenwald SA. Patellar resurfacing or retention in total knee arthroplasty: a prospective study of patients with bilateral replacement. J Bone Joint Surg. 1994;76-A:930–7.

Kesman TJ, Kaufman KR, Trousdale RT. Popliteus tendon resection during total knee arthroplasty: an observational report. Clin Orthop. 2011;469:76–81.

Kim BS, Reitman RD, Schai PA, et al. Selective patellar nonresurfacing in total knee arthroplasty. 10-year results. Clin Orthop. 1999;367:81–8.

Kim YH, Cho SH, Kim RS. Drainage versus nondrainage in simultaneous bilateral total knee arthroplasties. Clin Orthop. 1998;347:188–93.

Kim YH, Kim JS, Yoon SH. A recession of posterior cruciate ligament in posterior cruciate-retaining total knee arthroplasty. J Arthroplasty. 2008;23:999–1004.

Khan MS, Seon JK, Sone EK. Rational profile of lower limb and axis for tibial component alignment in varus osteoarthritic knees. J Arthroplasty. 2012;27:797–802.

Klatt BA, Goyal N, Austin MS, et al. Custom-fit total knee arthroplasty (OtisKnee) results in malalignment. J Arthroplasty. 2008;23:26–9.

Kobayashi T, Suzuki M, Sasho T, et al. Lateral laxity in flexion increases the postoperative flexion angle in cruciate-retaining total knee arthroplasty. J Arthroplasty. 2012;27:260–5.

Koo MH, Choi CH. Conservative treatment for the intraoperative detachment of medial collateral ligament from the tibial attachment site during primary total knee arthroplasty. J Arthroplasty. 2009;24:1249–53.

Krackow KA. Medial and lateral ligament advancement. In: Scuderi GR, editor. Surgical techniques in total knee arthroplasty. 1st ed. New York: Springer; 2002. p. 205–9.

Krackow KA, Jones MM, Teeny SM, et al. Primary total knee arthroplasty in patients with fixed valgus deformity. Clin Orthop. 1991;273:9.

Krackow KA, Mihalko WM. Flexion-extension joint gap changes after lateral structure release for valgus deformity correction in total knee arthroplasty: a cadaveric study. J Arthroplasty. 1999;14:994–1004.

Krackow KA, Mihalko WM. The effect of medial release on flexion and extension gaps in cadaveric knees: implications for soft-tissue balancing in total knee arthroplasty. Am J Knee Surg. 1999;12:222–8.

Laskin RS. Flexion space configuration in total knee arthroplasty. J Arthroplasty. 1995;10:657–60.

Laskin RS. Soft tissue balancing of the varus knee. In: Callaghan JJ, editor. The adult knee. 1st ed. Philadelphia: Lippincott Williams & Wilkins; 2003. p. 1217–22.

Laughlin RT, Werries BA, Verhulst SJ, et al. Patellar tilt in total knee arthroplasty. Am J Orthop. 1996;25:300–4.

Lavernia C, Contreras JS, Alcerro JC. The peel in total knee revision: exposure in the difficult knee. Clin Orthop. 2011;469:146–53.

Lee GC, Lotke PA. Management of intraoperative medial collateral ligament injury during TKA. Clin Orthop. 2011;469:64–8.

Lemon M, Packham I, Narang K, et al. Patellar tendon length after knee arthroplasty with and without preservation of the infrapatellar fat pad. J Arthroplasty. 2007;22:574–80.

Li C, Nijat A, Askar M. No clear advantage to use of wound drains after unilateral total knee arthroplasty: a prospective randomized, controlled trial. J Arthroplasty. 2011;26:519–22.

Lombardi AV. Soft tissue balancing of the knee-flexion. In: Callaghan JJ, editor. The adult knee. 1st ed. Philadelphia: Lippincott Williams & Wilkins; 2003. p. 1223–32.

Lombardi AV, Mallory TH, Maitino PD. Freehand resection of the patella in total knee arthroplasty referencing the attachments of the quadriceps tendon and patellar tendon. J Arthroplasty. 1998;13:788–92.

Lotke PA, Ecker ML. Influence of positioning of prosthesis in total knee replacement. J Bone Joint Surg. 1977;59-A:77–9.

Matsuda Y, Ishii Y, Noguchi H, et al. Varus-valgus balance and range of movement after total knee arthroplasty. J Bone Joint Surg. 2005;87-B:804–8.

Matsueda M, Gengerke TR, Murphy M, et al. Soft tissue release in total knee arthroplasty. Cadaver study using knees without deformities. Clin Orthop. 1999;366:264–73.

Matsumoto T, Muratsu H, Kubo S, et al. Soft tissue tension in cruciate-retaining and posterior-stabilized total knee arthroplasty. J Arthroplasty. 2011;26:788–95.

McMahon MS, Scuderi GR, Glashow JL, et al. Scintigraphic determination of patellar viability after excision of infrapatellar fat pad and/or lateral retinacular release in total knee arthroplasty. Clin Orthop. 1990;260:10–6.

Mihalko WM, Boyle J, Clark LD, et al. The variability of intramedullary alignment of the femoral component during total knee arthroplasty. J Arthroplasty. 2005;20:25–8.

Mihalko WM, Krackow KA. Posterior cruciate ligament effects on the flexion space in total knee arthroplasty. Clin Orthop. 1999;360:243–50.

Mihalko WM, Krackow KA. Anatomic and biomechanical aspects of pie crusting posterolateral structures for valgus deformity correction in total knee arthroplasty- cadaveric study. J Arthroplasty. 2000;15:347–53.

Miller MC, Zhang AX, Petrella AJ, et al. The effect of component placement on knee kinetics after arthroplasty with an unconstrained prosthesis. J Orthop Res. 2001;19:614–20.

Mullaji A, Shetty GM. Persistent hindfoot valgus causes lateral deviation of weight bearing axis after total knee arthroplasty. Clin Orthop. 2011;469:1154–60.

Nicoll D, Rowley DI. Internal rotational error of the tibial component is a major cause of pain after total knee replacement. J Bone Joint Surg. 2010;92-B:1238–44.

Nizard RS, Biau D, Porcher R, et al. A meta-analysis of patellar replacement in total knee arthroplasty. Clin Orthop. 2005;432:196–203.

Omonbude D, El Masry MA, O'Connor PJ, et al. Measurement of joint effusion and haematoma formation by ultrasound in assessing the effectiveness of drains after total knee replacement: a prospective randomised study. J Bone Joint Surg. 2010;92-B:51–5.

Onishi CS, Kaufman KR, Irby SE, et al. Effects of patellar thickness on compression and shear forces in total knee arthroplasty. Clin Orthop. 1996;331:283–90.

Pagnano MW, Hanssen AD, Lewallen DG, et al. Flexion instability after primary posterior cruciate retaining total knee arthroplasty. Clin Orthop. 1998;356:39–46.

Pagnano MW, Kelly MA. The intraoperative assessment of patellar tracking. In: Scuderi GR, editor. Surgical techniques in total knee arthroplasty. 1st ed. New York: Springer; 2002. p. 317–25.

Parker DA, Tsigaras H, Rorabeck CH. Surgical exposure for primary total knee arthroplasty. In: Callaghan JJ, editor. The adult knee. 1st ed. Philadelphia: Lippincott Williams & Wilkins; 2003. p. 1095–109.

Pavlou G, Meyer C, Leonidou A, et al. Patellar resurfacing in total knee arthroplasty: does design matter? A meta-analysis of 7075 cases. J Bone Joint Surg. 2011;93-A:1301–9.

Poilvache PL. The epicondylar axis for femoral component rotation. In: Scuderi GR, editor. Surgical techniques in total knee arthroplasty. 1st ed. New York: Springer; 2 p. 227–35.

Politi J, Scott R. Balancing severe valgus deformity in total knee arthroplasty using a lateral cruciform retinacular release. J Arthroplasty. 2004;19:553–7.

Rae PJ, Noble J, Hodgkinson JP. Patellar resurfacing in total condylar knee arthroplasty. Technique and results. J Arthroplasty. 1990;5:259–65.

Ranawat CS. The patellofemoral joint in total condylar knee arthroplasty. Pros and cons based on five- to ten-year follow-up observations. Clin Orthop. 1986;205:93–9.

Ranawat CS, Holden DS, Ranawat AS, et al. Soft tissue balancing of the valgus knee. In: Callaghan JJ, editor. The adult knee. 1st ed. Philadelphia: Lippincott Williams & Wilkins; 2003. p. 1207–16.

Rand JA. The patellofemoral joint in total knee arthroplasty. J Bone Joint Surg. 1994;76-A:612–20.

Reuben J, McDonald C, Woodard P, et al. Effect of patellar thickness on patellar strain following total knee arthroplasty. J Arthroplasty. 1991;6:251–8.

Ries MD, Rauscher LA, Hoskins S, et al. Intramedullary pressure and pulmonary function during total knee arthroplasty. Clin Orthop. 1998;356:154–60.

Ritter MA, Campbell ED. Postoperative patellar complications with or without lateral release during total knee arthroplasty. Clin Orthop. 1987;219:163–8.

Ritter MA, Keating EM, Faris PM. Clinical, roentgenographic and scintigraphic results after interruption of the superior lateral genicular artery during total knee arthroplasty. Clin Orthop. 1989;248:145–51.

Rodriguez-Merchan EC, Gomez-Cardero P. The outerbridge classification predicts the need for patellar resurfacing in TKA. Clin Orthop. 2010;468:1254–7.

Romero J, Stahelin T, Binkert C, et al. The clinical consequences of flexion gap asymmetry in total knee arthroplasty. J Arthroplasty. 2007;22:235–40.

Schindler OS. Patellar resurfacing in total knee arthroplasty. In: Scott WN, editor. Surgery of the knee. 5th ed. Philadelphia: Churchill Livingstone; 2011. p. 1161–90.

Scott RD. Primary total knee arthroplasty surgical technique. In: Scott RD, editor. Total knee arthroplasty. 1st ed. Philadelphia: Saunders; 2006. p. 20–38.

Scott RD, Chmell MJ. Balancing the posterior cruciate ligament during cruciate-retaining fixed and mobile-bearing total knee arthroplasty: description of the pull-out lift-off and slide-back tests. J Arthroplasty. 2008;23:605–8.

Scott RD, Volatile TB. Twelve years experience with posterior cruciate-retaining total knee arthroplasty. Clin Orthop. 1986;205:100–7.

Scuderi G, Scharf SC, Meltzer LP, Scott WN. The relationship of lateral releases to patella Viability in total knee arthroplasty. J Arthroplasty. 1987;2:209–14.

Seon JK, Song EK, Park SJ, et al. Rotational axes of the femoral component in total knee arthroplasty. J Korean Orthop Assoc. 2006;41:428–33.

Shih HN, Shih LY, Wong YC, et al. Long-term changes of the nonresurfaced patella after total knee arthroplasty. J Bone Joint Surg. 2004;86-A:935–9.

Smith AJ, Wood DJ, Li MG. Total knee replacement with and without patellar resurfacing: a prospective, randomized trial using the profix total knee system. J Bone Joint Surg. 2008; 90-B:43–9.

Sneppen O, Gudmundsson GH, Bunger C. Patellofemoral function in total condylar knee arthroplasty. Int Orthop. 1985;9:65–8.

Soudry M, Mestriner LA, Binazzi R, et al. Total knee arthroplasty without patellar resurfacing. Clin Orthop. 1986;205:166–70.

Stern SH, Moeckel BH, Insall JN. Total knee arthroplasty in valgus knees. Clin Orthop. 1991;273:5–8.

Stiehl JB. Tibial shaft axis for femoral component rotation. In: Scuderi GR, editor. Surgical techniques in total knee arthroplasty. 1st ed. New York: Springer; 2002. p. 236–9.

Stoeckl B, Nogler M, Krismer M, et al. Reliability of the transepicondylar axis as an anatomical landmark in total knee arthroplasty. J Arthroplasty. 2006;21:878–82.

Teeny SM, Krackow KA, Hungerford DS, et al. Primary total knee arthroplasty in patients with severe varus deformity: a comparative study. Clin Orthop. 1991;273:19–31.

Vail TP, Lang JE. Surgical techniques and instrumentation in total knee arthroplasty. In: Scott WN, editor. Surgery of the knee. 4th ed. Philadelphia: Churchill Livingstone; 2006. p. 1455–521.

Vail TP, Lang JE, Sikes III CV. Surgical techniques and instrumentation in total knee arthroplasty. In: Scott WN, editor. Surgery of the knee. 5th ed. Philadelphia: Churchill Livingstone; 2011. p. 1042–99.

van Jonbergen HP, Scholtes VA, van Kampen A, et al. A randomised, controlled trial of circumpatellar electrocautery in total knee replacement without patellar resurfacing. J Bone Joint Surg. 2011;93-B:1054–9.

Vanlommel J, Luyckx JP, Labey L, et al. Cementing the tibial component in total knee arthroplasty: which technique is the best? J Arthroplasty. 2011;26:492–6.

Verlinden C, Uvin P, Labey L, et al. The influence of malrotation of the femoral component in total knee replacement on the mechanics of patellofemoral contact during gait: an in vitro biomechanical study. J Bone Joint Surg. 2010;92-B:737–42.

Vince KG. Subvastus approach. In: Scuderi GR, editor. Surgical techniques in total knee arthroplasty. 1st ed. New York: Springer; 2002. p. 119–26.

Vince KG, Abdeen A, Sugimori T. The unstable total knee arthroplasty: causes and cures. J Arthroplasty. 2006;21(4 Suppl 1):44–9.

Wachtl SW, Jakob RP. Patellar osteotomy for lateral retinaculum decompression in total knee arthroplasty. Acta Orthop Scand. 2000;71:522–4.

Wai Hung CL, Wai Pan Y, Kwong Yuen C, et al. Interobserver and intraobserver error in distal femur transepicondylar axis measurement with computed tomography. J Arthroplasty. 2009;24:96–100.

Wakankar HM, Nicholl JE, Koka R, D'Arcy JC. The tourniquet in total knee arthroplasty. A prospective, randomized study. J Bone Joint Surg. 1999;81-B:30–3.

Walker PS, Soudry M, Ewald FC, et al. Control of cement penetration in total knee arthroplasty. Clin Orthop. 1984;185:155.

White RE, Allman JK, Trauger JA, et al. Clinical comparison of the midvastus and medial parapatellar surgical approaches. Clin Orthop. 1999;367:117–22.

Whiteside LA. Correction of ligament and bone defects in total knee arthroplasty of the severely valgus knee. Clin Orthop. 1993;288:234–45.

Whiteside LA. Exposure in difficult total knee arthroplasty using tibial tubercle osteotomy. Clin Orthop. 1995;321:32–5.

Whiteside LA. Selective ligament release in total knee arthroplasty of the knee in valgus. Clin Orthop. 1999;367:130–40.

Wolff AM, Hungerford DS, Krackow KA, et al. Osteotomy of the tibial tubercle during total knee replacement. J Bone Joint Surg. 1989;71-A:848–52.

Wood DJ, Smith AJ, Cllopy D, et al. Patellar resurfacing in total knee arthroplasty: a prospective, randomized trial. J Bone Joint Surg. 2002;84-A:187–93.

Worland RL, Jessup DE, Johnson J. Posterior cruciate recession in total knee arthroplasty. J Arthroplasty. 1997;12:70–3.

Xu C, Chu X, Wu H. Effects of patellar resurfacing on contact area and contact stress in total knee arthroplasty. Knee. 2007;14:183–7.

Yacoubian SV, Scott RD. Skin incision translation in total knee arthroplasty: the difference between flexion and extension. J Arthroplasty. 2007;22:353–5.

Yasgur DJ, Scuderi GR, Insall JN. Medial release for fixed-varus deformity. In: Scuderi GR, editor. Surgical techniques in total knee arthroplasty. 1st ed. New York: Springer; 2002. p. 189–96.

Yoshii T, Whiteside LA, Anouchi YS. The effect of patella button placement and femoral design on patellar tracking in total knee arthroplasty. Clin Orthop. 1992;275:211–9.

Young CF, Bourne RB, Rorabeck CH. Tibial tubercle osteotomy in total knee arthroplasty surgery. J Arthroplasty. 2008;23:371–5.

Zhang QD, Guo WS, Zhang Q, et al. Comparison between closed suction drainage and nondrainage in total knee arthroplasty: a meta-analysis. J Arthroplasty. 2011;26:1265–72.

Zhang LZ, Zhang XL, Jiang Y, et al. Lateral patellar facetectomy had improved clinical results in patients with patellar-retaining total knee arthroplasty. J Arthroplasty. 2012;27:1442–7.

5 TKA in Specific Conditions

5.1 Bone Defects

5.1.1 Introduction

Bone defects can be found in various disorders or conditions of the knee joint. In primary TKA, bone defects are commonly observed in the medial or posteromedial side of the tibia if there is a varus deformity due to severe degenerative arthritis or in the lateral condyle of the femur if there is a valgus deformity due to rheumatoid arthritis (RA) or traumatic arthritis, etc. Bone defects can also develop in case of osteonecrosis, after high tibial osteotomy or Charcot disease. During revision arthroplasty, bone defects are encountered in cases with infection and loosening, and they may also develop while removing the prosthesis and bone cement.

5.1.2 Classification

Bone defects are classified according to their site, size, and shape. They can be classified using a *simple and easy method into contained (cavitary) defect and uncontained (peripheral, segmental) defect*; a contained defect is a cavitary defect surrounded by an intact cortical or corticocancellous bone, and an uncontained or peripheral defect is a defect in which the cortical rim is deficient (Fig. 5.1).

However, the AORI (Anderson Orthopaedic Research Institute) classification, which classifies bone defects according to the size and shape in addition to the contained and uncontained defect, is the most widely used classification. *The AORI classification is systematic, and it can be applied to both the tibia and femur.* This classification can be made preoperatively based on the X-rays, but *it is more accurate to classify the bone defects intra- or postoperatively since the classification may change during operation.*

This classification is based on the condition of the bone defect in the metaphyseal segment. According to this classification, bone defects are divided into three types: type I, II, and III. Femoral defect is divided into F1, F2, and F3, while tibial defect is divided into T1, T2, and T3 (Fig. 5.2).

Type 1 defect, i.e., F1 or T1, has an intact metaphyseal bone and *refers to minimal bone defects that do not affect the stability of prosthesis. Type 2 defect, i.e., F2 or T2,* has an epiphyseal defect *of the cortical or cancellous bone.* If this type of bone defect is found only in one of the tibial or femoral condyle, it is classified as type 2A, whereas type 2B refers to bone defects in both condyles. *Type 3 defect, i.e., F3 or T3, has a deficient metaphyseal segment, and generally the collateral ligaments or the patellar tendon has been detached from the bone or has been injured* since the main parts of the femoral condyle or the tibial plateau are missing.

The major differentiation between the type 2 and type 3 defects is whether the joint stability can be maintained by the usual bone reconstruction methods alone or not. *Anatomically, the femoral defect distal to the epicondyle is type 2, and the femoral defect proximal to the epicondyle is type 3. The tibial defect proximal to the fibular head is type 2 and that distal to the fibular head is type 3. In type 1 defect, patients have little deformity or instability, whereas the patients with a type 2 defect have a varus or valgus deformity, and those with a type 3 defect always have instability due to insufficient ligamentous structures.*

Bone defects may also occur in the patella, but they are excluded from the AORI classification.

However, the AORI classification is sometimes not practical as it does not consider huge cavitary defects which are frequently encountered during revision surgery. *Hospital for Special Surgery (HSS) introduced a new classification, which divides bone defects into cystic, epiphyseal, cavitary, and segmental defects in the cancellous bone.* This method of classification is more practical for determining the bone reconstruction method during revision surgery. *The cystic defect is a small contained defect and does not affect the stability of prosthesis; bone cement is used if the diameter of the defect is 5 mm or smaller, and bone graft is performed if the diameter of the defect is greater than 5 mm. The epiphyseal defect is a bone defect involving the cortical bone of the epiphysis or metaphysis and may affect the stability of*

W. Cho, *Knee Joint Arthroplasty*,
DOI 10.1007/978-3-642-39389-1_5, © Springer-Verlag Berlin Heidelberg 2014

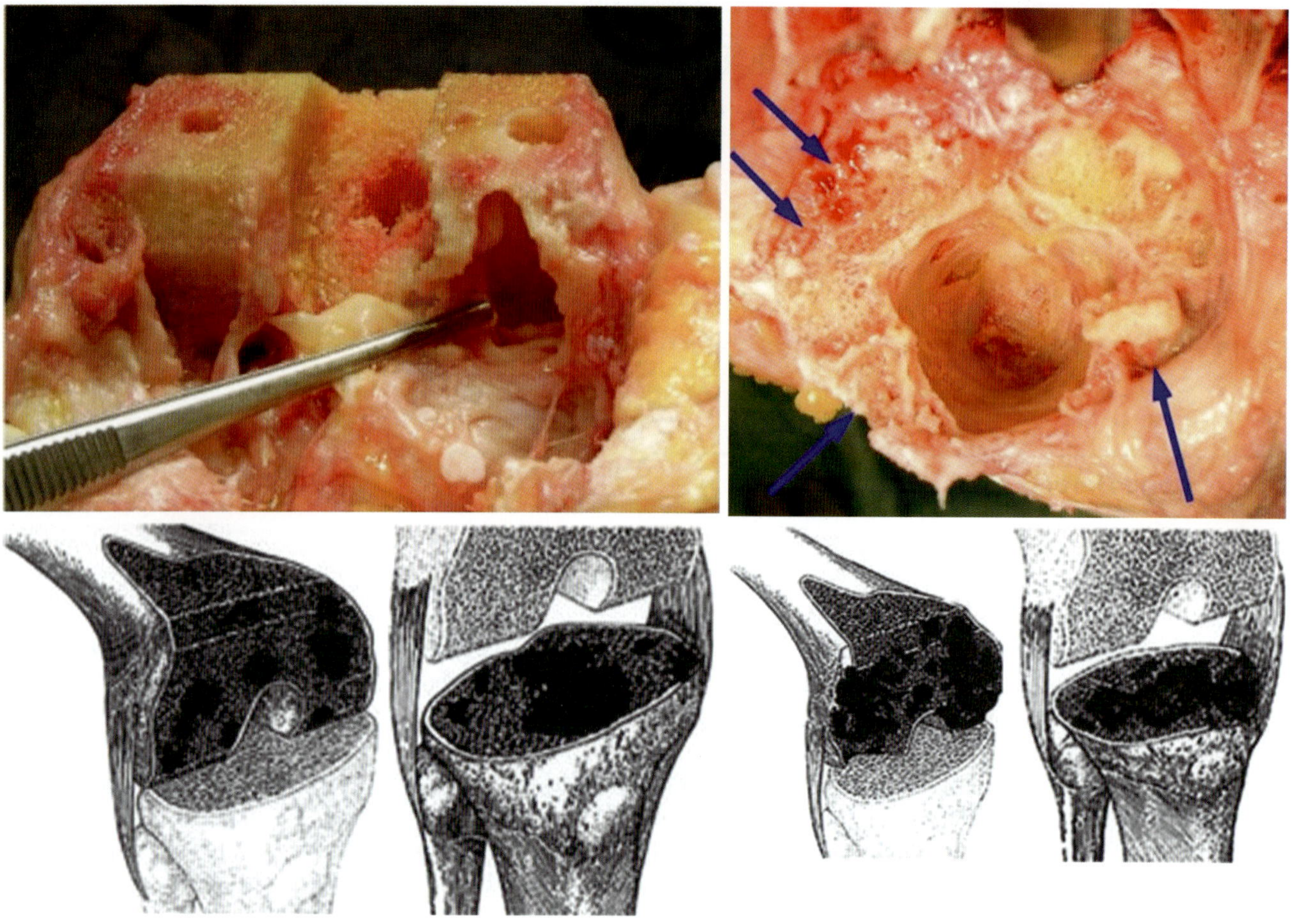

Fig. 5.1 Contained and uncontained (peripheral) defect

prosthesis. Usually there is a wedge-shaped defect on the medial tibial plateau, and *it is observed when there is a varus deformity. This type of bone defect can be reconstructed using metal augments, and an extension stem may be needed in some cases. Cavitary defect involves a severe loss of the cancellous bone although the cortical wall remains intact,* and it is caused due to severe osteolysis, infection, or during removal of the prosthesis with a violent force. *It affects the stability of prosthesis, and hence, strut allografts or impaction of morcellized grafts with extension stem or trabecular system may be required. Segmental defect is a combined epiphyseal and cavitary defect, and it may be required to use allografts or hinged prosthesis.*

5.1.3 Diagnosis

In primary TKA, the diagnosis of bone defect can be made relatively easily on the simple preoperative X-rays, and the classification of bone defect rarely changes when the operation has been performed properly. The AORI type I defect may not be detected on the simple X-ray. In the type II defect, there is an accompanying varus or valgus deformity of the knee joint on weight-bearing A–P X-rays. The knee joint may also show slight subluxation. In primary osteoarthritis, the bone defect is generally on the posteromedial side of the tibia. On careful observation, two joint lines can be seen on the A–P view, and these lines are seen more clearly on the lateral X-rays (Fig. 5.3). In femoral defects, the femoral condyle shows some flattening on the A–P and the lateral view, and this finding becomes more obvious when lines are drawn along both the condyles on the lateral view. In type III defect, the bony defect is clearly seen, and the deformity is marked on the simple X-ray. The instability is more prominent on weight bearing or stress X-ray.

In revision TKA, it is not easy to make the diagnosis of bone defect on simple X-ray. In osteolysis or loosening, bone defect is often masked because of the overlap of bony contour. *CT or three-dimensional (3D) CT is often needed in revision cases.* Also, the bone defect classification can change during or after the operation since implant removal may have an effect on the extent of bone defect.

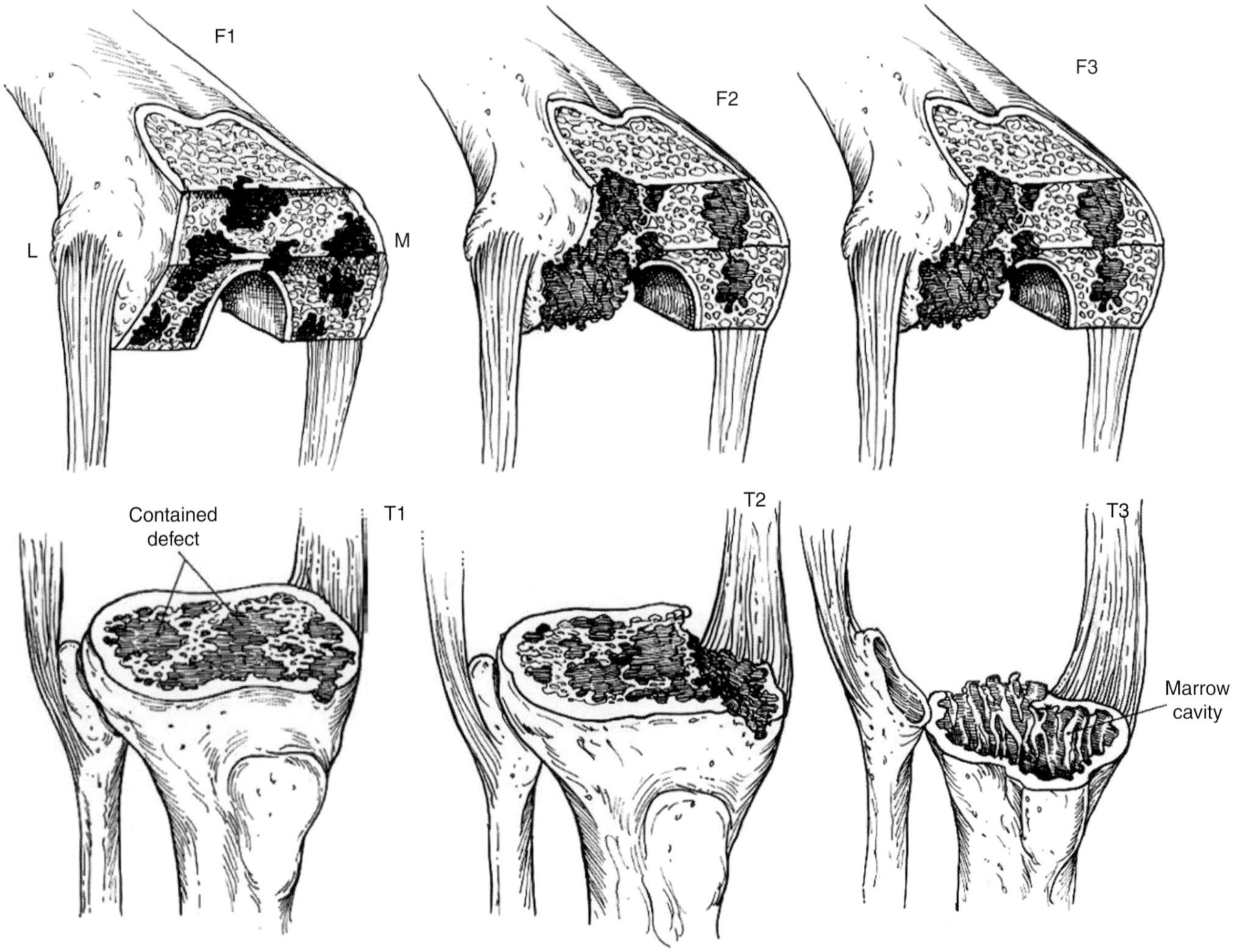

Fig. 5.2 The AORI bone defect classification

5.1.4 Principles and Methods of Treatment

The purpose of bone defect reconstruction is to achieve implant stability with good alignment, maintain the joint line, and achieve an adequate ligament balance. The principles of treatment depend on the type and size of bone defect, but other factors such as patient's age, activity, or life expectancy are also considered.

When bone defects are divided into contained and peripheral defects, *the contained defect is reconstructed using* either *morcellized cancellous autogenous or allogeneic bone grafts* or by *filling the defect with bone cement if it is a small defect*. Whereas structural allografts or trabecular system may be needed for larger contained defects. Scott emphasized that a *bone defect caused by a large cystic cavity in rheumatoid arthritis or osteoarthritis (OA) should be filled with bone graft after curettage.* He stated that when a cystic defect is filled with bone cement, there is a risk of developing loosening due to progressive bone resorption.

In a peripheral defect, several methods such as metal augmentation, bone graft, custom-made prosthesis, *tumor prosthesis*, or APC (allograft prosthesis composite) can be used according to the size of bone defect.

Principles of treatment *according to the AORI classification* are as follows: *In a type 1 defect, it is only required to fill the defect with a bone graft or bone cement. In a type 2 defect, it is required to use bone cement, metal augment, or bone graft*, and extension stem may be required to prevent subsidence or migration of the prosthesis. *Type 3 defect can be reconstructed with bone graft alone (Fig. 5.4), bone graft along with metal augmentation or trabecular system, and a constrained type or hinged prosthesis may be used if the implant stability seems doubtful. In severe bone defects, the use of tumor prosthesis* or custom-made prosthesis can be considered.

I agree with the above principles of treatment, and I would like to describe the methods in more detail.

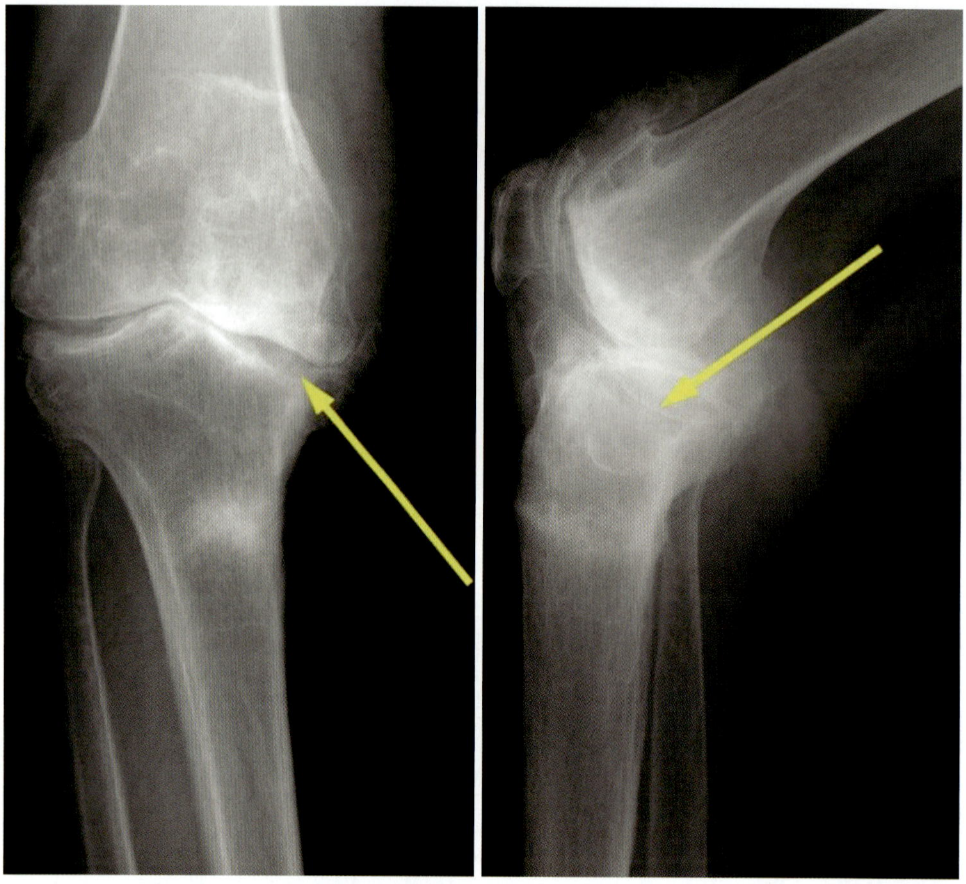

Fig. 5.3 X-ray of the bone defect in the tibia (*arrow*)

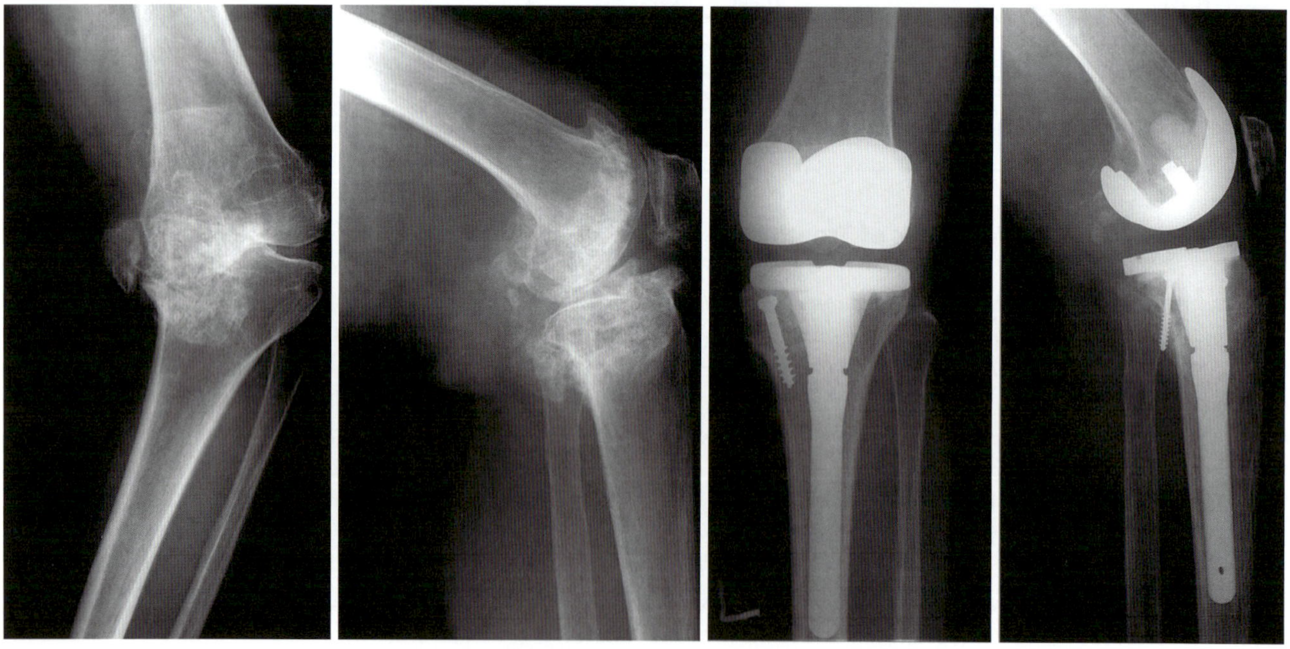

Fig. 5.4 AORI T3 defect reconstructed using structural allograft

5.1.4.1 Cementing

Cementing is recommended *when the bone defect is smaller than 5 mm in depth regardless of whether it is a contained defect or a peripheral defect*. Chen and Krackow demonstrated that cementing is mechanically as strong as metal augmentation in smaller bone defects since the cement fills the defect completely. *Cementing is not recommended in relatively younger and active patients*. Considering

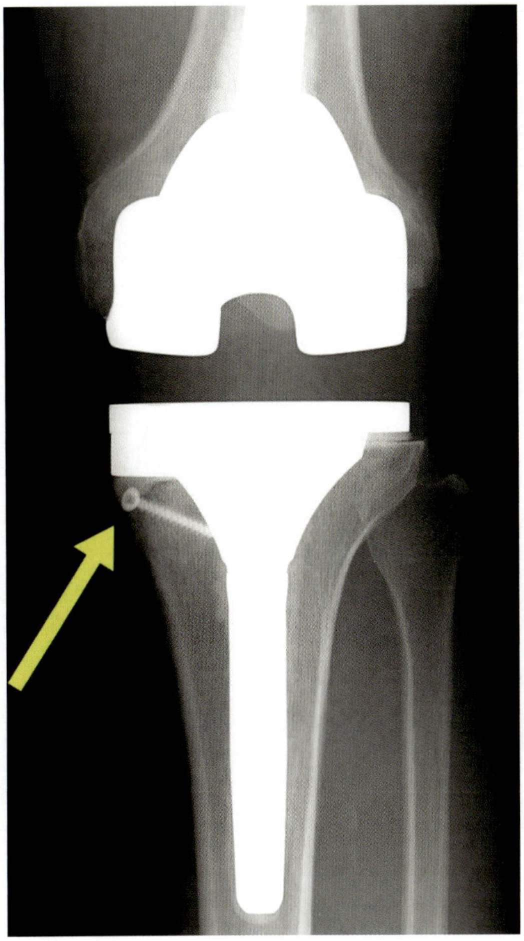

Fig. 5.5 An X-ray of cement with screw augmentation technique

revision surgery, cement is mechanically weaker than bone graft, and bony incorporation occurs easily in younger patients.

When there is a slightly larger peripheral bone defect, cementing and screw augmentation techniques may be used. Ritter and Harty found that cement with screw augmentation showed superior clinical results than those in cement without screw augmentation. Scott introduced screw augmentation in the distal part of the femur and when the appropriate length of screws is used, they can maintain proper alignment as well as strengthen the cement fixation. The technique requires insertion of screws into the bone and covering them with cement. The use of titanium cancellous screws is recommended, and it is necessary to ensure that the screws do not protrude from the cement (Fig. 5.5).

On the other hand, according to Brooks et al., *cementing of larger bone defects worsens the clinical results, and radiolucent lines appear beneath the cement.* The reason for this is that larger lumps of cement cause thermal necrosis, infection, and fibrous membrane formation. However, Pagnano et al. insisted that osteolysis is the result of poor cementing technique, and they emphasized the importance of proper cementing technique.

It is important not to make a wedge-shaped cut but to make a step cut on the host bone so as to reduce the shear force, especially in a peripheral defect. Chen and Krackow experienced 100 % failure when cement was formed into a wedge shape.

5.1.4.2 Metal Augmentation

Metal augment is convenient and simple to use. Brand et al. observed good results using metal augments without radiolucent lines after 5–6 years of midterm follow-up.

There are two types of metal augments, wedge or flat block (rectangular) type for the tibial defect and single unit that augments the anterior, distal, and posterior defects simultaneously or separate blocks that augment the femoral defect according to their location.

Wedge Type

The wedge type of metal augment is an earlier model, and its major benefit is preservation of more bones, since most of the bone defects are wedge shaped. However, *more time is needed* to perform osteotomy for an accurate engagement of the augment into the defect. *Another drawback of the wedge type* of metal augment is that the augment is *under shear force instead of compressive force* (Fig. 5.6). For this reason, Windsor et al. recommended the use of an extension stem with a wedge-shaped augment.

Block Type

On the other hand, *although a little more bone resection is required for using the block type* of metal augment, *it is easier to apply, and it is mechanically more durable than the wedge type* of augment. This finding was confirmed in studies by Fehring et al. and Cho et al.

The fixation of metal augment onto the implant is done either by using screws or cement. Cement fixation can reduce metal corrosion; however, rigid fixation cannot be achieved, and changes in the position of the augment can occur. Screws can provide rigid fixation between the augment and the implant, but they may cause corrosion due to metal interaction. Hence, it is desirable to use both the fixation methods.

Extension stem is needed to a lesser extent with the *block type* of metal augment than with the wedge type, but *it is desirable to use an extension stem when a thicker augment is used or when the stability of prosthesis is doubtful due to osteoporosis.*

Trabecular System

If a cavitary defect is huge, a *metal trabecular system* may be used to reconstruct the bone defect. *It is made of porous tantalum and is designed for bony ingrowth. The advantage of the trabecular system is that the incidence of infection is reduced and bone resorption does not occur.* Its disadvantage is that the surgical technique is not easy as morcellized bone graft

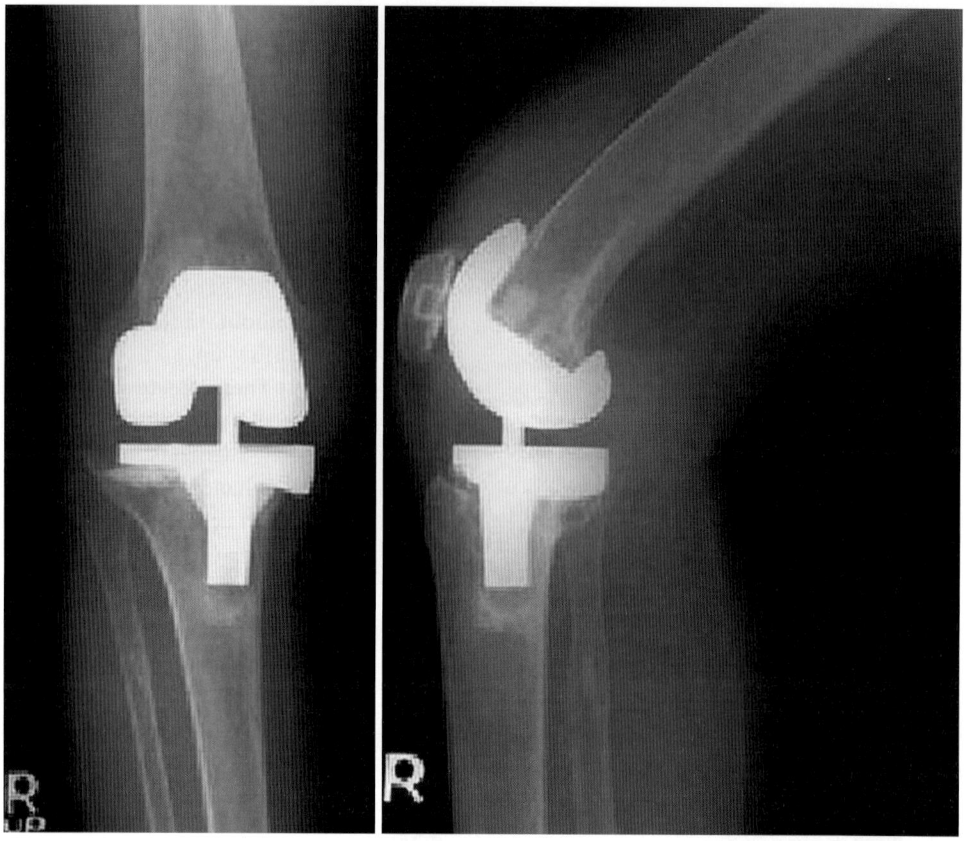

Fig. 5.6 X-rays showing loosening in wedge type of metal augment

may be needed sometimes for tight fitting, and its removal is very difficult during revision surgery. There are various sizes and shapes of the trabecular system according to the shape of the bone defect. Choosing the correct size and shape of the trabecular system is also a very important procedure.

5.1.4.3 Bone Graft

An autogenous graft, allograft, or both can be used in combination as a bone graft. *Once the bone graft is incorporated, it is the most biologic* reconstruction. This is the reason why bone graft is recommended for younger and more active patients, even though the bone defect is mild. Dorr et al. stated that the use of a bone graft is indicated when surface defects are more than 50 % and are deeper than 5 mm in one condyle.

A contained defect can be treated with morcellized cancellous graft, but a peripheral defect requires a structural graft. Peripheral defect can be reconstructed using impaction allograft with wire mesh.

Autograft

Autogenous bone can be obtained from the osteotomized bones; however, only a *limited amount of bone* is available.

Morcellized cancellous autogenous graft is commonly used to fill a small bone defect or it is used in combination

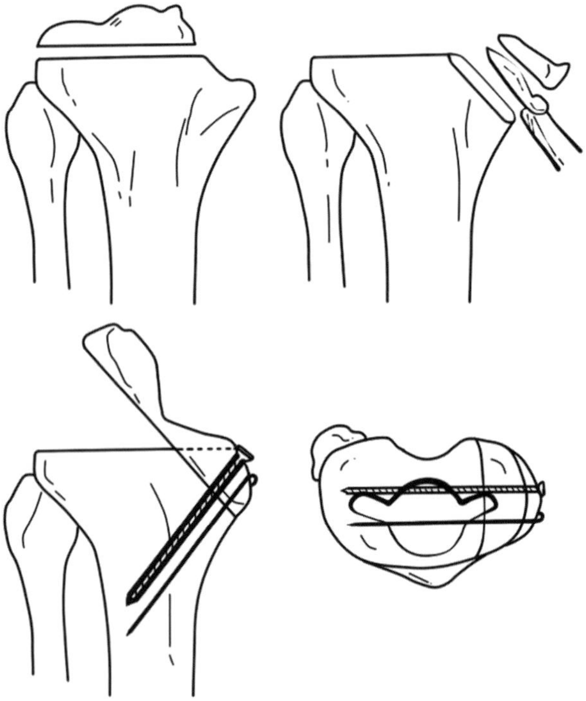

Fig. 5.7 Autograft in the proximal tibia using resected femoral bone

with allograft. Bones from the distal femur can be used in case of a wedge type of bone defect in the tibia, but autogenous bone is often not suitable for structural bone graft because it is too small for achieving stable fixation (Fig. 5.7), and the bone quality is poor due to sclerotic changes. Iliac bone can also be used, but it can cause donor site morbidity, and its mechanical strength is not adequate when the shape and direction of the graft are not compatible with the host trabecular system.

Allograft

Although the *allograft has a lower capacity for osteoinduction than the autograft*, it has excellent osteoconduction function. Bony incorporation of the allograft can occur, although it takes a longer time than that of the autograft.

Although the allograft has the potential to transmit infectious diseases, it is most commonly used for large bone defects since the required amount of bone can be obtained easily. The femoral head is the most commonly used allograft, while the other bones are also available for this purpose. The femoral head is spherical in shape and can be cut to adapt to the shape and thickness of the proximal tibial and distal femoral defects. The allogeneic bone should be freeze dried in order to reduce immune reactions.

The problem with the use of allograft is that it occasionally collapses when it fails to incorporate into the host bone. Also, the allograft undergoes creeping substitution after revascularization, and this process may cause nonunion if it occurs too slowly, or a fracture may develop if it occurs too rapidly. Even after bone union has been achieved, *if the graft bone is too large, it acts as an inert material causing fatigue fracture over time due to limited remodeling*.

Bone Graft Techniques

A few factors are *important for* enhancing the incorporation of the bone graft. *First, good alignment of the implant must be ensured. Second, cancellous to cancellous interface contact should be achieved. Third, rigid fixation should be established. Fourth, interposition of cement between the graft and host bone should be avoided. Lastly, the sclerotic bone should be drilled to cause bleeding*. However, some surgeons do not recommend drilling of the sclerotic bone since the sclerotic bone plays an important role in providing bony support.

Contact

The complete removal of soft tissues and foreign bodies is as important as avoiding contact of the cortical allograft to the cancellous host bone. The contact surfaces of the graft bone and the host bone should be even and gap-free; hence, an osteotomy should be performed such that the grafted bone fits accurately on the host bone, or morcellized bone should be used to fill the gap between the bone graft and the host bone.

Size and Shape

When the morcellized graft is to be used, the bone should be broken into pieces smaller than 5 mm. The structural graft has to be fixed with K-wires or metal screws, and hence *the size of bone must be large enough, at least 1 cm in thickness in every plane*. If it is smaller than this, the grafted bone can get fractured during fixation. However, if an allogeneic bone is too big in size, it results in problems of union or incorporation and is likely to collapse. *The bone graft itself should provide stability by its own shape, and it is recommended that the host bone should be prepared in a reverse trapezoid shape or step cut so as to prevent shear force* (Fig. 5.8).

When using the femoral head, the acetabular reamer can be used to prepare the recipient site so as to match it with the femoral head.

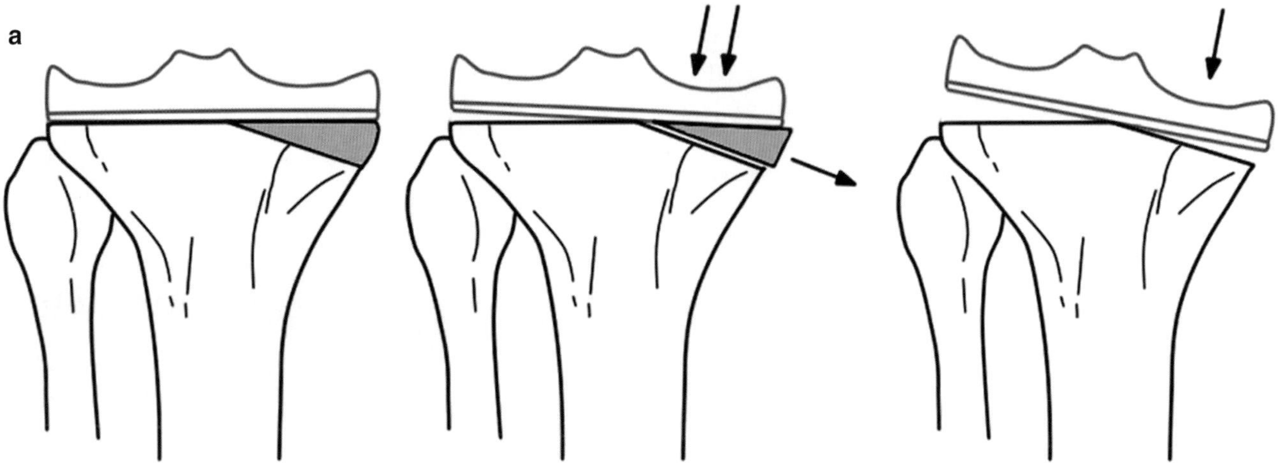

Fig. 5.8 Ideal shape of the bone graft. The bone graft should not be as shown in the *top* (**a**) *figures*, but it should be as shown in the *bottom* (**b**, **c**) *figures*

Fig. 5.8 (continued)

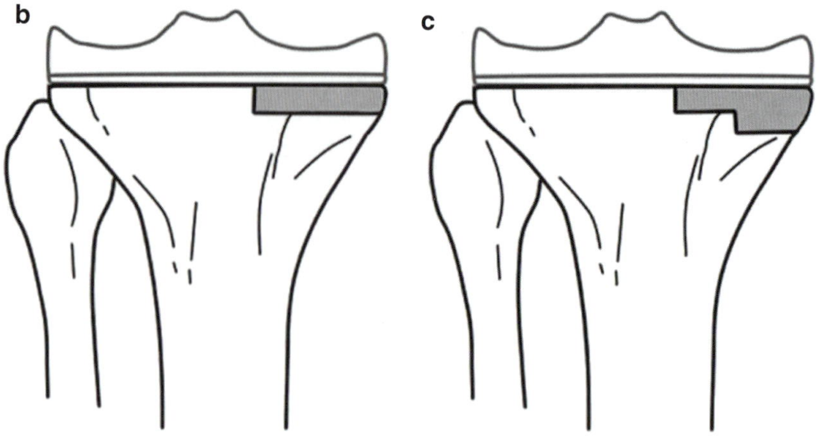

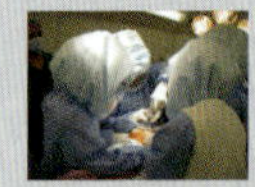

Author's Method

In case of a severe segmental bone defect in the tibia, I use the allograft with "the bone in the host bone" method, with which some portion of the patellar tendon and the collateral ligament can be preserved. Allogeneic tibial bone graft can be used in tibial defect just like APC (allograft prosthetic composite), but this allograft does not engage into the host tibia due to the similarity in size of the medullary canal. So there are

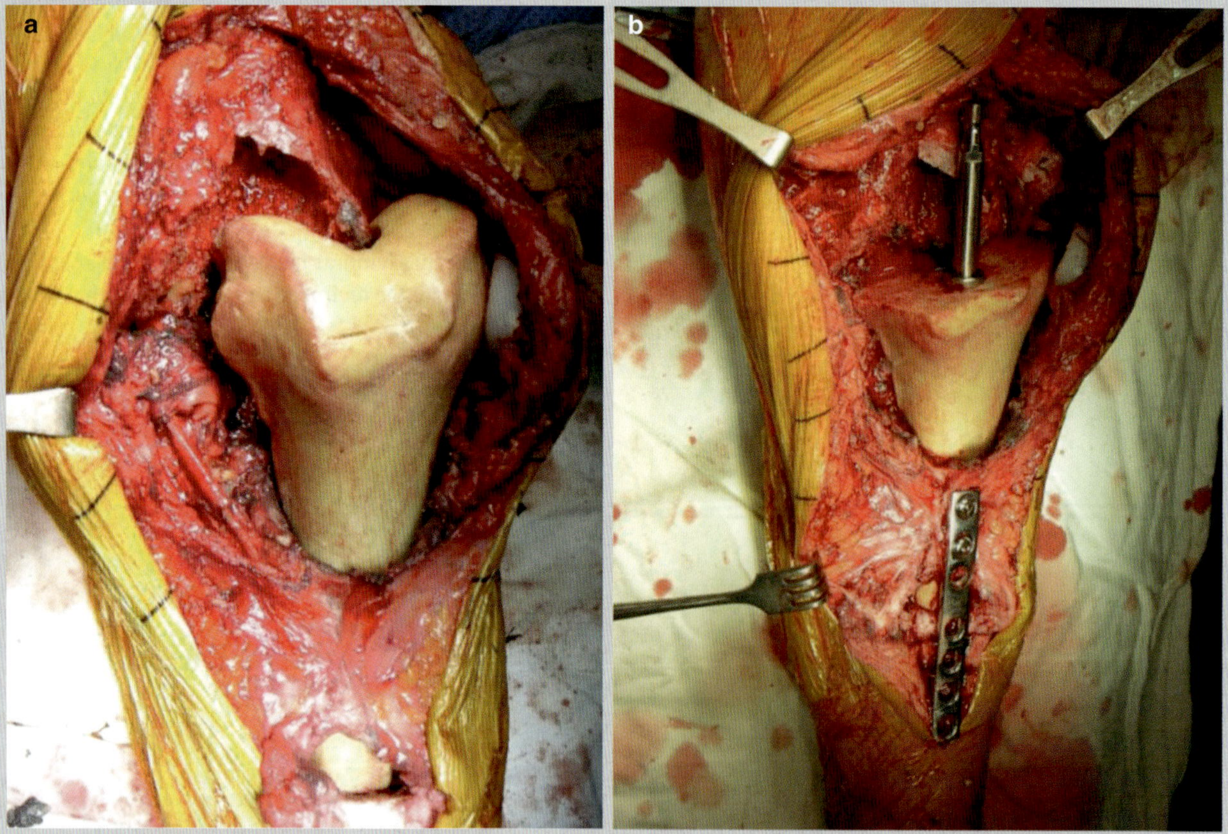

Fig. 5.9 (**a**) Allograft with the whole distal part of femur inserted into the tibia in the reverse direction for reconstructing a severe segmental defect in the tibia. (**b**) Plate fixation and reaming. (**c**) Replacement. (**d**): Postoperative X-ray

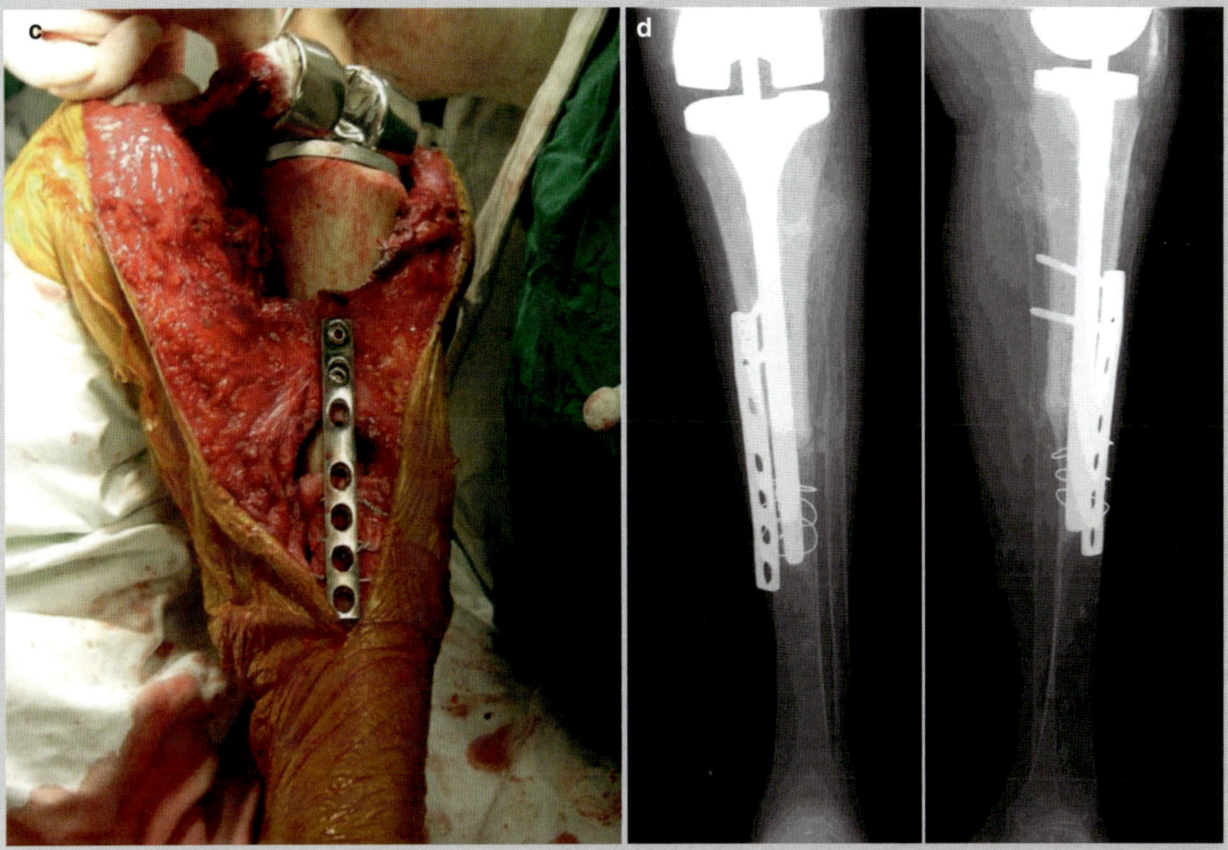

Fig. 5.9 (continued)

many difficulties in fixation of the allograft bone to the host bone. As the diameter of femoral diaphysis is smaller than that of tibial metaphysis, inserting the distal part of femur into the tibial metaphysis in the reverse direction is possible (Fig. 5.9). Since the femoral condyle articulates with the tibial plateau, the cut surface of the femoral condyle matches well with that of the tibial plateau.

Fixation of Bone Graft

Before *morcellized bone grafting*, a stem or guide rod is inserted into the intramedullary canal so that the morcellized bone fragments do not enter into the medullary canal. After *impaction*, carefully remove the stem or the rod, and the prosthesis is inserted (Fig. 5.10). Cement coating on the surface is optional.

Technically, morcellized bone grafting is relatively easier to perform in the tibia, but it may scatter when used in the femoral side even when it is coated with cement. Hence, the bone graft should be handled with care until the prosthesis is inserted.

A structural graft can be fixed by various methods. K-wires are not recommended for use due to insecure fixation and chances of migration unless they are being used for temporary fixation. Metal screws can be fixed in an oblique or vertical direction. In any case, the screws should not inhibit prosthesis insertion, so it is recommended to place a reamer inside the canal and aim the drill in the direction such that the screws do not interfere with implant insertion. Plate and screws can be used for further fixation.

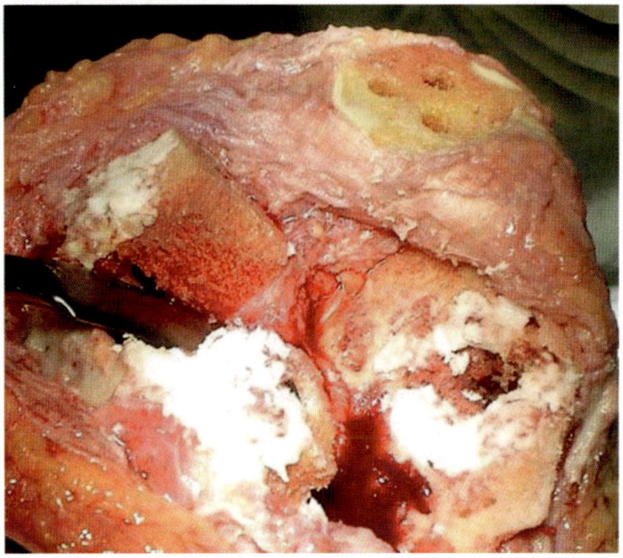

Fig. 5.10 Morcellized bone graft coated with cement

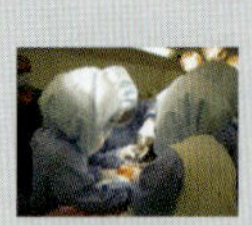

Author's Method

While performing morcellized bone graft, I usually release the tourniquet after impaction of the morcellized bone graft in order to allow hematoma formation which prevents the scattering of bone fragments, instead of coating the graft with bone cement.

Revision surgery takes longer time than primary TKA, and twice tourniquet time is usually required. Hence, I release the tourniquet at the time of morcellized bone grafting even though it is not until the time limit of the first tourniquet time.

Sequence of performing morcellized grafting is as follows: fill the defect with a morcellized bone graft, insert the trial implant for impaction, and release the tourniquet so that the blood will flow into morcellized bones to form hematoma. This hematoma holds the morcellized bone fragments together and blocks the penetration of cement into the bone fragments (Fig. 5.11).

As the hematoma has a limited adherence effect, it is recommended to ask the assistant to press the periphery of graft with his/her hands when the prosthesis is being inserted so that the morcellized bone graft is not squeezed out.

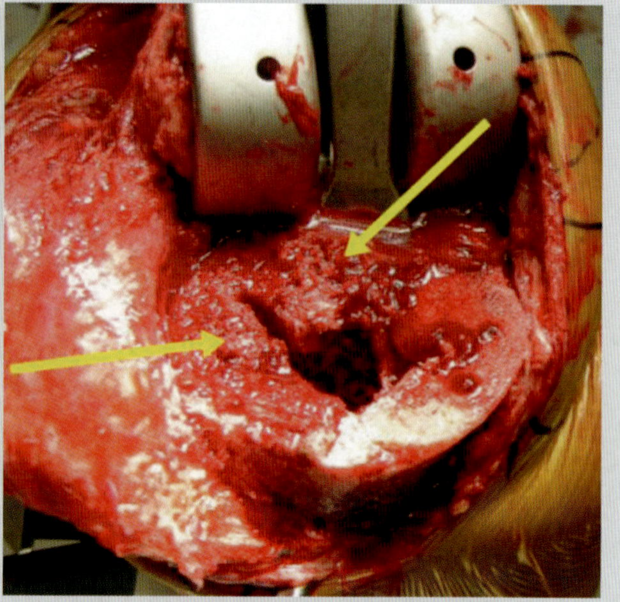

Fig. 5.11 Defect is filled with morcellized bone graft and tourniquet is released. Cancellous bone is held in its place by hematoma

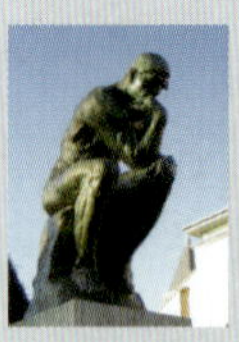

Author's Opinion

I have a strong doubt about the function and role of allogeneic bone graft.

The advantage of allogeneic bone graft is physiological bone reconstruction. Hence, I performed allogeneic bone grafting in the case in which the bone defect could not be reconstructed using metal augments. I found very disappointing findings during re-revision surgeries of patient in whom allogeneic bone graft was used. The allogeneic bone graft appeared just like an inert bone mass rather than a living bone, and the bone quality was also poor. I had the opinion that allogeneic bone graft was not better than bone cement.

On the other hand, I have experience of filling large bone defects with cement. Clinically, the patient showed no specific complications at the 3-year follow-up. Considering that the use of allogeneic bone graft is associated with the risk of disease transmission, prolonged operation time, incorporation failure and increased costs, the routine use of allogeneic bone in reconstruction of bone defects should be reconsidered.

I have developed a new cementing technique, which is a modification of screw augmentation. After preparing the host bone with a burr, I insert multiple cancellous screws at the defect site. The screw heads are located just beneath the implant. Cement is filled at the site of screw insertion and extension stem is used for additional fixation. This technique is useful in the elderly and less active patients. The advantages of this technique are that it is easy to perform, it is cost-effective, there is no risk of disease transmission, and early weight bearing can be allowed (Fig. 5.12).

5.1.5 Surgical Methods of Each Bone Defect

5.1.5.1 Tibial Defect

Tibial defect may exist on the lateral side in case of a valgus deformity, revision, or infection. However, the most frequent tibial defect in primary arthroplasty is located on the medial side.

In case of a small contained defect, the surface is drilled and the defect is filled with cement or morcellized cancellous graft, and if the defect is large, strut cancellous grafting is performed.

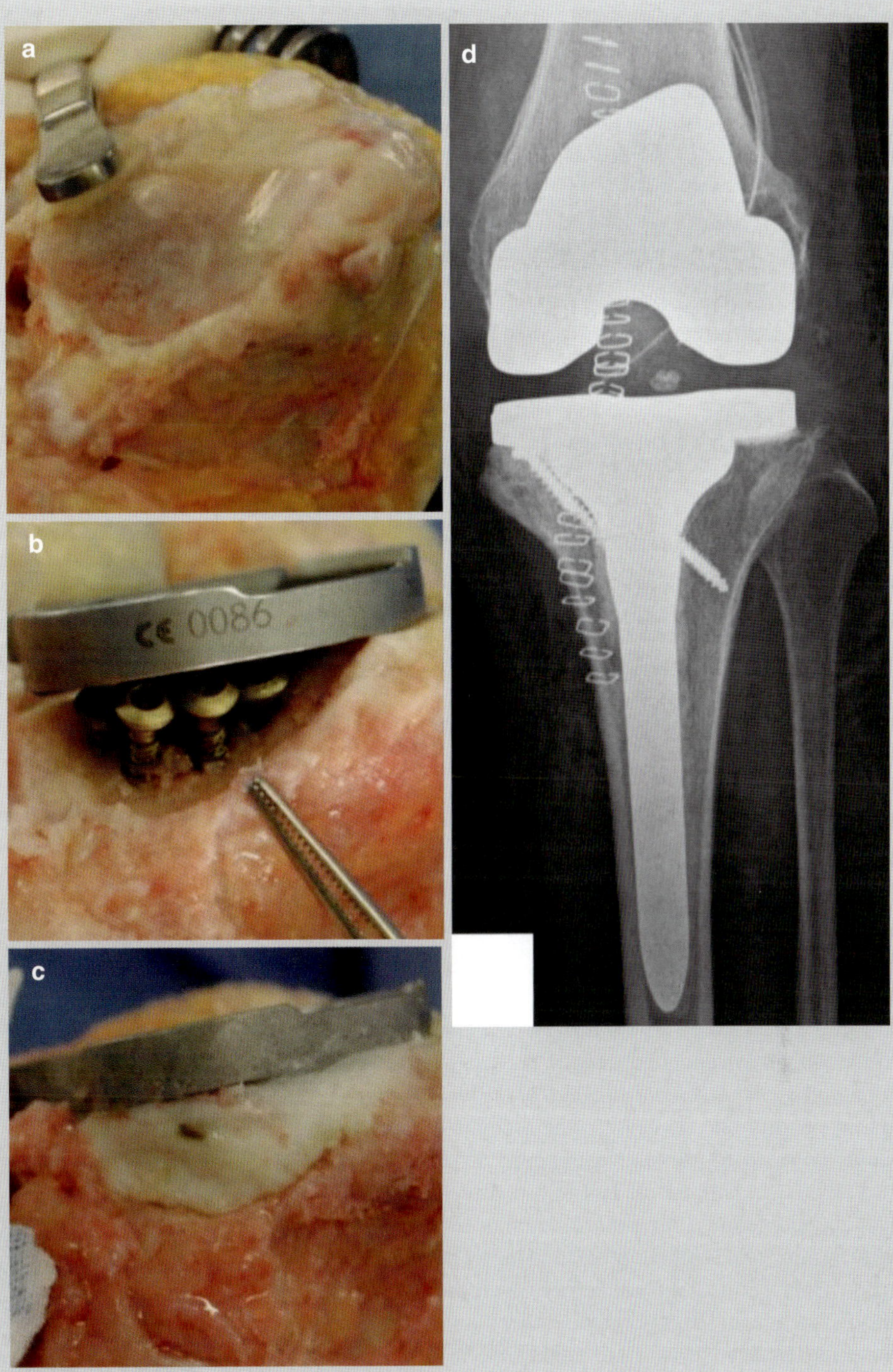

Fig. 5.12 Bone defect reconstruction with cement using multiple screws augmentation. (**a**) Bone defect. (**b**) After multiple screw insertion. (**c**) After cement fixation. (**d**) Postoperative X-ray

For a peripheral defect, the size of the defect is measured and a solution according to the size of the defect is determined. If the real defect is less than 5 mm, it can be reconstructed by cementing alone or cementing with screw augmentation. If the defect is confined to the epiphysis (real defect less than 10 mm), it can be reconstructed with a metal augment. If the real defect is larger than 10 mm, an allograft is needed. As the osteotomy level from the articular surface is different between medial and lateral condyle, real defect implies the defect needed to be reconstructed. When extension stem is used, the posterior slope should be 0°, since the angle of most of the extension stems is designed perpendicular to the tibial plate.

In case of large cavitary defect, trabecular metal augment can be used (Fig. 5.13).

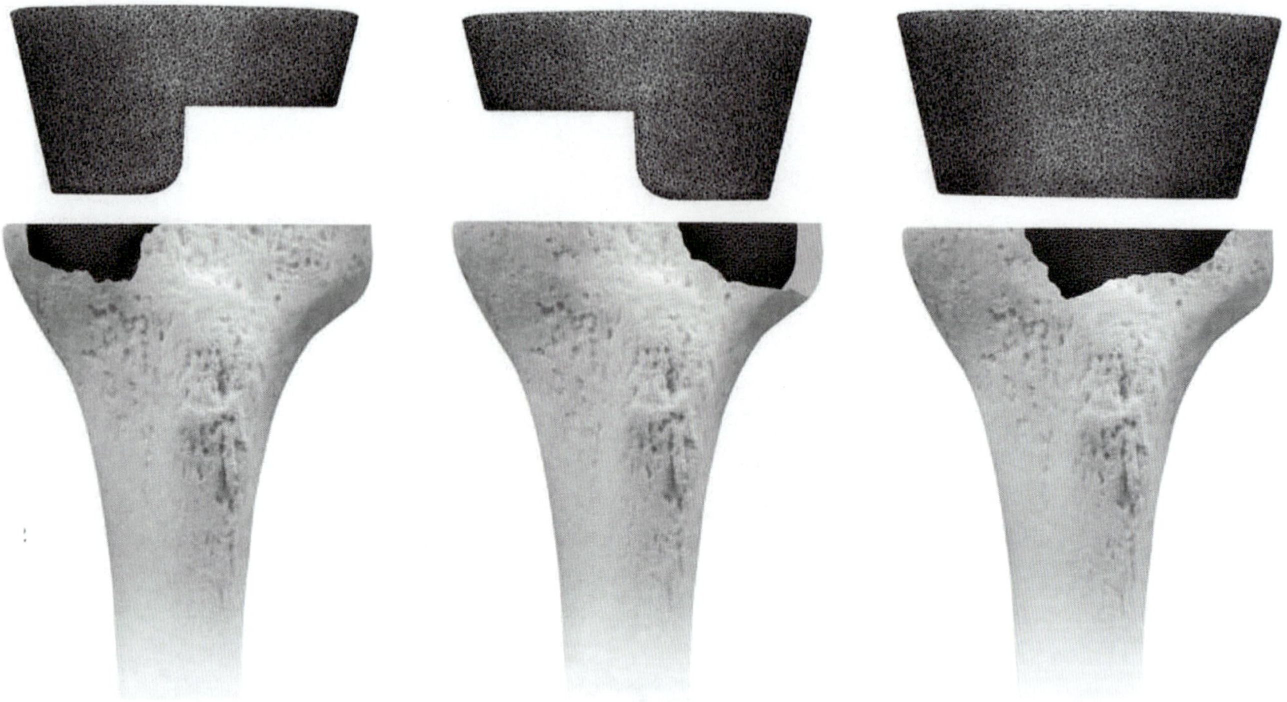

Fig. 5.13 Trabecular metal augment on tibial cavitary defect

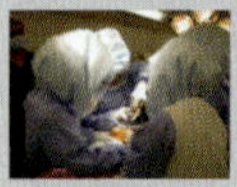

Author's Method

My principles for reconstructing the peripheral defect in the tibial side are as follows:

On the true *A–P X-rays, I draw a straight line at right angles to the mechanical axis of the tibia at a virtual resection point (subchondral bone) of the medial condyle.* Based on this line, I measure the amount of bone that would be resected from the lateral condyle (Fig. 5.14).

I divide the amount of possible bone resection from lateral condyle into four groups: 8 mm or less, 9–12 mm, 13–22 mm, and 23 mm or more, and then I decide how to reconstruct the medial tibial defect. The reason why I use the distance from lateral condyle rather than real defect is that this distance is easier and practical to use. Assuming that about 8 mm of osteotomy level is noted in ordinary TKA, 8 mm subtracted from measured distance is the real defect.

When less than 8 mm of lateral osteotomy is expected, it is considered to be normal. And when *bone resection* is expected to be another 4 mm, namely, *up to 12 mm*, either I do an 8–9 mm osteotomy and do cementing of the medial defect or I perform a *12 mm osteotomy* of the lateral condyle, and I use a thicker spacer without medial augmentation (Fig. 5.15).

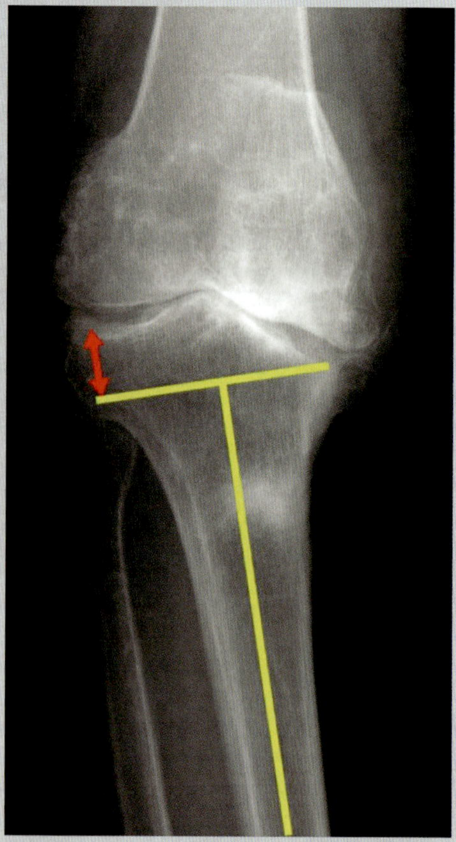

Fig. 5.14 Method for measuring the expected lateral resection in the tibia

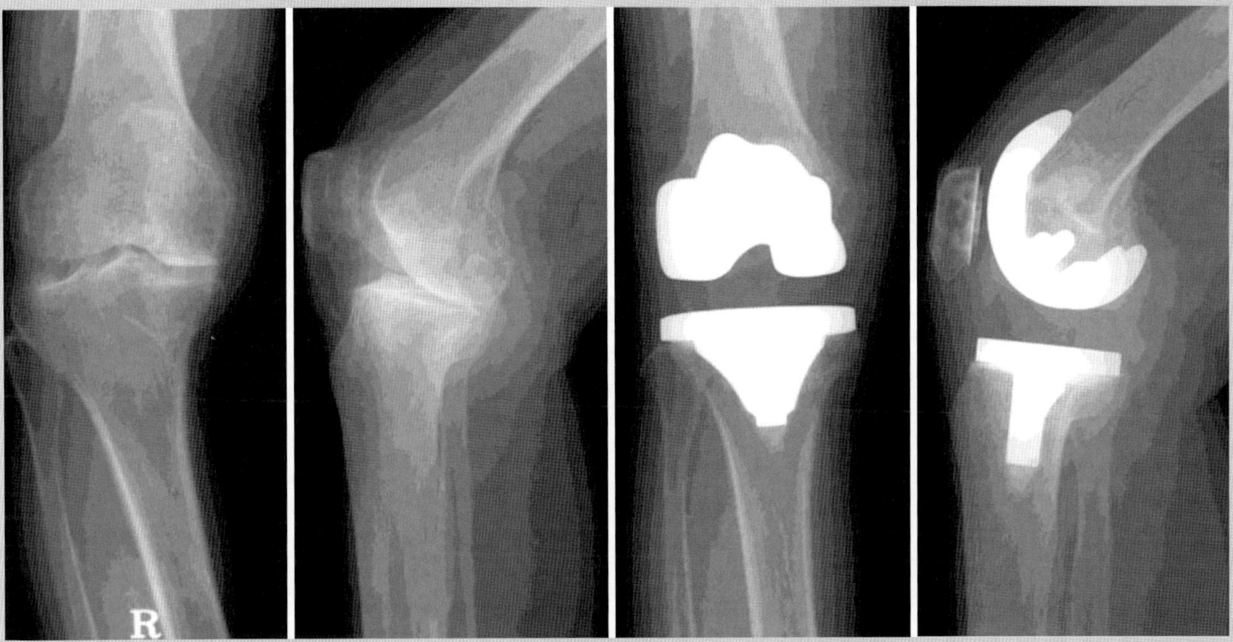

Fig. 5.15 Additional osteotomy and use of thicker PE for T1 defect

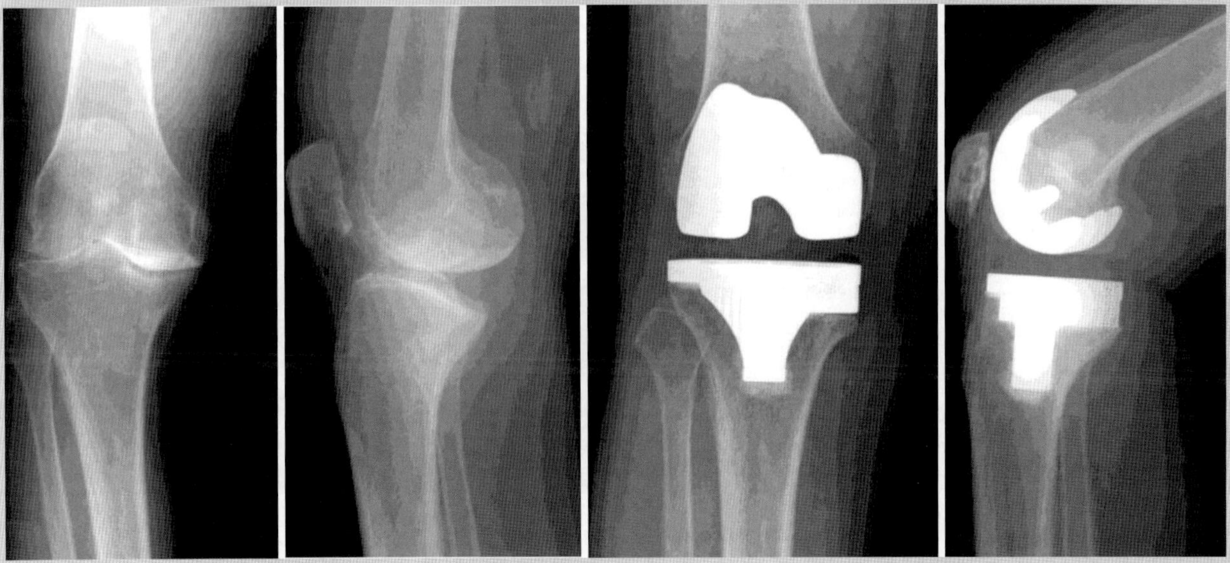

Fig. 5.16 Use of a metal augment in a T2 defect

Cases in which lateral resection is expected to be up to 13–22 mm, it may be classified into AORI T2. This means that there is a *5–10 mm of real bone defect*, and it is *reconstructed using a metal augment*. The reason why the use of this method is limited to 22 mm is that most of the metal augments can cover up to 10 mm, and a metal augment combined with bone graft is not recommended in case of more than 10 mm of a real bone defect (Fig. 5.16).

If the lateral resection is expected to be more than 22 mm, it can be classified into AORI T3 with a real bone defect of 10 mm or larger than 10 mm. In this case, the use of a structural allograft or tumor prosthesis may be considered.

The reconstruction of tibial defect can be summarized as follows (Fig. 5.17):

(a) Expected lateral resection of 8 mm or lesser → Routine method without augmentation
(b) Expected lateral resection of 9–12 mm → Cement augmentation or more bone cutting and using thicker PE

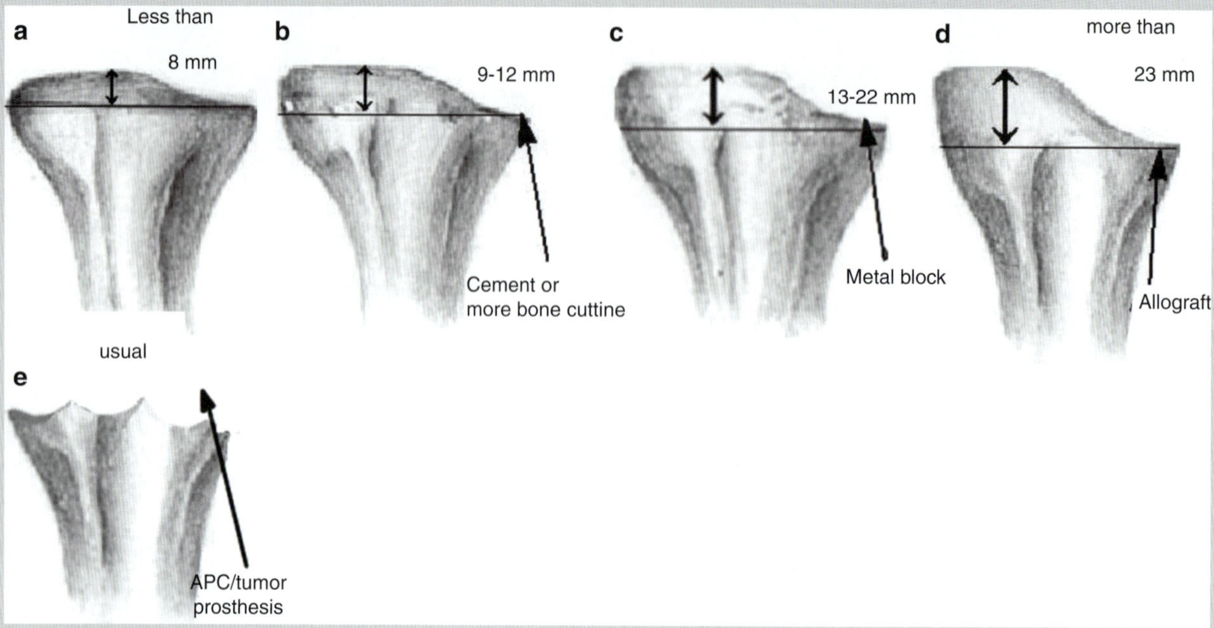

Fig. 5.17 My principles for treatment of the tibial defect

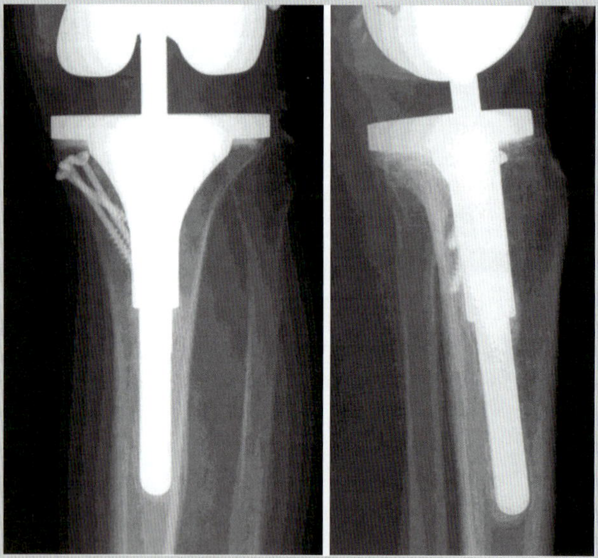

Fig. 5.18 Graft fixation using screws for strut graft

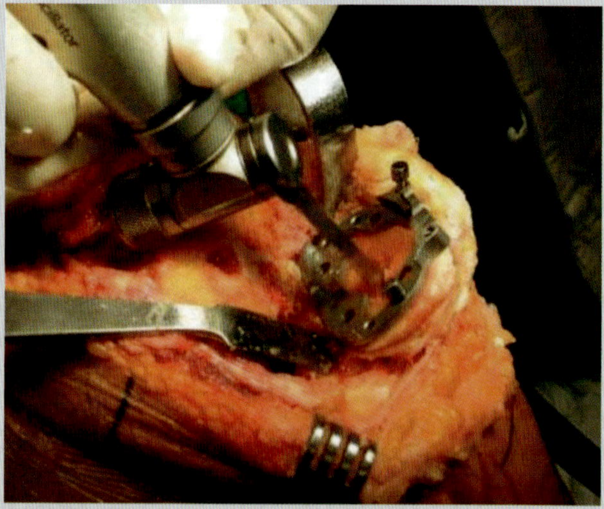

Fig. 5.19 Sawing before keel punching to prevent fracture of grafted bone

(c) Expected lateral resection of 13–22 mm → Metal augmentation
(d) Expected lateral resection of 23 mm or greater → Allograft
(e) Massive defect → Trabecular augmentation (cavitary)/tumor prosthesis

When using structural allograft on the tibial plateau, I prefer to use 4.0 mm cancellous screws to fix the bone graft. The shape of the bone graft is designed so as to facilitate compressive force, and the gap between the allograft and the host bone is filled with morcellized bone. Special techniques are used while inserting the screws, e.g., screw fixation with the *stem guide inside the medullary canal and countersinking the screw head to prevent protrusion of screws* (Fig. 5.18). *If the bone graft is large, oblique insertion of screws or buttress plating* can be considered. To prevent a fracture of the grafted bone during implantation of prosthesis, *I enlarge the keel site with a saw* before using the keel punch (Fig 5.19).

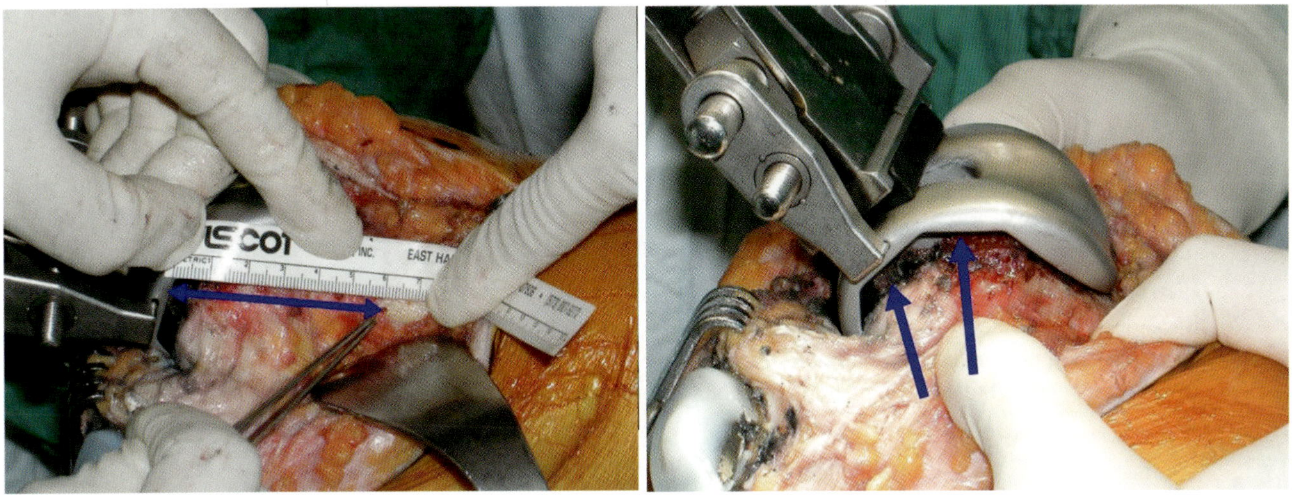

Fig. 5.20 Measuring the joint line before removing the femoral component in revision TKA (*left*). The trial femoral implant is inserted up to the joint line which is determined by the drill hole made before removal of the implant, and the gap between the implant and the bone (*arrows*) is the size of the bone defect (*right*)

Special care should be taken for the correct positioning and rotational alignment of the tibial prosthesis as the grafted bone appears different from the normal bone and may adversely affect implant positioning. For positioning and *rotational alignment, the tibial tuberosity should be used as the landmark, or the dynamic method can be used for* checking the patellar tracking while flexing and extending the knee joint repeatedly. If this is not done, the prosthesis is likely to be inserted in the internal rotation position, and this may cause patellar maltracking or restrict the flexion motion.

For ensuring *stability of the bone graft, the use of an extension stem* and cementing *is recommended* in AORI type 3 bone defect, although opinions of surgeons vary in terms of cementing around the stem.

5.1.5.2 Femoral Defect

Reconstruction of the femoral bone defect is different from that of the tibial bone defect in several aspects.

First, the anatomy of the femur is complex, and it is often difficult to make an accurate diagnosis of the site and size of the femoral defect on simple X-rays. Second, the joint line should be preserved as much as possible. The tibial defect can be reconstructed up to a certain level, and the gap can be adjusted using different PE thicknesses, whereas in case of the femoral defect, a more accurate reconstruction is required in order to maintain the joint line and to balance flexion and extension gaps. *Third, rotational alignment should be determined at the time of bone reconstruction.* In almost all cases, the anatomical landmarks are lost due to the bone defect and ordinary osteotomy instruments cannot be used. When determining the rotational axis, the use of the posterior condylar axis is difficult and less reliable due to the bone defect. The external rotation should be based on the transepicondylar axis or Whiteside's line, but very often it may be impossible to use these parameters. Therefore, *it is a good option to set external rotation using the ligament tension technique.*

The key to bone defect reconstruction is preservation of the joint line and balance the flexion/extension gap, and the amount of bone defect is measured based on the joint line. The landmarks for determining the joint line include the inferior pole of the patella, fibular styloid process, tibial tuberosity, and femoral epicondyles. The X-rays of contralateral knee joint and the pre-marked joint line before removing the implant in revision surgery (this has been described in Chap. 9) can be of great help. The position of the inferior pole of the patella changes during flexion and extension motion which causes the surgeons to make mistakes. The use of fibular styloid process is also difficult as it is located far posteriorly and laterally, while the use of the tibial tuberosity is ambiguous as it is too broad. *It is known that the joint line is about 25 mm distal to the lateral epicondyle and 30 mm distal to the medial epicondyle.* It is about 20 mm proximal to the tibial tubercle and 14–16 mm distal to the PCL insertion. *When the trial implant is inserted at the level of the joint line, the gap between the trial implant and the host bone is the size of the bone defect* (Fig. 5.20).

The method of reconstructing the femoral defect is not very different from that of the tibial defect. An *F1 defect is filled with autogenous slice bone graft or cement.* Resection of the distal portion can be done occasionally according to the gap discrepancy. *In F2 defect, filling the bone defect with metal augment is a better option than distal bone resection.* However, cementing is not recommended as it can cause malalignment. For an *F3 defect, an allograft is required,* while tumor prosthesis may also be used in case of a massive bone defect.

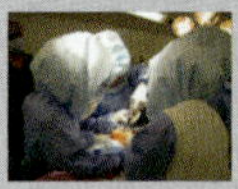

Author's Method

Based on these principles, my method of reconstruction of the femoral defect is as follows (Fig. 5.21):

(a) Bone defect of 2 mm or less → Joint line elevation or slice bone graft
(b) Bone defect of 4 mm or less → Distal bone graft or more resection and metal augmentation
(c) Bone defect of 5–10 mm → Metal augmentation
(d) Bone defect of 11 mm or greater → Allograft
(e) Massive bone defect → Trabecular augmentation (cavitary) or tumor prosthesis or APC

When a screw is inserted in the distal to the proximal direction for the fixation of bone graft, countersinking is performed so that the screw head does not interfere with the implantation (Fig. 5.22). Whereas washers provide a more rigid fixation in fixation from the lateral side. I also use the buttress plate when the bone graft is large. In this case, like in the case of tibia, I insert a trial implant before drilling for ascertaining the accurate direction of the screws.

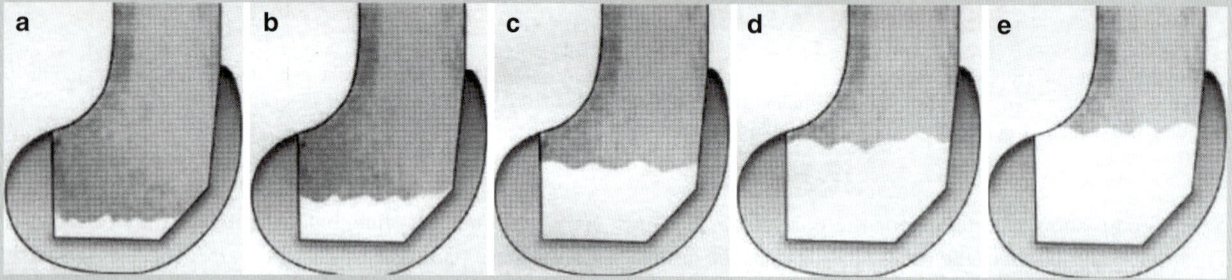

Fig 5.21 My principles for reconstruction of the femoral defect. (**a**) Less than 2 mm → joint line elevation or bone graft. (**b**) Less than 4 mm → slice bone graft or more resection and metal augment. (**c**) 5–10 mm → metal augmentation. (**d**) More than 11 mm → allograft. (**e**) Massive defect → tumor prosthesis or APC

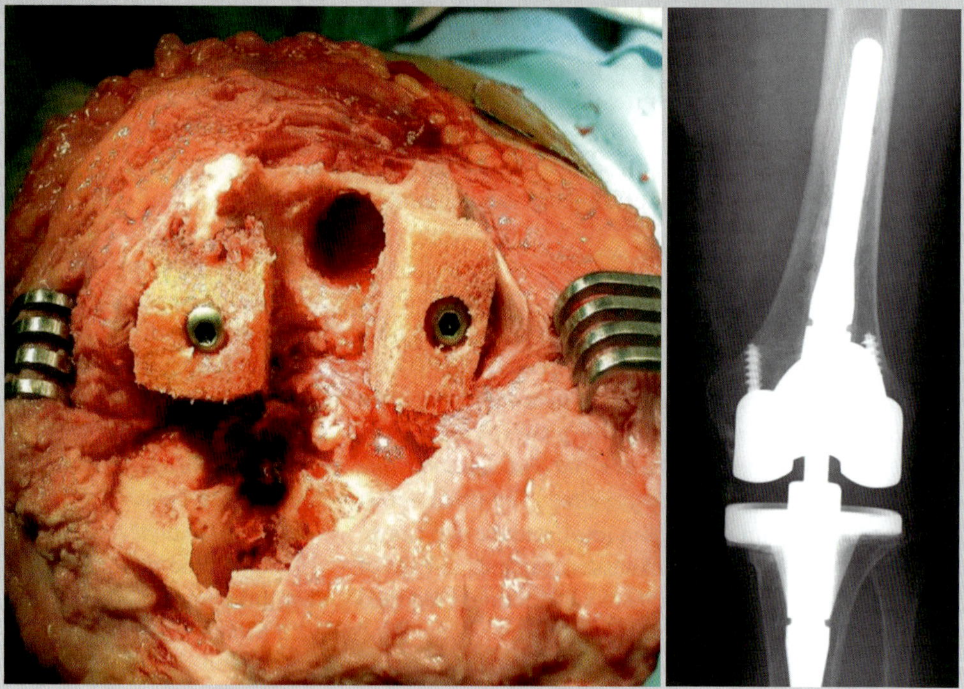

Fig. 5.22 Femoral bone graft fixed with cancellous screws

Anterior femoral defect is not included in the AORI classification although it is found in almost all cases of revision surgery. It occurs due to stress shielding of the anterior part, or its occurrence is inevitable during implant removal. The defect in this portion can be filled with cement, bone graft, or metal augment. Dennis *recommended a cementing technique as the bone graft tends to be resorbed due to stress shielding*.

Posterior femoral defect can be treated with metal augment, if the defect is large. If the defect is small, it can be filled with cement. In this case, careful attention should be paid to prevent internal rotation of the femoral component.

For stabilization of the implant and bony incorporation, the use of an extension stem can be considered. Extension stem is useful not only for secure fixation, but also for correct alignment. The length of the stem differs according to the method of bone reconstruction and whether cement fixation or cementless fixation is done. When cementless fixation is used, the length of the stem should be at least 100 mm.

When applying the extension stem, a few things need to be considered. First, most of the femoral extension stems have the angle set at 5° or 7° in coronal plane, and hence the distal osteotomy should be done at this angle. Therefore, it is meaningless to calculate the angle between the anatomical and mechanical axis on femoral A–P X-ray preoperatively. *Second, the extension stem should not be too thick.* In most of the cases, the portal site of the *extension* stem in the intercondylar area is broad. If medullary reaming is done according to this width, *periprosthetic fracture is likely to occur postoperatively due to endosteal thinning in the diaphysis.* Reaming of the medullary canal for IM nailing in fracture treatment does not cause serious problems even though there is endosteal thinning as the IM nail extends beyond the site of reaming. However, the extension stem ends at the site of reaming in the diaphyseal area in TKA and may act as stress riser leading to fracture. *Lastly, an offset stem may be needed to prevent anterior angulation due to anterior femoral defect and lower position of extension stem which is a common pitfall during revision TKA.*

5.1.5.3 Patellar Defect

Patellar defect occurs when there is a bone cyst, in case of severe patellofemoral arthritis due to long-standing patellar maltracking or in case of revision.

The management of patella defect is dictated by the thickness of more than half of the patellar surface after osteotomy. If this thickness is more than 11 mm, then the patellar defect can either be drilled without resurfacing, or the defect can be filled with cement along with resurfacing of patella. If more than half of the patellar surface has a *thickness of less than 10 mm after osteotomy, one of the non-resurfacing, biconvex patellae or inset patellae can be chosen* (Fig. 5.23). Hanssen stated that pain and function improved after patelloplasty in a huge defect in which bone graft is done, and the graft site is covered with soft tissues. Currently, *trabecular metal augmentation* has been introduced as a method for *reconstruction of a severe bone defect of the patella.* Nasser et al. and Ries et al. reported that they could improve function and reduce anterior knee pain by using the *trabecular metal* augment in patients with severe bone defect (Fig. 5.24). Another method for reconstructing a severe patellar bone defect is the K-wire insertion and cementing technique. *Resection patelloplasty* by trimming of the remaining bone is performed when there is only a cortical shell of bone remaining. Pavizi et al. observed that this procedure delivers better results than patellectomy or patellar resurfacing. However, Barrack et al. demonstrated that about one-third of the patients experienced anterior knee pain and showed poor satisfaction due to difficulty on stair climbing.

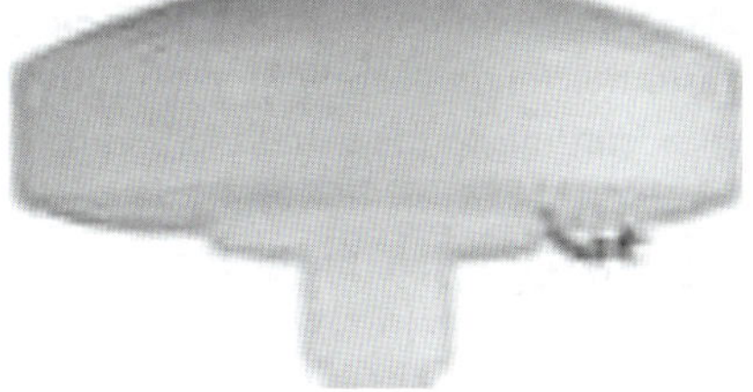

Fig. 5.23 Biconvex patellar component (Smith & Nephew, Richards, TN)

Vince et al. introduced *gull-wing sagittal osteotomy* and bone grafting of the anterior part of the patella in case only a thin cortical shell of bone was remaining (Fig. 5.25).

Buechel introduced the subsynovial iliac graft by using the synovial envelope for augmenting the bone after resection (Fig. 5.26).

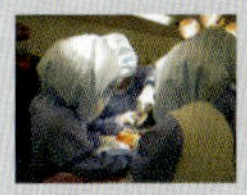

Author's Method

I replace the patella whenever the remaining bone in more than half of the patellar surface is more than 10 mm in thickness. I drill the sclerotic bone and fill the defect with cement. In case of a larger defect, I either perform patelloplasty and use the trabecular system, or I do not resurface the patella.

I have performed gull-wing osteotomy in a patient with vertical fracture of the patella. The result was promising in this special case.

5.2 Deformity

Almost all knee joints have a deformity to a greater or lesser extent preoperatively, so clearly it is the degree of deformity that matters. Deformity can be classified into intra-articular and extra-articular deformity based on the site of deformity. There are different surgical techniques for correction of the intra-articular and extra-articular deformities. When doing correction of deformity, leg length discrepancy may develop, which results in poor clinical outcome. Lang et al. reported that about 83 % of knees measured showed an increase in limb length after TKA. Preoperative varus alignment was associated with an average lengthening of 5.2 and 8.4 mm lengthening in valgus deformity.

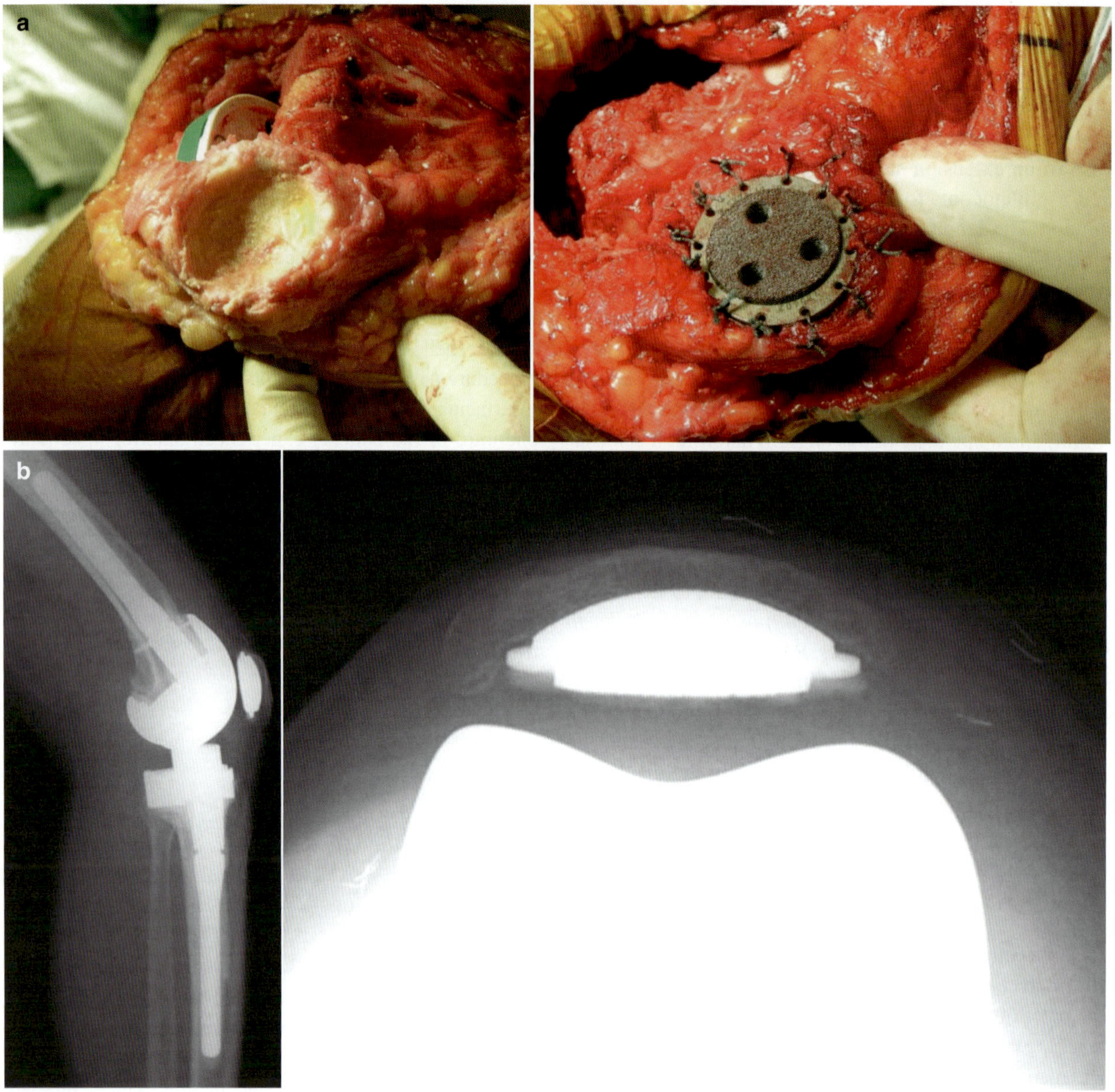

Fig. 5.24 Patellar resurfacing using trabecular metal augment. (**a**) Operative findings while using trabecular metal augment (**b**) Postoperative X-rays

5.2.1 Intra-articular Deformity

This type of deformity is largely caused due to a bone defect or laxity/contracture of the ligamentous tissues. However, in most cases these two types of deformities occur in combination.

The surgical techniques for the correction of deformity have already been described in Sect. 5.1 and in the "Ligament Balancing" section, but I think that it is necessary to briefly review them here.

5.2.1.1 Varus Deformity

In the coronal plane, 4°–7° valgus of the femorotibial angle is considered normal, and a valgus angle of 3° or lesser is considered as a varus deformity, which is coincident with the mechanical axis of less than 0°.

The principle of treatment varies according to the degree and cause of the deformity. If the deformity is mild, the method of treatment is similar to the usual osteotomy and medial release. In moderate deformity, the semimembranosus or pes anserinus tendon is released carefully. Osteotomy is performed according to the usual method of aligning the mechanical axis. If the varus deformity is severe, it should first be ascertained whether the deformity is a *dynamic deformity or static deformity*. Dynamic deformity is purely due to a lax LCL and it is obvious while walking. *A lateral thrust or lateral instability is a common finding when the varus deformity is caused due to lax lateral structures*. This

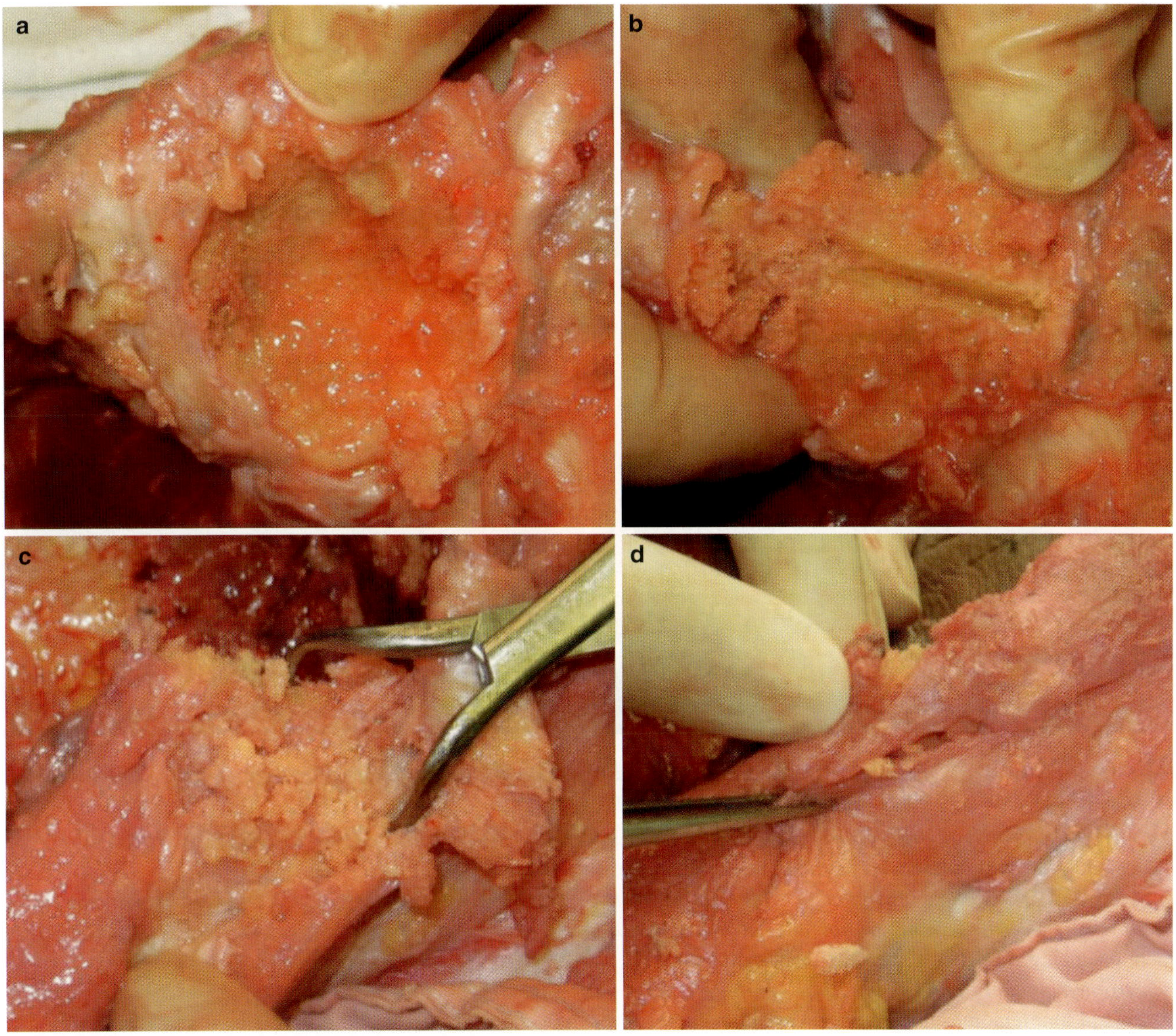

Fig. 5.25 Gull-wing sagittal osteotomy. (**a**) Cavitary defect of patella, (**b**) vertical osteotomy is done, (**c**) morcellized bone graft on the anterior side of patella. (**d**) The graft is sealed with surrounding soft tissue

condition can be detected on the preoperative weight bearing or stress X-rays (Fig. 5.27). *This type of deformity can be corrected by a medial release and by using a thicker PE. On the other hand, static deformity* is accompanied by a bone defect and a contracture of medial soft tissues. *This type of varus deformity* is mostly caused due to *a bone defect* of the medial tibial condyle, which leads to secondary contracture of the medial soft tissues. Therefore, *ligament balancing should be done simultaneously with the reconstruction of bone defect.*

There are a few technical tips for the correction of varus deformity. First, the cartilage of the medial femoral condyle may be worn out. So, it is necessary to verify the alignment from time to time to prevent varus alignment during femoral osteotomy. It is also necessary to increase the amount of external rotation when the varus deformity is severe. Second, *balance in extension is critical* for the varus deformity, while balance in flexion is critical for the valgus deformity. In other words, imbalance in extension causes more problems as a result of instability due to varus deformity, whereas valgus deformity causes more problems in flexion due to contracture of soft tissues. Third, in *patients who have had a severe varus deformity since their young age constitutional varus deformity due to such as Blount disease, less correction of deformity is preferable*. Otherwise, the patients may fail to adapt to the corrected neutral alignment and suffer from inconvenience or discomfort. Magnussen et al. analyzed the patients with preoperative varus deformities and reported that residual postoperative varus deformity after TKA is not associated with lower International Knee Society (IKS)

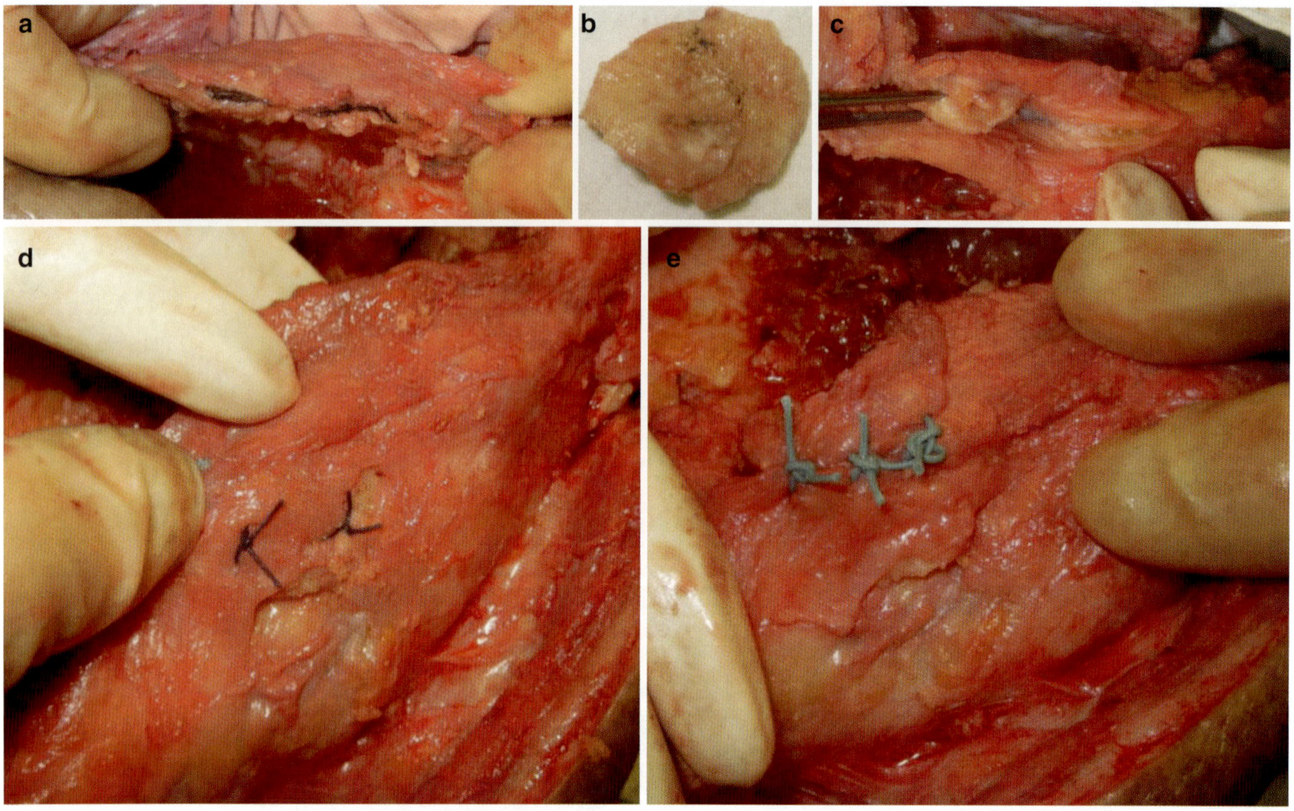

Fig. 5.26 Subsynovial iliac graft. (**a**) Split the soft tissue on the patella area. (**b**) Iliac bone is harvested. (**c**) Insertion of the harvested bone into the gap. (**d**) The bone is fixed with vertical suture. (**e**) After completion of the graft

scores and increased failure rate, provided the tibial component varus is avoided. Fourth, *joint instability is likely to occur when the varus deformity is not fully corrected.* If ligament balancing cannot be achieved by any of the methods, a *constrained implant should be used.*

Lateral tibiofemoral subluxation and rotational deformity may develop after correction of a severe varus deformity. Over-release of the medial soft tissues evokes lateral tightening when PE thickness is adapted to the widened medial gap. In such a case, the insertion of the popliteal tendon can be partially released from its femoral attachment to avoid postoperative painful snapping on the lateral aspect of the knee joint.

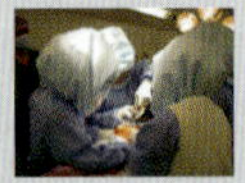

Author's Method

I always sacrifice the posterior cruciate ligament (PCL) and release the medial soft tissues until balance is achieved in a severe varus deformity. In many cases, I experienced that the ligament balancing cannot be achieved without complete release of the medial collateral ligament (MCL). Despite of complete detachment of MCL, the implant itself provides stability, and the soft tissues become bound up due to scarring in a balanced state, which eliminates the instability. After balancing has been achieved, the joint motion improves, and stress on the medial part of the knee joint is reduced. If mild instability develops postoperatively, I prescribe brace fitting for 6 weeks until healing of the detached MCL is achieved.

What is most important in complete medial release is that alignment should not be in valgus and the gap in the contralateral side (the lateral side) should neither be tight nor loose. A tight lateral gap further increases the widening on the medial side due to seesaw effect, and a loose lateral gap causes instability on both sides.

I have no experience of procedures such as lateral reefing or advancement, and I believe that it is neither absolutely necessary to perform these procedures nor are these procedures successful. If overcorrection causes an imbalance, I use the constrained type of prosthesis.

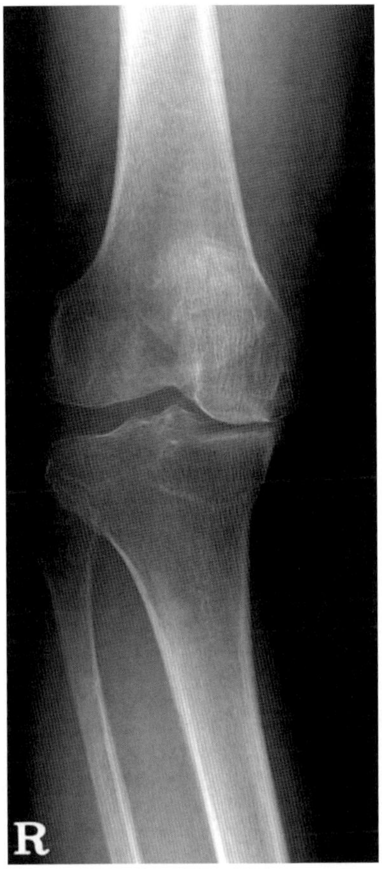

Fig. 5.27 Varus deformity due to lateral instability. Deformity is the result of instability rather than bone defect

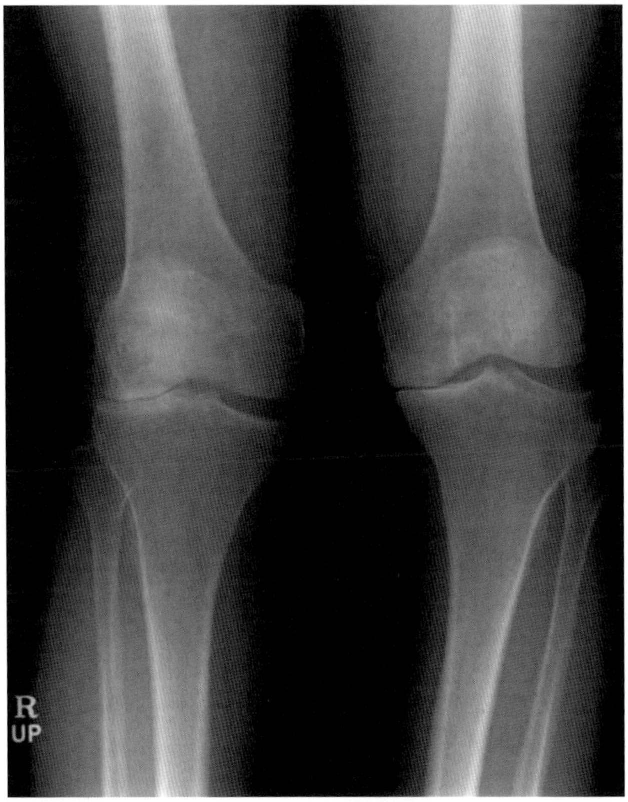

Fig. 5.28 Windblown knees

5.2.1.2 Valgus Deformity

A valgus deformity is generally caused due to rheumatoid arthritis or post-traumatic arthritis. Ranawat et al. demonstrated that about 10 % of the patients of total knee joint arthroplasty fall into this category. A valgus deformity is sometimes found in both knee joints, but there also is a condition called "*windblown knees*" in which one knee has a valgus deformity and the other knee has a varus deformity (Fig. 5.28). *The mechanism for windblown knees is that the valgus knee pushes the other knee in a high adduction moment* and causes a varus deformity of the other knee joint.

The valgus deformity has more functional disturbance due to more difficulties in walking and provokes more cosmetic problems. Valgus deformity is not found frequently, and hence beginners would face a completely different situation from that of a varus deformity from ligament release to osteotomy.

The common findings of a valgus deformity are as follows: first, the MCL is lax and lateral soft tissue structures are contracted; second, there often is an accompanying lateral bone atrophy or defect usually in the femur; third, it is also accompanied by the patellofemoral problems. Patellar dysplasia, patellar subluxation, and patella alta may also coexist. The knee joint tends to become unstable due to the MCL relaxation and hyperextension.

Therefore, in a *valgus deformity, it is required to release the contracted lateral soft tissues, align the knee through bone resection or reconstruction, and correct the patellofemoral malalignment. The degree of deformity* is commonly classified as mild if the valgus is less than 10°, moderate if the valgus is less than 20°, and severe if the valgus is greater than 20°, and *step by step soft tissue release is recommended according to the degree of deformity*.

Insall suggested releasing the iliotibial band at Gerdy's tubercle and releasing the soft tissues from the lateral condylar area of the femur in a mild deformity, and followed by resecting the iliotibial band and intramuscular septum in a moderate to severe deformity.

Buechel recommends paramedial arthrotomy when there is a valgus deformity less than 8° and lateral arthrotomy when the valgus deformity is greater than 8°. He recommends performing subperiosteal elevation of the ITB from Gerdy's tubercle in cases with a mild valgus deformity less than 8° as a first step and proceeding to the second step if valgus deformity becomes 0° with a varus stress and returns to the valgus state between 5 and 8° without stress. The second step is subperiosteal elevation of the lateral collateral ligament (LCL) and popliteus tendon, while the proximal portion is attached to the femur. If the valgus deformity cannot be corrected after the second step, he recommends proceeding to the third step to perform subperiosteal elevation of the LCL and biceps femoris complex at the fibular head or resection of the proximal portion of the fibular head.

Krackow classified the valgus deformity into three types. Type I involves lateral femoral bone loss, lateral soft tissue contractures, and intact medial soft tissues. Type II is type I with lengthened medial soft tissues. Type III is severe valgus deformity with malpositioning of the proximal tibial joint line. He suggested advancement of MCL in type II deformity.

It is controversial as to which ligament should be released first and how much release should be performed. Since *the iliotibial band (ITB) is the main structure that can cause the deformity, some surgeons emphasize that it should be released first and the popliteus tendon and the LCL should be retained until the very end*, if possible. By releasing ITB, primary correction of the deformity is accomplished by eliminating the main cause of deformity, and the possibility of injury to the peroneal nerve due to excessive retraction is reduced. Releasing can be done by performing pie crust technique, a transverse cut, Z-plasty, or periosteal elevation, and the level of release can be about 8–10 cm above the joint line, at the level of the joint line, or at the Gerdy's tubercle.

On the other hand, others emphasize that the LCL and the popliteus tendon should be released first from the femur based on the theory that releasing the shorter and closer ligaments affects the gap discrepancy between the medial and lateral sides to a lesser extent in flexion, whereas the longer ligaments open up the gap wider in flexion.

In a severe deformity, it is necessary to release the posterolateral capsule as well as the iliotibial band, along with the LCL and the popliteus tendon. If the LCL and popliteus tendon are not released sufficiently, ligament balance cannot be achieved, and this is similar to medial release in which complete release of the MCL is required until ligament balance is established. The LCL should be completely released by cutting the ligament or through periosteal elevation. Other methods include the lateral cruciform retinacular release. It is also possible to perform sliding osteotomy of the lateral femoral condyle or perform fibular head resection.

Some surgeons suggested minimal soft tissue management and using the constrained type, since there are so many complications due to extensive soft tissue release. Easley et al. reported that primary constrained condylar knee arthroplasty in the elderly patients with valgus knee resulted in significant pain relief and improved function.

It is also controversial whether *peroneal nerve exploration* is needed during soft tissue release. In fact, the reason to release the LCL on the femoral side is to reduce the incidence of peroneal nerve injury as much as possible, hence it

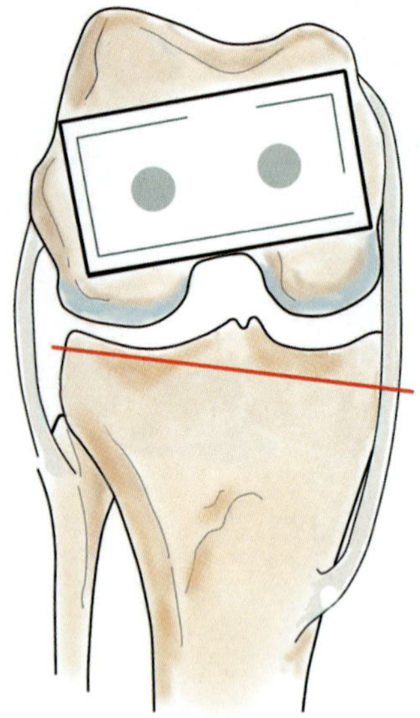

Fig. 5.29 Flexion gap with external rotation in a valgus deformity

is *more acceptable that exploration is not necessary* unless there is a severe deformity with a flexion contracture.

The *osteotomy* is performed as usual *following the ordinary classic method of aligning with the mechanical axis. And then the valgus deformity is automatically corrected after ligament balancing*. However, distal osteotomy of femur should not be done excessively from the beginning as there is atrophy of the lateral femoral condyle. It needs to be done carefully in order to maintain the balanced joint gap. *Conservative femoral and tibial resections are performed, when the deformity is combined with recurvatum or medial soft tissue stretching. Thus, soft tissue balancing can be achieved without elevating the joint line or creating a too large extension gap*. Scott emphasized that less than 5° of valgus osteotomy should be done to reduce the tension of the medial side even though the difference between the anatomical and mechanical axes exceeds 5°.

With respect to the amount of external rotation of the femur, the rotation becomes inaccurate when it is determined using the posterior condylar axis. As there is atrophy of the lateral femoral condyle, the medial condyle would be cut more to open the medial side in flexion when the transcondylar method is used (Fig. 5.29). *When the ligament tension technique is used, the femur may be in a neutral rotation or in mild internal rotation. However, if* there is not too much internal rotation and *the patellar tracking is good, this may be acceptable*.

As many cases have problems of patellofemoral alignment, *the incidence of lateral retinacular release is very high*; Griffin et al. reported an incidence of lateral retinacular release ranging from about 62 to 100 % in valgus deformity. Hence, they recommended the use of constrained type of prosthesis from the beginning rather than excessive soft tissue release in severe valgus deformity in the aged patients with limited activity in order to reduce the morbidity and complications such as peroneal nerve palsy or instability.

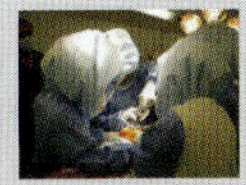

Author's Method

I have been able to correct most of the valgus deformities with a medial approach. This approach encounters little difficulties when an ordinary midline skin incision and medial parapatellar arthrotomy are extended.

Osteotomy is performed according to the classical alignment method.

In terms of ligament release, I sacrifice the PCL routinely. The sequence of release, although it varies according to the degree of deformity, begins with the popliteus tendon and the LCL complex in a mild deformity. If the snapping phenomenon occurs at 30° of flexion during testing of the knee motion, it means that there is an iliotibial band contracture. I perform an additional ITB release in this case at the most tight site.

If the deformity is severe, I release the iliotibial band first. Without release of ITB in severe valgus deformity, the deformity cannot be corrected. The level of release can be either at the Gerdy's tubercle by periosteal elevation in very severe cases, or just above the patella in moderate cases. I have tried the pie crust technique to release the lateral structure, but it usually failed due to either inadequate release or over-release.

Although the transepicondylar axis is the standard for determination of external rotation, I use the ligament tension technique to balance the mediolateral gap in flexion. Hence, in a valgus deformity, I always perform tibial osteotomy first. This may reduce the amount of external rotation that may cause patellofemoral maltracking. If patellofemoral maltracking occurs in spite of lateral retinacular release, I correct the maltracking by lateral positioning and more external rotation of the tibial component.

5.2.1.3 Flexion Contracture

Flexion contractures may develop due to the long-term morbidity associated with degenerative or rheumatoid arthritis. When the motion is limited due to pain, the posterior joint capsule and hamstrings become contracted, which is more common in inflammatory diseases. On the other hand, inflammation often causes bone defects due to condylar erosion, which paradoxically leads to flexion instability.

Spurs are also one of the most common causes of flexion contractures. The posterior spurs not only limit flexion, but they also limit extension as they tether the joint capsule. Spurs in the intercondylar notch interfere with mobility of the cruciate ligaments thereby causing a flexion contracture.

Preoperative X-rays might show obliteration of the joint space just like an ankylosed joint, and the bones appear larger than their actual size because of the magnification caused due to the shorter distance between the tube and the flexed knee joint. Therefore, the selection of implant size should be done carefully.

Most of the patients who have had walking difficulties since a long time would often have accompanying osteoporosis (Fig. 5.30).

Flexion contracture imposes more stress on the posterior side of the prosthesis resulting in sinking and wear on the posterior side of PE. Also more quadriceps power is needed during walking. In this sense, flexion contracture is more problematic than limited flexion on walking, and hence the knee joint should be fully extended if possible. Flexion contracture less than 10° may be acceptable, but flexion contracture more than 15° needs to be corrected.

If there is a mild flexion contracture, stretching can be performed preoperatively to relieve the flexion contracture as much as possible. If flexion contracture is severe, serial casts

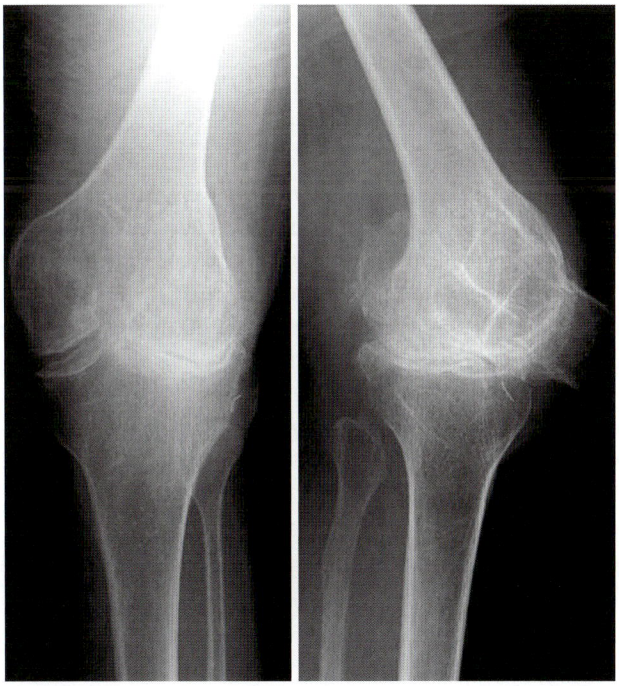

Fig. 5.30 X-ray of a flexion contracture

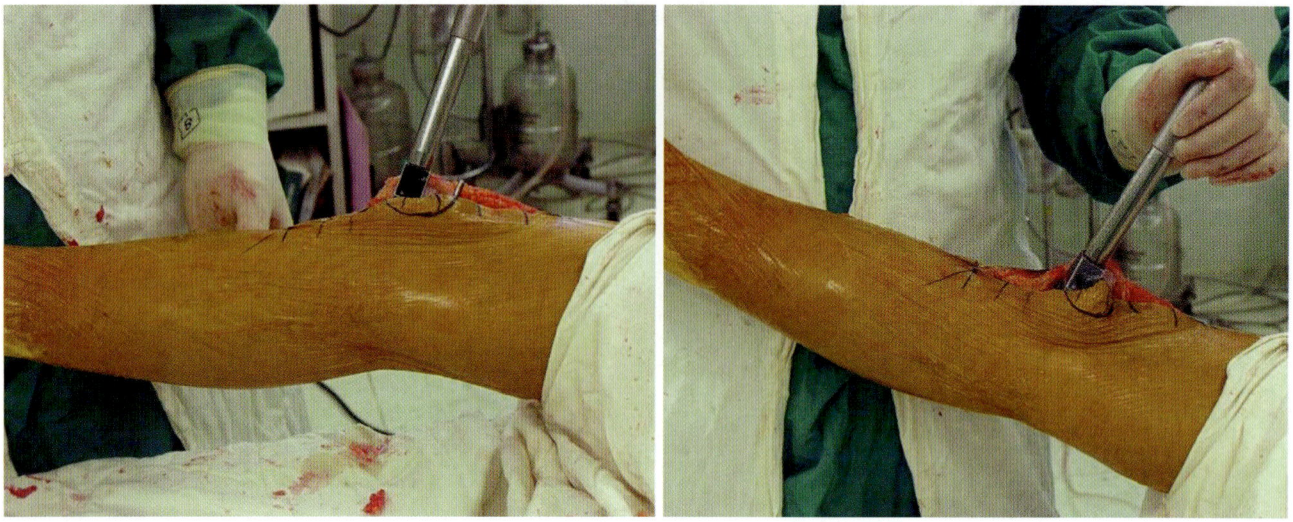

Fig 5.31 Difference in the flexion contracture before and after 2 mm more distal femoral resection

have been applied in the past, but it is not recommended as it is painful, may cause cast sores, and has a high probability of recurrence of the deformity.

It is also controversial as to whether the flexion contracture should be completely corrected intraoperatively. Dorr et al. and Tanzer et al. observed that flexion contracture of less than 10° can be relieved by rehabilitation, and Chung et al. also reported that a residual flexion contracture of about 17° disappeared postoperatively. Mitsuyasu et al. reported that a flexion contracture of more than 15° can be improved postoperatively, but the flexion contracture still persisted at 3 months after surgery. This concept of gradual correction of the flexion contracture varies according to the type of disease; in case of rheumatoid arthritis, the flexion contracture tends to reduce slowly; however, it would remain unchanged in osteoarthritis. When the flexion contracture is relieved postoperatively, flexion instability may develop progressively due to simultaneous increase of flexion gap. On the other hand, Firestone et al. found that the residual flexion contracture is likely to progress when the PCL is retained. Berend et al. and Tew and Forster stated that *the goal should be to achieve full extension during operation.*

With respect to the surgical techniques, flexion contracture means soft tissue contracture of the posterior capsule or a narrow extension gap. Hence, the surgical technique is directed towards the removal of posterior spur, posterior release, increase in the extension gap, and decrease in the posterior tibial slope.

For application of different surgical techniques, flexion contractures are classified into three categories according to their degree: less than 15°, 15°–30°, and more than 30°. *If the flexion contracture is less than 15°, removing the posterior spurs and performing soft tissue release properly* are adequate enough to eliminate the flexion contracture. It is recommended to *use a one-size larger femoral prosthesis so as to reduce the flexion gap and use a thinner PE*, or just use a one-size thinner PE since a little wider flexion gap is permitted. *If the flexion contracture is between 15° and 30°, release of the soft tissues on the posterior side*, including the PCL and posterior capsule, and peeling off the origin of gastrocnemius muscle should be tried. If the flexion contracture persists even after soft tissue release, a simple and effective method is to *widen the extension gap by performing an additional distal femoral resection.* More distal cutting can be done from the beginning without soft tissue release so as not to cause soft tissue injury. It is known that *2 mm of distal resection is equivalent to about 15° increase in extension (Fig. 5.31). However, more than 6 mm of resection is not recommended as this would elevate the joint line*, and the collateral ligaments may be injured.

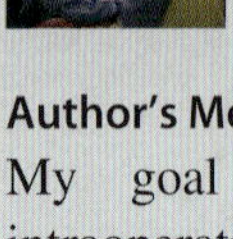

Author's Method

My goal is to relieve the flexion contracture intraoperatively.

If the flexion contracture is less than 15°, I perform posterior release. To ensure that the neurovascular tissue in the posterior space is not injured, I make a hole in the posterior capsule with scissors at the notch portion and resect the soft tissues close to the bone step by step while palpating the tight structures (Fig. 5.32).

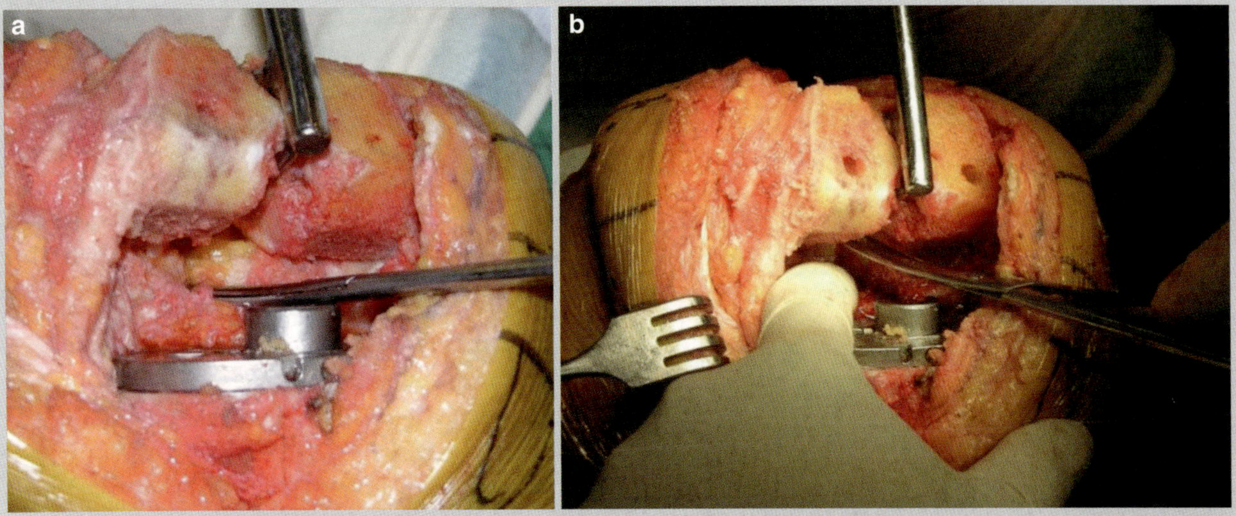

Fig. 5.32 Posterior soft tissue release. (**a**) Making a hole beneath the notch area. (**b**) After subperiosteal elevation through the hole, insert the index finger and release the tight structures

When performing brisement after posterior release, I use a one-size thinner PE for the PS type. This is because the post blocks the extension force. If a one-size thinner PE is used, hyperextension occurs during brisement. After this, I insert the appropriate-sized PE.

If there is a flexion contracture between 15° and 30°, I perform a little more distal femoral resection so as to widen the extension gap rather than performing capsular or gastrocnemius muscle release. I think too much soft tissue release is harmful for the posterior part of the knee joint. With an additional 2–4 mm of distal femoral resection, more than 20° of extension can be achieved. With an additional resection of the distal femur, the length of the limb will be shortened, the quadriceps power will be weakened, and the joint line will be elevated slightly. However, these problems are not that critical, and it is better than leaving the flexion contracture uncorrected.

If the flexion contracture is more than 30°, it is not always possible to use the best method for its correction, and hence we may need to choose the second best method. In other words, it may be impossible to extend the knee completely without sacrificing the knee joint kinematics. Patients who have been suffering from rheumatoid arthritis since a long time are likely to have a flexion contracture of more than 60°. The goal is to achieve a less flexion contracture and a more stable knee joint. Preoperative stretching, manipulation, and serial casting can be considered in a severe flexion contracture caused due to an acute inflammatory process.

We need to decide *whether to correct the deformity in one stage or in two stages*. The two-stage method consists of the release of the hamstrings and posterior capsule followed by traction or serial casting in the first stage. The advantage of this method is that it slowly extends the posterior neurovascular structures, and hence the risk of neurovascular complications is decreased. The drawback of this method is that two operations are required, which may increase the risk of infection and may cause instability. Furthermore, the flexion contracture may not be completely corrected with this method.

If the operation is done in one stage, we should be cautious so as not to damage the neurovascular structures. The key factor is to achieve complete release of the posterior soft tissues and to maximize the extension gap. The patients who have been unable to walk for a longer duration due to a severe flexion contracture always have accompanying osteoporosis. *Forceful extension without releasing the posterior soft tissues and without ensuring a sufficient extension gap would cause compression fracture of the anterior portion of the tibial plateau resulting in anterior slope of the tibial prosthesis*. The use of constrained type is inevitable in most of the cases.

If the flexion contracture persists in spite of performing the above-mentioned technique, maintaining the epidural anesthesia and using the serial cast method can be done postoperatively. Besides, modification of CPM and heel elevation are used for relieving flexion contracture postoperatively.

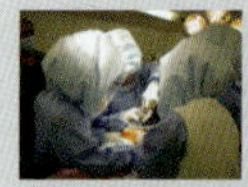

Author's Method

In case of a severe flexion contracture, I suggest the method of widening the extension gap so as to release the flexion contracture.

First, I do more distal cutting up to 6–8 mm on the femoral side and resect the tibial plateau as much as possible. Here, "as much as possible" indicates that the ligament tissues are protected and the remaining tibial plateau is not too small. When I do osteotomy in this manner, I can achieve the desired extension gap, but at the same time there is inevitably a much wider flexion gap with respect to flexion and extension gap balancing. There is a need to find a way to decrease the flexion gap. The solution is to choose a femoral prosthesis as large as possible. Here, "as large as possible" indicates that the femoral component corresponds to the size of tibial prosthesis and causes relatively lesser overhanging of the prosthesis on the femoral side. By using a larger implant, the flexion gap becomes narrow (Fig. 5.33). Resection of the posterior condyle is less than that in the usual osteotomy, and in some cases, the posterior condyle of the femur is not resected at all, or the posterior part should sometimes be reinforced with a metal augment. I use a constrained prosthesis if the joint shows gross instability due to the discrepancy between the flexion and extension gaps.

This technique may shorten the limb, but the limb will still be longer than that with a flexion contracture preoperatively. There will be lesser damage to the neurovascular structures due to less stretching on the posterior side of the knee joint.

These methods may cause problems in knee joint kinematics due to changes in the joint line and discrepancies between the size of the tibial and femoral components. However, I think that it is much better than having a severe flexion contracture.

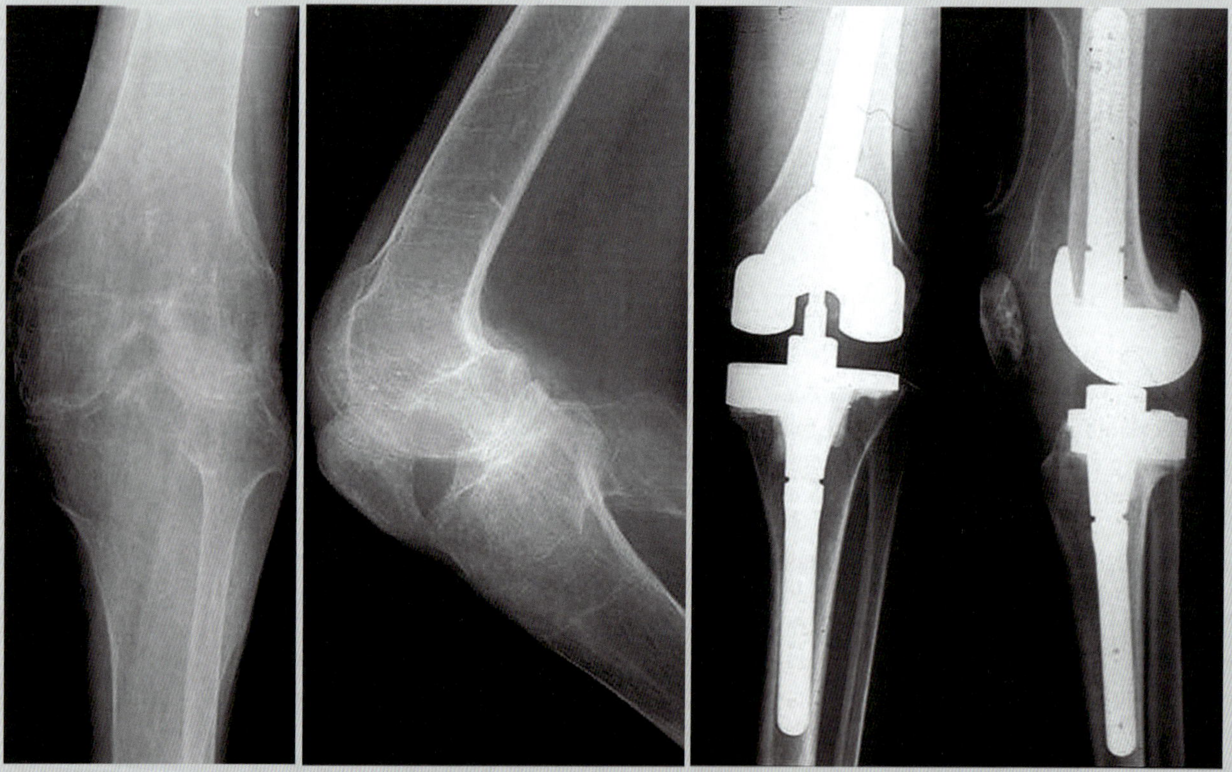

Fig. 5.33 A severe flexion contracture and postoperative X-ray after correction

5.2.2 Extra-articular Deformity

Extra-articular deformity is caused by malunion, sequelae of high tibial osteotomy, or when a patient has a history of osteomyelitis, physeal injury, or metabolic bone disease since his/her young age, etc. If there is a femoral or tibial deformity, secondary osteoarthritis is likely to develop.

Angular deformity may be a varus, valgus, recurvatum, or procurvatum deformity and is often accompanied with a certain degree of rotational deformity. Regardless of the causes, it is most important to establish correct limb alignment for the long-term survival of an artificial knee joint, and *it is highly recommended to correct the deformity at the actual site of deformity*.

If we try to correct a severe extra-articular deformity intra-articularly, the osteotomy can be oblique from medial to lateral in the coronal plane or from anterior to posterior in the sagittal plane. Extra-articular correction requires an additional surgery and may cause complications such as nonunion and infection. Therefore, it is necessary to decide whether an intra-articular correction is possible or if the correction needs to be done at the site of the deformity. *In general, extra-articular correction is needed when bone resection seems to extend to the epicondylar attachment of the collateral ligaments during intra-articular correction*. If correction is done at the site of the deformity, it should be decided whether it will be a one-stage or a two-stage operation.

The tibial deformities are easier to correct than the femoral deformities as the tibial deformity causes less gap balancing problem.

An improved clinical outcome was achieved with the use of the navigation system compared to the conventional technique, because in the conventional technique an extramedullary alignment device would be required due to a tortuous medullary canal.

5.2.2.1 Intra-articular Correction

Although not recommended, *intra-articular correction may be performed for an extra-articular angular deformity which is not very severe* since it is easier to perform. However, *it is impossible to perform intra-articular correction if the angular deformity is more than 20° or the difference between the anatomical and mechanical axis of the femur is more than 13° in the coronal plane*. According to Wang et al., an *angular deformity of* approximately *15° in the sagittal plane can be treated with intra-articular correction*. In other words, intra-articular correction should not be performed for a severe extra-articular deformity for which an osteotomy of the femoral epicondyle is needed. If we try to save the femoral epicondyle, the alignment may change or discrepancy may occur in the flexion and extension gaps. More deformities can be corrected by the intra-articular method when an offset stem is used in addition to metal augmentation or bone graft on the contralateral side of deformity, or constrained or custom-made prosthesis is used after sacrificing the collateral ligaments.

Since skin necrosis or other complications may occur when soft tissues are released extensively, care should be taken to prevent the development of these complications. *When intra-articular correction is performed, soft tissue balancing is just as important as the osteotomy. The closer is the apex of the deformity to the joint line, the greater is the effect on soft tissue balancing*. Sacrificing of the PCL is inevitable, and the contracture should be completely released. If soft tissues are not balanced after this procedure, the use of a constrained prosthesis along with an extension stem should be considered. However, it is often very difficult to use the extension stem due to the deformity.

An extramedullary guide is very often needed for alignment, and *C-arm is prepared for verification of the alignment*. In any case, the mechanical axis line should be drawn on preoperative X-ray. Anatomical axis, unlike the mechanical axis, is often impossible to draw on the preoperative X-ray and may not always be needed as an intramedullary guide may not be used. The navigation system, of course, provides more convenience and accuracy to the surgeon in cases with deformity.

There are three methods of correction according to the site and shape of deformity. *First, when an intramedullary guide cannot be used due to a gradual deformity, the mechanical axis and two lines perpendicular to it at the most distal point of the both articular surfaces are drawn. The difference in the amount of resection medially and laterally is calculated*. When the cutting plane is determined, distal osteotomy of the difference between the medial and lateral condyle is done step by step considering the flexion and extension gap balance. The axis is confirmed by an extramedullary method (Fig. 5.34a). Second, if the angular deformity is at some distance from the joint, a *shorter intramedullary guide can be inserted upto the deformed site. The mechanical axis and the axis of the medullary guide are drawn, and the angle between the two axes* is measured. *Osteotomy is done along the short intramedullary guide according to the difference in the two axes* (Fig. 5.34b).

Third, *if the angular deformity is not very severe*, an imaginary anatomical axis through which a medullary guide can pass is drawn on the preoperative X-ray. The angle between this line and the mechanical axis is calculated. *A shorter intramedullary guide which can pass through the medullary canal is inserted*, and osteotomy is done according to this angle. In this method, we should keep in mind that the portal of medullary guide is not at the center of the joint, but it is the point where the imaginary anatomical line meets the condyle. So, the portal may be shifted far away from the center of the joint (Fig. 5.34c).

When performing an osteotomy, anterior and posterior angular deformities in the sagittal plane should also be corrected. The focus of *osteotomy in sagittal plane should be based on the flexion–extension motion and patellofemoral mechanism rather than alignment with the mechanical axis. So anatomy of the distal femur and proximal tibia is more important than mechanical axis.*

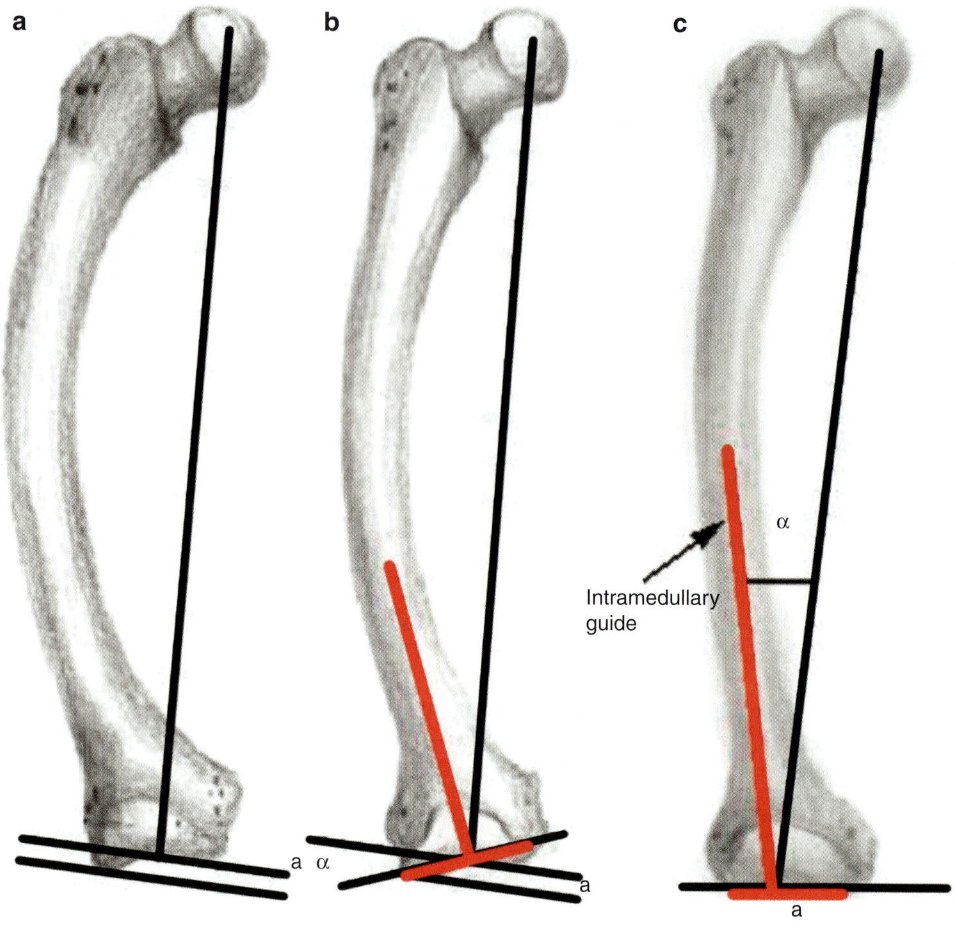

Fig. 5.34 Method of correction according to the site and shape of deformity. (**a**) Gradual deformity. Check the difference of bone cutting between medial and lateral femoral condyle according to the mechanical axis (Resect more lateral condyle of that difference.). (**b**) The method of using a shorter intramedullary guide when the deformity is at the lower level. (**c**) Correction in case of minimal and gradual deformity. Guide rod is inserted as much inside as possible. The portal of guide rod is located far laterally from the center (α is the resection angle and *a* is the point along which an intramedullary guide is inserted)

The C-arm is prepared in severe angular deformity, and the axis is checked intraoperatively from time to time using the Bovie line (Fig. 5.35).

5.2.2.2 Meta-diaphyseal Correction

If intra-articular correction is impossible, extra-articular osteotomy is required in order to correct the deformity. The point of the osteotomy is not where the angular deformity is located, but it is the point where the axes of the proximal and distal parts meet.

The method of correction can be one staged or two staged. The *one-stage method* of correction is *cost-effective and less time-consuming, and autogenous bone obtained from the osteotomy during TKA is available*. The drawback of this method of correction is that it is surgically demanding and there is a risk of skin necrosis. When the one-stage operation is performed using the navigation system, the following sequence of operation has been recommended by Mason et al.: first, osteotomy of the normal site (tibial cut first in femoral deformity); second, ligament balancing in extension; third, corrective osteotomy of the deformed site according to alignment; fourth, fixation of osteotomy site; and lastly, TKA procedure on femoral side.

The two-stage method of correction is relatively easy to perform, but it takes longer time until bone healing is achieved. In case of a severe deformity, Rand experienced poor results along with many complications after a two-stage arthroplasty, whereas Mann et al. compared the results of the two-stage knee replacement with those of the one-stage knee replacement and found that there was not much difference in the results between the two methods. However, they pointed out that infection was the most serious complication associated with the two-stage arthroplasty.

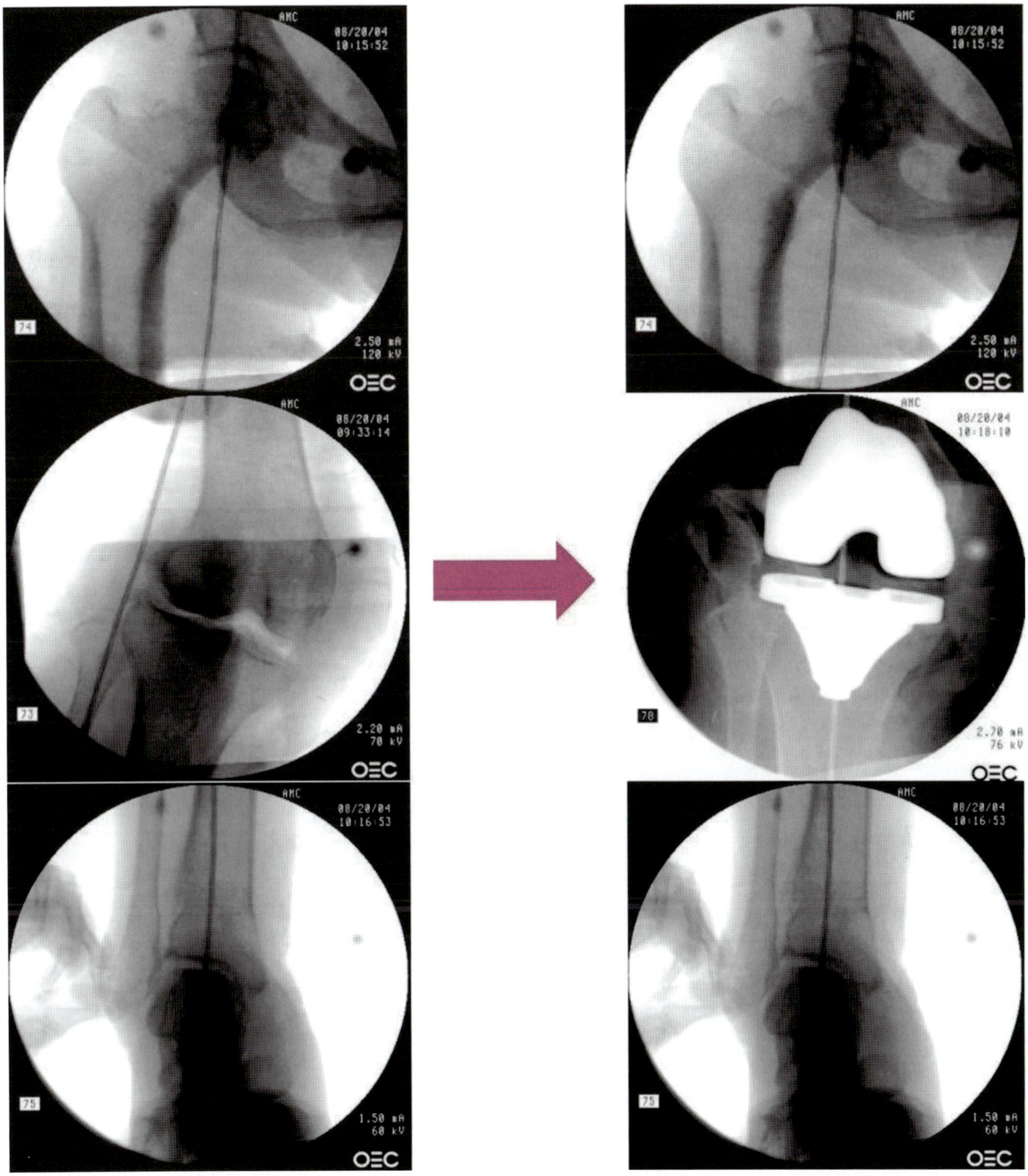

Fig. 5.35 Checking the alignment intraoperatively using the Bovie line

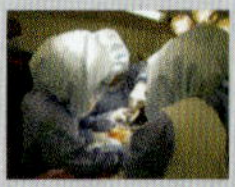

Author's Method

I try to correct the deformity intra-articularly whenever it is possible, and I prefer drawing a line perpendicular to the mechanical axis so as to know the required amount of bone resection of the medial and lateral condyles. When excessive bone is likely to be resected, I resect less distal bone and try to reconstruct the defect either by using a bone graft or a metal augment.

When intra-articular correction is impossible, I recommend the one-stage operation, in which corrective osteotomy and arthroplasty are performed simultaneously. After osteotomy of the deformed bone at the intended site is performed, I insert a medullary guide temporarily by which the deformity is corrected automatically. The angular deformity is corrected just like in the open wedge method, and then a buttress plate is fixed to the bone with the trial stem inserted into the medullary canal.

Usually there are no difficulties in inserting screws in the metaphyseal area, and 2–3 screws can be inserted in the diaphyseal area, although it is not very easy to do so. I perform the usual arthroplasty, and I fill the osteotomy site with the bone obtained from the TKA procedure.

I usually use an extension stem, which plays the role of an IM nail. Since the screws are inserted with the trial stem at the site, they do not interfere with implant insertion. I always prepare the C-arm to check the alignment during operation (Fig. 5.36).

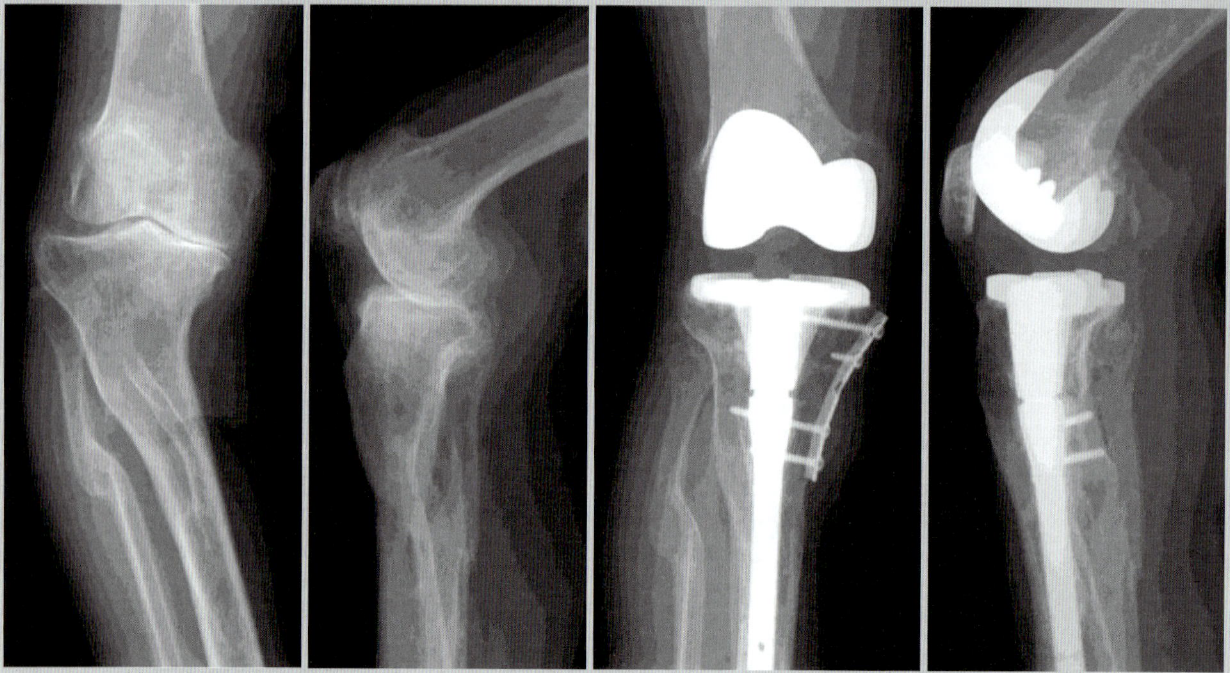

Fig. 5.36 One-stage angular deformity correction and arthroplasty. Preoperative and postoperative X-rays

5.3 Ankylosis

Limping is more prominent in ankylosis of the knee joint than in that of the hip joint. It is not certain how much limitation of motion (LOM) should be regarded as ankylosis. Ankylosis literally means the absence of joint motion. Clinically, ankylosis means limited joint motion that interferes with daily activities of living. More than 65° of flexion is necessary for level walking, and more than 95° of flexion is needed for stair walking. If the patient has a flexion contracture of more than 10°, the gait pattern changes, and more energy is needed for walking. Considering this aspect, the arc of motion from 10° to 95° can be classified into ankylosis. Clinically, *if patient has a flexion contracture of more than 20° and less than 70° of flexion, surgical intervention is needed in order to improve the ROM.*

If the knee joint is ankylosed, it is almost impossible to go up and down the stairs, very difficult to get into a car, sit down on the floor, or sit on the traditional oriental toilet bowl. Therefore, an increased ROM is of critical importance in these patients.

5.3.1 Indication

An ankylosed knee may be suitable for young active laborers. But young patients who do not engage in laborious work are a good indication for conversion to a mobile knee joint for a better social life.

Unlike the hip joint, it is relatively easy to do a fusion (arthrodesis) of the knee joint when complications develop after total joint replacement. Therefore, the range of indications for conversion to a mobile knee joint is wider than that for the hip joint.

However, *the knee joint is very superficial with a very little soft tissue envelope and is more prone to develop wound infection and subsequent deep infection. The patients may not achieve the desired ROM, and the knee joint may not function properly due to the extensor weakness. Therefore, the indication of conversion of the ankylosed knee joint to a mobile knee joint should be selected very carefully.*

Naranja et al. reviewed the results of a multicenter study in the patients who underwent conversion of ankylotic knee to TKA. The average range of motion increased from 7° of flexion contracture to 62° of flexion in patients with complete ankylosis of the knee joint. Short-term complications were seen in 24 % of patients, and major long-term complications such as infection and loosening developed in 35 % of patients, and the patient satisfaction rate was 29 %. Kim et al. also reported that an average flexion motion of 78° could be achieved using a posterior-stabilized knee, but half of the patients showed skin necrosis. Cho et al. reported that about 19 % of patients required revision arthrodesis due to deep infection.

While performing the operation, it is important to know the patient's level of expectations, because satisfaction tends to increase with lowering of the expectations. The patients should be informed that the goal for the range of motion is about 90° of flexion, and joint fusion may be needed if complications develop.

The prerequisite for the operation is the continuity of the extensor mechanism, i.e., the patella, patellar tendon, and quadriceps tendon should be intact. Sonography or MRI is helpful in detecting the extensor defect. Tendon allograft may be used for the deficiency of the extensor mechanism, but this makes the operation too complicated and weakens the quadriceps power. If the extensor mechanism is incompetent, it is recommended not to convert the ankylotic knee joint to a mobile knee joint.

5.3.2 Prognostic Factors

Prognosis may vary according to the skin condition, causative factors of ankylosis, degree and position of ankylosis, and the duration of ankylosis.

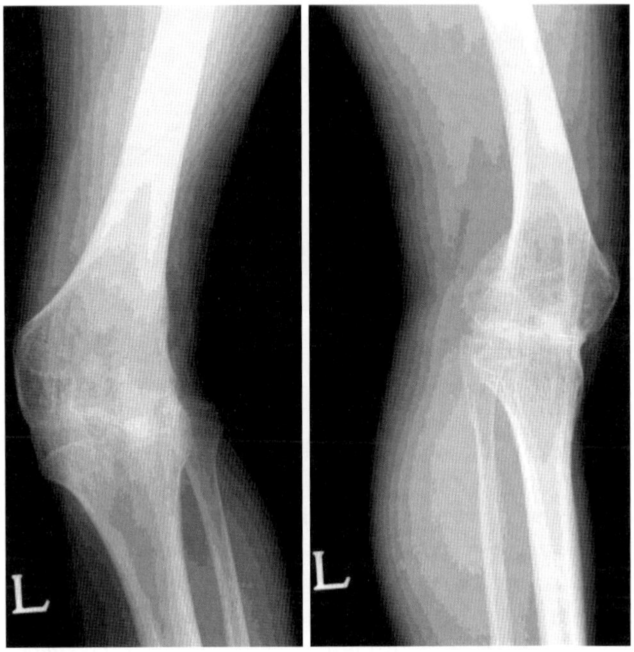

Fig. 5.37 Complete ankylosis with no visible joint line

If the skin condition is poor, the skin may not be closed after the main procedure. Tension at the incision site causes skin necrosis and infection and reduces the ROM due to the difficulties during the postoperative rehabilitation period. For improving the skin yield, tissue expanders are often used. Cho et al. experienced satisfying results using tissue expanders.

With respect to the causes of ankylosis, ankylosis caused due to degenerative arthritis is neither serious nor difficult to pay special attention to it. Ankylosis caused due to inflammatory diseases, such as rheumatoid arthritis, is often associated with deformities at other sites, ankylosis of the other joints, and is accompanied by osteopenia which makes the operation more difficult. In case of ankylosis caused due to infection, usually there is coexisting intra- and extra-articular fibrosis and joint destruction. Extensive surgical procedures may provoke reactivation of infection. Patients who have ankylosis due to prior knee joint surgery or those who underwent knee joint fusion show anatomical changes in the bone, joint, and tendons. The knee joint may show instability or progressive limited ROM postoperatively due to scar contracture.

The degree of ankylosis is classified into complete ankylosis and incomplete ankylosis. Complete ankylosis is further classified into fibrous ankylosis and bony ankylosis (Fig. 5.37).

Incomplete ankylosis is classified as severe when the ROM is less than 45°, moderate when the ROM is between 45° and 70°, and mild when the ROM is between 70° and 90°. The methods of surgery and prognosis vary greatly

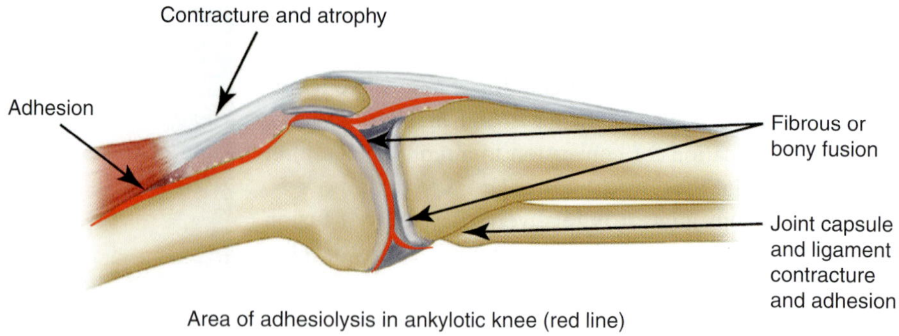

Fig. 5.38 Extensor mechanism problem in ankylotic knee. It is often associated with adhesion, contracture, and atrophy of the extensor mechanism

according to the severity of ankylosis. Of course, it is more difficult to perform the operation and the prognosis is poorer in cases with more severe ankylosis.

The angle of ankylosis has a critical impact. If there is ankylosis in flexion state, it is relatively easy to perform the operation, even though there is a possibility of postoperative extension lag. If ankylosis is in extension state, it is accompanied by quadriceps shortening. Ancillary procedures for the extensor mechanism would cause motion limitation and extensor weakness.

Another factor to be taken into consideration is the duration of ankylosis. If the duration of ankylosis is not very long, a good ROM can be expected by adhesiolysis and brisement. A longer duration of ankylosis would lead to degeneration of muscles, tendons, and ligaments causing weakening of the muscle power and joint instability.

5.3.3 Surgical Techniques

The *problems* confronted during conversion of ankylotic knee joint to mobile knee joint include *abnormal skin condition* which requires careful preparation and handling, *difficulty in ligament balancing due to weakening and adhesion of the surrounding ligaments and other soft tissues, difficulty in achieving the desired ROM due to extensor contracture and adhesion, possibility of the use of tendon allograft* to compensate for the insufficient ligament, and *high risk of neurovascular injury* during osteotomy (Fig. 5.38).

In case of mild ankylosis, the operative procedure is generally the same or is a little more difficult than that in the usual arthroplasty. In moderate to severe ankylosis, the procedure is more complicated as it is difficult to evert the patella, to treat the extensor mechanism, to release the soft tissues, and to balance the flexion and extension gaps. In any case, the surgical technique for incomplete ankylosis is less demanding compared to that for complete ankylosis.

Harwin emphasized that brisement under anesthesia before arthrotomy is helpful in reduction of the extensor contracture. *After arthrotomy, resection of the fibrous tissues between the patella and the supracondylar area of the femur should be performed first.* If the patella cannot be everted, it is recommended to perform *lateral retinacular release in advance or just retract the patella laterally. When lateral retinacular release* is planned, *it should be considered in conjunction with quadricepsplasty* which may be needed later.

It is important to achieve maximum ROM before osteotomy. All tissues that restrict the ROM should be resected or released by adhesiolysis.

After adhesiolysis, *brisement* should be performed. In cases with long duration of ankylosis, however, it may be impossible to achieve the desired ROM without ancillary procedures for the extensor mechanism. If excessive force is applied during *this procedure, avulsion fracture of quadriceps or patellar tendon may occur. This is a serious complication* since healing of the tendon is delayed or is impossible due to the interruption of blood supply. Therefore, it is necessary to prevent this complication during brisement. *If the ROM is insufficient even after adhesiolysis, quadricepsplasty or tibial tubercle osteotomy should be considered.* Quadricepsplasty is performed if the ROM is less than 60°–70°. In such a case, a rectus snip is done first, if it has not been done before. If the ROM is still restricted after a rectus snip, V–Y plasty for lengthening of the quadriceps tendon or tibial tubercle osteotomy can be considered. These sequential procedures may be harmful to the soft tissues. When poor ROM is expected with a rectus snip alone, it is recommended to do V–Y plasty or tibial tubercle osteotomy from the beginning.

Osteotomy is the same as that in the usual total knee arthroplasty since the shape of bone is relatively well preserved.

Complete ankylosis in *extension* is associated with extensor contracture, and fibrous or bony union is often observed between the patella and the femoral condyle. The first step is to separate the patella from the bone by soft tissue release in case of fibrous fusion and by osteotomy in case of bony union. Adhesiolysis after arthrotomy is also required for complete ankylosis in extension, and the methods have been described just before in moderate and severe ankylosis and in Sect. 5.2.1.3.

In case of bony fusion, the joint line is hardly seen. The osteotomy line can be traced according to the patella and the tibial tuberosity, or by comparing with an X-ray of the sound side. While performing osteotomy of the far posterior part, it is advisable not to use a saw or an osteotome in order to protect the nerves and vessels. With an intact posterior cortex, the bone is opened by using a flexion force to separate the two bones (osteoclasis). After osteotomy, careful release of the soft tissues in the posterior part of the joint should be done using a periosteal elevator until the fatty tissues are visible.

Since the cruciate and collateral ligaments are not reliable in cases with long-standing ankylosis, the use of the CR type is not recommended, even when the ligaments look healthy to the naked eyes. The constrained type should be considered for correction of the medial and lateral instability.

The use of a smaller femoral implant is recommended as a wider flexion gap is needed for ankylosis in extension. Although usual method is to perform femoral osteotomy first, a few surgeons recommend to perform osteotomy of the proximal tibia first for determination of femoral external rotation and for securing joint stability in flexion.

Tibial osteotomy is performed using the extramedullary method, and the *level of resection is determined by lowering the osteotomy jig click by click*. It is also important to maintain the joint line. *The amount of distal resection of the femur is also done gradually click by click while observing the gap balance*. External rotation of femur is determined by the ligament tension method, and the anterior reference system is recommended for adjusting the flexion gap.

Tibial prosthesis should not be implanted in internal rotation. Ankylosis is often associated with rotational deformity, so it is recommended to determine the rotational alignment of the tibial prosthesis using the dynamic method by performing flexion and extension repeatedly rather than using the anatomical landmark.

Patellar replacement is not recommended if the patella is too small due to the long duration of ankylosis or in case of patella baja which causes impingement of the patella onto the spacer. A thinner patella helps to improve ROM and patellar tracking provided the bone is not broken.

Trial implant is inserted and the ROM is checked. If the ROM is unsatisfactory, gentle manipulation is tried again, and the causes for restricted flexion motion should be checked and addressed appropriately.

Complete ankylosis in flexion needs same method of adhesiolysis as with ankylosis in extension, especially in the posterior compartment. Special care should be taken so as not to decrease the extension gap. To prevent postoperative extensor lag, injuring the extensor mechanism is best avoided, and sewing the medial capsule with distal advancement is recommended.

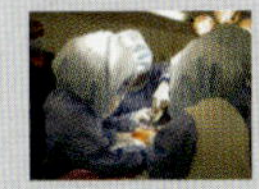

Author's Method

Preoperatively, I check the skin condition first. If the skin yield is not good, I consult a plastic surgeon, and the use of a tissue expander is considered for making the skin more pliable.

Paramedial arthrotomy is done. After arthrotomy, the quadriceps tendon is elevated, and adhesiolysis is done to mobilize the patella. The adhesiolysis is performed right up to the proximal femur. The thick fibrous tissue along the patellar tendon is removed. To prevent disruption of the extensor mechanism, tension band suturing is done by making a transverse hole across the tibial tuberosity distally and by using the modified Bunnell suturing on the quadriceps tendon proximally. This tension band suture is left in situ for postoperative rehabilitation (Fig. 5.39). While performing brisement, I place my fingers under the quadriceps tendon. If I perceive excessive tension on my fingers, I do a rectus snip or V–Y quadriceps turndown.

In fibrous union, I resect the fibrous tissues gradually. In bony union, I perform osteoclasis.

Osteotomy is done starting from the tibia and is gradually increased click by click to ensure the adequate joint space.

I use the anterior reference system for femoral osteotomy, as it is easy to adjust the flexion gap. Femoral external rotation is determined by the ligament tension technique, and tibial rotation is determined by the dynamic method. During this procedure, special attention is paid to patellar tracking.

If the intended range of motion is not achieved after insertion of the tibial component, I first try brisement followed by insertion of a one-size thinner PE, or I use the constrained type of implant.

Patellar treatment is decided according to the condition of the patellar bone stock.

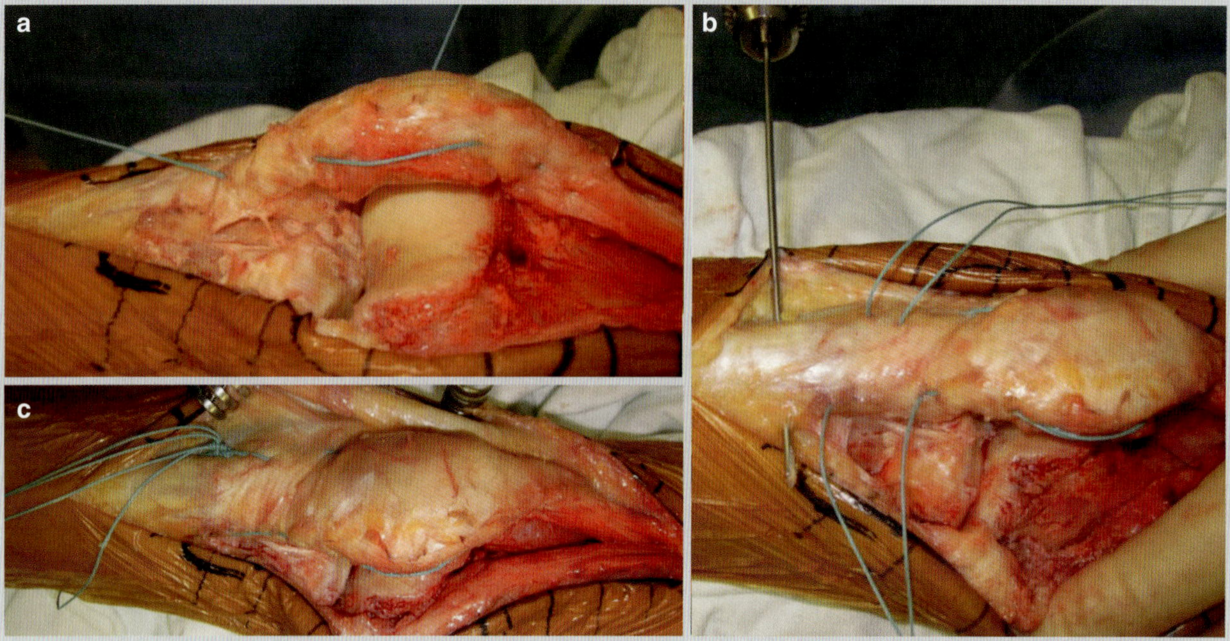

Fig. 5.39 Tension band technique from the quadriceps tendon to the distal part of the tibial tuberosity. (**a**) Modified Bunnell suture on the quadriceps tendon. (**b**) The sutures are passed through a hole which is made distal to tibial tuberosity. (**c**) The suture is tied

5.4 Miscellaneous Conditions and Diseases

5.4.1 Osteopenia

Patients who need TKA often have accompanying osteopenia. This is because most of the patients are elderly women who have several predisposing factors for osteopenia such as decreased activity due to pain in the knee joint and long history of medications due to comorbidity. It is not necessary to include osteopenia under special conditions for arthroplasty; however, I would like to describe this condition here as there are many factors to be considered during the operation.

Clinically, osteopenia is defined as reduction of the bone mass which increases the risk of fracture. Osteoporosis is a more severe form of osteopenia. It is generally accepted that the definition of osteoporosis is the BMD below 2.5SD compared to that in a young adult. If there are findings suggestive of osteoporosis on the plain X-ray, it should be considered that the bone mass has been decreased by about 30–50 %. For the knee joints, Li and Nilsson reported that the average BMD measured at 5 mm below the joint line was 0.81 ± 0.30 g/cm^2, and the migration of prosthesis increased when the average BMD was below 0.60 g/cm^2.

Most of the times, patients with osteopenia do not simply have loss of the bony substance. The skin is thin and fragile, and wound healing is difficult. The ligaments and tendinous structures are so weakly anchored to the bone that they can easily be detached or stripped off during the operation (Fig. 5.40).

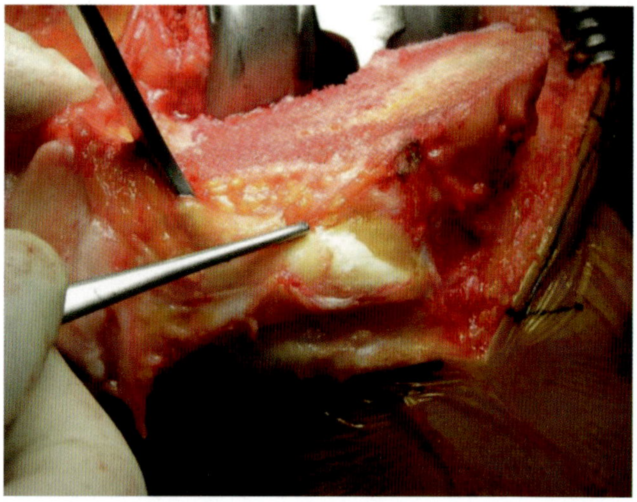

Fig. 5.40 Patellar tendon is likely to be stripped off due to osteopenia

These problems of the soft tissues and bones should be considered together during the operation. *Excessive retraction of skin and soft tissues should be avoided during the operation, and it is sometimes necessary to protect the patellar tendon so as not to strip it off.*

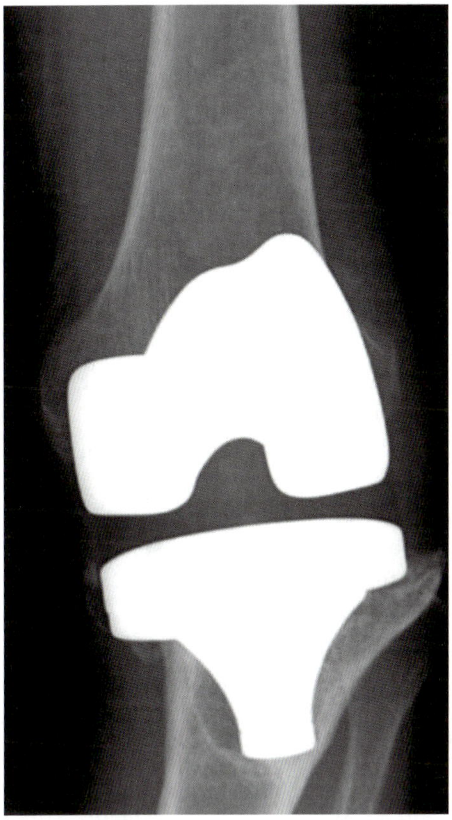

Fig. 5.41 X-ray of loosening without use of extension stem in patient with osteopenia

When choosing the prosthesis, the constrained type should be avoided if possible since it has a high risk of loosening, and the use of an *extension stem should be considered* when the fixation is not stable.

When the bones are weak, they may break easily during the operation. Special care should be taken so as *not to cause a fracture intraoperatively and avoid anterior notching of the femoral condyle as it may cause a periprosthetic fracture postoperatively*.

If there is malalignment or instability, the incidence of loosening may increase postoperatively, and this is the reason why alignment is more important in osteopenia (Fig. 5.41). Baldwin and Rubinstein stated that the success of TKA depends on how strongly the bone supports the prosthesis and fixation stability to resist stress, which is directly related to bone quality.

In fact, the tibial prosthesis moves slightly in the lateral direction after the operation. Petersen et al. demonstrated that patients with higher BMD showed less migration of the tibial prosthesis. Hence, the use of cement is critical in patients with osteopenia. Rand et al. reported that patients with osteopenia do not show good clinical outcomes when cement has not been used. Sugita et al. showed that using cement does not increase the incidence of loosening provided good alignment of the prosthesis has been achieved even in cases with severe osteopenia, and *they emphasized the importance of alignment as well as cementing technique*.

However, Li and Nilsson found that a phenomenon developed in which one part of the prosthesis sank down and the other part was lifted up when cement was not used in cases with mild osteopenia, and there was no difference in the incidence of migration of the prosthesis even with cementing. They also found that the incidence of migration of the prosthesis increased up to postoperative 6 weeks until stability had been established in case of cementless fixation, whereas the incidence of migration of the prosthesis was minimal at first, and it increased after postoperative 6 weeks with cemented fixation. Lee et al. also emphasized that cementing is not recommended, although it is not contraindicated, if stable fixation can be established using an extension stem in the patients with osteopenia. Therbo et al. concluded that the need for revision surgery did not increase in cases with osteopenia just because of non-cementing.

Forceful exercises or too early full weight bearing during rehabilitation can also cause a fracture of the osteoporotic bone postoperatively. It is necessary to protect the joint by brace fitting during the early rehabilitation period in cases with severe osteopenia, or if a minor fracture develops during the operation.

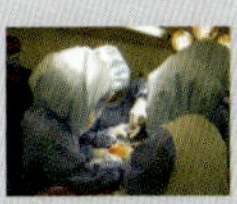

Author's Method

I make a slightly longer skin incision than usual to prevent excessive retraction of the skin and soft tissues. I routinely protect the patellar tendon from being stripped off by using a pin or a patellar tendon protector before eversion of the patella.

I try my best to avoid anterior notching of the distal femur during osteotomy and pay more attention to the alignment. I follow the principle of not using a constrained implant as far as possible. I use an extension stem when the fixation is not stable enough with the usual method, when a thick metal augment has been used or when a minor fracture has occurred during the operation.

I use cement in all cases without exception. I do not recommend pulsatile lavage for patients with osteopenia because it increases the risk of thermal necrosis since the cement penetrates more than the recommended depth (2–3 mm). I close the skin very carefully and use paper bandage instead of cotton bandage to minimize the skin problem.

During rehabilitation, I recommend the patients to avoid vigorous exercises and slow down the rehabilitation program. I also prescribe brace fitting and medication for osteoporosis in severe cases.

5.4.2 Previous Knee Operation

In the patients who have undergone knee operation previously, the operative procedure of the TKA may have to be altered from that of the usual TKA. Previous knee operations include arthroscopic surgery, open ligament surgery, high tibial osteotomy, open reduction and internal fixation of fracture, and arthrodesis.

5.4.2.1 Arthroscopic Surgery

A simple arthroscopic examination or meniscal surgery does not interfere with the surgical procedure of TKA. There is only a small incision scar, no change in the bony structure of the knee joint, and no serious adhesions of the soft tissues. However, it is necessary to consider the possibility of infection. There will not be any problems if arthroplasty is performed after careful assessment of the possibility of infection.

5.4.2.2 Ligament Surgery

If an operation has been performed on the ligament, the considering factors are incision scar, instability, or limited ROM. Usually the fixtures used for ligament surgery can be easily removed intraoperatively, and it is best to remove all such fixtures.

If the joint has been opened before, the condition and location of the scar should be checked. Incision scars are mostly midline, paramedial, medial, or lateral. If it is a midline or paramedial incision, the incision should be made along the previous scar. If it is medial or lateral incision, *the new incision should be at least 7 cm away from the previous scar*. It is generally believed that there will not be any problem even if the new incision is very close to the previous scar when the previous operation has been performed more than 10 years ago, but it is still important to follow this principle in order to prevent skin necrosis.

If the collateral ligaments are not in a good condition despite of reconstructive surgery, the best method for the ligament balancing must be chosen, or the use of a constrained implant should be considered according to the degree of instability.

5.4.2.3 Fracture Surgery

Fracture near the joint may cause problems with respect to the *incision scar or soft tissue problem, bone defect due to bony necrosis and nonunion or malunion, ankylosis or instability, and possibility of occult infection*. Zelicof et al. analyzed that arthroplasty for post-traumatic arthritis due to fractures showed poor clinical results and was associated with a higher risk of deep infection. The procedures for TKA after fracture treatment vary according to whether it is a shaft fracture or an articular fracture.

Shaft Fracture

If the operation was performed on the shaft, the incision scar may be of little importance.

A decision should be taken regarding *whether to remove the internal fixtures* and the timing of their removal. If it is decided not to remove the fixtures, the procedures for TKA are the same except for the use of an extramedullary guide. Since most of the patients want the fixtures to be removed, they can be removed as long as bony union is confirmed. Some surgeons recommend waiting for at least six months after removal of the internal fixtures for performing TKA, because the bone may be weakened after removal of the implant. Although Reis proposed preventive IM nailing after the removal of plate and screws, it may be better not to remove the fixtures rather than performing IM nailing.

Stem extension may be considered after the removal of plate and screws. When performing reaming, care should be taken so as not to perform over-reaming which will make the cortical bone thinner, and such a site can act as a stress riser to cause a fracture. The risk of fracture increases if the length of the stem is not at least 3–4 cm longer than the last screw hole.

Metaphyseal and Articular Fracture

Skin incision can be made along the previous scar, but a new incision is needed as most of the surgeons prefer to use the medial or lateral approach for open reduction and internal fixation. If it is a medial or lateral incision scar, the principles of skin incision for TKA are the same as have been described before. Hence, *it is recommended to make a midline incision in fracture surgery for elderly patients for a possible subsequent arthroplasty*.

If the fracture has been treated using the Ilizarov technique, it is necessary to be even more careful to decide operation since occult infection may be reactivated postoperatively.

All internal fixtures used for an articular fracture should be removed. If there is bone union at the fracture site, procedures are just the same as in the usual arthroplasty. *If there is nonunion or there is a possibility of bone necrosis, it will be accompanied by bone defect*. In such a case, arthroplasty is needed mostly due to the failure of fracture treatment. The knee joint may be swollen and soft tissues may be weakened since an adequate time has not passed after the fracture surgery to allow healing of the surgical trauma of the soft tissue.

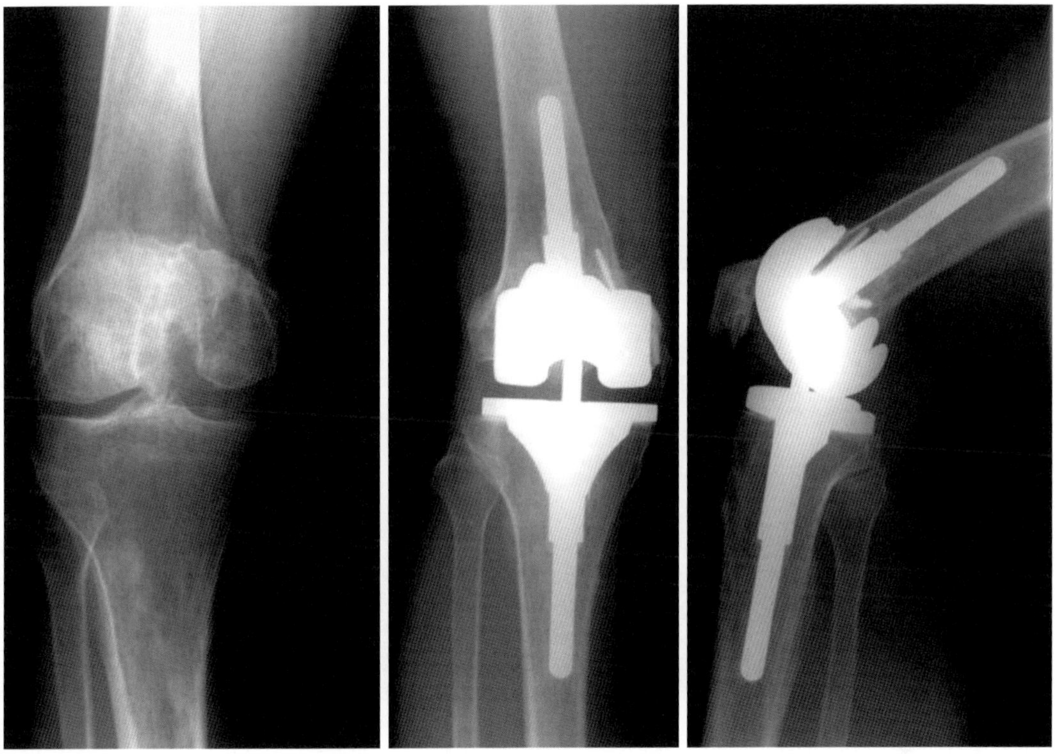

Fig. 5.42 Arthroplasty for nonunion of the distal femur. The *left X-ray* shows nonunion of the medial femoral condyle. The *right X-ray* shows bone union by reduction of fragment and bone grafting after TKA

It is necessary to decide whether to retain or remove the bony fragments. *If the bony fragments are large and attached to the soft tissues, internal fixation of the fragment and bone grafting can be performed*. The fixtures should not interfere with the insertion of the prosthesis. In patients with an open fracture or bone necrosis, it is recommended to remove the bony fragments and reconstruct the bone defect (Fig. 5.42).

If there is *malunion*, there might be an angular deformity combined with rotational deformity of the bone. If open reduction has been performed, the angular deformity is usually not severe. TKA can be performed as usual while watching for the development of rotational deformity. When performing distal femoral osteotomy, in particular, the flexion and extension gaps should be balanced. The ligament tension technique is preferred since the bone fragment may have twisted thereby causing a rotational deformity.

5.4.2.4 High Tibial Osteotomy (HTO)

The surgical procedure can differ according to the osteotomy method and depending on how well the osteotomy was performed. In open wedge osteotomy, it is easy to perform the operation since the deformity is not severe. However, removal of the relatively large fixtures is needed. In closed wedge osteotomy, the surgical procedure is not easy as it is usually accompanied by deformity, shortening, and bone defect.

Many factors should be considered while performing TKA in patients who have had a high tibial osteotomy. First, the previous incision scar should be considered. Second, patella eversion or retraction is difficult due to the scar contracture. Third, the metaphyseal bone is weak after removal of the internal fixtures. Fourth, a bone defect may be encountered. Fifth, deformities may have occurred due to osteotomy. The top of the tibia is short, shifted to the lateral side, and there is accompanying genu recurvatum, rotational, or valgus deformity. Sixth, there is accompanying patella baja in almost all cases. Finally, instability may coexist (Fig. 5.43).

An accurate evaluation of the preoperative X-ray is very important for detecting nonunion or stress fracture, state of correction (overcorrection or undercorrection), height of the medial and lateral tibial plateau, posterior slope of the tibial plateau, patellar height and tracking, and instability of the joint.

The previous incision scar is generally transverse, oblique, or longitudinal on the lateral side. If the previous scar is transverse, it is desirable to make an incision perpendicular to it. If it is vertical, the previous incision can be extended proximally and distally, and arthrotomy can be performed medially. If the surgeon has experience with the lateral approach, this approach can be used. A short oblique incision from the fibular head to the tibial tuberosity can be ignored.

It is often difficult to evert the patella due to patella baja or fibrosis after osteotomy. Most of the times, lateral retinacular release is performed in advance, or the patella is retracted laterally without eversion. It may also be necessary to perform V–Y quadricepsplasty or tibial tubercle osteotomy in order to provide a better surgical exposure.

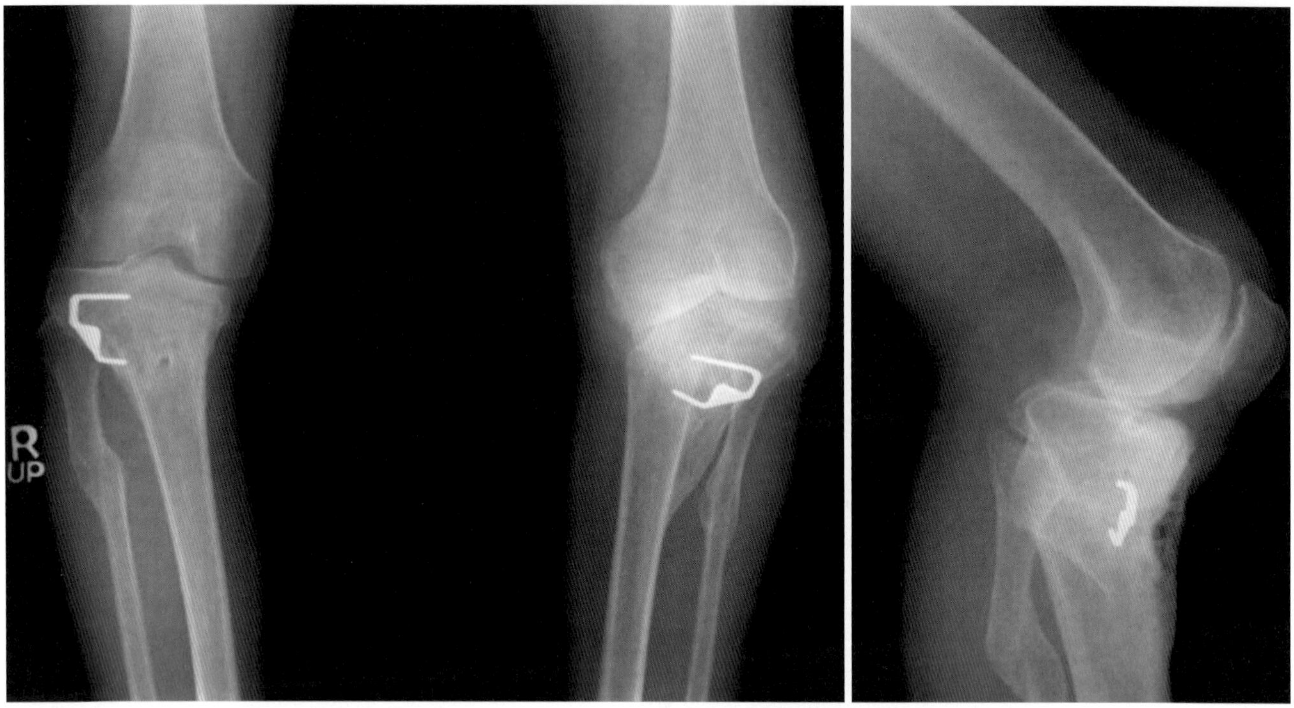

Fig. 5.43 Changes in the knee joint after HTO

Although it is *not always necessary to remove the staples or other fixtures* used for high tibial osteotomy, it is recommended to remove them if they cause any hindrance during prosthesis insertion. However, it is not that easy to remove these fixtures as expected because they may be buried or hidden deep inside the bone. Removal of fixtures should be done very carefully in order to save as much cortical bone as possible. If a bone defect develops, bone grafting may be needed. In some cases, these fixtures may be removed 4–6 weeks before arthroplasty.

Above all, the presence of *valgus deformity due to overcorrection* should be taken into consideration. With a valgus deformity, collateral ligament balancing is difficult not only in extension but also in flexion due to the rotational deformity. In such a situation, mediolateral balance in flexion should be achieved even at the cost of internal rotation of the femoral component. The patellar maltracking can be corrected later by lateral positioning and more external rotation of the tibial prosthesis.

The proximal portion of the tibia may have shifted laterally. To solve this problem, a smaller prosthesis can be placed more medially or an offset stem can be used (Fig. 5.44).

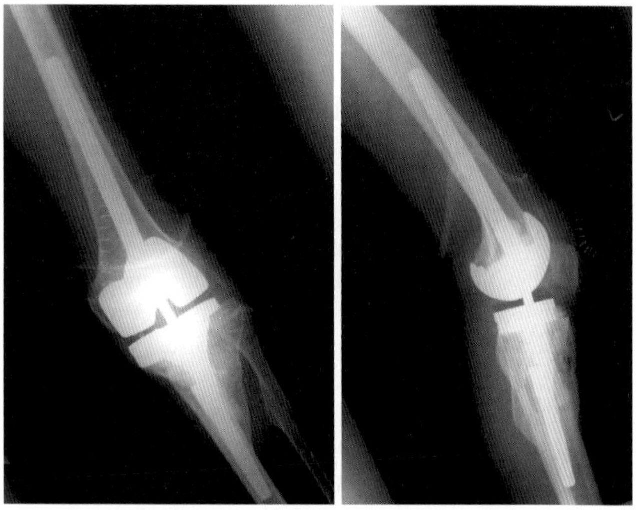

Fig. 5.44 Operation performed using an offset stem for a patient with previous HTO

Shortening of the proximal tibia can also cause problems. The best possible efforts should be taken to maintain the joint line and minimize the lateral bone resection for better support of the tibial prosthesis. In cases with anterior inclination of the tibial plateau or *genu recurvatum*, a posterior slope should be avoided during tibial osteotomy so that the flexion gap does not become too wide. Nelson and Windsor strongly recommended preoperative X-ray templating to determine the amount of bone resection and alignment for an accurate osteotomy.

Patellar replacement should also be done carefully. In cases with *patella baja*, less osteotomy of the distal femur and more osteotomy of the proximal tibia can be considered. However, this is not a simple decision to make since this procedure weakens the proximal portion of the tibia. In case of PE impingement, the patella may not be replaced, or *a smaller patellar component can be placed a little higher, and a beveled PE should be used in order to minimize impingement.*

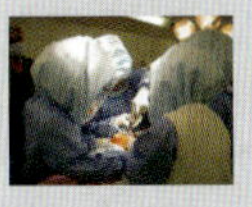

Author's Method

My principle of arthroplasty after a high tibial osteotomy is as follows: First, a careful skin incision is made. Second, I always remove the fixtures used for osteotomy. Third, the PS type of prosthesis is used. This is because the PCL is usually nonfunctional, or it has already been degenerated, and it is difficult to correct a severe deformity with the PCL being retained. *Fourth, I minimize the lateral and posterior osteotomy of the tibia* and perform bone grafting for reconstruction of the bone defect, if any. *Fifth, an offset stem is sometimes used for stable fixation, and sixth, patella replacement is carefully considered. Finally, I use the constrained prosthesis when instability is noted.*

In severe genu recurvatum deformity, I perform "derotational autogenous grafting." Before performing the tibial osteotomy, I trim the articular cartilage and subchondral bone with saw. Proximal osteotomy is done with a lesser degree than intended slope. The wedge-shaped slice of the bone that is obtained by the osteotomy is placed in a reverse direction as a bone graft (Fig. 5.45).

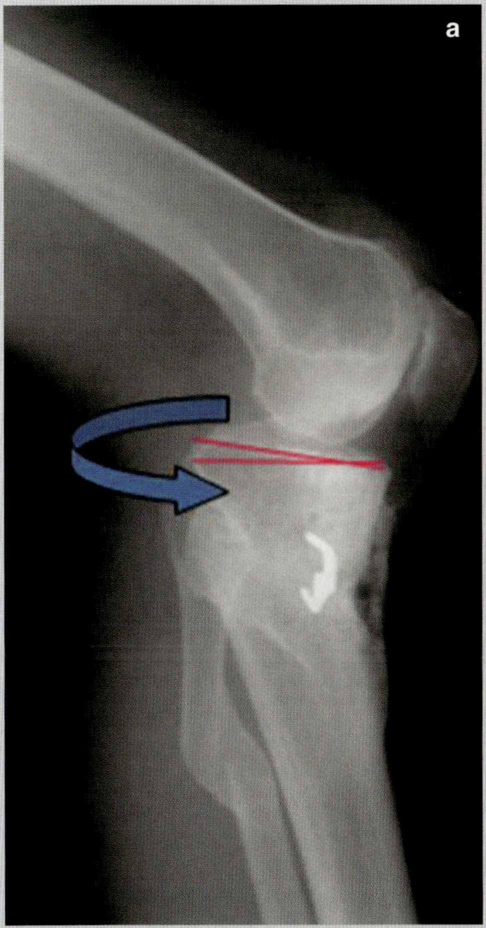

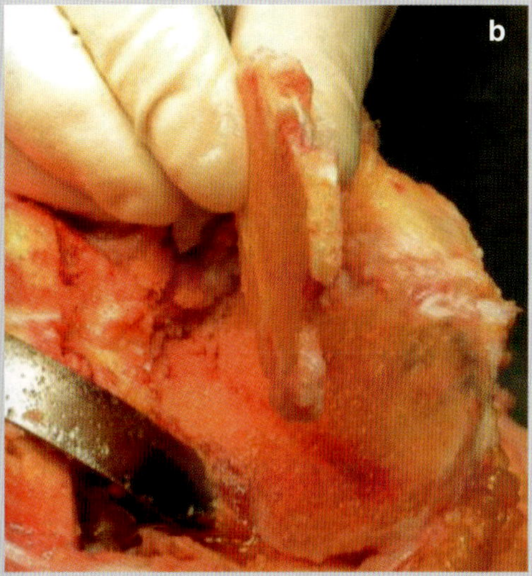

Fig. 5.45 Derotational autogenous grafting in a severe genu recurvatum deformity. (**a**) Preoperative lateral X-ray. *Red lines* indicate the osteotomy line. (**b**) Wedge-shaped slice of the bone from proximal tibial osteotomy. (**c**) *Arrows* indicate the slice of the bone placed in a reverse direction. (**d**) Postoperative lateral X-ray

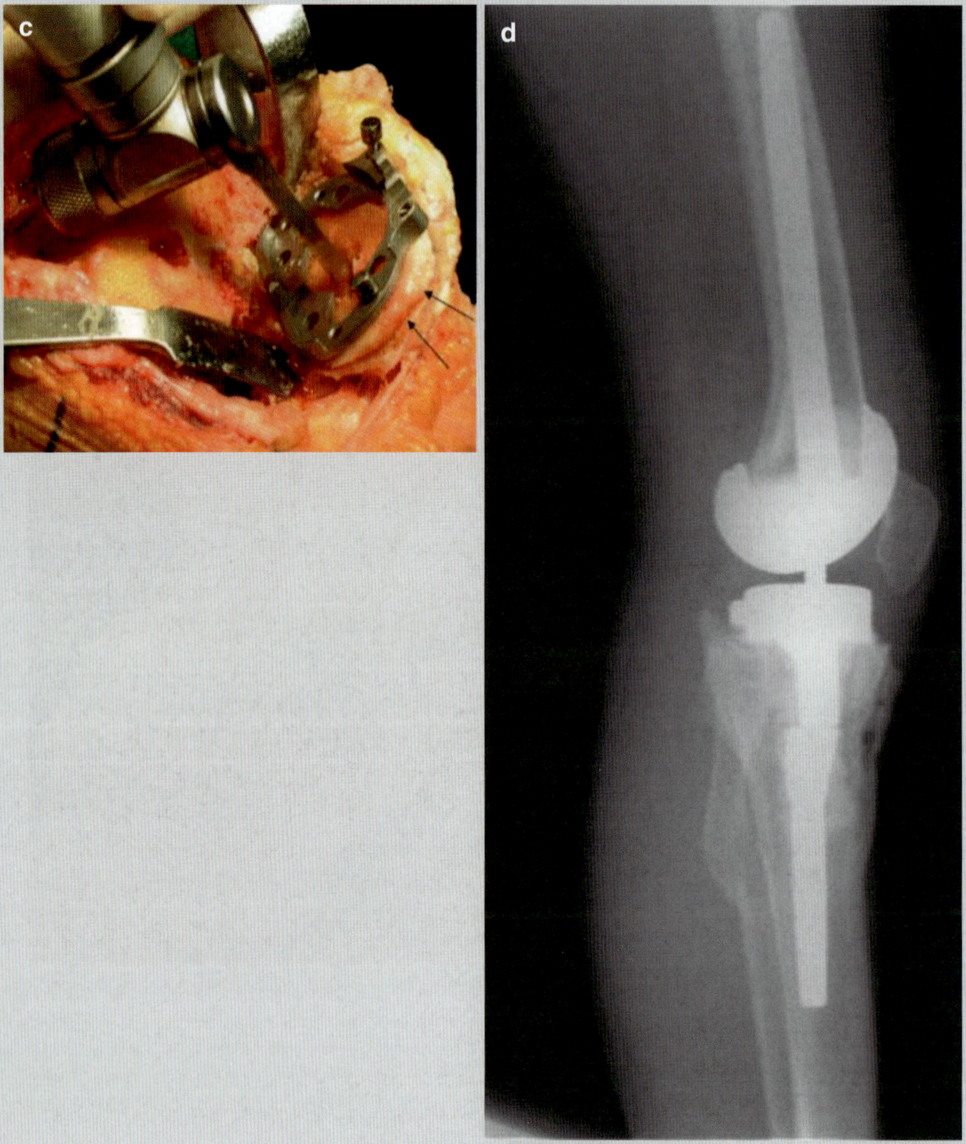

Fig. 5.45 (continued)

The possible postoperative complications include skin necrosis, malalignment, instability, limited motion, patellar subluxation, avascular necrosis of the patella, and patellar tendon rupture.

The result of TKA after failed HTO is not as satisfactory as that of the usual TKA. Haslam et al. followed up the patients who received TKA due to failed high tibial osteotomy for an average of 12 years and concluded that many patients had a limited flexion motion and a high incidence of revision surgery.

5.4.3 Ankylotic Hip

TKA is relatively contraindicated in ankylotic hip since the knee replacement alone will not restore function to allow normal walking. In rare cases, TKA is performed when there is ipsilateral or contralateral hip joint ankylosis. *If possible, THA should be performed first* before performing TKA. Rittmeister et al. emphasized that *TKA should be performed after THA* as an ankylotic hip is one of the causes for poor prognosis of TKA due to the mechanical changes leading to early wear and loosening.

If the hip joint has been ankylosed since a long time, the patients will suffer from pain due to degenerative changes in the joints proximal and distal to the hip joints. Some patients also complain of referred pain in the knee joint. This referred pain is not relieved after TKA. As the pain is competitive, the patient may feel more referred pain when the pain in the knee joint is subsided.

When performing TKA in a case with an accompanying ankylotic hip, two factors should be considered: first, the position of ankylosis and second, the condition of the other joints around the hip such as the spine, sacroiliac joint, and the hip joint of the contralateral side. Romness and Morrey stated that *appropriate positioning and good alignment of the hip joints is the most important prognostic factor for TKA.* Roberts et al. described that for achieving good results of TKA, the fused hip joint should be in a position of flexion at less than 25°, 0° abduction, and external rotation of less than 5°, and the leg length discrepancy should not be greater than 2 cm.

During the TKA operation in a case with an accompanying ipsilateral ankylotic hip, it is very difficult to check the alignment and soft tissue balance. Therefore, the operation table should be prepared such that the patient's leg can drop down.

Even if the patient has a mild deformity of the hip joint, he may undergo hip replacement in the future. Hence, the current position of the hip joint as well as the physiologic mechanical alignment should be considered concomitantly in aligning the knee joint axis.

In an ankylotic hip, a mobile-bearing joint which automatically corrects malrotation can be used. However, it is associated with a higher risk of PE dislocation.

The early postoperative complications include limited ROM and ankylosis of the knee joint. Garvin et al. recommended scheduled rehabilitation programs.

5.4.4 Miscellaneous Diseases

5.4.4.1 Rheumatoid Arthritis

Rheumatoid arthritis (RA) is the second most common indication for knee arthroplasty, and hence it is not a very special condition. However, I would like to describe TKA in cases with RA here since some special points need to be considered other than those in TKA for osteoarthritis.

Difference Between RA and OA

There are several differences between RA and OA.

The first difference is that RA occurs at a relatively younger age and involves several joints. Therefore, a comprehensive treatment plan needs to be established considering the medical conditions and conditions of the other joints. RA would simultaneously affect the ipsilateral hip joint. Here again, it is *recommended to perform the operation on the hip joint first.* There are several reasons for doing so. The first reason is that the radiating pain from the hip joint often has an adverse effect on TKA. The second reason is that the patient might prefer not to undergo the hip surgery after the knee surgery since the postoperative pain following TKA is extreme, which may discourage the patient to undergo another arthroplasty. The third reason is that it is not easy to perform the knee exercises in the presence of hip joint pain, and the hamstring muscle may develop a contracture after THA, which has an adverse effect on the TKA. The fourth reason is that brisement can also be performed to relieve the knee flexion contracture while the patient is under anesthesia for the hip surgery. Finally, operating on the knee joint without correcting the deformity of the hip joint affects the long-term survival of TKA.

The second difference is that RA is a chronic debilitating disease that causes other medical comorbidities due to long-term medications. The patient may have poor cardiopulmonary and renal function due to the long-term use of analgesics and anti-inflammatory drugs. Also, RA is a progressive disease, and more number of patients complain of pain with the passage of time.

Third, the patient's activity is decreased, and in some cases, the patient is bedridden for a long time. *The skin, soft tissues, and bones around the knee joint are weak and may not show good healing.*

The fourth difference is that the soft tissues or bony structures are often deformed which makes the surgery more difficult, and the prognosis is poorer than that in OA. Laskin reported the 10-year follow-up results which demonstrate that the tibial loosening was very common because of the incorrect positioning of the tibial component, and the incidence of infection was high. Although the postoperative prognosis of RA has been reported to be the same or better compared to that of osteoarthritis by some authors, this is only because the patients with RA perform lesser activity. The results of surgery are actually not as good as to those in OA.

Fifth, the risk of postoperative infection is very high.

Finally, providing anesthesia is difficult since there are accompanying cervical and lumbar spinal lesions.

Considering Factors

Skin

The skin is thin, fragile, and can be easily lacerated, and so it should be handled very carefully from incision to closure. *If the incision is too short, the skin will be tense, and wound problem is also likely to develop.* For wound healing, the length of the incision should be sufficient.

Soft Tissues

As the lesion in RA originates from the synovium, *synovectomy can reduce pain and delay the progress of the disease. The PCL is surrounded by the synovium and it may be weakened or it may get resorbed if it is retained, and hence it is recommended to sacrifice the PCL and use the PS type.* Laskin and O'Flynn experienced that revision rate was increased due to PCL deficiency when CR type prosthesis was used in patients with RA, and they recommended the use of a PS type of prosthesis.

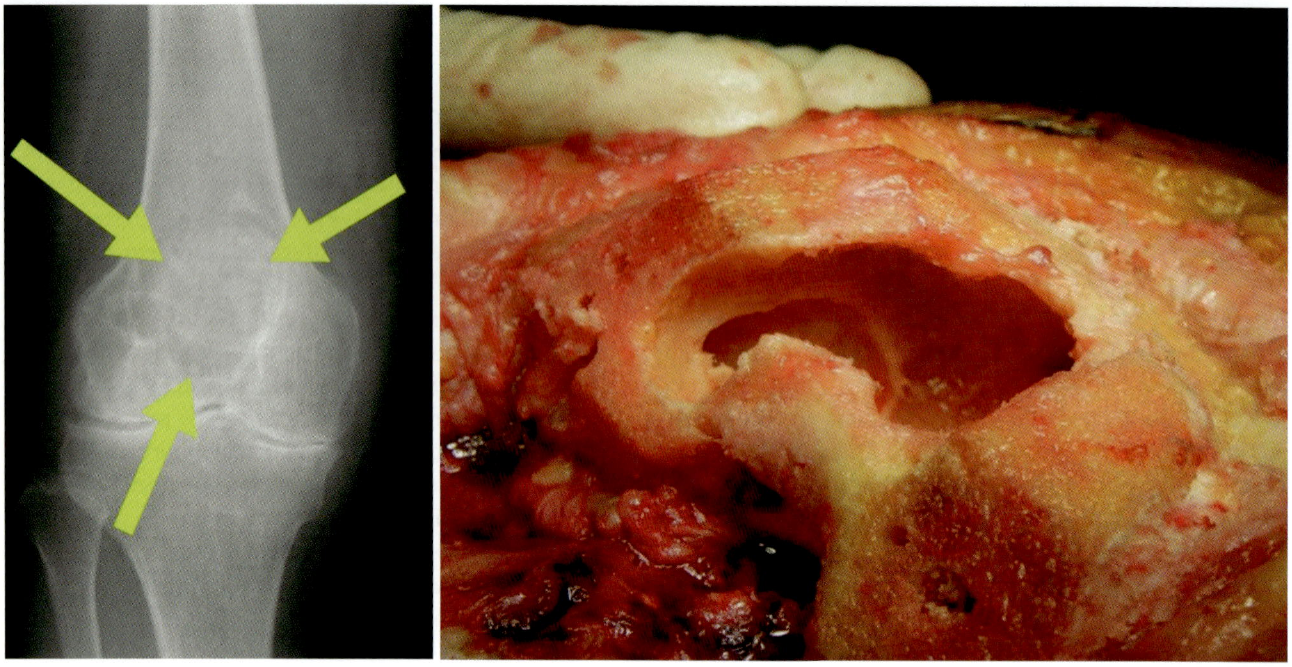

Fig. 5.46 X-ray and surgical finding of a bone cyst in rheumatoid arthritis

Since the other ligaments are also very weak, careful attention should be paid so as to avoid the development of intra- and postoperative instability. *The tendon may easily be stripped off at the insertion site*. If the patellar tendon is stripped off, the healing is difficult due to poor vascularity. *Therefore, it is advisable to fix a pin or use a protector so as to prevent* this occurrence.

Bony Structure

The bony structure in RA is often *associated with atrophy and osteopenia*. Since the landmarks may be altered due to a deformity or atrophy, *it is recommended to use the transepicondylar axis or ligament tension method for the external rotation of the femur*.

An avulsion fracture may occur even by gentle retraction due to weakened bone. Tough and incautious surgical techniques can easily cause an intercondylar fracture or a depression fracture.

Anterior notching of the femur is best avoided as it predisposes to a fatigue fracture postoperatively. It is not uncommon to find a very *big cyst, and failing to perform curettage and bone grafting will lead to inflammatory progression followed by loosening* (Fig. 5.46).

For the stability of the prosthesis, *cementing and stem extension are recommended in cases with severe osteopenia*.

As the patellar lesions have a tendency to progress, *patellar resurfacing is recommended*. Steinberg et al. reported that the remaining cartilage of the patella can cause recurrence of arthritis.

Deformity

RA is often *accompanied by a valgus deformity, flexion contracture, or limited ROM*. Valgus deformity is also associated with lateral femoral condylar atrophy, lateral soft tissue contracture, and patellofemoral malalignment.

The degree of flexion contracture varies according to the duration and progression of the inflammatory reaction of the soft tissues. Special techniques are not required if the degree of flexion contracture is mild, but correction of deformity may be needed before or during the operation, or a two-stage operation may be required if the degree of flexion contracture is severe. The posterior slope of the tibia can also aggravate the flexion contracture, so it is advisable not to make too much posterior slope.

Patellofemoral malalignment increases the incidence of lateral retinacular release.

Postoperative Care

As there is a high risk of infection postoperatively, it is recommended to administer prophylactic antibiotics for slightly longer duration than usual.

As RA often involves the other joints, an attempt should be made to achieve more flexion for better function, and *special attention should be paid in order to prevent recurrence of the flexion contracture*.

The bone is prone to fractures, and hence *vigorous ROM exercises are prohibited*. In some cases, brace fitting may be needed for the knee joint. Due to arthritis of the upper limbs, the brace, walker, and crutches should be more stable, more comfortable, and better fitting than those used ordinarily.

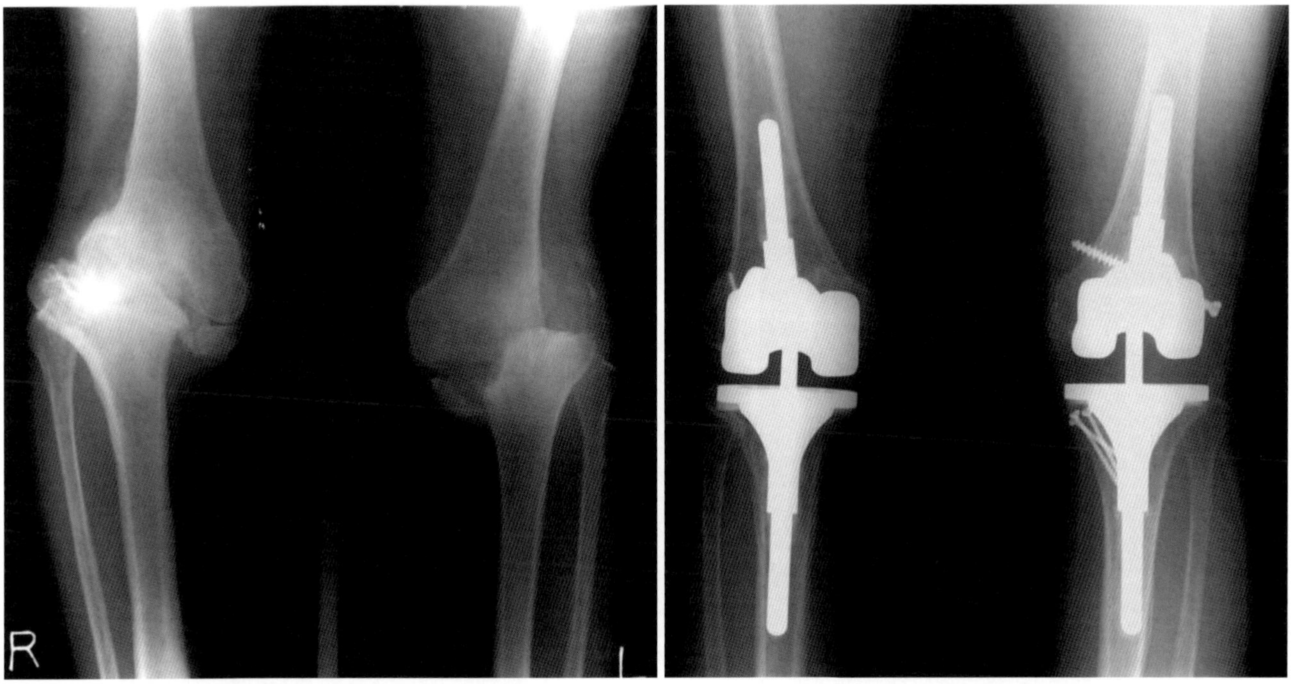

Fig. 5.47 TKRA for the Charcot joint

5.4.4.2 Charcot Joint

Charcot joint is a type of arthritis associated with progressive bony and ligament destruction due to consistent and repeated trauma as a result of an underlying neurologic disorder. *In contrast to the assumption that the patients do not feel any pain, about half of the patients suffer from pain as deep sensation and loss of proprioception are affected mostly.*

It is controversial whether Charcot joint is an indication for TKA. Even though the operation may be successful, the prognosis may worsen due to the lack of sensation. Hence, even if the arthritic changes appear to be serious on X-ray, it is *recommended not to perform TKA if the patient can walk with brace fitting.*

The problems involved in TKA for Charcot joint are first, there is a marked bone defect; second, the joint is unstable; third, the remaining bony structures are not normal; and fourth, rehabilitation is difficult due to the loss of sensation.

An allogeneic graft is needed since there is usually a severe bone defect, and the bone graft should be securely fixed. A constrained prosthesis is often needed due to ligament instability. Refer to Sect. 5.1 for the methods used for reconstructing the bone defect. It is often needed to use an extension stem for stable fixation of the prosthesis (Fig. 5.47).

The prognosis of TKA in Charcot joint depends on the degree of the bone defect and instability. Parvizi et al. and Soudri et al. reported relatively good results provided the patients were selected appropriately. While Kim et al. *reported that although TKA is not contraindicated in Charcot joint. They experienced too many complications and the results were not very good.*

5.4.4.3 Paget's Disease

Problems regarding Paget's disease in TKA consist of two aspects, general and regional. Paget's disease is a progressive disease with high-output cardiac failure which increases the blood circulation and causes excessive bleeding intra- and postoperatively. Regionally, achieving alignment is difficult due to the gradual deformity of femur and tibia, and abnormal bone property such as coexisting osteopenia and sclerosis easily causes a fracture postoperatively. In particular, the posterior slope of the tibial plateau is so marked that it may inadvently lead to excessive resection of the anterior portion.

Generally, the PS type or constrained type is used with an extension stem, and cementing is recommended for fixation.

5.4.4.4 Hemophilic Arthritis

Hemophilia causes arthritis by involving the synovium and cartilage due to recurrent intra-articular bleeding. Many patients show a flexion contracture, and a valgus and external rotation deformity. It is often associated with intra-articular fibrosis and muscular contracture. The patient is at a high risk of postoperative infection.

Mostly, the PS type with cementing is recommended.

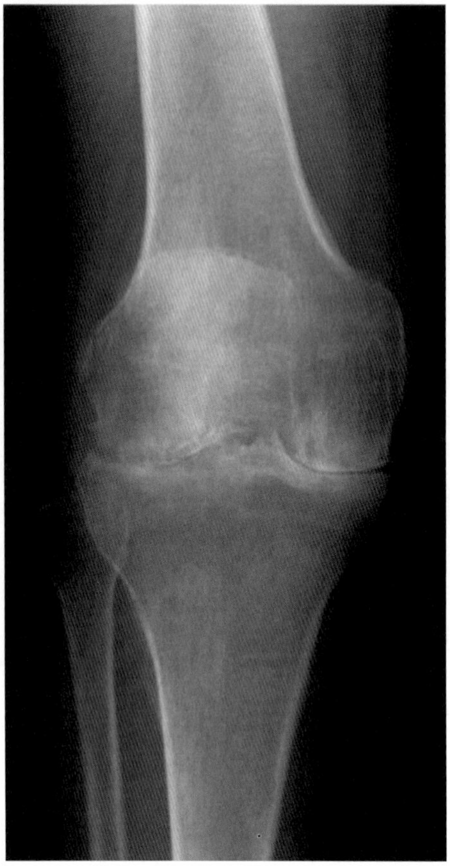

Fig. 5.48 Arthritis in a patient with hemophilia

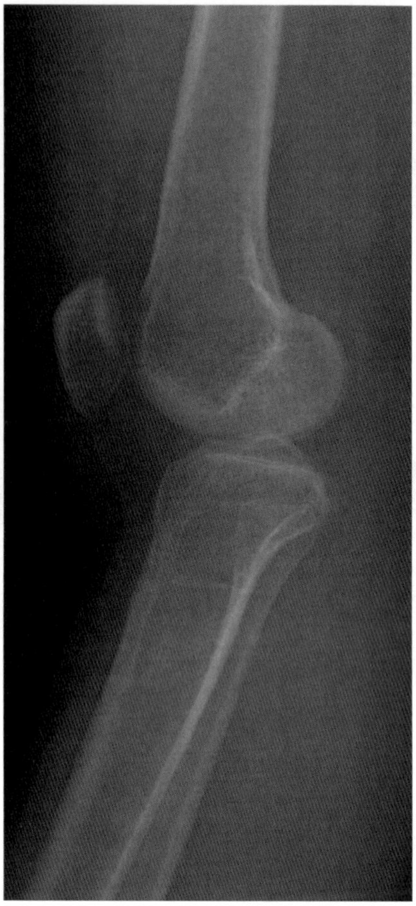

Fig. 5.49 Anterior slope in genu recurvatum

It is necessary to provide the deficient coagulation factors intra- and postoperatively. The coagulation factors should be transfused up to the 100 % level preoperatively, up to the 75 % level until postoperative day 5, up to the 50 % level until postoperative day 10, and up to the 25 % level until postoperative day 15 (Fig. 5.48).

5.4.4.5 Polio Sequelae

Before planning the operation, it is necessary to decide whether or not to perform the TKA considering the patient's muscular strength, deformity of the other joints, and length discrepancy of the lower limbs. *Muscular strength for knee extension and flexion should be at least grade IV. Shortening of the lower limbs by more than 3 cm or a serious ankle deformity should be corrected in advance.*

The factors to be considered for TKA are first, extensor mechanism is weakened thereby causing genu recurvatum and joint instability; second, the joint mechanics are altered; third, the tibia shows an external rotation deformity with instability on the lateral side; fourth, there is atrophy and shortening of the lower limbs; and finally, there is a coexisting bone deformity in the other sites such as the foot.

There are several options available for treating the genu recurvatum deformity (Fig. 5.49): first, less distal osteotomy of the femur for correcting the recurvatum deformity; second, the use of a rotating hinged prosthesis in patients with less than antigravity quadriceps strength; third, repositioning of the collateral ligaments more proximally and posteriorly to recreate the optimal tension; fourth, the use of brace postoperatively; and finally to leave the joint in 10–15° genu recurvatum state. But the last method has high incidence of loosening.

Generally, the PS type or constrained type with an extension stem and cementing is recommended. However, the use of an extension stem is sometimes not possible due to accompanying bony atrophy.

5.5 Tumor Prosthesis

5.5.1 Indication

Tumor prosthesis is used as *one of the methods for limb salvage* when there is a *malignant tumor* around the knee joint. *The Enneking type 2A is the best indication for the use of a*

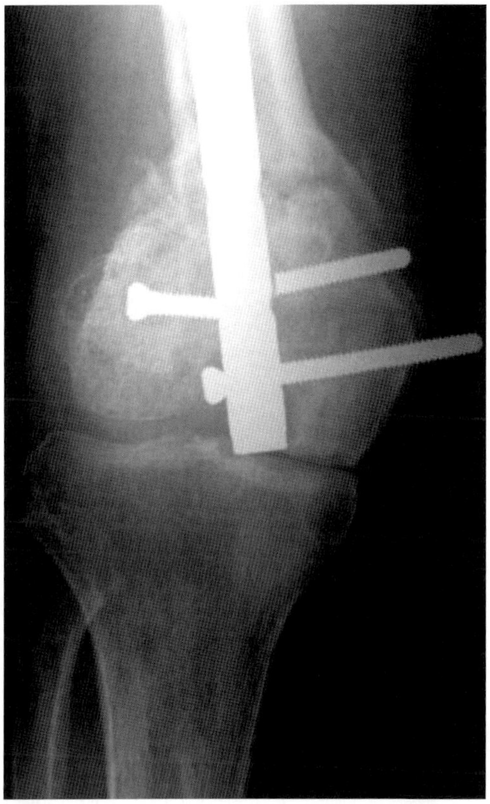

Fig. 5.50 X-ray of the patient showing nonunion of distal femur. This can be an indication for the use of a tumor prosthesis

tumor prosthesis, but it can also be used in type 2B using chemotherapy preoperatively for reducing the size of the tumor or after clarifying the boundaries. Amputation is the treatment of choice in case of neurovascular involvement; however, limb salvage operation can be performed along with reconstruction of vessels and nerves by microsurgery. *Even if the tumor is not malignant*, a huge benign tumor can be an indication for the use of a tumor prosthesis if a constrained prosthesis cannot be used despite of a massive bone graft.

In case of *nonunion* around the joint, the basic principle is to perform bone grafting and promote union of the fracture. Tumor prosthesis may be used *if fracture union is expected to take a longer time or the acceptable level of function cannot be expected even after the union (Fig. 5.50). When there is a periprosthetic fracture*, tumor prosthesis may be considered in cases of severe comminution with prosthetic loosening.

In cases of severe bone defect in re-revision, custom-made prosthesis or APC (allograft prosthetic component) can be used, but it is very expensive, and the function is not very good compared to that of the tumor prosthesis. Wunder et al. stated that the results of tumor prosthesis were far superior to those of APC in case of re-revision.

5.5.2 Type and Composition

All the tumor prostheses are linked type, which connects the femoral component to the tibial component by implant itself to achieve ligament stability. Kotz system, MUTARS (Modular Universal Tumor and Revision System-Munster), and Endo knee are the currently available prostheses (Fig. 5.51). Kotz system is a hinge joint that allows only flexion and extension, whereas MUTARS and Endo knees are the rotating hinge types that allow rotation.

Most of the tumor prostheses including the Kotz system are of the modular type which have an anchorage piece, a connecting part, and an articular portion. The configuration of the articular portion is different according to whether the lesion is located in the femur or in the tibia, and patellar resurfacing is optional.

5.5.3 Surgical Techniques

5.5.3.1 Biopsy and Excision

The success of tumor prosthesis depends on meticulous excision of the tumor, coverage of the prosthesis, maintenance of the length, rotational alignment, and appropriate handling of the extensor mechanism. Even if the first item, excision of the tumor, is limited to malignant tumor, the other factors are very important for the long-term survival and prognosis of tumor prosthesis.

Tumor removal should be carefully planned from the time of biopsy. When the biopsy is performed, it is necessary to take into consideration the possibility of contamination by tumor cells. The skin incision should be selected carefully for the subsequent limb salvage operation, and the biopsy *should not pass across the muscle planes*. It is recommended to perform a biopsy through the vastus lateralis muscle because vastus medialis is stronger than vastus lateralis. However, some surgeons prefer to perform a biopsy through the vastus medialis muscle. Also, *the biopsy should be done at the site where the tumor is the most active which is usually at the periphery and not at the center of tumor where only necrotic tissues can be found*.

Tourniquet can be used for biopsy or limb salvage operation, but the limb should not be exsanguinated in order to avoid dissemination of tumor cells.

Radical excision is the best choice for eradication of the tumor. Since it is impossible to retain the neurovascular tissues, it is meaningless to salvage the limb by radical excision. Therefore, a *wide excision* is performed most commonly. The main neurovascular tissues should be protected while removing the posteriorly located tumor. Nerves may be sacrificed in certain cases; however, amputation can be considered if the tumor has invaded the main vessels.

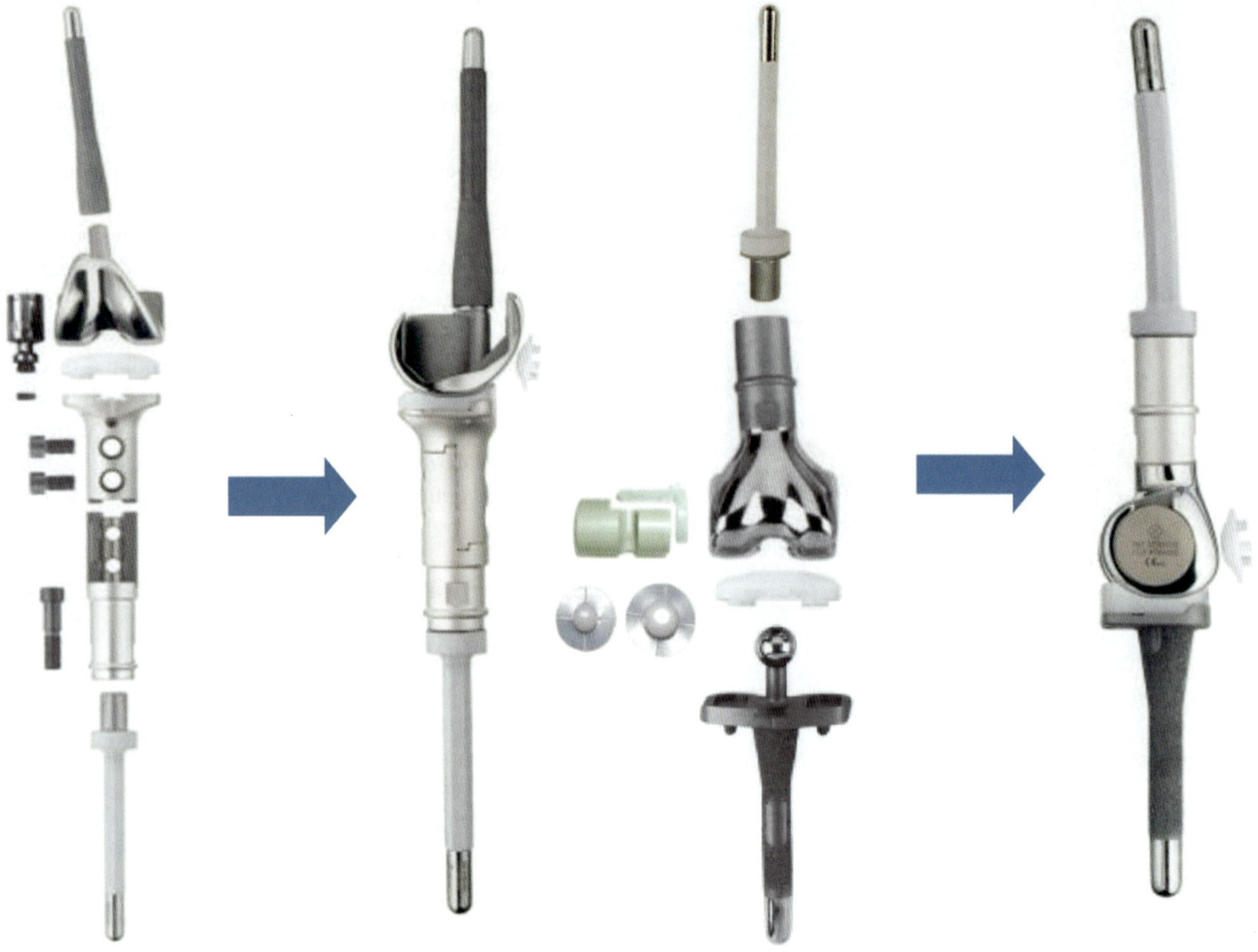

Fig. 5.51 Various components of a tumor prosthesis (MUTARS system, Implantcast, Buxtehude, Germany)

A no-touch technique is recommended in order to prevent the spread of tumor cells and contamination of the healthy tissues by the tumor cells. For the meticulous removal, tumor-free resection margins should be confirmed on frozen section.

How much bone should be removed is a controversial issue. The invasion of tumor cells can be detected using bone scan and MRI. Some authors state that up to 5 or 7 cm of bone should be removed from the margin of the lesion on bone scan or up to 3 cm away from the lesion when anticancer therapy has been performed. Currently however, the standard is *removal of bone 5 cm proximal (femur) or distal (tibia) to the lesion on MRI.*

To maintain the length, the distance can be measured from the articular surface to the resection site before performing bone resection. Bone resection is performed perpendicular to the shaft so as to establish good contact between the prosthesis and the bone. The marrow tissues are curetted after resection, and the specimen should be sent for histological confirmation of tumor cells.

5.5.3.2 Implantation

Kotz System

If there is a lesion in the femur, the length of the bone to be resected is measured so as to determine the length of the prosthesis, and the linea aspera is used as a guide for rotation.

When reaming for the anchorage piece, the fixation may become loose if its diameter is too small, but using a too-thick piece can also cause problems. Most of the times, the medullary canal of the resection area is wider than the proximal part in the femur, and reaming according to the size of the medullary canal of the resection area causes endosteal thinning at the end of the stem thereby acting as stress riser of a fracture.

The anchorage piece has a flange for more stable fixation by using three cortical screws. However, some surgeons insert only one screw to achieve only rotational stability of the prosthesis as rigid fixation causes stress shielding leading to osteolysis (Fig. 5.52). Bone grafting may also be performed at the junction between the resected bone and the tumor prosthesis in order to prevent osteolysis (Fig. 5.53).

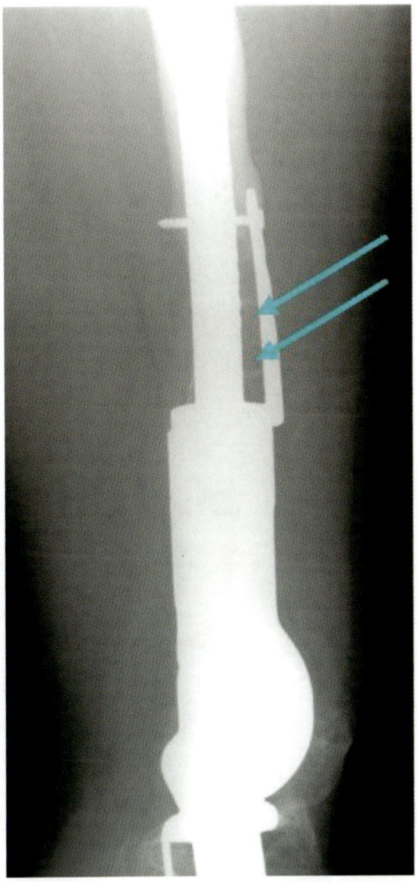

Fig. 5.52 Stress shielding with the Kotz system. The *arrow* indicates the stress shield effect

The tibial portion can be treated in a manner similar to that in the usual arthroplasty; however, *rotational alignment is very important*. The bone about 5 mm from the articular surface is resected, and the point of rotation is slightly medial to the tibial tuberosity or parallel to both posterior condyles.

The fixation of the tibial prosthesis is enhanced with nuts and bolts through the wings on both the sides. The wings are tightened, and the ends of the bolts should be cut short so as not to irritate the soft tissues.

If there is a lesion in the tibia, tibial resection of appropriate length is performed, rotational alignment should be established, the anchorage piece is fixed, and the prosthesis with a modular system of equal length as that of the resected bone is inserted. For rotational alignment, it helps to make a marking before performing the resection.

When the bone is resected distal to the tibial tuberosity, the *patellar tendon may occasionally be too short* to anchor to the prosthesis. *In such a case, autograft or allograft ligament augmentation may be done for reinforcement*. The case in which a gastrocnemius flap is used, the patellar tendon can be sutured to the flap.

If the *skin and soft tissue envelope is poor* due to wide resection of soft tissues, *the implant can be covered by a flap of the medial head of gastrocnemius*. It is recommended to consult a plastic surgeon for the skin coverage.

Femoral prosthesis is inserted with the rotation adjusted to the posterior condylar axis (Fig. 5.54).

After fixation of both the components, the ring type PE is inserted and the components are connected.

MUTARS System

MUTARS is a rotating hinge type of prosthesis and it is conceptually similar to the Kotz system, and the surgical technique is nearly the same for both types. It has two types: prosthesis for the femoral defect and for the tibial defect depending on the location of major bone defect.

On the site of the main defect, the implant consists of an anchorage piece, a connecting part as an option of extension piece, and the articular portion. The anchorage piece on the femoral side has no anterior flange which is present in the Kotz system for screw fixation. The junction between the anchorage piece and the articular portion is serrated so as to allow readjustment of rotation of the articular portion even after fixation of the anchorage piece. The tibial component has two pegs for additional rotational stability instead of the bolts and nuts in Kotz system. The PE is snap fit type, and it should be inserted in posterior to anterior direction for fitting.

The joint is a modified ball and socket type. A column-shaped bearing is interposed between the two components, which allows rotational motion providing varus and valgus constrain at the same time (Fig. 5.51).

Endo System

Endo-Model Modular Knee Prosthesis System is basically similar to the ordinary constrained prosthesis. However, it allows for rotation which is restricted by the capsule and ligaments. The joint part of the femur is relatively anatomical, and the stem axis is fixed at 6°, and cementing is optional. Modular extension stem is used for restoration of length, and the length of the stem varies from 50 to 280 mm. The metaphyseal part has a special segment for cement augmentation so that it can be used as a tumor prosthesis. The joint part and the extension stem are connected together with screws.

Operative procedure for Endo system includes soft tissue dissection, bony resection, extensor mechanism treatment, and prosthesis coverage, which are the same as in the other types of tumor prosthesis. The amount of external rotation of the femur and the tibia is similar to that in the usual arthroplasty.

5.5.4 Results

Results of tumor prosthesis vary among surgeons. This is because the recurrence rate and metastasis vary according to the type of tumor. Besides, the amount of soft tissue

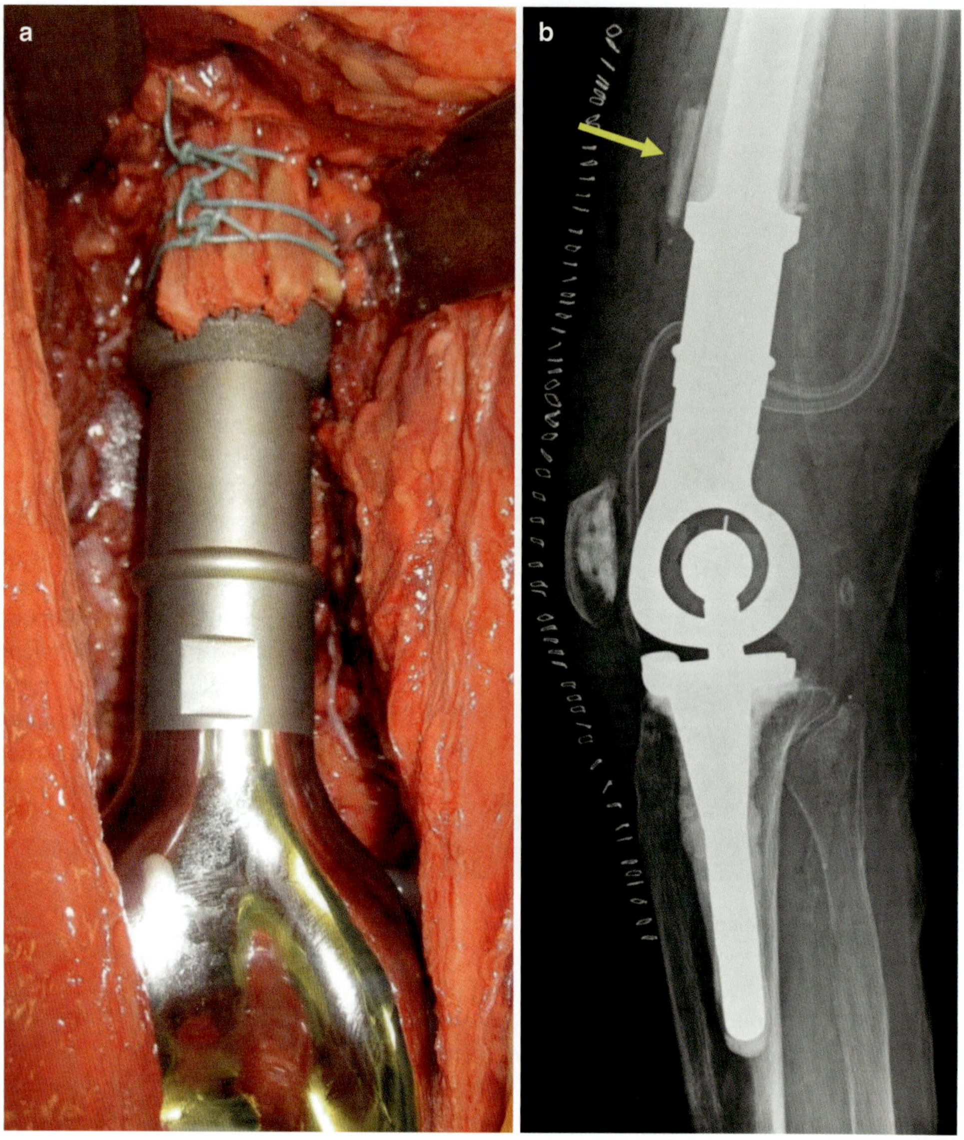

Fig. 5.53 Bone grafting on the anchorage piece. (**a**) Match stick autogenous bone is grafted at the junction between host bone and tumor prosthesis and tied with nonabsorbable suture. (**b**) Postoperative X-ray. *Arrow* indicates autogenous bone

removed, postoperative treatment and the type of prosthesis used are also the important prognostic factors.

Patients' dissatisfaction after surgery is related to limited motion, weakness of the extensor mechanism, cosmetic issues, etc. Tsuboyama et al. reported that a good extensor mechanism can be achieved when more than 40 % of the quadriceps muscle power was remaining, and Kendall et al. emphasized that the quadriceps muscle power should be reinforced with transfer of semimembranosus or semitendinosus muscles to maintain a good extension power.

With respect to the *postoperative complications*, Kawai et al. reported the results of an 8-year follow-up study. In their analysis, the *femoral prosthesis loosening was the most common* occurrence *followed by fracture of the implant and infection in that order*. The factors that had a negative impact on these complications included male gender, the amount of bone resection (40 % or greater), and cement fixation. However, Plotz et al., Grimer et al., and Kaste et al. reported that infection and breakdown of the prosthesis were as common as loosening of the prosthesis.

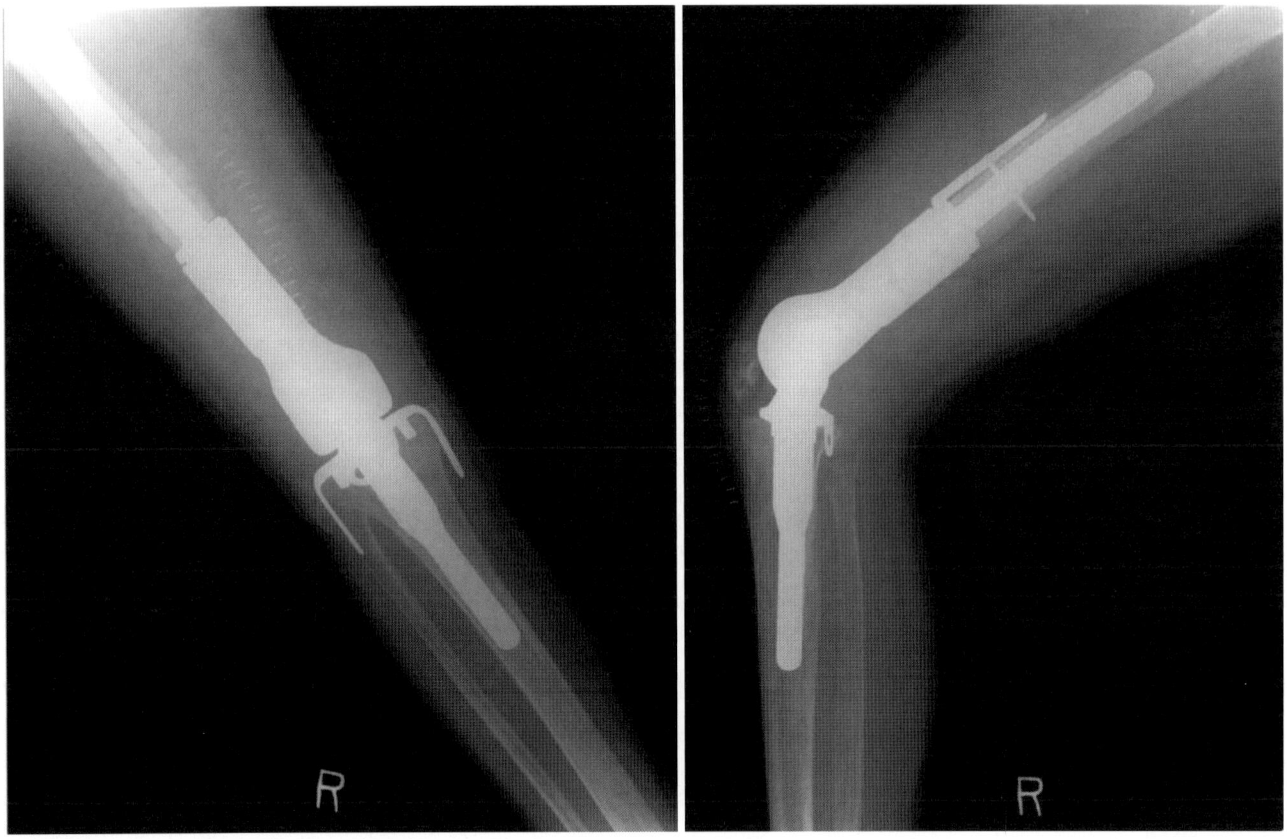

Fig. 5.54 Arthroplasty using the Kotz system

Bibliography

Aglietti P, Buzzi R. Correction of combined deformity. In: Scuderi GR, editor. Surgical techniques in total knee arthroplasty. 1st ed. New York: Springer; 2002. p. 216–23.

Aglietti P, Windsor RE, Buzzi R, et al. Arthroplasty for the stiff or ankylosed knee. J Arthroplasty. 1989;4:1–5.

Bae DK, Song SJ, Yoon KH, Noh JH. Long-term outcome of total knee arthroplasty in Charcot joint: a 10- to 22-year follow-up. J Arthroplasty. 2009;24:1152–6.

Baldini A, Aglietti P. Correction of fixed deformities with total knee arthroplasty. In: Scott WN, editor. Surgery of the knee. 5th ed. Philadelphia: Churchill Livingstone; 2011. p. 1100–7.

Baldwin JL, Rubinstein RA. The effect of bone quality on the outcome of ingrowth total knee arthroplasty. Am J Knee Surg. 1996;9: 45–50.

Barrack RL, Matzkin E, Ingraham R, Engh G, Rorabeck C. Revision knee arthroplasty with patellar replacement versus bony shell. Clin Orthop. 1998;356:139–43.

Berend KR, Lombardi Jr AV, Adams JB. Total knee arthroplasty in patients with greater than 20 degrees flexion contracture. Clin Orthop. 2006;452:83–7.

Bhan S, Malhotra R, Kiran EK. Comparison of total knee arthroplasty in stiff and ankylosed knees. Clin Orthop. 2006;451:87–95.

Bowne JA, Pagnano MW. Patellar revision. In: Scott WN, editor. Surgery of the knee. 5th ed. Philadelphia: Churchill Livingstone; 2011. p. 1375–80.

Brand MG, Daley RJ, Ewald FC, Scott RD. Tibial tray augmentation with modular metal wedges for tibial bone stock deficiency. Clin Orthop. 1989;248:71–9.

Brooks PJ, Walker PS, Scott RD. Tibial component fixation in deficient tibial bone stock. Clin Orthop. 1984;184:302–8.

Buechel FF. A sequential three-step lateral release for correcting fixed valgus knee deformities during total knee arthroplasty. Clin Orthop. 1990;260:170–5.

Burns BS, Lachiewicz PF. Total knee replacement in special situation. In: Callaghan JJ, editor. The adult knee. 1st ed. Philadelphia: Lippincott Williams & Wilkins; 2003. p. 1273–83.

Chen F, Krackow KA. Management of tibial defects in total knee arthroplasty. A biomechanical study. Clin Orthop. 1994;305: 249–57.

Cho SH, Jeong ST, Park HB, et al. Two-stage conversion of fused knee to total knee arthroplasty. J Arthroplasty. 2008;23:476–9.

Cho WS, Park JH, Kim JH, et al. Total knee arthroplasty in stiff knee. J Korean Knee Soc. 2003;15:1–9.

Cho WS, Park SS, Kim JH, et al. Treatment of tibial bone defect in primary TKA. J Korean Knee Soc. 1999;11:13–9.

Chung HK, Choi CH, Choi YJ, et al. Total knee replacement in severe flexion contracture. J Korean Orthop Assoc. 1997;32: 1039–46.

Dennis DA. Structural allografting in revision total knee arthroplasty. Orthopedics. 1994;17:849–51.

Dennis DA. Revision knee arthroplasty. How I do it. In: Insall JN, editor. Surgery of the knee. 3rd ed. New York: Churchill Livingstone; 2001. p. 1934–41.

Dorr LD, Ranawat CS, Sculco TA, et al. Bone graft for tibial defects in total knee arthroplasty. Clin Orthop. 1986;205:153–65.

Easley ME, Insall JN, Scuderi GR, et al. Primary constrained condylar knee arthroplasty for the arthritic valgus knee. Clin Orthop. 2000;380:58–64.

Engh GA. The difficult knee: severe varus and valgus. Clin Orthop. 2003;416:58–63.

Engh GA, Herzwurum PJ, Parks NL. Treatment of major defects of bone with bulk allograft and stemmed components during total knee arthroplasty. J Bone Joint Surg. 1997;79-A:1030–9.

Fehring TK, Peindl RD, Humble RS, et al. Modular tibial augmentations in total knee arthroplasty. Clin Orthop. 1996;327:207–17.

Firestone TP, Krackow KA, Davis JD, Teeny SM, Hungerford DS. The management of fixed flexion contractures during total knee arthroplasty. Clin Orthop. 1992;284:221–7.

Fullerton BD, Browngoehl LA. Total knee arthroplasty in a patient with bilateral Charcot knees. Arch Phys Med Rehabil. 1997;78: 780–2.

Garvin KL, Pellicci PM, Windsor RE, et al. Contralateral total hip arthroplasty or ipsilateral total knee arthroplasty in patients who have a long-standing fusion of the hip. J Bone Joint Surg. 1989;71-A:1355–62.

Griffin FM, Scuderi GR, Insall JN. Lateral release for fixed-valgus deformity. In: Scuderi GR, Tria AJ, editors. Knee arthroplasty handbook. 1st ed. NewYork: Springer; 2006. p. 41–56.

Grimer RJ, Carter SR, Tillman RM, et al. Endoprosthetic replacement of the proximal tibia. J Bone Joint Surg. 1999;81-B: 488–94.

Gupta R. A short history of neuropathic arthropathy. Clin Orthop. 1993;296:43–9.

Haddad FS, Bentley G. Total knee arthroplasty after high tibial osteotomy. A medium-term review. J Arthroplasty. 2000;15:597–603.

Hanssen AD. Patellar revision: bringing back the bone. Orthopedics. 2003;26:977–8.

Harwin SF. Revision arthroplasty. How I do it. In: Insall JN, Scott WN, editors. Surgery of the knee. 3rd ed. New York: Churchill Livingstone; 2001. p. 1967–74.

Haslam P, Armstrong M, Geutjens G, Wilton TJ. Total knee arthroplasty after failed high tibial osteotomy long-term follow-up of matched groups. J Arthroplasty. 2007;22:245–50.

Hockman DE, Ammeen D, Engh GA. Augments and allografts in revision total knee arthroplasty: usage and outcome using one modular revision prosthesis. J Arthroplasty. 2005;20:35–41.

Hoeffel D, Rubash HE. Osseous deficiency in total knee replacement and revision: femur. In: Callaghan JJ, editor. The adult knee. 1st ed. Philadelphia: Lippincott Williams & Wilkins; 2003. p. 1185–97.

Hofmann AA, Kane KP. Total knee arthroplasty after high tibial osteotomy. Orthopedics. 1994;17:887–90.

Hungerford DS. The effect of extra-articular deformity on the femoral component. In: Scuderi GR, editor. Surgical techniques in total knee arthroplasty. 1st ed. New York: Springer; 2002. p. 640–4.

Insall JN, Easley ME. Surgical techniques and instrumentation in total knee arthroplasty. In: Insall JN, editor. Surgery of the knee. 3rd ed. New York: Churchill Livingstone; 2001. p. 1553–620.

Kaste SC, Neel MN, Rao BN, et al. Complications of limb-sparing procedures using endoprosthetic replacements about the knee for pediatric skeletal sarcomas. Pediatr Radiol. 2001;31:62–71.

Kawai A, Lin PP, Boland PJ, et al. Relationship between magnitude of resection, complication, and prosthetic survival after prosthetic knee reconstructions for distal femoral tumors. J Surg Oncol. 1999;70:109–15.

Kendall SJH, Singer GC, Briggs TWR, et al. A functional analysis of massive knee replacement after extra-articular resections of primary bone tumors. J Arthroplasty. 2000;15:754–60.

Khakharia S, Nett MP, Hajnik CA, et al. Complications of total knee arthroplasty. In: Scott WN, editor. Surgery of the knee. 5th ed. Philadelphia: Churchill Livingstone; 2011. p. 1293–319.

Kim YH, Cho SH, Kim JS. Total knee arthroplasty in bony ankylosis in gross flexion. J Bone Joint Surg. 1999;81-B:296–300.

Kim YH, Kim JS, Oh SW. Total knee arthroplasty in neuropathic arthroplasty. J Bone Joint Surg. 2002;84-B:216–9.

Kim YH, Oh SH, Kim JS. Conversion of a fused knee with use of posterior stabilized total knee prosthesis. J Bone Joint Surg. 2003;85B:1047–50.

Krackow KA. Medial and lateral ligament advancement. In: Scuderi GR, editor. Surgicaltechniques in total knee arthroplasty. 1st ed. New York: Springer; 2002. p. 205–9.

Krackow KA, Jones MM, Teeny SM, et al. Primary total knee arthroplasty in patients with fixed valgus deformity. Clin Orthop. 1991;273:9–18.

Krackow KA, Mihalko WM. Flexion-extension joint gap changes after lateral structure release for valgus deformity correction in total knee arthroplasty: a cadaveric study. J Arthroplasty. 1999;14:994–1004.

Lang JE, Scott RD, Lonner JH, Bono JV, et al. Magnitude of limb lengthening after primary total knee arthroplasty. J Arthroplasty. 2012;27:341–6.

Laskin RS. The classic: total condylar knee replacement in patients who have rheumatoid arthritis. A ten-year follow-up study. Clin Orthop. 2008;466:2589–96.

Laskin RS. Soft tissue balancing of the varus knee. In: Callaghan JJ, editor. The adult knee. 1st ed. Philadelphia: Lippincott Williams & Wilkins; 2003. p. 1245–58.

Laskin RS, O'Flynn HM. The Insall Award. Total knee replacement with posterior cruciate ligament retention in rheumatoid arthritis. Problems and complications. Clin Orthop. 1997;345: 24–8.

Lee GC, Sanchez-Sotelo J, Berry DJ. Total knee arthroplasty in patients with Paget's disease of bone at the knee. J Arthroplasty. 2005;20:689–93.

Li MG, Nilsson KG. The effect of the preoperative bone quality on the fixation of the tibial component in total knee arthroplasty. J Arthroplasty. 2000;15:744–53.

Lotke PA, Cook EA. Total knee arthroplasty for patients with prior knee arthrodesis. In: Scuderi GR, editor. Surgical techniques in total knee arthroplasty. 1st ed. New York: Springer; 2002. p. 627–31.

Lotke PA, Simon RG. Flexion contracture in total knee arthroplasty. In: Scuderi GR, editor. Surgical techniques in total knee arthroplasty. 1st ed. New York: Springer; 2002. p. 210–5.

Magnussen RA, Weppe F, Demey G, et al. Residual varus alignment does not compromise results of TKAs in patients with preoperative varus. Clin Orthop. 2011;469:3443–50.

Maheshwer CB, Mitchell E, Kraay M, et al. Revision of the patella with deficient bone using a biconvex component. Clin Orthop. 2005;440:126–30.

ManIII JW, Scuderi GR, Insall JN. Total knee replacement with associated extra-articular angular deformity of tibia. In: Scuderi GR, editor. Surgical techniques in total knee arthroplasty. 1st ed. New York: Springer; 2002. p. 645–8.

Mason JB, Fehring TK. Management of extra-articular deformity in total knee arthroplasty with navigation. In: Scott WN, editor. Surgery of the knee. 5th ed. Philadelphia: Churchill Livingstone; 2011. p. 1232–9.

McDonald DJ, Sim FH. Total hip arthroplasty in Paget's disease. A follow-up note. J Bone Joint Surg. 1987;69-A:766–72.

Meding JB, Keating EM, Ritter MA, et al. Total knee arthroplasty after high tibial osteotomy. Clin Orthop. 2000;375:175–84.

Mitsuyasu H, Matsuda S, Miura H, et al. Flexion contracture persists if the contracture is more than 15° at 3 months after total knee arthroplasty. J Arthroplasty. 2011;26:639–43.

Mont MA. Total knee arthroplasty after high tibial osteotomy. Clin Orthop. 1994;299:125–30.

Montgomery WH, Insall JN, Haas SB, et al. Primary total knee arthroplasty in stiff and ankylosed knees. Am J Knee Surg. 1998;11: 20–3.

Moran MC. Functional loss after total knee arthroplasty for poliomyelitis. Clin Orthop. 1996;323:243–6.

Mullaji AB, Padmanabhan V, Jindal G. Total knee arthroplasty for profound varus deformity: technique and radiological results in 173 knees with varus of more than 20 degrees. J Arthroplasty. 2005; 20:550–61.

Naranja RJ, Lotke PA, Pagnano MW, et al. Total knee arthroplasty in a previously ankylosed or arthrodesed knee. Clin Orthop. 1996;331: 234–7.

Nasser S, Poggie FA. Revision and salvage patellar arthroplasty using a porous tantalum implant. J Arthroplasty. 2004;19:562–72.

Nelson CL, Windsor RE. Total knee arthroplasty following high tibial osteotomy. In: Scuderi GR, editor. Surgical techniques in total knee arthroplasty. 1st ed. New York: Springer; 2002. p. 601–9.

Nett MP, Scuderi GR. Revision of aseptic failed total knee arthroplasty. In: Scott WN, editor. Surgery of the knee. 5th ed. Philadelphia: Churchill Livingstone; 2011. p. 1327–45.

Pagnano MW, Scuderi GR, Insal JN. Patellar component resection in revision and reimplantation total knee arthroplasty. Clin Orthop. 1998;356:134–8.

Pagnano NE. Management of bone defect. In: Scott WN, editor. Surgery of the knee. 4th ed. Philadelphia: Churchill Livingstone; 2006. p. 1799–813.

Parvizi J, Marrs J, Morrey BF. Total knee arthroplasty for neuropathic (Charcot) joints. Clin Orthop. 2003;416:145–50.

Pavizi J, Seel MJ, Hanssen AD, Berry DJ, Morrey BF. Patellar component resection arthroplasty for the severely compromised patella. Clin Orthop. 2002;397:356–61.

Petersen MM, Nielsen PT, Lebech A, et al. Preoperative bone mineral density of the proximal tibia and migration of the tibial component after uncemented total knee arthroplasty. J Arthroplasty. 1999;14:77–81.

Plotz W, Rechl H, Burgkar R, et al. Limb salvage with tumor endoprostheses for malignant tumors of the knee. Clin Orthop. 2002;405:207–15.

Ranawat AS, Ranawat CS, Elkus M, et al. Total knee arthroplasty for severe valgus deformity. J Bone Joint Surg. 2005;87-A Suppl 1: 271–84.

Ranawat CS, Holden DS, Ranawat AS, et al. Soft tissue balancing of the valgus knee. In: Callaghan JJ, editor. The adult knee. 1st ed. Philadelphia: Lippincott Williams & Wilkins; 2003. p. 1207–16.

Rand JA. Bone deficiency in total knee arthroplasty. Use of metal wedge augmentation. Clin Orthop. 1991;271:63–71.

Reis MD. Prophylactic intramedullary femoral stem during total knee arthroplasty with simultaneous femoral plate removal. J Arthroplasty. 1998;13:718–21.

Richards CJ, Garbuz DS, Pugh L, et al. Revision total knee arthroplasty: clinical outcome comparison with and without the use of femoral head structural allograft. J Arthroplasty. 2011;26: 1299–304.

Ries MD. Porous tantalum patellar augmentation: the importance of Residual bone stock. Clin Orthop. 2006;452:166–70.

Ritter MA, Harty LD. Medial screws and cement: a possible mechanical augmentation in total knee arthroplasty. J Arthroplasty. 2004;19:587–9.

Rittmeister M, Starker M, Zichner L. Hip and knee replacement after long standing hip arthrodesis. Clin Orthop. 2000;371: 136–45.

Roberts CS, Fetto JF. Functional outcome of hip fusion in young patient: follow-up study of 10 patients. J Arthroplasty. 1990;5: 89–96.

Romness DW, Morrey BF. Total knee arthroplasty in patients with prior ipsilateral hip fusion. J Arthroplasty. 1992;7:63–70.

Scott RD. Total knee arthroplasty in severe varus deformity. In: Scott RD, editor. Total knee arthroplasty. 1st ed. Philadelphia: Saunders; 2006. p. 39–44.

Scott RD. Total knee arthroplasty in severe valgus deformity. In: Scott RD, editor. Total knee arthroplasty. 1st ed. Philadelphia: Saunders; 2006. p. 45–53.

Scott RD. Stiffness before and after total knee arthroplasty. In: Scott RD, editor. Total knee arthroplasty. 1st ed. Philadelphia: Saunders; 2006. p. 63–8.

Scott RD. Flexion contracture associated with total knee arthroplasty. In: Scott RD, editor. Total knee arthroplasty. 1st ed. Philadelphia: Saunders; 2006. p. 69–73.

Scott RD. Total knee arthroplasty after osteotomy. In: Scott RD, editor. Total knee arthroplasty. 1st ed. Philadelphia: Saunders; 2006. p. 74–82.

Scott RD. Total knee arthroplasty in rheumatoid arthritis. In: Scott RD, editor. Total knee arthroplasty. 1st ed. Philadelphia: Saunders; 2006. p. 83–8.

Scott RD. Bone stock deficiency in total knee arthroplasty. In: Scott RD, editor. Total knee arthroplasty. 1st ed. Philadelphia: Saunders; 2006. p. 89–99.

Sculco TP. Management of stiff knee. In: Callaghan JJ, editor. The adult knee. 1st ed. Philadelphia: Lippincott Williams & Wilkins; 2003. p. 1333–40.

Sheth DS, Oldfield D, Ambrose C, et al. Total knee arthroplasty in hemophilic arthropathy. J Arthroplasty. 2004;19:56–60.

Silva M, Luck Jr JV. Long-term results of primary total knee replacement in patients with hemophilia. J Bone Joint Surg. 2005;87-A: 85–91.

Soudry M, Binazzi R, Johanson NA, et al. Total knee arthroplasty in Charcot and Charcot like joints. Clin Orthop. 1986;208:199–204.

Steinberg J, Sledge CB, Noble J, et al. A tissue-culture model of cartilage breakdown in Rheumatoid arthritis: quantitative aspects of proteoglycan release. Biochem J. 1979;180:103–412.

Su EP, Perna M, Boettner F, et al. A prospective, multi-center, randomized trial to evaluate the efficacy of cryopneumatic device on total knee arthroplasty recovery. J Bone Joint Surg. 2012;94-B Suppl 11:153–6.

Sue CK, Michael NN, Bhaskar NR, et al. Complications of limb-sparing procedures using endoprosthetic replacements about the knee for pediatric skeletal sarcomas. Pediatr Radiol. 2001;31:62–71.

Sugita T, Umehara J, Sato K, et al. Influence of tibial bone quality on loosening of the tibial component in total knee arthroplasty for rheumatoid arthritis: long term result. Orthopedics. 1999;22: 213–5.

Tadao T, Reinhard W, Wolfgang D. Knee function after operation for malignancy of the distal femur. Acta Orthop Scand. 1993;64:673–7.

Tanzer M, Miller J. Natural history of flexion contracture. Clin Orthop. 1989;248:129–34.

Tarabichi S, Tarabichi Y. Can an anterior quadriceps release improve range of motion in the stiff arthritic knee? J Arthroplasty. 2010;25:571–5.

Teeny SM, Krackow KA, Hungerford DS, et al. Primary total knee arthroplasty in patients with severe varus deformity. A comparative study. Clin Orthop. 1991;273:19–31.

Tew M, Forster IW. Effect of knee replacement on flexion deformity. J Bone Joint Surg. 1987;69-B:395–9.

Therbo MM, Peterson JE, Varmarken CA, et al. Influence of preoperative bone mineral content of the proximal tibia on revision rate after uncemented knee arthroplasty. J Bone Joint Surg. 2003;85-B: 975–9.

Tsuboyama T, Windhager R, Dock W, et al. Knee function after operation for malignancy of the distal femur. Quadriceps muscle mass and knee extension strength in 21 patients with hinged endoprostheses. Acta Orthop Scand. 1993;64:673–7.

Vail TP, Lang JE, Sikes III CV. Surgical techniques and instrumentation in total knee arthroplasty. In: Scott WN, editor. Surgery of the knee. 5th ed. Philadelphia: Churchill Livingstone; 2011. p. 1042–99.

Vince KG, Blackburn DC, Ortaaslan SG, et al. "Gull wing" osteotomy of the patella in total knee arthroplasty. J Arthroplasty. 2000; 15:254–9.

Vince KG, Long W. Revision knee arthroplasty. The limits of press fit medullary fixation. Clin Orthop. 1995;317:172–7.
Wang JW, Chen WS, Lin PC, et al. Total knee replacement with intra-articular resection of bone after malunion of a femoral fracture: can sagittal angulation be corrected? J Bone Joint Surg. 2010;92-B: 1392–6.
Whiteside LA. Correction of ligament and bone defects in total knee arthroplasty of the severely valgus knee. Clin Orthop. 1993;288: 234–45.
Windsor RE, Insall JN, Vince KG. Technical considerations of total knee arthroplasty after proximal tibial osteotomy. J Bone Joint Surg. 1988;70-A:547–55.
Wolff AM, Hungerford DS, Pepe CL. The effect of extraarticular varus and valgus deformity on total knee arthroplasty. Clin Orthop. 1991;271:35–51.
Wunder JS, Leitch K, Griffin AM, et al. Comparison of two methods of reconstruction for primary malignant tumors at the knee: a sequential cohort study. J Surg Oncol. 2001;77:87–99.
Yoshino N, Takai S. Total knee arthroplasty after failed tibial osteotomy. In: Callaghan JJ, editor. The adult knee. 1st ed. Philadelphia: Lippincott Williams & Wilkins; 2003. p. 1265–71.
Yoshino S, Fujimori J, Kajino A, et al. Total knee arthroplasty in Charcot's joint. J Arthroplasty. 1993;8:335–40.
Zelicof SB, Scuderi GR, Vince KG, et al. Total knee arthroplasty in post-traumatic arthritis. Orthop Trans. 1988;12:547–8.

6 Unicompartmental Knee Arthroplasty

If arthritis is confined to one compartment of the knee joint, it may be difficult to decide whether to perform unicompartmental knee arthroplasty (UK) or TKA. This is because widely varying results of UK have been reported in the literature. There has been renewed interest in UK after Repicci introduced the minimally invasive techniques for UK. UK has certain advantages over TKA, and good results can be achieved in well-selected patients.

Generally, UK refers to medial or lateral unicondylar knee replacement, but patellofemoral arthroplasty (PFA) performed for patellofemoral arthritis can also be classified into unicompartmental arthroplasty. Hence, I have included patellofemoral arthroplasty in this chapter.

Although concomitant replacement of the medial compartment and the patellofemoral joint cannot be termed as unicompartmental knee arthroplasty in the strict sense, the basic concept for it came from unicompartmental knee arthroplasty. Hence, I have briefly described bicompartmental knee arthroplasty in the last section of this chapter.

6.1 Unicompartmental Knee Arthroplasty

6.1.1 Introduction

Arthritis confined to one compartment of the knee joint or a small chondral lesion in one compartment of the knee joint can be treated by chondroplasty, chondrocyte transplantation, osteochondral graft, high tibial osteotomy (HTO), UK, or TKA.

UK offers many advantages such as higher early success rate and good function since the healthy tissues are preserved. Recently better results have been reported due to the improvement in surgical techniques and development of new prostheses. The incidence of UK was 6–8 % of all TKAs performed in the USA in 2008.

6.1.1.1 UK vs. HTO

A comparison of UK with HTO revealed that *HTO is indicated in relatively younger, more active, and heavier patients,* whereas *UK is indicated in relatively slender patients below 60 years of age or above 80 years of age and who are less active.*

UK has a good initial success rate and has minimal complications, whereas *HTO causes less improvement in pain and the prognosis following HTO worsens rapidly over time.* However, *the advantage of HTO is that it allows the patients to retain their own joints and achieve a better ROM postoperatively than that after UK. Bone graft or metal augmentation may not be required in* revision of a failed HTO to TKA, *although it is not easy to perform revision to TKA.* Stukenborg et al. reported that the 10-year survival rate of UK was 77 % and that of HTO was 60 %.

6.1.1.2 UK vs. TKA

The advantage of UK in comparison with TKA is that healthy tissues are retained. As a result, *UK provides more normal knee mechanics, and hence greater ROM and better proprioception can be expected.* The operation time is shorter, and morbidity and length of hospital stay are reduced. *However, aligning the axis is more difficult in UK than in TKA and malalignment may cause adverse effects on the adjacent part of the knee joint. Therefore, more skill is required for performing UK since the scope for an error is very narrow.*

Many reports revealed that the clinical results of the two operations are similar. *In terms of function, UK shows better results than TKA, yet TKA provides better pain relief and increased survival rate.* Newman et al. reported that UK showed better results than TKA at the first 5-year follow-up. Noticewala et al. reported that the patients who underwent UK showed higher SF-12 physical and mental score component, and better WOMAC scores than TKA. However, Lyons et al. reported that even though UK showed higher postoperative scores, the changes of scores between UK and TKA is similar in both groups. It means that the preoperative status of UK patients is better than TKA. McAuley et al. demonstrated that *revision after UK is easier than revision after TKA.* However, Padgett et al. stated that when UK was performed as compartment replacement instead of surface

W. Cho, *Knee Joint Arthroplasty*,
DOI 10.1007/978-3-642-39389-1_6,

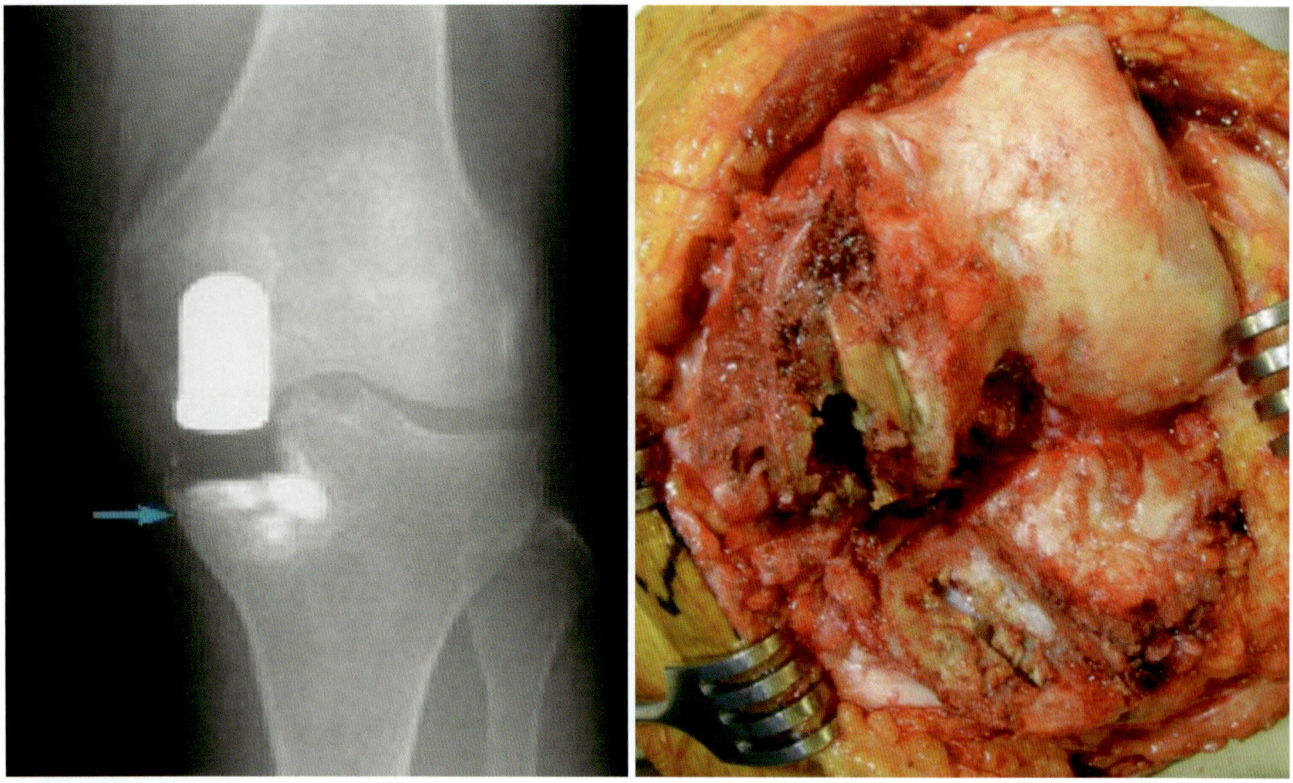

Fig. 6.1 Bone defect due to failure of unicondylar arthroplasty. *Left*: Bone defect in failed UK on X-ray as indicated by the *arrow*. *Right*: Intraoperative finding

replacement, 26 % of patients who underwent UK showed bone defects, and bone grafting or metal augmentation was needed in many cases, thereby *making the revision a bit difficult to perform*. Furthermore, Lai and Rand reported that the results of revision after UK were not any better than those after TKA due to the high incidence of loosening. In this respect, some authors are more in favor of TKA than UK (Fig. 6.1). *However, the current techniques using surface replacement demonstrate that the results of conversion of failed UK to TKA are similar to those after primary TKA.*

6.1.2 Implant

6.1.2.1 History

Historically, the first modern UK was designed by McKeever in the 1950s; it was a type of hemiarthroplasty of the tibial surface with metals and the main cause of failure was loss of the femoral cartilage. In 1970s, Marmor solved this problem by performing femoral resurfacing simultaneously and this was the first type of cemented UK. The femoral part was made of stainless steel and the tibial part was totally made of PE (polyethylene). It was designed so as to retain as much bone as possible. The new version of the St. George Sledge type has a biconvex metal femoral component and a PE tibial component.

Brigham added metal bars on the inner side of the femoral prosthesis for ensuring rotational stability and increased the width of the femoral prosthesis to reduce the incidence of subsidence. The tibial component was made of metal-backed PE. However, it was proved later that the metal-backed PE increased the wear rate. The Oxford type was developed in the late 1970s. In this type, the mobile congruous design of PE in the shape of a meniscus was adopted so as to reduce the wear and loosening. There are other types such as Miller–Galante and Repicci UK (Fig. 6.2).

6.1.2.2 Design

The design of the prosthesis varies according to the degree of conformity, whether it is fixed bearing or mobile bearing and whether it has an all-poly or a metal-backed PE tibial component.

With respect to conformity, the incidence of loosening increases as the conformity increases and the incidence of wear increases as the conformity decreases after UK, which is similar to that after TKA. The design with round femoral condyles and flat tibia increases the stress concentration, thereby increasing the wear rate, and causes joint instability as a result of gradual weakening of the ACL (anterior cruciate ligament), which further increases the wear rate. Since a smaller diameter of the posterior condyle and a flat PE tend to increase the wear rate, most of the current designs have a

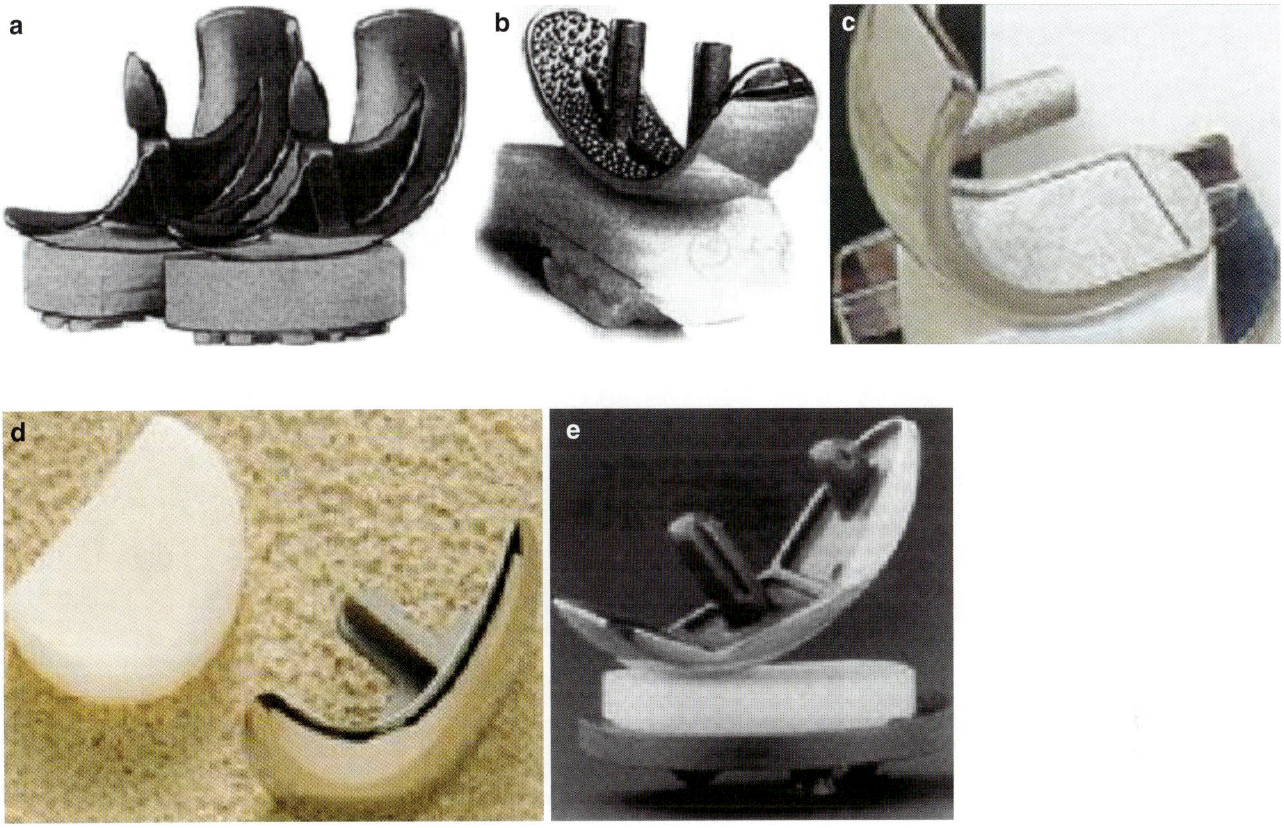

Fig. 6.2 Various types of unicompartmental knee prostheses. (**a**) Marmor modular knee, (**b**) George Sledge unicompartmental replacement, (**c**) Oxford unicompartmental meniscal knee replacement, (**d**) Repicci II, (**e**) Miller-Galante unicompartmental prosthesis

larger diameter of the posterior condyle with an adequate degree of conformity to the PE. Earlier designs had a narrower femoral prosthesis, thereby causing subsidence, whereas in the *current designs, the width of the femoral prosthesis is maximized so that it can cover the articular surface as much as possible.*

Mobile-bearing PE was developed so as to *decrease the wear and loosening*. This design has more advantages compared to the fixed-bearing design. *The added advantage of mobile-bearing PE in UK is that it allows for resurfacing, which reduces the amount of bone resection as well.* However, *the drawbacks of this design are that the operation is more difficult to perform, more resection of the anterior portion of the tibia* is required, the *PE may not move*, and *joint instability such as PE dislocation can occur.*

Cementless type of UK has been designed, but micromotion of the prosthesis makes bony ingrowth difficult. Therefore, the cemented type of prosthesis is currently preferred.

Femoral Component

The design of the femoral component varies according to the width, the curvature of condyles, and the method used to reinforce the fixation of the prosthesis. *The current design aims to restore anatomy of the posterior condyle so as to cover the posterior condyle fully and to taper the anterior femoral edge below the subchondral bone* so as to reduce the chances of patellar impingement.

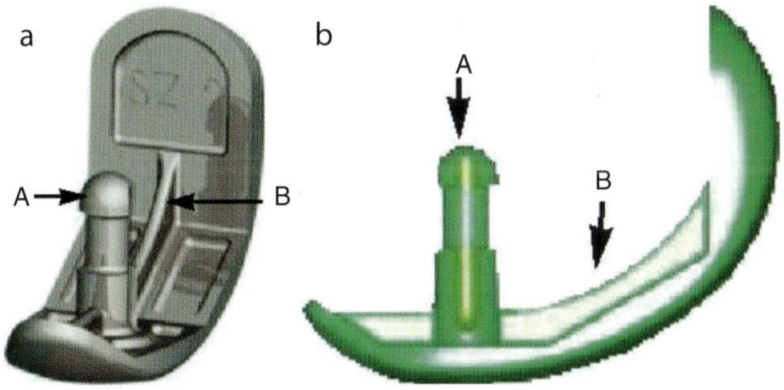

Fig. 6.3 The design for improving fixation of the femoral prosthesis. It has a lug (**a**) and a fin (**b**)

For fixation, a fin, pod, or lug is used. For rotational stability, some designs have two lugs, a metal bar or a cruciform groove (Fig. 6.3). In general, relatively small fixation lugs appear to be sufficient as long as there are two lugs or some type of a fin is present to ensure rotational stability.

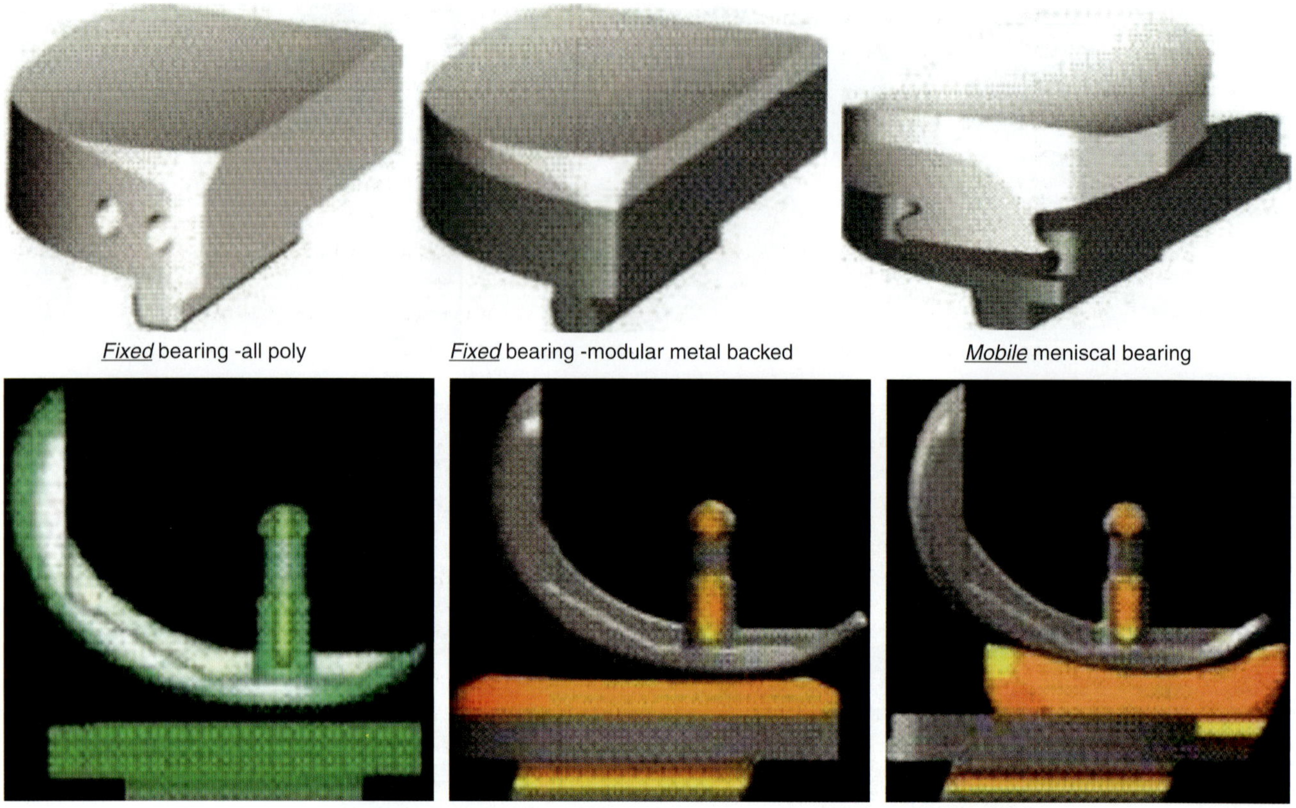

Fig. 6.4 Various types of tibial prostheses

Tibial Component

The shape of the tibial component should be as anatomical as possible. Even with the use of theoretically optimized designs, a maximum of 76 % of the implant edge lay on cortical bone. Hence, personalized implants will play an important role in the future.

The earlier form of the tibial component was all-poly tibial component, and metal-backed PE was developed later. Metal-backed PE has the advantage of even load distribution, and the PE is exchangeable when it has worn out. On the other hand, the drawback of metal-backed PE is that the PE has to be thinner. There are many debates between the advantages and drawbacks of all-poly and metal-backed PE. *The thickness of PE should be at least 6 mm at the thinnest portion regardless of the type of PE so as to reduce the wear. If the PE is thinner than 6 mm, it not only increases the wear rate, but the wear particles are also precipitated in the cartilage of other parts of the joint, causing progression of arthritis.*

Currently, designs that minimize bone resection through surface replacement have been developed in order to make revision easier. In these designs, the thickness of PE has been reduced, and this causes the same problems as those with the use of metal-backed PE (Fig. 6.4).

Mobile-bearing PE has been designed to reduce the wear and loosening.

6.1.3 Indications

UK has been *indicated in aged patients with unicompartmental arthritis who are slim and relatively inactive.* However, *the indications for UK can be widened by dividing the patients into two groups. The first group comprises of the relatively younger and nonobese patients* who regard the UK as the *first operation that will be followed by a subsequent arthroplasty. The second group comprises of the patients above 80 years of age with life expectancy of less than 10 years, who can benefit from the short operation time, early recovery, and low morbidity.* Spontaneous osteonecrosis of the knee (SPONK) which is the necrosis confined to the subchondral bone on MRI can be a good indication for UK. Laskin demonstrated that UK could be performed in about 15 % of the patients requiring TKA.

The preoperative ROM should be at least between 10° and 90°, the medial collateral ligament should be intact, and there should *not be more than 5° of varus deformity or 10° of valgus deformity on standing X-ray.*

If the joint has subluxation of 3 mm or more or there is a *so-called kissing lesion (Fig. 6.5) wherein the femoral notch and the tibial spine overlap* due to instability of the femorotibial joint, *it should not be considered as an indication for UK. However, some surgeons perform UK in spite of the kissing lesion.*

Dennis et al. emphasized the importance of the ACL in UK. If the function of the ACL is inadequate, it has an adverse effect on UK and causes weakening of the muscle power or loss of function progressively. It also causes wear in the anterior portion of the prosthesis due to load concentration on this part on weight bearing. In terms of the mechanical aspect, Argenson expressed the same opinion stating that a *healthy ACL is needed to maintain normal knee function*. In his research using videofluoroscopy, he showed that −0.8 mm of femoral rollback occurred after medial resurfacing and −2.5 mm of femoral rollback occurred after lateral resurfacing in the ACL-deficient patients. Goodfellow et al. also reported that unhealthy or injured ACL contributed to a failure rate that was greater than ten times. Therefore, if there is instability of the collateral ligament or ACL on anterior–posterior and varus–valgus stress X-rays, it is a contraindication for UK.

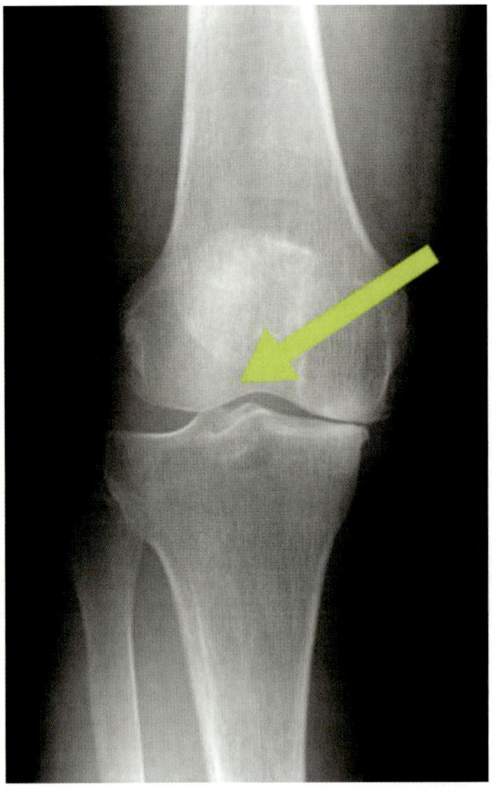

Fig. 6.5 Kissing lesion (*arrow*)

There are different theoretical perspectives on the *patellar lesion* with respect to the indication for UK. Generally it is accepted that *UK is not indicated if there is exposed patellar subchondral bone, although minimal chondromalacia is not a big problem*. However, Beard et al. and Kang et al. reported that the results were not very different even for severe patellar arthritis if there was no bone defect.

UK *is known to be a relatively contraindicated* in patients with *rheumatoid arthritis or other inflammatory arthritis* because they have progressive inflammatory changes in the other compartment and it may be associated with relaxation of the ligament tissues. *Although UK is relatively contraindicated in obese patients, a recent* study has found no correlation between weight and outcomes. Since the wear is more related to activity than to weight, obesity itself may not be a contraindication. *Some surgeons do not recommend lateral compartment arthroplasty in obese patients since the result is not as good as that of medial arthroplasty.*

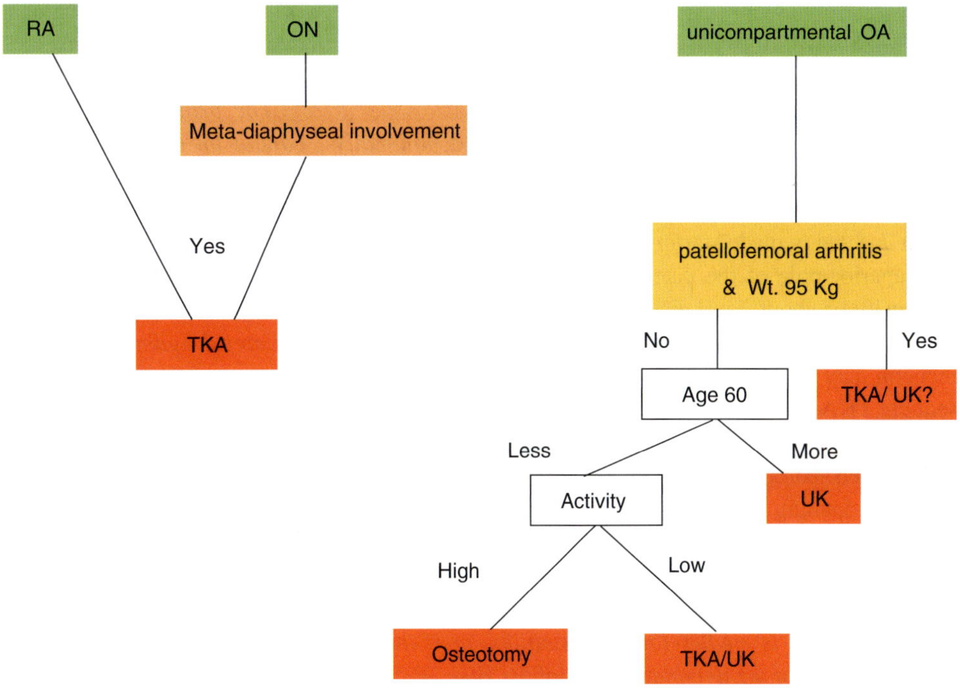

Fig. 6.6 Algorithm for indications of unicondylar arthroplasty

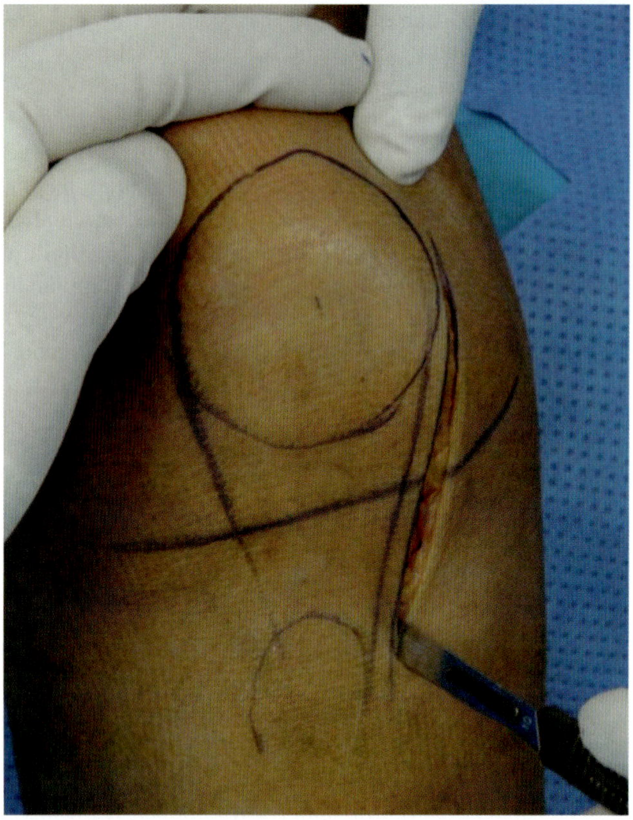

Fig. 6.7 Skin incision for MIS in UK (Courtesy of MH Song)

UK is *contraindicated in* patients with *osteonecrosis* because they are mostly young and loss of fixation may occur due to extensive bone necrosis (Fig. 6.6).

6.1.4 Surgical Technique

6.1.4.1 Approach

Although the ordinary TKA approach can be used, *minimally invasive surgery (MIS) is currently recommended.* In case of medial replacement, a parapatellar skin incision measuring about 7–8 cm is made starting from about 1 cm proximal to the superior pole of the patella and extending to the tibial tuberosity or about 2 cm distal to the joint line. Although a lateral skin incision is often made for lateral UK, a midline incision may be chosen considering the possibility of a subsequent TKA that might be performed in the future.

Arthrotomy is done paramedially and the quadriceps tendon is often spared (Fig. 6.7).

When opening the knee joint, care should be taken so as not to damage the ACL, medial collateral ligament, and the anterior horn of the lateral meniscus.

If there are pathology on anterior or posterior cruciate ligaments, there is medial–lateral instability, or if there is severe arthritis of the unreplaced part of the knee joint or of the patellofemoral joint, TKA should be performed instead of UK. The arthritis in the unreplaced part of the knee joint should not be greater than grade II and patellofemoral arthritis should not be greater than grade IV.

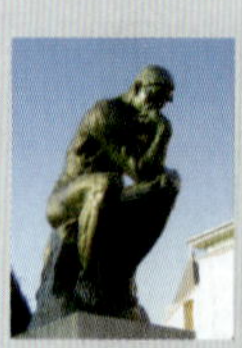

Author's Opinion

Good results can be expected after minimally invasive UK if the patients are selected carefully and the operation is done by an experienced surgeon. Since alignment and soft tissue balancing are important, minimally invasive UK is recommended for balancing the soft tissues naturally.

However, minimally invasive UK has some accompanying problems; the operation is wholly dependent on the comfort level and experience of the surgeons in working on the posterior side due to limited exposure. Hence, a learning curve is needed for performing minimally invasive UK. However, I think faster recovery and less morbidity override these drawbacks.

6.1.4.2 Soft Tissue Procedure

The meniscus should be resected, and the spur in the intercondylar notch, in the periphery of the tibia and femur, should be removed. In medial replacement, it is possible to achieve a certain level of passive correction of the varus deformity by removing the spur on the medial side of the tibia (Fig. 6.8).

The principles of ligament balancing followed in TKA cannot be applied to UK. The medial collateral ligament should be released till the retractor can just be inserted. If the medial collateral ligament needs to be released to a greater extent, it can cause joint instability and progressive arthritis of the unreplaced, i.e., lateral part of the knee joint. Hence, TKA should be considered instead of UK if the medial collateral ligament needs to be released to a greater extent because of the varus deformity.

6.1.4.3 Osteotomy

Osteotomy can either be performed first on the femur or on the tibia.

If osteotomy is performed first on the femur, an intramedullary guide is used for femoral osteotomy. On the other hand, if osteotomy is performed first on the tibia, spacer block is used for femoral osteotomy in relation to tibial osteotomy. Whiteside suggested that the use of an intramedullary

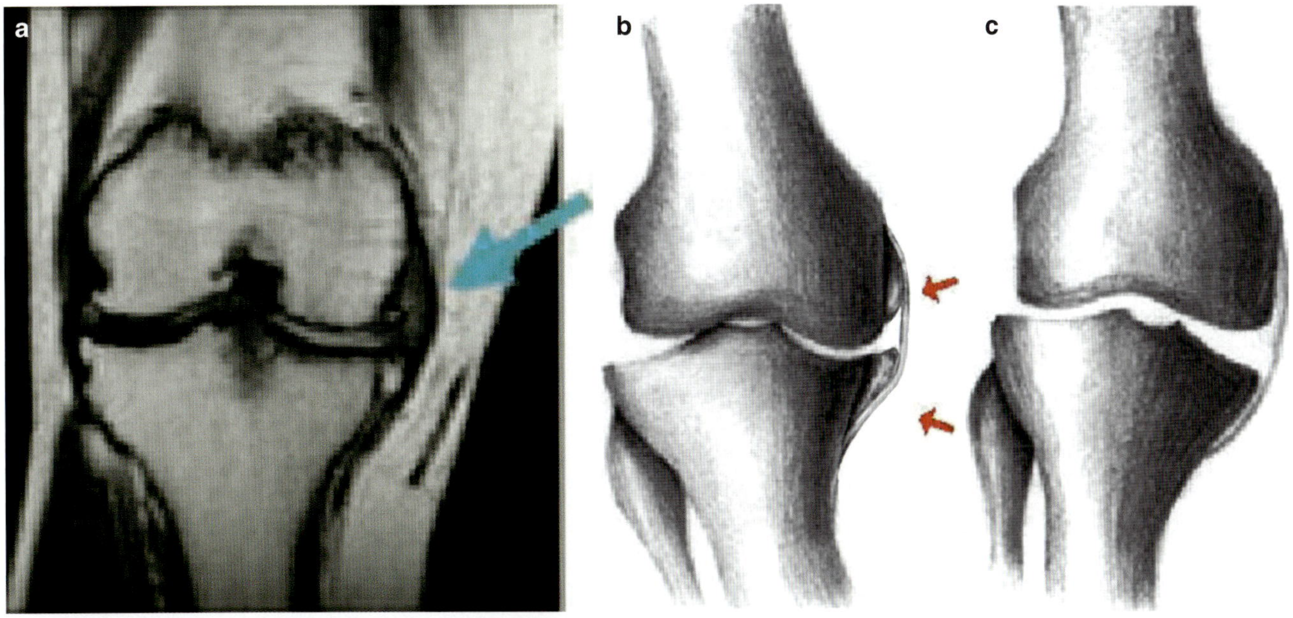

Fig. 6.8 The influence of the spur on the medial side on ligament balancing. (**a**) Influence of the spur on the collateral ligament on MRI, (**b**) illustration, (**c**) effect of collateral ligament release after removal of the spur

guide on the femoral side is more accurate than the extramedullary one and yields higher reproducibility. *In any case, an attempt should be made to preserve as much bone as possible. The femur should be aligned with the mechanical axis in extension and it should be perpendicular to the tibia in flexion. Overcorrection should be avoided at any cost.* Some authors recommend undercorrection because 4°–7° valgus femorotibial angle according to the mechanical axis imposes excess load on the lateral side.

If the femur is resected first, reamer for an intramedullary guide is inserted just above the intercondylar notch where the PCL is attached. The knee is flexed by 90° and the intramedullary guide which is attached the distal femoral cutting guide is inserted such that the guide is parallel to the tibial cutting surface or perpendicular to the tibial axis (Fig. 6.9).

For distal resection, gradual resection is done by every millimeter up to the first 6 mm with the angle adjusted preoperatively, and an additional 2 mm can be resected if the valgus angle exceeds 6°. This technique can help to increase the extension gap and decrease the valgus deformity without performing additional osteotomy of the tibia. However, Scuderi recommended more tibial resection as more distal resection of the femur only exaggerates the deformity and increases the chances of loosening. Posterior condyle should be resected as much as possible so that the posterior space is not too narrow.

The A–P size of the implant is important; a *larger implant should be chosen if the size of the implant is in between sizes*; however, about 1 mm of cutting surface of the articular portion should be left uncovered (Fig. 6.10). Therefore, *it is recommended to do osteotomy with the larger implant size first. The prosthesis should fully cover the distal articular surface so that the articular cartilage does not articulate with the tibial component on weight bearing, and the junction between the articular cartilage and the prosthesis should be smooth so that the patella can move smoothly.* Intraoperative

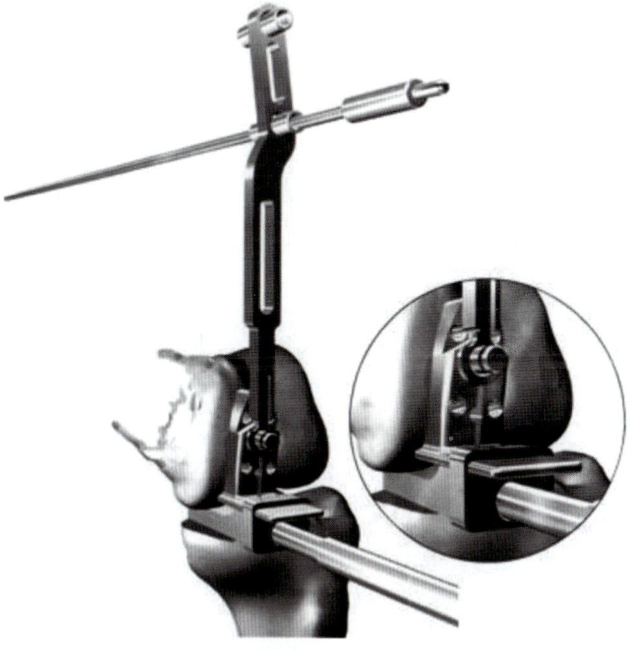

Fig. 6.9 Guide for performing femoral osteotomy

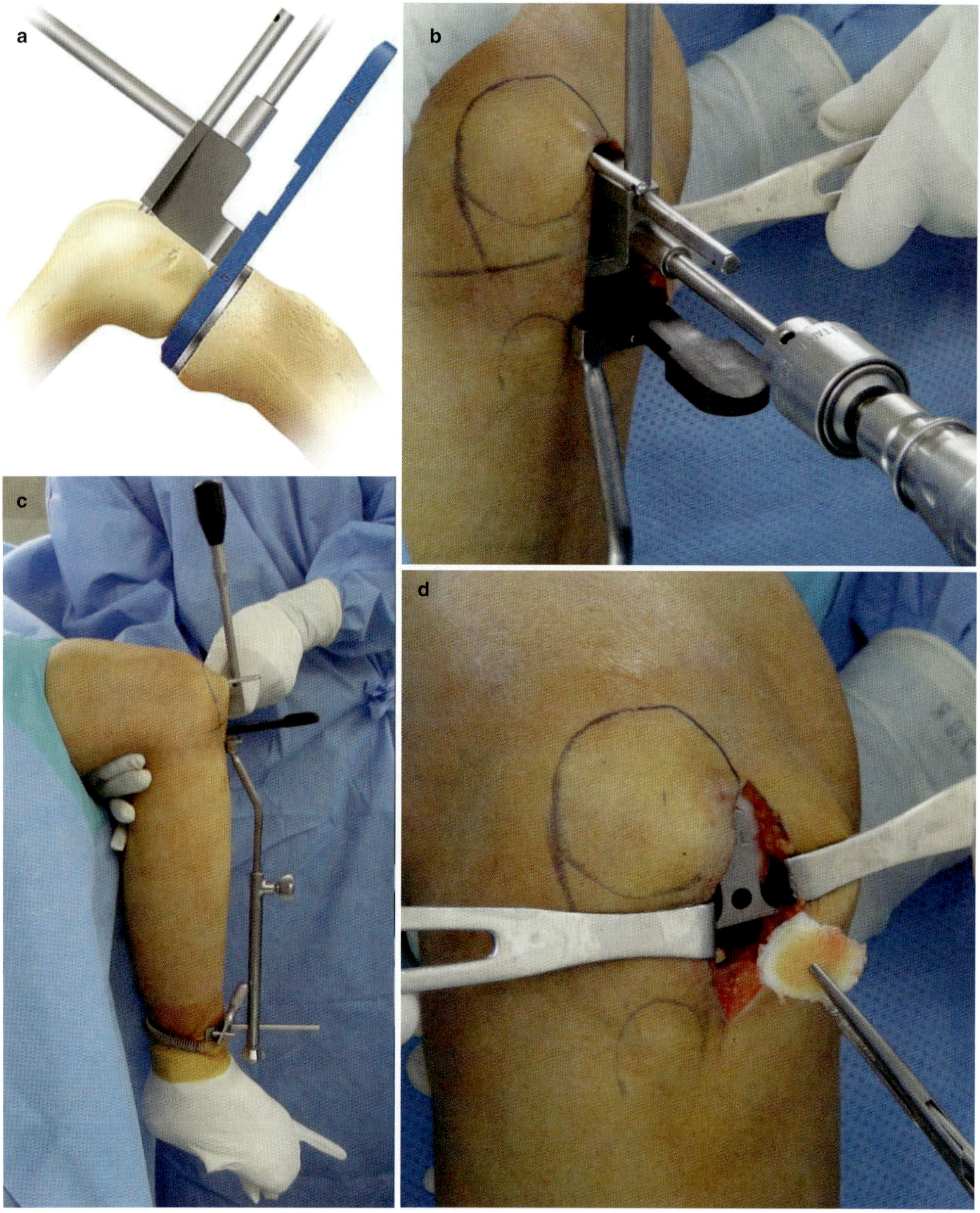

Fig. 6.10 Posterior femoral osteotomy (Courtesy of MH Song/ Biomet, Warsaw, IN). (**a**, **b**) Posterior cutting instrument in place. (**c**) Checking the alignment with the posterior cutting instrument. (**d**) Removing the bone fragment after posterior cutting

reference of coverage is the *"tide mark," which is the junction of the anterior and distal femoral condyles* (Fig. 6.11). However, *it is recommended to use a slightly smaller femoral prosthesis for lateral replacement as larger prosthesis can cause more problems in the patellofemoral joint.*

The femoral prosthesis should not protrude distally so as not to interfere with patellar tracking. This technical error is commonly caused by performing too little distal osteotomy and malpositioning of the prosthesis. *The femoral prosthesis should be placed in the center of the tibial prosthesis upon extension*, and then the femoral slope is matched with that of the tibia.

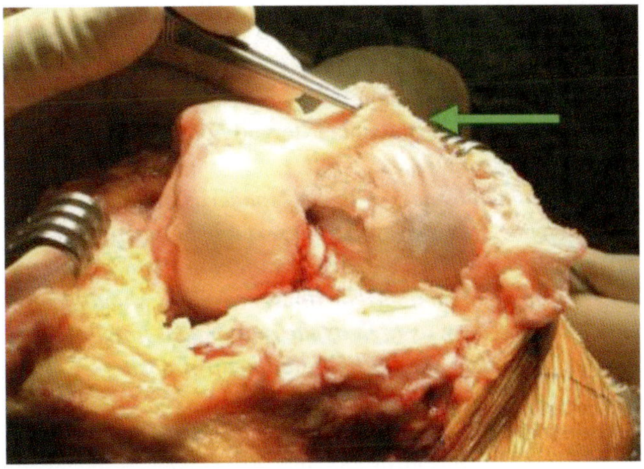

Fig. 6.11 Tide mark

If the femoral prosthesis is too close to the intercondylar notch, there will be medial subluxation of the tibia, thereby causing edge loading on PE, or there will be impingement of the femur on the tibial spine. To prevent this occurrence, the femoral prosthesis can be shifted on the medial side for medial UK, and the tibial prosthesis can be shifted slightly on the medial side for lateral UK. *The trial implant which can cover the most of the bone leaving a 1 mm of exposed bone is inserted.*

To set the rotation, the joint is gradually extended from 90° of flexion to flexion angles of 60°, 30°, and 0°. *Rotational alignment is closely related to the wear in UK. So the prosthesis should be slightly externally rotated, but this should not be more than 5°* (Fig. 6.12).

Tibial resection is performed using an extramedullary guide and the procedures are the same as those used for TKA. *The medial osteotomy is done until the subchondral bone is resected* at the deepest point, and in the lateral UK, 8–10 mm of bone is resected. *During osteotomy, overcorrection is not recommended as it can cause subluxation of the joint and progressive arthritis in the unreplaced part of the knee joint.*

Each surgeon has a different opinion about the degree of osteotomy, but *undercorrection by 2°–3° is recommended by most surgeons so that the mechanical axis passes through the medial one-third of the medial condyle* (Fig. 6.13). Gulati

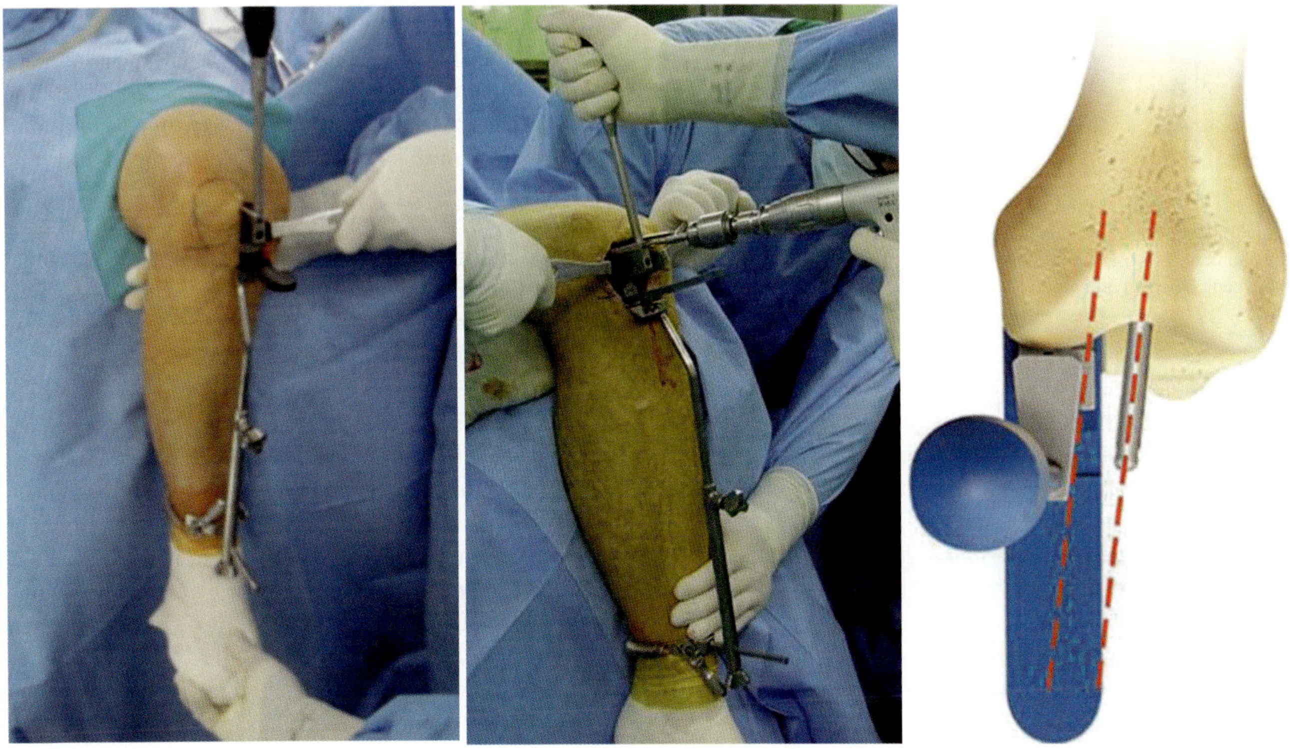

Fig. 6.12 Size and rotation of the femoral prosthesis (Courtesy of MH Song/ Biomet, Warsaw, IN)

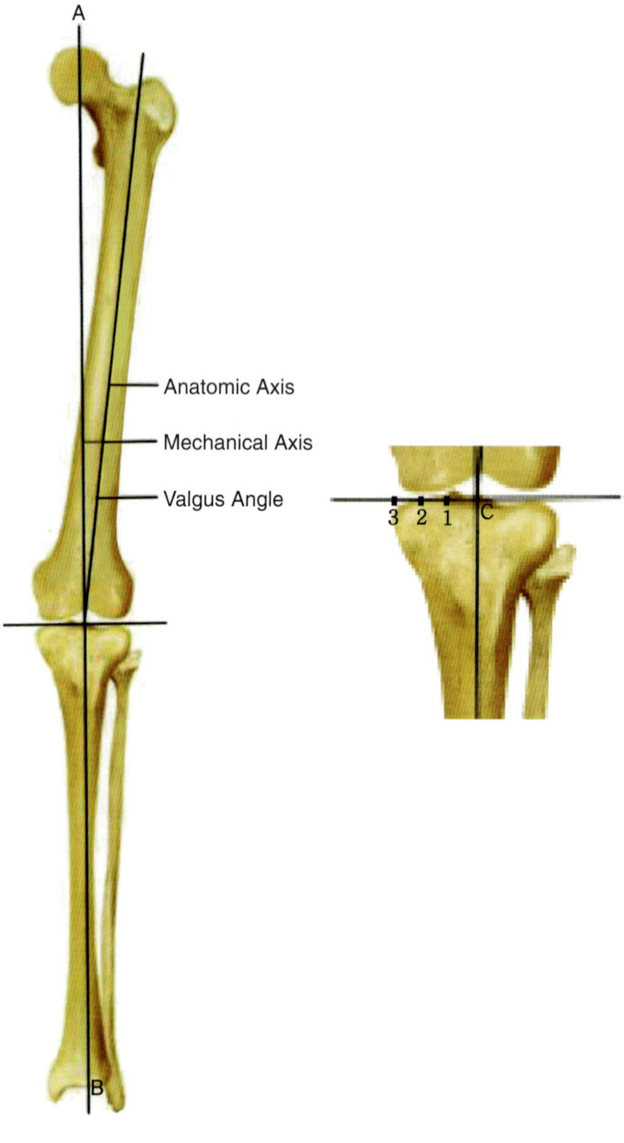

Fig. 6.13 The ideal point at which the mechanical axis drops on the tibial plateau. (**a**, **b**) Mechanical axis, best zone: The point at which the mechanical axis of the femur meets the tibial plateau at the point between center (**c**) and medial 1/3

et al. demonstrated that a mild varus deformity does not significantly affect the clinical results or survival rate. However, a varus deformity greater than 5° increases the possibility of a rotational deformity and increases the wear rate and cartilage damage in the lateral condyle.

Anterior–posterior slope should be between 0° and 10°; however, a 3°–5° slope is preferable according to the preoperative slope.

Vertical osteotomy is done as close to the tibial spine as possible, but up to a point where the cruciate ligaments are not injured (Fig. 6.14).

The size of the tibial prosthesis may be independent to the size of the femoral prosthesis and should be large enough. However, there should not be any overhanging on the posterior and the medial sides. *The A–P length of the tibial plateau sometimes differs from the mediolateral width especially in the female knee joints. So, different sizes of implants are tried to determine the most appropriate implant size.*

The tibial rotation is determined by the joint motion. *The rotational alignment of the tibia should be checked by extending the knee with the patella in situ. If the rotational alignment of the tibia is determined without the patella in situ, the tibia tends to rotate externally and the rotational alignment may not coincide with the real rotation.* However, Pennington et al. stated that the *tibial prosthesis should be fixed in 10°–15° internal rotation in lateral UK* because of the "screw home" movement. If malrotation exists, the quadriceps contraction forces rotate the tibia externally or the tibia may subluxate laterally.

In UK, the thickness of the PE spacer is of utmost importance. Hence, it is necessary to insert a trial implant for testing the thickness of the spacer, the femorotibial alignment, and the range of motion. The tibial prosthesis should generally be at the level as high as the anatomical tibial plateau, and its alignment should be in the neutral position without overcorrection.

Ligament balancing should be examined when the knee is fully extended, flexed to 45° and 90° flexion, respectively. *The medial part neither should be opened by more than 2 mm nor should it be too tightened by the valgus stress test.* If the ligament is lax or there is a varus or valgus deformity of the knee joint, it is necessary to adjust the thickness of the PE or that of the tibial component (all poly). If the joint space is too tight, the tibia is likely to subluxate laterally and the wear rate can increase. *Flexion can be performed up to about 120°. If 120° of flexion cannot be achieved, the tibia can be resected a little more.*

The tibia first technique is commonly used in mobile-bearing joint. An extramedullary guide is used for tibial resection. For fixation of the alignment guide, *fixation lateral to the sagittal plane and predrilling are recommended to avoid a possible stress fracture of the medial plateau.* Conservative tibial resection up to 8–10 mm from the normal lateral tibial plateau is to be done. For joint line preservation, the amount of resection should be calculated. For example, if bone loss is 2 mm, total loss is 5 mm (cartilage 3 mm + 2 mm). When an 8 mm thick component is planned for use, 3 mm of bone (component 8 mm − total loss 5 mm) is resected. *Even though the anatomical posterior slope is known to be 10°, posterior slope greater than 7° is not recommended since it causes ACL strain.*

Femoral osteotomy is done using the gap technique and then the spacer block is used to balance the extension gap for femoral resection. The spacer block should slide with little resistance. When tibial resection is less than 2 mm at the peripheral bone level, it may result in a little tight gap in flexion. Fitz and Scott recommended a little more resection of the posterior femoral condyle instead of more tibial resection. In this procedure, the axis should be aligned to the mechanical axis in extension and the femoral component should be aligned at right angle to the tibial component.

After osteotomy, the trial implant is inserted, and alignment of the tibial and femoral components is checked first and followed by the assessment of patellar tracking.

6.1.4.4 Fixation

In minimally invasive surgery, the key to fixation is proper removal of posterior cement (Fig. 6.15). To remove the cement effectively, some surgeons place a gauze on the posterior side just before cementing. Too much application of the cement to prosthesis should be avoided. Generally, it is preferred to perform *cementing of the tibial component first followed by cementing of the femoral component.*

6.1.5 Postoperative Care

Postoperative care after UK is the same as that after TKA, and postoperative recovery after UK can be a little faster than that after TKA. CPM can be started in the recovery room or postoperative 2–3 days after removal of Hemovac. Active exercises are started early so as to achieve at least 90° of flexion in a week. The patient can be allowed to walk within 3 days, walk without walker or clutches in 2 weeks, and return to normal daily activities within 6 weeks postoperatively.

6.1.6 Complications

Early complications after UK such as deep vein thrombosis and infection are the same as those after TKA. Infection after UK has been reported in only 0.1–0.7 % of patients, which is slightly lower than that reported after TKA.

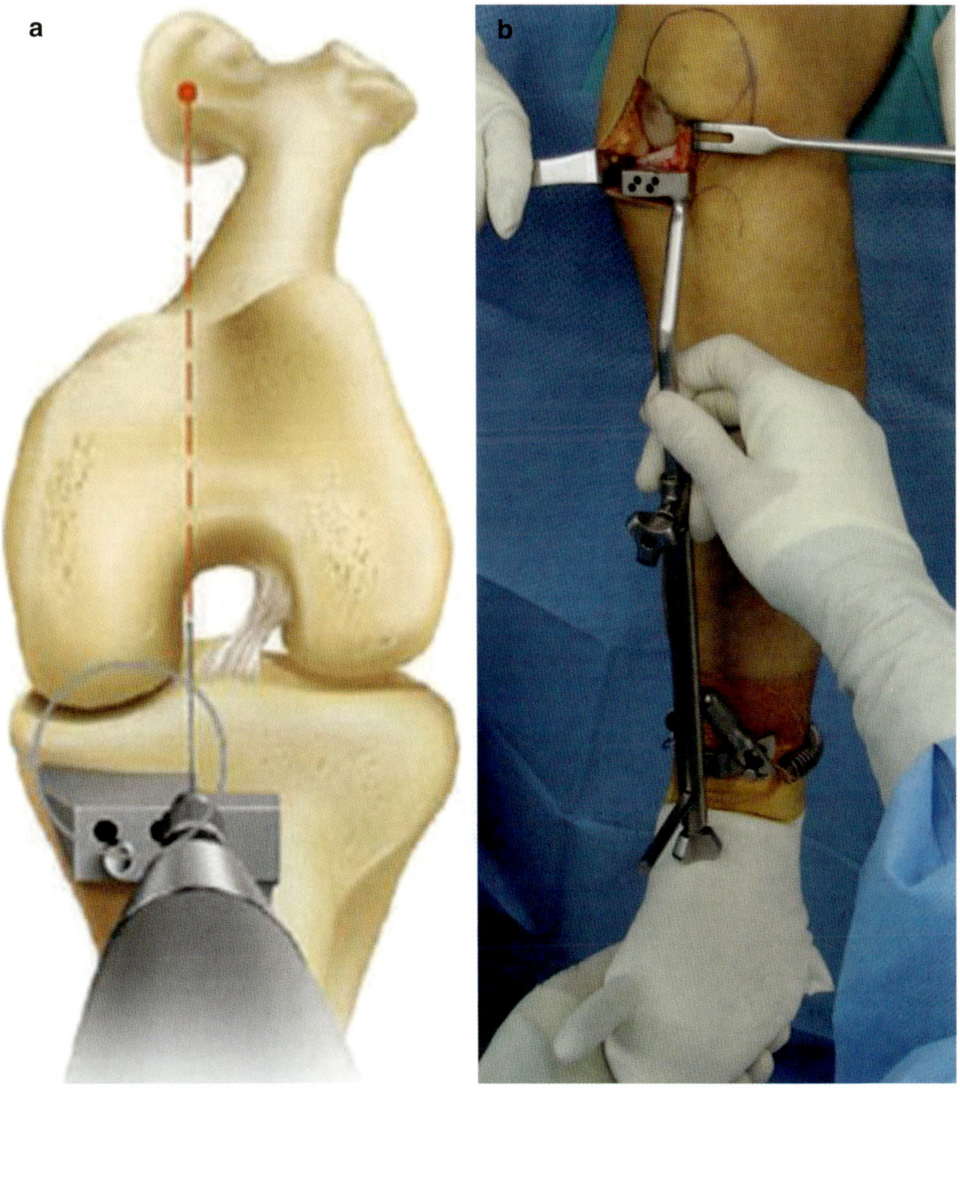

Fig. 6.14 Tibial osteotomy (Courtesy of MH Song/ Biomet, Warsaw, IN). The diagrams of this page show the aligning method (**a**) and fixation of cutting guide (**b**). The left diagrams of next page show the overview of tibial osteotomy (**c**, **d**). The *right photograph* shows the operative procedure of osteotomy for the alignment and tibial osteotomy

c

d

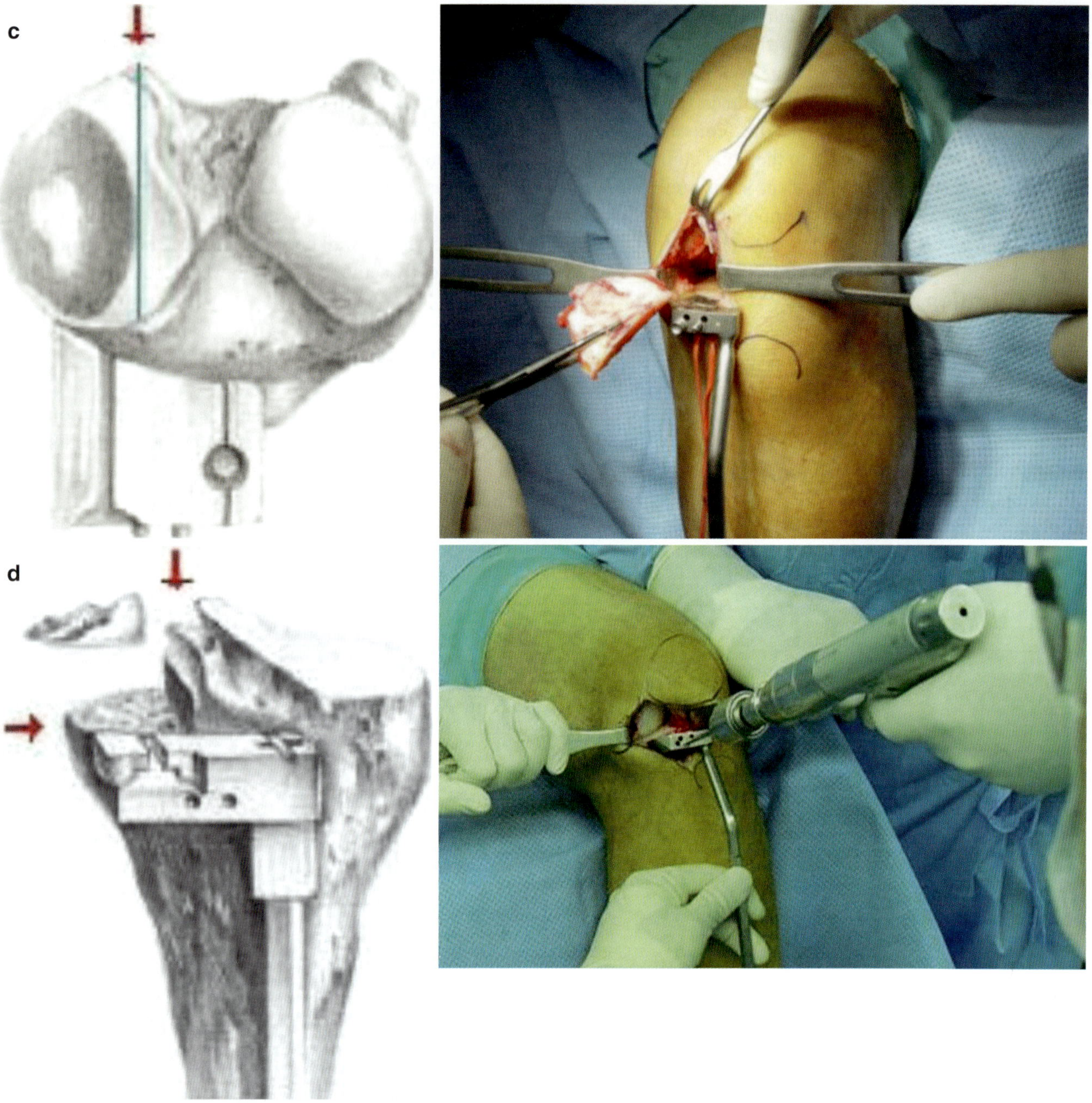

Fig. 6.14 (continued)

The most common mid- to long-term complications include *arthritis of the unreplaced part of the knee joint or of the patellofemoral joint due to overcorrection of the varus deformity. Other complications include wear, subsidence or loosening of the prosthesis, break down of the prosthesis, and PE dislocation*.

In terms of the incidence, most authors reported that *arthritis of the unreplaced part of the knee joint* is the most common, while others reported that the *PE wear* is the most common. Such differences occur due to the difference in *selection of patients, selection of the prosthesis, and surgical technique* including overcorrection, malalignment, and malpositioning. Bae et al. reported that the *selection of the prosthesis is the most* important factor and the wear of the prosthesis was the most common finding for the Microloc prosthesis.

As in TKA, the radiolucent area in UK is also divided into several zones to determine the site and degree of loosening (Fig. 6.16). *If each zone has 2 mm or greater radiolucency and there is cement fracture or subsidence of the prosthesis, these should be considered as signs of clinical loosening.* Kalra et al. reported that radiolucent line at the tip of the femoral peg was significantly associated with loosening of the femoral component.

Dislocation of the meniscal bearing has been reported in meniscal-bearing UK. Gunther et al. stated that dislocation occurs more frequently after lateral UK than after medial UK, because the lateral collateral ligament is in a more relaxed state when the knee is flexed. Gunther suggested a few guidelines to prevent dislocation after lateral UK: first, the lateral parapatellar approach should be used; second, the popliteus tendon should be cut and the remaining soft tissues in the posterolateral space should be removed; and finally, the flexion and extension gaps should be carefully balanced. Song et al. reported the occurrence of intra- and postoperative *tibial condylar fractures*.

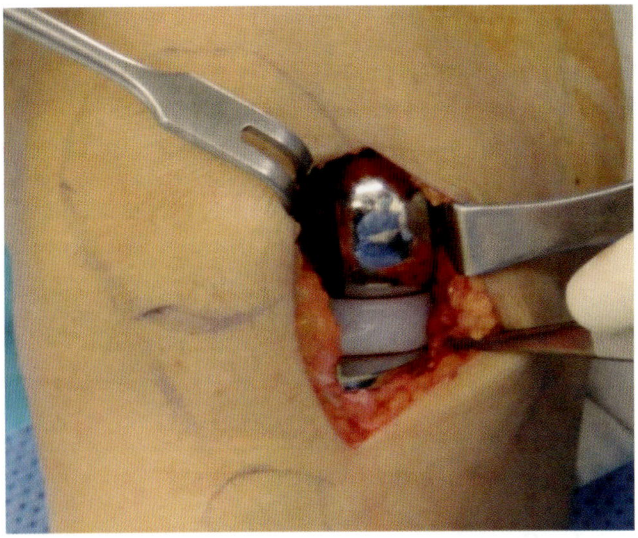

Fig. 6.15 After fixation of the prosthesis (Courtesy of MH Song)

In addition to the above complications, pain relief may not be achieved due to overactivity, and in about 10 % of these cases, pain is due to *pes anserinus bursitis*. Once pes anserinus bursitis has been diagnosed, hydrocortisone can be injected with local anesthetics to relieve the symptoms.

6.1.7 Prognosis

Every surgeon has a significantly different opinion about the results and prognosis of UK.

This is because *the results and prognosis vary according to the indication, type of prosthesis used, and surgical techniques*.

Early UK did not show a good prognosis, and the common causes of poor prognosis were inappropriate selection of patients, problems with the prosthesis, and poor surgical techniques. Laskin reported that patient's satisfaction rate was 65 % and Insall and Walker also reported that UK was not very successful in 42 % of the patients in 1970s. The results improved progressively since 1970, as the surgeons selected the patients carefully and the surgical techniques as well as the design and materials of the prostheses improved. Marmor reported 70 % satisfaction among his patients. Scott and Cobb reported a 10-year survival rate of 85 % and the survival rate decreased by about 1 % per year for 10 years, which *decreased markedly after 10 years*. Argenson et al. reported that they recently (in 2002) achieved very satisfying results in 92 % of the patients and the 10-year survival rate reached up to 94 %. Murray et al. and Berger et al. reported a 10-year survival rate of as high as 98 %.

In comparison between mobile-bearing and fixed-bearing UK, Parratte et al. reported that the number of overcorrections and the number of radiolucencies were statistically higher in mobile-bearing UK. However, survivorship between two groups showed no demonstrable difference.

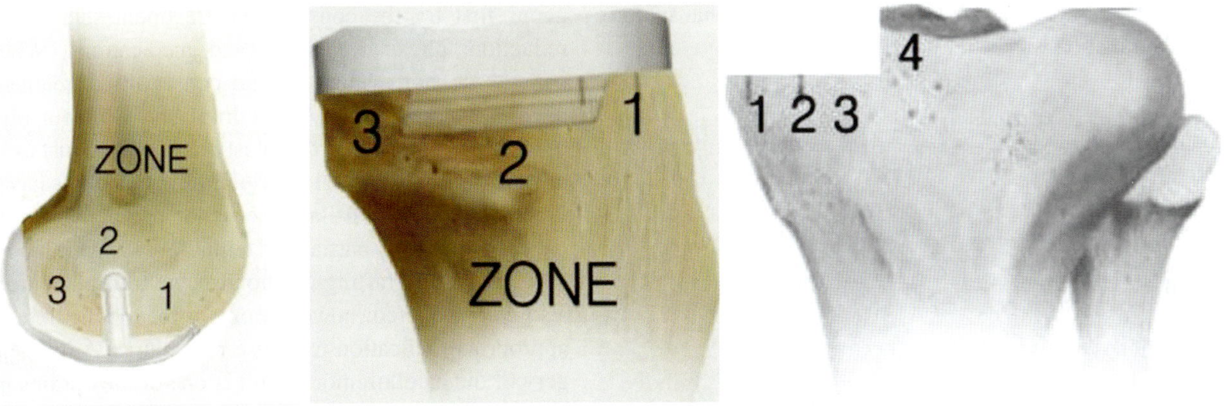

Fig. 6.16 Zones to describe radiolucent area in unicondylar arthroplasty

Comparison between medial UK and lateral UK revealed that the medial UK was performed in 85–95 % of the cases. Some authors have reported good results with lateral UK, but *it is a generally accepted fact that lateral UK is more often associated with arthritis and loosening of the prosthesis than medial UK*. Gunther et al. reported that the 10-year survival rate in lateral UK was 67 %, whereas Ashraf et al. reported that the 10-year survival rate in lateral UK was 83 % and half of the revisions were performed due to arthritis of the medial side. The failure rate of lateral UK was higher using mobile-bearing Oxford UK prosthesis. Based on this result, *the fixed-bearing implant seems to be more appropriate for lateral UK*. Streit et al. reported that the risk of dislocation using mobile-bearing UK prosthesis in lateral compartment is higher than fixed-bearing UK. To avoid this complication, they recommended not to elevate the lateral joint line. Lustig et al. achieved an excellent success rate with fixed-bearing UK on the lateral side.

Comparison between minimally invasive surgery and conventional surgery revealed that *morbidity and early results were better after minimally invasive surgery*. Muller et al. reported that the HSS score and ROM were better after minimally invasive surgery although these were not statistically significant and the number of patients with an extension lag was significantly higher after conventional surgery. At the 8-year follow-up, Romanowski and Repicci evaluated 136 UKs which were performed through a mini-incision. The revision rate was 7 % including technical errors in 3 of 10 cases of revision. This result is poorer than that of conventional incision. This means that UK is less tolerant to component malpositioning compared to that after TKA. In terms of the position of the prosthesis, abnormal position was more often seen after minimally invasive surgery. But Price et al. and Carlsson et al. *stated that no statistically significant difference was seen in component malpositioning between conventional surgery and minimally invasive surgery at the long-term follow-up*. Pandit et al. reported the results of a minimum 5-year follow-up of 1,000 cases of Oxford phase 3 UK using a minimally invasive surgical approach. The 10-year survival rate was 96 % and it was comparable to that achieved after a conventional surgery, and the function was better in MIS.

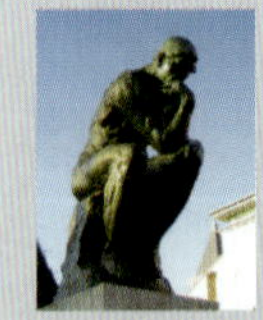

Author's Opinion

I think good results can be expected after UK if the indication for UK is selected carefully and the operation is performed correctly. UK is best indicated in old and less active patients with unicompartmental arthritis, but the range of indication may be widened to include the younger patients who may need a subsequent TKA after a few years.

In my opinion, the indication and surgical technique are the most important prognostic factors.

The surgical techniques in UK have a greater importance and are more difficult than those in TKA and hence a learning curve is needed. With respect to the approach, a minimally invasive surgery seems to be better than the conventional approach in balancing the soft tissues and reducing the morbidity. To reduce the complications of minimally invasive surgery, I think correct osteotomy as well as cement removal in the posterior part of the joint should be done properly.

Current reports show a very good survival rate of UK; however, it is still lower compared to that of TKA because of three reasons: first, the activity is almost unrestricted; second, arthritis progresses in the nonreplaced part of the joint; and third, there are not many surgeons who have experience with this operation.

It is known that revision of UK is easier than that of TKA. However, it is not so easy to reconstruct the defect without bone grafting or metal augmentation if the implant is not surface-replacement type, since the bone defect on one side of the femoral and tibial condyles is too extensive as compared to the unreplaced part.

6.2 Patellofemoral Arthroplasty

6.2.1 Overview

Some patients complain of anterior knee pain or functional disturbance limited to the patellofemoral joint. Most surgeons first try the conservative treatment such as weight reduction, physical therapy, and medications. When the patients do not respond to the conservative treatment, an operation is considered. Chondroplasty with spur removal, drilling, and abrasion arthroplasty can be done just as for the other arthritic lesions. However, these procedures have limitations since the cartilage does not regenerate and some patients show only partial and temporary symptomatic relief. Osteochondral grafting or chondrocyte transplantation may also be considered; however, only a focal bone defect is an appropriate indication for these procedures. Alignment surgery of the patellofemoral joint is one of the options in case of maltracking of the patella. Tibial tubercle elevation may yield temporary improvement. Patellectomy also has limitations since the muscular strength becomes weak and nutrition to the femoral trochlea is obliterated. Furthermore, the operative procedures of TKA can be compromised after patellectomy.

Hence, it is difficult to determine the ideal method of treatment which is suitable *for the patients with arthritis confined to the patellofemoral joint. Patellofemoral arthroplasty has been suggested as an alternative method for treatment of patellofemoral arthritis.*

6.2.2 Design

McKeever developed a patellar resurfacing prosthesis using Vitallium in the 1950s, but many patients complained of pain not only in the patella but also in the femoral trochlear area. Therefore, in the 1970s, Bechtol, Aglietty, Lubinus, and Richards et al. developed a modern type of prosthesis that resurfaces both the trochlea and the patella.

There are numerous specific design features of the trochlear components including the sagittal radius of curvature, proximal extension of the trochlear component, mediolateral width, and constraint of the trochlear groove. There are also inlay and onlay prostheses. The onlay device is more suitable for a larger variation in trochlear geometries.

The early types of prostheses had an anatomical shape for the trochlea and the patella and were classified as the first-generation prostheses. These first-generation prostheses had a trochlea with an obtuse curvature and a shorter anterior flange on the sagittal plane, and a narrow trochlear groove on the axial plane. With *this design, the prosthesis was similar to a constrained type of prosthesis and it was less forgiving for operation, leading to early failure.* Due to the obtuse curvature and a shorter anterior flange, it was difficult to implant the prosthesis flush with the surrounding articular cartilage. The trochlear prosthesis was often implanted in a flexed position, due to which the anterior flange tended to lift off at the femoral cortex to cause snapping or catching during knee motion. As the trochlear groove was narrow on the axial plane, even a minor error could cause maltracking. The patellar prosthesis had an anatomical form, but it was not very compatible because the shape of the patella is different in every patient. The patients with degenerative changes in the patella showed more deformity of the patella, thus making it difficult to design a standard form of patellar prosthesis.

In the current *second-generation prostheses, the trochlear portion was converted into a longer anterior flange with a rather perpendicular curvature and a wider trochlear groove which is less constraining for better tracking of the patella during flexion. Also, design of the trochlear notch portion is changed so as neither to hinder the ACL movement nor to impinge on the tibia.* Aglietti et al. designed a dome-shaped patella on the basis of biomechanics, since the anatomically shaped patella could not be applied universally in all patients. Patellar instability was decreased in these newer designs. The mobile type of patella was another available option.

Lonner reported the results of a comparative study which demonstrated that the failure rate of 17 % with the first-generation prostheses was decreased to 4 % with the second-generation prostheses. Hollinghurst et al. reported the results of the second-generation Avon prosthesis which suggested that the sagittal plane mechanics were just as good as normal.

In terms of products, the Autocentric Patellofemoral Prosthesis (Medinov, Roanne, France), Lubinus (Link, Hamburg, Germany), and Richards I (Smith & Nephew Richards, Memphis, TN) were classified into the first-generation prostheses which had a shorter anterior flange, narrower trochlear groove, and an obtuse curvature. The later designs of the Richards II (Smith & Nephew Richards, Memphis, TN), Low-Contact Stress Patellofemoral Joint (DePuy Orthopedics, Warsaw, IN), Natural-Knee II Patellofemoral Joint (Zimmer, Warsaw, IN), and Avon (Stryker/Howmedica Osteonics, Mahwah, NJ) were classified into the second-generation prostheses. The trochlear component is made of cobalt chromium and the patellar component is made of polyethylene (Fig. 6.17).

6.2.3 Indication

The indication for PFA is advanced osteoarthritis confined to the patellofemoral joint (Outerbridge grade IV) with severe pain in the retropatellar area or functional disturbance that has not improved after more than 6 months of conservative treatment. Detailed history taking of the problem, meticulous physical examination, and X-ray should be performed for making a decision regarding the operation, and MRI may be useful for evaluating patellofemoral arthritis. Functional disturbances are problems associated with going up and down the stairs, staying seated for a long time, and pain and difficulty during standing up and squatting. A history of patellar fracture or dislocation and failure of the other operations are also good indications for PFA. However, these indications are not applicable to many patients, and it is assumed that only about 2–3 of 100 cases of TKA would meet these criteria.

Surgeons have significantly different opinions regarding the appropriate age for PFA; Lubinus, Arciero et al., and Toomey et al. agreed that PFA is better indicated in patients older than 60 years of age, whereas Blazina et al. and Lonner recommended patellofemoral arthroplasty (PFA) for patients younger than 60 years of age and TKA for patients older than 60 years of age, since aged patients are more likely to show concomitant degeneration of the femorotibial joint.

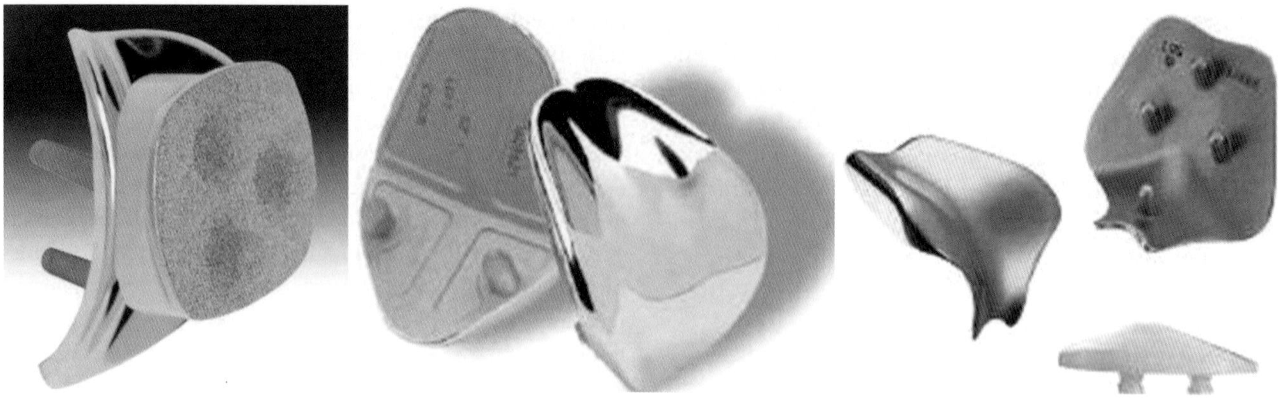

Fig. 6.17 Types of trochlear prostheses. Low-Contact Stress Patellofemoral joint (DePuy, Warsaw, IN). Natural-Knee II Patellofemoral joint (Zimmer, Warsaw, IN). Avon Patellofemoral joint (Stryker, Allendale, NJ)

In case of inflammatory arthritis, chondrocalcinosis, and limited ROM, it is best not to perform PFA. PFA is also contraindicated in case of malalignment or maltracking of the patella that cannot be corrected by the operation. In such cases, it is advisable to correct these problems and observe the clinical course before performing PFA.

PFA is also contraindicated in laborious workers who do not wish to limit their activities or in those who play sports. PFA may not be contraindicated in patients who are obese or who have ACL deficiency, but there is a high possibility of failure in these cases.

6.2.4 Surgical Technique

Midline skin incision and paramedial arthrotomy or a subvastus approach may be used in PFA as in TKA. The length of the incision in PFA may be shortened compared to that in TKA, but it should be adequate enough to evert the patella and observe the inside of the joint, although some surgeons do not evert the patella. Care must be taken so as not to injure the meniscus during arthrotomy.

If there is inflammatory arthritis, chondrocalcinosis, or degenerative changes in the tibiofemoral joint, it is recommended to perform TKA instead of PFA.

When removing the spurs, it is particularly important to perform a notchplasty so as to smoothen this area.

The trochlea should be resected as suggested in each implant's manual, but there are a few common guidelines. First, the *trochlea should be rotated externally by 3–6° along the transcondylar axis, or external rotation should be based on Whiteside's line or transepicondylar axis* in order to improve patellar tracking. The trochlea may be placed 1–2 mm to the lateral side, but the trochlear groove should be in alignment with the anatomical axis of the femur. Second, the *trochlear coverage should be as large as possible without overhang.* The notch portion should not overhang and the trochlea should not extend to the weight-bearing area so as not to cause impingement onto the tibia. In order to achieve this, the end of the trochlear prosthesis should be about 3–5 mm proximal to the notch. Third, *too much of the subchondral bone should not be removed for surface replacement.* About 3–4 mm of the anterior cortex of the femur is removed, or a high-speed burr can be used so that the prosthesis does not protrude or sink down. The prosthesis should be flush with the surrounding cartilage.

Patellar resurfacing is performed in the same manner as that in TKA. There are two types, inset and onset patella. In particular, the thickness of the patella should remain the same as its preoperative thickness, and the patella should be slightly shifted towards the medial side. In onset patella, the bone that is not covered with the prosthesis should be beveled.

After bone resection, a trial implant is used to check patellar tracking and to examine whether there is patellar tilt, subluxation, or catching. If necessary, lateral retinacular release or realignment operation can be performed. Generally, *tracking is considered to be good, when the medial facet of the patella contacts the medial trochlea and the medial femoral condyle through the full range of motion by the "no-thumb technique."*

Cementing is recommended to prevent loosening; however, some surgeons do not use cement for patellar fixation (Fig. 6.18).

6.2.5 Postoperative Care

Postoperative rehabilitation is in the manner similar to that after TKA and it is slightly faster than that after TKA.

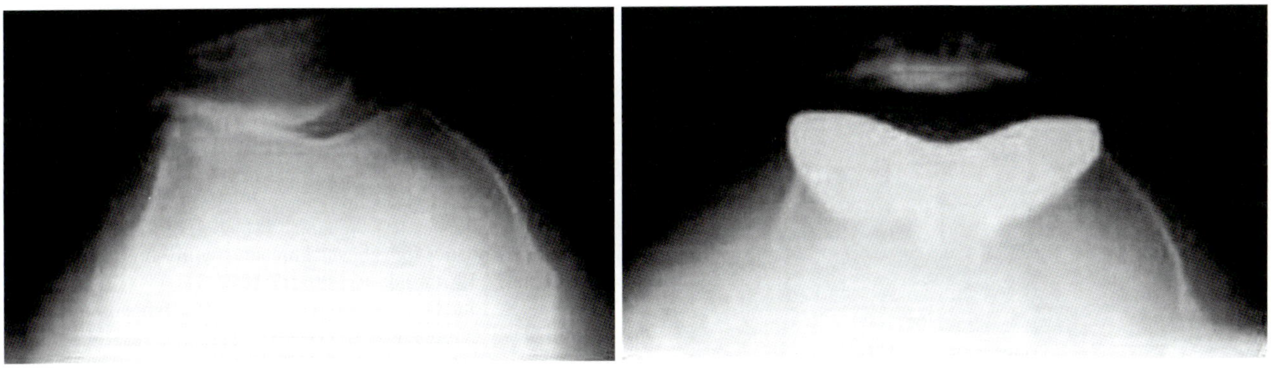

Fig. 6.18 Preoperative and postoperative X-rays of patellofemoral arthroplasty

ROM exercises including CPM may be started immediate postoperatively and weight bearing can be permitted when the pain becomes tolerable.

6.2.6 Complications

Complications include persistent pain, maltracking, catching or snapping, extension lag, limited ROM, persistent swelling, giving way, and tibiofemoral arthritis. Loosening occurs in less than 1 % of cases when cement is used. Among the complications, *arthritis of the unreplaced part of the joint is the most common complication.*

The causes of these complications include inappropriate selection of patients, design defect of the prosthesis, and poor surgical techniques. *The most common cause of complications is poor surgical techniques combined with design defect of the prosthesis.* As mentioned above, minor surgical errors with the use of the first-generation prosthesis lead to maltracking, malpositioning of the prosthesis, and catching or snapping.

6.2.7 Prognosis

There are many different reports regarding the prognosis of PFA; *some reports are encouraging, while the others are disappointing.* However, the results are gradually improving with the development of the prosthesis.

Many authors have reported good and excellent results up to 85 % at the short-term and midterm follow-up; Argenson et al. reported that 84 % of cases showed satisfying results and the 16-year survival rate was 58 % based on the midterm follow-up. When the Avon prosthesis was used, Odumenya et al. reported a 5-year survival rate of 100 % and Ackroyd et al. reported a 5-year survival rate of 95.8 %. However, Tauro abandoned this operation because of the poor results with the use of the Lubinus prosthesis. The success rate was only 45 % and the 8-year survival rate was only 65 %.

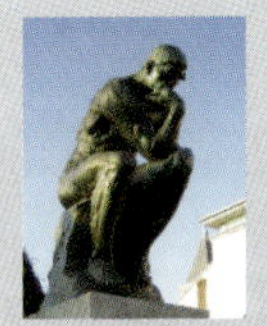

Author's Opinion

I have no experience of patellofemoral arthroplasty.

However, I believe that it may be indicated in relatively younger patients who have severe patellofemoral arthritis with pain and functional disturbance which is not improved by conservative treatment. Patients should be selected carefully since the prosthetic design and surgical techniques are not yet very popular and experience is needed.

It is important to sincerely discuss this treatment option with the patients and explain to them that conversion to TKA may be needed if complications do develop.

In this respect, it is recommended not to perform this operation when patients have high expectations, and I personally recommend TKA for patients above 60 years of age.

6.3 Bicompartmental Knee Arthroplasty

When there is a medial condylar lesion and patellofemoral arthritis, most of the surgeons prefer TKA. But some surgeons perform UK and PFA separately or they use a single-piece femoral component that comprises of the femoral trochlear groove and the medial femoral condyle (Fig. 6.19). Although this is not unicompartmental arthroplasty, I will briefly describe it here.

The indication for bicompartmental knee arthroplasty is pain in the medial tibiofemoral joint associated with patellofemoral symptoms. Mild lateral tibiofemoral pain is

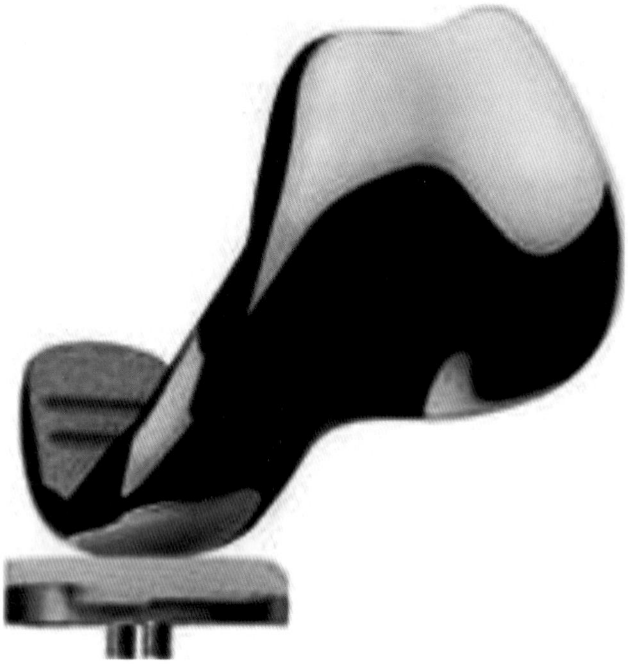

Fig. 6.19 Bicompartmental prosthesis (Deuce: Smith & Nephew, Memphis, TN)

acceptable in the patients older than 75 years of age, although it is not ideal.

The deformity should not exceed 10° of varus or 10° of flexion contracture and all ligaments should be clinically intact. CT image may be needed for the operation using the single-piece patellofemoral component.

The procedure can be performed through a limited, or minimally invasive surgical approach. The operation is technically demanding. Even 1 mm of offset may lead to patellofemoral symptoms.

The advantages of bicompartmental knee arthroplasty include preservation of the normal ligaments of the knee joint, less-invasive surgery, and a rapid postoperative recovery.

Unfortunately, *the clinical results* of bicompartmental knee arthroplasty *have never been better than those of TKA*.

Bibliography

Ackroyd CE, Chir B. Development and early results of a new patellofemoral arthroplasty. Clin Orthop. 2005;436:7–13.

Ackroyd CE, Newman JH, Evans R, et al. The Avon patellofemoral arthroplasty: five-year survivorship and functional results. J Bone Joint Surg Br. 2007;89-B:310–5.

Aglietti P, Insall JN, Walker PS, et al. A new patellar prosthesis. Design and application. Clin Orthop. 1975;107:175–87.

Amis AA, Senavongse W, Darcy P. Biomechanics of patellofemoral joint prostheses. Clin Orthop. 2005;436:20–9.

Arciero FA, Toomey HE. Patellofemoral arthroplasty. A three to nine year follow-up study. Clin Orthop. 1988;236:60–71.

Argensen JN. Unicompartmental knee arthroplasty. An European perspective. In: Scott WN, editor. Surgery of the knee. 4th ed. Philadelphia, PA: Churchill Livingstone; 2006. p. 1421–9.

Argenson JN, Benkeddache YC, Aubaniac JM. Modern unicompartmental knee arthroplasty with cement. J Bone Joint Surg Am. 2002;84-A:2235–9.

Argenson JN, Guillaume JM, Aubaniac JM. Is there a place for patellofemoral arthroplasty? Clin Orthop. 1995;321:162–7.

Argenson JN, Komistek RD, Aubaniac JM, et al. In vivo determination of knee kinematics for subjects implanted with a unicompartmental arthroplasty. J Arthroplasty. 2002;17:1049–54.

Argenson JN, Murray D, Coon TM, et al. Unicompartmental knee arthroplasty: international roundtable discussion. In: Scott WN, editor. Surgery of the knee. 5th ed. Philadelphia, PA: Churchill Livingstone; 2011. p. 1005–9.

Argenson JN, Parratte S. Unicompartmental knee arthroplasty: A European perspective. In: Scott WN, editor. Surgery of the knee. 5th ed. Philadelphia, PA: Churchill Livingstone; 2011. p. 996–1004.

Ashraf T, Newman JH, Evans RL, et al. Lateral unicompartmental knee replacement. J Bone Joint Surg. 2002;84-B:1126–30.

Bae DK, Yoon KH, Ko BW, et al. Survivorship of unicompartmental knee replacement. J Korean Knee Soc. 2001;13:1–7.

Barnes CL, Scott RD. Unicompartmental knee replacement. In: Scott WN, editor. The knee. 1st ed. St. Louis, MO: Mosby;1994. p. 1097–103.

Barrett WP, Scott RD. Revision of failed unicompartmental knee arthroplasty. J Bone Joint Surg Br. 1987;69-A:1328–31.

Beard DJ, Pandit H, Gill HS, et al. The influence of the presence and severity of pre-existing patellofemoral degenerative changes on the outcome of the Oxford medial unicompartmental knee replacement. J Bone Joint Surg Br. 2007;89-B:1597–601.

Berend KR, Morris MJ, Skeels MD, et al. Perioperative complications of simultaneous versus staged unicompartmental knee arthroplasty. Clin Orthop. 2011;469:168–73.

Berger RA, Nedeff DD, Barden RM, et al. Unicompartmental knee arthroplasty. Clinical experience at 6-to 10-year follow-up. Clin Orthop. 1999;367:50–60.

Blazina ME, Fox JM, Del Pizzo W, et al. Patellofemoral replacement. 1979. Clin Orthop. 2005;436:3–6.

Carlsson LV, Albrektsson BE, Regner LR. Minimally invasive surgery vs conventional exposure using the Miller-Galante unicompartmental knee arthroplasty: a randomized radiostereometric study. J Arthroplasty. 2006;21:151–6.

Cartier P, Sanouiller JL, Khefacha A. Long-term results with the first patellofemoral prosthesis. Clin Orthop. 2005;436:47–54.

Christensen NO. Unicompartmental prosthesis for gonarthrosis. A nine-year series of 575 knees from a Swedish hospital. Clin Orthop. 1991;273:165–9.

Dennis BD, Komistek R, Scuderi GR, et al. In vivo three-dimensional determination of kinematics for subjects with a normal knee or a unicompartmental or total knee replacement. J Bone Joint Surg Am. 2002;83-A:104–5.

Fehring TK, Berend KR, Hofmann S, et al. Advanced technologies in performing total knee arthroplasty: roundtable discussion. In: Scott WN, editor. Surgery of the knee. 5th ed. Philadelphia, PA: Churchill Livingstone; 2011. p. 1283–92.

Fitz W, Scott RD. Unicompartmental total knee arthroplasty. In: Scott WN, editor. Surgery of the knee. 4th ed. Philadelphia, PA: Churchill Livingstone; 2006. p. 1408–20.

Fitz W, Scott RD. Unicompartmental knee arthroplasty. In: Scott WN, editor. Surgery of the knee. 5th ed. Philadelphia, PA: Churchill Livingstone; 2011. p. 988–95.

Fitzpatrick C, Fitzpatrick D, Lee J, et al. Statistical design of unicompartmental tibial implants and comparison with current devices. Knee. 2007;14:138–44.

Furnes O, Espehaug B, Lie SA, et al. Failure mechanisms after unicompartmental and tricompartmental primary knee replacement with cement. J Bone Joint Surg Am. 2007;89-A:519–25.

Gesell MW, Tria Jr AJ. MIS unicondylar knee arthroplasty: surgical approach and early results. Clin Orthop. 2004;428:53–60.

Goodfellow JW, Kershaw CJ, DA Benson MK, et al. The Oxford knee for unicompartmental osteoarthritis. J Bone Joint Surg Br. 1988;70-B:692–701.

Gulati A, Pandit H, Jenkins C, et al. The effect of leg alignment on the outcome of unicompartmental knee replacement. J Bone Joint Surg Br. 2009;91-B:469–74.

Gunther T, Hurray DW, Miller R, et al. Lateral unicompartmental arthroplasty with Oxford meniscal knee. Knee. 1996;3:33–9.

Hollinghurst D, Stoney J, Ward T, et al. In vivo sagittal plane kinematics of the Avon patellofemoral arthroplasty. J Arthroplasty. 2007;22:117–23.

Inglis G. Unicompartmental arthroplasty of the knee. J Bone Joint Surg Br. 1984;66-B:682–4.

Insall JN, Walker P. Unicondylar knee replacement. Clin Orthop. 1976;120:83–5.

Jamali AA, Rodrick DJ, Malberg MI, et al. Unicompartmental knee arthroplasty. In: Callaghan JJ, editor. The adult knee. 1st ed. Philadelphia, PA: Lippincott Williams and Wilkins; 2003. p. 1111–34.

Kalra S, Smith TO, Berko B, et al. Assessment of radiolucent lines around the Oxford unicompartmental knee replacement: sensitivity and specificity for loosening. J Bone Joint Surg Br. 2011; 93-B:777–81.

Kang SN, Smith TO, Sprenger De Rover WB, et al. Pre-operative patellofemoral degenerative changes do not affect the outcome after medial Oxford unicompartmental knee replacement. J Bone Joint Surg Br. 2011;93-B:476–8.

Kendrick BJ, Rout R, Bottomley NJ, et al. The implications of damage to the lateral femoral condyle on medial unicompartmental knee replacement. J Bone Joint Surg Br. 2010;92-B:374–9.

Kennedy W, White R. Unicompartmental total knee arthroplasty of the knee: postoperative alignment and its influence on overall results. Clin Orthop. 1991;271:96–100.

Kennedy WR, White RP. Unicompartmental arthroplasty of the knee. postoperative alignment and its influence on overall results. Clin Orthop. 1987;221:278–85.

Kooijman HJ, Driessen APPM, van Horn JR. Long-term results of patellofemoral arthroplasty. J Bone Joint Surg Br. 2003;85-B:836–40.

Lai CH, Rand JA. Revision of failed unicompartmental total knee arthroplasty. Clin Orthop. 1993;287:193–201.

Laskin RS. Unicompartmental tibiofemoral resurfacing arthroplasty. J Bone Joint Surg Am. 1978;60-A:182–5.

Laskin RS. Unicompartmental knee replacement: some unanswered questions. Clin Orthop. 2001;392:267–71.

Levine WN, Ozuna RM, Scott RD, et al. Conversion of failed modern unicompartmental arthroplasty to total knee arthroplasty. J Arthroplasty. 1996;11:797–801.

Lonner JH. Patellofemoral arthroplasty: pros, cons, design considerations. Clin Orthop. 2004;428:158–65.

Lonner JH. Patellofemoral arthroplasty. In: Scott WN, editor. Surgery of the knee. 4th ed. Philadelphia, PA: Churchill Livingstone; 2006. p. 1440–54.

Lonner JH. Patellofemoral arthroplasty. In: Scott WN, editor. Surgery of the knee. 5th ed. Philadelphia, PA: Churchill Livingstone; 2011. p. 1010–20.

Lotke PA, Lonner JH, Nelson CL. Patellofemoral arthroplasty: the third compartment. J Arthroplasty. 2005;20 Suppl 2:4–6.

Lubinus HH. Patella glide bearing total replacement. Orthopedics. 1979;2:119.

Lustig S, Elguindy A, Servien E, et al. 5- to 16-year follow-up of 54 consecutive lateral unicondylar knee arthroplasties with a fixed-all polyethylene bearing. J Arthroplasty. 2011;26:1318–25.

Lyons MC, MacDonald SJ, Somerville LE, et al. Unicompartmental versus total knee arthroplasty database Analysis: is there a winner? Clin Orthop. 2012;470:84–90.

Marmor L. The modular knee. Clin Orthop. 1973;94:242–8.

Marmor L. Unicompartmental knee arthroplasty. Ten- to 13-year follow-up study. Clin Orthop. 1988;226:14–20.

McAuley JP, Engh GA, Ammeen DJ. Revision of failed unicompartmental knee arthroplasty. Clin Orthop. 2001;392:279–82.

Mullaji AB, Sharma A, Marawar S. Unicompartmental knee arthroplasty: functional recovery and radiographic results with a minimally invasive technique. J Arthroplasty. 2007;22:7–11.

Muller PE, Pellengahr C, Witt M, et al. Influence of minimally invasive surgery on implant positioning and the functional outcome for medial unicompartmental knee arthroplasty. J Arthroplasty. 2004;19:296–301.

Murray DW, Goodfellow JW, O'Connor JJ. The Oxford medial unicompartmental arthroplasty: a ten-year survival study. J Bone Joint Surg Br. 1998;80-B:983–9.

Newman JH, Ackroyd CE, Shah NA. Unicompartmental or total knee replacement? Five-year results of a prospective, randomised trial of 102 osteoarthritic knees with unicompartmental arthritis. J Bone Joint Surg Br. 1998;80-B:862–5.

Noticewala MS, Geller JA, Lee JH, et al. Unicompartmental knee arthroplasty relieves pain and improve function more than total knee arthroplasty. J Arthroplasty. 2012;27 Suppl 8:99–105.

Odumenya M, Costa ML, Parsons N, et al. The Avon patellofemoral joint replacement: Five-year results from an independent centre. J Bone Joint Surg Br. 2010;92-B:56–60.

Padgett DE, Stern SH, Insall JN. Revision total knee arthroplasty for failed unicompartmental replacement. J Bone Joint Surg Am. 1991;73-A:186–90.

Pandit H, Jenkins C, Gill HS, et al. Minimally invasive Oxford phase 3 unicompartmental knee replacement: results of 1000 cases. J Bone Joint Surg Br. 2011;93-B:198–204.

Parrattte S, Pauly V, Aubaniac JM, et al. No long-term difference between fixed and mobile medial unicompartmental arthroplasty. Clin Orthop. 2012;470:61–8.

Pennington DW, Swienckowski JJ, Lutes WB, et al. Lateral unicompartmental knee arthroplasty: survivorship and technical considerations at an average follow-up of 12.4 years. J Arthroplasty. 2006;21:13–7.

Perkins TR, Gunekle W. Unicompartmental knee arthroplasty. J Arthroplasty. 2002;17:293–7.

Price AJ, Webb J, Topf H, et al. Rapid recovery after Oxford unicompartmental arthroplasty through a short incision. J Arthroplasty. 2001;16:970–6.

Rachala SR, Sierra RJ. Unicompartmental, bicompartmental, or tricompartmental arthritis of the knee: algorithm for surgical management. In: Scott WN, editor. Surgery of the knee. 5th ed. Philadelphia, PA: Churchill Livingstone; 2011. p. 1026–8.

Repicci J, Eberle R. Minimally invasive surgical technique for unicondylar knee arthroplasty. J South Orthop Assoc. 1999; 8:20–7.

Riddle DL, Jiranek WA, McGlynn FJ. Yearly incidence of unicompartmental knee arthroplasty in the United States. J Arthroplasty. 2008;23:408–12.

Romanowski MR, Repicci JA. Minimally invasive unicondylar arthroplasty: eight-year follow-up. J Knee Surg. 2002;15:17–22.

Schai PA, Thornhill TS, Scott RD. Total knee arthroplasty with the PFC system. J Bone Joint Surg Br. 1998;80-B:850–8.

Scott RD. Unicompartmental knee arthroplasty. In: Scott RD, editor. Total knee arthroplasty. 1st ed. Philadelphia, PA: Saunders; 2006. p. 123–8.

Scott RD, Cobb AG. Unicompartmental knee arthroplasty, eight to twelve year follow-up with survivorship analysis. Clin Orthop. 1991;271:96–100.

Scuderi GR, Tria AJ. Minimally invasive surgery for unicondylar arthroplasty of the knee. In: Scott WN, editor. Surgery of the knee. 4th ed. Philadelphia, PA: Churchill Livingstone; 2006. p. 1430–9.

Song MH, Kim BH, Ahn SJ, et al. Early complications after minimally invasive mobile-bearing medial unicompartmental knee arthroplasty. J Arthroplasty. 2009;24:1281–4.

Streit MR, Walker T, Bruckner T, et al. Mobile-bearing lateral unicompartmental knee replacement with the Oxford domed tibial component: an independent series. J Bone Joint Surg Br. 2012;94-A: 1356–61.

Stukenborg-Colsman C, Worth CT, Lazovic D, et al. High tibial osteotomy versus unicompartmental joint replacement in unicompartmental knee joint osteoarthritis; 7-10-year follow-up prospective randomised study. Knee. 2001;8:187–94.

Swank M, Stulberg SD, Jiganti J, et al. The natural history of unicompartmental arthroplasty: an eight year follow-up study with survivorship analysis. Clin Orthop. 1993;286:130–42.

Swienckowski JJ, Pennington DW. Unicompartmental knee arthroplasty in patients sixty years of age or younger. J Bone Joint Surg Am. 2004;86-A Suppl 1:131–42.

Tauro B, Ackroyd CE, Newman JH, et al. The Lubinus patellofemoral arthroplasty. A five to ten year prospective study. J Bone Joint Surg Br. 2001;83-B:696–701.

van Jonbergen HP, Werkman DM, Barnaart LF, et al. Long-term outcomes of patellofemoral arthroplasty. J Arthroplasty. 2010;25: 1066–71.

Vince KG, Cyran LT. Unicompartmental knee arthroplasty: new indications, more complications? J Arthroplasty. 2004;19 Suppl 1: 9–16.

Whiteside LA. Making your next unicompartmental knee arthroplasty last: three keys to success. J Arthroplasty. 2005;20 Suppl 2:2–3.

7 Postoperative Management

Postoperative management of TKA can greatly affect the prognosis of TKA. I have used the term "management" instead of "treatment" because I would like to describe all the relevant factors including the physical, psychological, and social factors.

Psychological and physical changes occur postoperatively and these changes vary from patient to patient. Therefore, there should be a standard treatment protocol and the rehabilitation program should be designed so as to meet each patient's needs as well.

The postoperative management includes recovery from anesthesia after the operation, pain control, wound care, rehabilitation exercises, ambulation, leisure, and occupational training. These management protocols vary according to the length of hospital stay which is somewhat different from country to country due to the socioeconomic circumstances.

Patients should be informed regarding the various problems that they would encounter after discharge from the hospital such as the duration of pain, the type of rehabilitation therapy they must undergo, as well as the activities they can perform and they should not do.

7.1 Postoperative Care

The protocol and contents of postoperative care can vary according to the length of hospital stay, because intensity of rehabilitation is quite different between that at home and at hospital.

The Beth Israel Medical Center divided postoperative care into three phases. Phase I is up to 1 week after operation for restoration of early function. Phase II is between week 2 and week 5 for restoration of progressive function. Phase III is between week 6 and week 8 for restoration of advanced function.

The purpose of Phase I postoperative care is that the patient should be able to get out of bed, regain balance, walk alone using a walker, and achieve more than 90° of flexion. The purpose of Phase II postoperative care is to improve the muscular strength and proprioception in the operated limb, maximize the functions at home, and achieve 0–110° of motion. The purpose of Phase III postoperative care is that the patient should be able to walk without a cane, do household work, and achieve 0–120° of motion.

The Beth Israel Medical Center's rehabilitation program includes the details regarding the postoperative care, but there are some difficulties in many aspects for adopting this rehabilitation program in Oriental patients because of the differences in the length of hospitalization, rehabilitation facilities, and lifestyle.

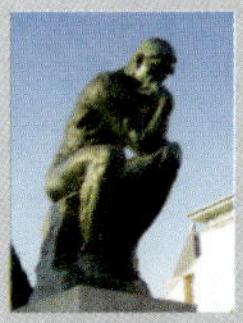

Author's Opinion

I divide the rehabilitation period into early, midterm, and late stages: The early stage is until Hemovac is removed, the midterm stage is until the stitches are removed, and the late stage is until postoperative 3 months.

I prefer this rehabilitation program because careful monitoring is required for ascertaining the patient's general condition until Hemovac is removed and the wound condition should be carefully observed until the stitches are removed. After the stitches are removed till postoperative 3 months, the patient should self-monitor his/her knee condition.

It is generally accepted that Hemovac should be retained for no longer than 2 days, because the risk of infection increases if it is retained for more than 2 days postoperatively. Therefore, the early stage starts immediately after the operation until the 2nd postoperative day.

W. Cho, *Knee Joint Arthroplasty*,
DOI 10.1007/978-3-642-39389-1_7, © Springer-Verlag Berlin Heidelberg 2014

Generally, stitch removal is done between postoperative 10 and 14 days. Hence, the midterm stage is generally considered from the third postoperative day until postoperative 2 weeks. Management during the midterm stage may be somewhat different according to the hospitalization period. In the United States where the cost of hospitalization is high, most patients are admitted for only 3–4 days. Whereas patients in some Oriental countries are discharged within a week or even a month after several rehabilitation therapies have been performed since the cost of hospitalization is not very high in these countries. When the length of hospital stay is short, postoperative care is provided by a home care nurse until stitch removal, and patients themselves should be able to self-monitor their own knee condition thereafter.

7.1.1 Early Stage

7.1.1.1 Care in the Recovery Room

Vital Signs

The purpose of immediate postoperative care is to monitor and maintain the patient's vital signs. After the patient recovers from anesthesia, he/she is transferred to the recovery room. First step is to check the patient's vital signs and consciousness. If the patient's vital signs are unstable, an attempt should be made to correct them immediately and an anesthesiologist should be consulted for identifying the cause of the problem. If the patient does not recover from anesthesia, the anesthetic record should be reviewed in order to identify the causes and to determine the next procedure that should be performed. This is done completely by the anesthesiologist.

After this, the amount of blood drained into Hemovac should be checked. *If it exceeds 200 cc per hour for several hours, the first step is to lock Hemovac and the elastic bandage* is applied more *tightly*. The knee joint is flexed to 30° *and any evidence of vascular compromise should be looked for*. The elastic bandage should be released if there is severe pain due to excessive compression or there are signs of compartment syndrome. If the amount of bleeding does not decrease and the vital signs drop, transfusion should be initiated and the use of a hemostatic agent should be considered. *If the amount of bleeding exceeds 400 cc per hour, an angiography should be performed for preparation of the revision surgery*. However, angiography may be skipped in emergent cases in the hospital where angiography takes a long time.

Neurovascular Assessment

Once the patient recovers from anesthesia, *he/she should be asked to move the great toe for checking the peroneal nerve function*. This is a very important step for differentiating between intraoperative peroneal injury and pressure palsy which develop postoperatively. If a peroneal nerve palsy is detected, it should be reviewed whether any surgical procedure was performed that may have damaged the peroneal nerve. This is very rare in usual TKA, but in cases of a severe valgus deformity, flexion contracture, or ankylotic knee, an exploration can be considered in case of any doubt.

Peroneal nerve palsy that is noticed immediately after the operation is likely to be related to the surgical trauma, but pressure nerve palsy may also develop in the knee that was operated first, due to the tight elastic bandaging or incorrect posture during the second operation in case a simultaneous operation is performed.

If there are signs of multiple nerve palsies, tourniquet palsy or compartment syndrome due to excessive bleeding should be suspected.

7.1.1.2 Care in the Ward

General Care

Once the patient returns to the ward, he or she is placed in the correct position with special care taken for the operated knee. The patient is comfortably laid with the neck in the extended position to keep the airway open. It is recommended to support the ankles with water bags so that the knees are not bent too much, thereby preventing a flexion contracture. The use of an air mattress or water mattress is recommended to prevent bedsores if the patient is obese, is not willing to move, or has history of steroid abuse.

The first step is to recheck the vital signs to confirm that patient's general condition is stable. It should also be checked whether the lines and attachments such as the IV route, Foley catheter, and Hemovac are working properly.

The peroneal nerve function is checked once again. In fact, a tight elastic bandage or incorrect posture could be the most common cause of peroneal nerve palsy when the patient is not fully conscious. Hence, the condition of the peroneal nerve should be checked from time to time in the ward especially in the early stage. If peroneal nerve palsy occurs, the elastic bandage is released without exposing the wound and the knee should be bent at 30°–60°. Pressure palsy may recover normally in a few days to several weeks. The recovery time seems to be related to the duration of compression. Exploration is not needed in most of the cases.

Hydration is very important especially in aged patients. Hence, the intake and output should be checked strictly in order to prevent pulmonary edema or dehydration due to excessive or insufficient fluid administration respectively.

It is also necessary to remove the sputum by coughing *to prevent atelectasis or pneumonia*. Deep breathing is encouraged and an inspirometer is useful for the patients.

Oral intake can be started from wetting the lips with a damp gauze when the patient is willing to start oral intake.

Blood Management

Maintaining an adequate postoperative hemoglobin (Hb) level is necessary for improving the patient's general condition, for preventing medical comorbidity and for promoting wound healing.

Stulberg and Zadzilka suggested that the *blood management program should be based on patient-specific strategy (PSS)* and can vary from surgeon to surgeon or from hospital to hospital.

Keating and Ritter found that the Hb level drops by an average of 3.9 g/dl in case of single knee arthroplasty and by an average of 5.4 g/dl in case of simultaneous knee arthroplasty, and about half of the patients need transfusion after TKA.

The blood management protocol is divided into three stages: preoperative, intraoperative, and postoperative stage.

Preoperative management includes administration of erythropoietic agent and autotransfusion. Currently, the most popular *erythropoietic agent is epoetin alfa* (recombinant human erythropoietin). If the Hb level is between 10 and 13 g/dl, 40,000 units can be injected subcutaneously at 3 weeks, 2 weeks, and 1 week prior to the operation. *It is recommended to give epoetin alfa concomitantly with 200–300 mg of iron and 1 mg of folic acid* daily to prevent iron deficiency disorder caused by the erythropoietic activity.

Autotransfusion, the technique in which the patient's blood is harvested preoperatively for transfusion, can also be used. However, this method has many limitations and its effect is controversial. If the patient has anemia before the operation, harvesting the blood can worsen the anemia. Hatzidakis et al. *did not recommend autotransfusion if the Hb level was below 13 g/dl.* Since the erythropoietic activity after blood harvesting is not as active as expected, the preoperative Hb level decreases. Fred emphasized that not more than 2 units of blood should be harvested. Also, *autotransfusion activates the immune reaction, thereby increasing the risks of allogeneic transfusion reaction*, and the autotransfusion process is inconvenient for the patient.

Another drawback of autotransfusion is that the blood is harvested 3–5 weeks prior to the operation during which *the number of red blood cells can decrease*. Also, the patients should be asked to stop taking any medications which can give rise to a bleeding tendency.

Intraoperative methods include hypotensive anesthesia, blood salvage and hemodilution, and use of a topical hemostatic agent or specialized cautery. Hypotensive anesthesia can cause hypoxia in the tissues, which can lead to the development of complications. It increases the risks of cardiovascular and cerebrovascular complications, and it also increases the incidence of deep vein thrombosis. *Mild acute normovolemic (isovolemic) hemodilution* is a method in which more than 1,000 cc of blood is collected preoperatively and the ECF is temporarily substituted with crystalloid or colloid fluids. It is indicated in patients whose Hb level is higher than 10 g/dl and when the operation is expected to last for a longer time and more than 1,000 cc of blood loss is likely.

Topical hemostatic agents include thrombin, collagen and fibrin glue, or antifibrinolytic agents such as aprotinin. However, there are reports that the use of these agents increases the incidence of deep vein thrombosis. Cho et al. reported that the initial bleeding can be reduced by synovial injection of norepinephrine.

Administration of *tranexamic acid* can reduce the blood loss and blood transfusion requirement. Tranexamic acid reduces postoperative bleeding by maintaining fibrin activity through the bonding with plasminogen which is related to thrombolysis. Clinically, it is effective when an antithrombotic agent is used or in hemophilia patients in whom there is a deficiency of fibrin formation. It is administered just before the operation or before deflation of the tourniquet. It cannot reduce the bleeding if it is administered after postoperative 24 h. Lin et al. reported that they could reduce the blood loss after minimally invasive TKA by single intraoperative injection of tranexamic acid.

Postoperative management includes either no use or modification in the usage of Hemovac, allogeneic transfusion, and reinfusion of drained blood.

The insertion of Hemovac is closely related to the amount of bleeding. Parker et al. and Song et al. reported that *the amount of bleeding and transfusion could be decreased by not using Hemovac*, and Shen et al. also stated that clamping Hemovac during the first 4 postoperative hours reduced the amount of bleeding and the need for transfusion.

The most widely used method is allogeneic transfusion. *However, allogeneic transfusion has a number of potential adverse effects such as disease transmission, allergic reactions, fluid overload, infection, or immunosuppression.* The most important factor in the prediction of blood transfusion requirement is the preoperative Hb level; the lower the preoperative Hb level, the more the need for blood transfusion. Generally, *transfusion requirement and amount* of blood *are determined in relation with the amount of bleeding and Hb level.* If the Hb level drops below 10 g/dl or the amount of bleeding exceeds 1,000 cc, blood transfusion is required. When *blood transfusion is to be done, packed cells are the best choice.* It is known that one pint transfusion is meaningless, and therefore transfusion of at least 2 pints is recommended. However in practice, only 1 pint is given in many cases. Some authors suggest platelet-rich plasma transfusion for decreasing the postoperative bleeding.

Reinfusion of drained blood or cell salvage method is also available and the methods for reinfusion vary according to the filtering mechanism. The drained blood contains bone and soft tissue debris, bone marrow, activated coagulation factors, etc. The small particles less than 40 μm can pass the filter and enter into the blood stream. As a result, complications such as febrile episodes and coagulation deficiency can occur. Reinfusion within 6 h can minimize these complications. The known problem associated with reinfusion is the defect in the anticoagulation factor, but Jensen et al. reported that the amount of allogeneic transfusion could be decreased by reinfusion of the blood from Hemovac and there was no defect in the anticoagulation factor.

Kourtzis et al. introduced the Aegion protocol, which comprised of a combination of these pre- and postoperative methods depending on the hemoglobin level and expected blood loss. With this method, allogeneic transfusion requirement could be reduced by 94 % without any adverse effect during postoperative care of TKA. Slappendel and Dirksen also reported that allogeneic transfusion requirement could be reduced by 80 % using a similar method.

Pain Management

Epidural block or PCA (patient-controlled analgesia) is the most frequently used method for pain control; however, the problem with PCA is that it may cause dyspnea, lethargy, urinary dysfunction, or nausea. It is important to use strong analgesics to relieve pain as much as possible. Hartrick et al. used a single epidural norepinephrine infusion to relieve the pain, whereas Szczukowski et al. and Hunt et al. reported that they could relieve the pain and decrease the amount of narcotic use by blocking the femoral or sciatic nerve.

Local anesthetic agents have also been tried intraoperatively; Vendittoli et al., Busch et al., and Cho et al. found that the initial pain could be reduced by injecting local anesthetics around the soft tissues before closure. Some surgeons mix these agents with steroids. Joo et al. compared the effect between intra-articular injection of multimodal drug and a placebo. The cocktail injection contained bupivacaine, morphine, methylprednisolone, and epinephrine. The results revealed that multimodal drug injection did not improve patient satisfaction, range of motion, or blood loss compared with that in the placebo group.

In spite of these trials, the pain will still be severe for the first 2–3 postoperative days. The pain increases when the patient moves or when there is a swelling, and it decreases when the patients elevate the limb, an ice pack is applied, and the movement is restricted. Ice pack has an anti-inflammatory action since the release of prostaglandin E2 is sensitive to temperature. Also decreased blood flow by cryotherapy is not accompanied by decreased oxygen saturation as the metabolic activity is reduced. Hence, pharmaceutical as well as cryo-methods is performed concomitantly to relieve the pain.

Some patients believe that analgesic agents can delay the healing process, and hence, they hesitate to use them; however, there is no supporting evidence for this concept. Since the patients may experience drowsiness, nausea, and lethargy with the use of opioid analgesics, it is necessary to monitor them regularly.

Currently the preemptive pain control method is widely accepted. The basic concept is that it is probably easier to prevent the pain than to eradicate it and prevention of the initial postoperative pain makes the subsequent pain management simpler. Preemptive analgesia limits the sensitization of the nervous system in response to painful stimuli and blocks the transmission of noxious afferent impulses from the peripheral nervous system to the spinal cord and brain. Opioids, nonsteroidal anti-inflammatory drugs, and COX II inhibitors (multimodal) are commonly used before operation.

Close observation is needed when extreme pain is experienced from the first postoperative day (pain from day 1 onwards). It strongly suggests the acute infection.

Other Medications

It is recommended to *use anticoagulants* for preventing deep vein thrombosis (DVT). It has been reported that thrombosis is not very common among the oriental population. However, when DVT develops, the hospital is legally liable. Therefore anticoagulants should be used in all high-risk patients unless they have coagulopathy. This is further described in Chap. 8.

Prophylactic antibiotics can be used longer than usual in the patients who are at risk of infection; this is also described in Chap. 8.

Wound Evaluation

It is not necessary to check the wound until Hemovac is removed, and it is also acceptable to check the wound after a day or 2 days after removal of Hemovac. However, *it may be necessary to check the wound on the first postoperative day if there is the risk of developing skin necrosis due to tight closure, poor skin condition, or previous operation scar.*

If blood is seen on the outside of the gauze, there is a possibility of an increased risk of ascending infection and so the gauze should be changed immediately.

Rehabilitation

If the patient wants to change his/her position, the patient should be allowed to do so and he/she should also be allowed to get on a wheelchair with help.

Even in the early phase, the patient should begin isometric exercises when the pain becomes tolerable. The quadriceps setting exercise or ankle pump can be started in the lying down position to promote blood circulation and to prevent weakening of muscular strength.

7.1.2 Midterm Stage

The focus of management from the time of Hemovac removal until the removal of stitches is monitoring the patient's general condition, wound care, and rehabilitation.

7.1.2.1 General Condition

Although the most risky period has passed, there are a few risk factors in this stage as well.

The most important risk factor is still the cardiopulmonary problem. If the patient complains of chest pain or dyspnea, it may be due to a fresh episode of angina or myocardial infarction, aggravation of preexisting *cardiopulmonary problem*, pulmonary edema due to overhydration, or pulmonary embolism. Careful monitoring of the patient is needed immediately to initiate appropriate treatment.

If the patient shows central nervous system symptoms such as disorientation, unconsciousness, or paralysis of limbs, *fat embolism or cerebral infarction* can be suspected. However, it should be checked first whether the pain control medications are being administered in excess. It is necessary to consult a neurologist and brain CT is ordered if needed. If there is no definite lesion on brain CT, the patient's condition may return to normal in a week.

Pain management is still important during this stage. Some patients experience more severe pain temporarily after the discontinuation of PCA. If there is swelling over the operated lower limbs and the pain is accompanied by mild fever, the work-up for DVT is needed. In case of thrombosis, a physician is consulted for initiation of heparin treatment.

Routine checkup such as CBC and urinalysis is checked immediate postoperatively and on the 3rd postoperative day or before discharge. Chemical tests are helpful for detecting toxic hepatitis which may have developed due to anesthesia and pain medications.

Other general symptoms are *voiding disorders, anorexia, insomnia, mild fever, etc.* Voiding disorder is generally temporary, but some patients develop an atonic bladder which requires an insertion of a urinary catheter and a few days of training. Most patients experience anorexia due to pain, lethargy, nausea, or insomnia. As wound healing is closely related to nutrition, it is important to restore the patient's appetite, although it is not very easy to do so. Antiemetics would be of help in some patients. If anorexia persists, it is sometimes necessary to provide nutrition through the IV route. Anorexia may also be caused due to gastritis, activation of peptic ulcer, or abdominal pain. If the symptoms persist for days, it is recommended to consult a physician.

Insomnia is caused due to postoperative pain, changes in the environment, etc. Since sleep is important for the patient's psychological and physical condition, hypnotics should be given so that the patient gets sufficient sleep. Hypnotics are also prescribed on discharge as sleeplessness often persists for a long time after discharge.

If the patient has fever, appropriate management should be initiated considering all the possibilities such as absorption fever, drug side effects, reaction to transfusion, thrombosis, pneumonia, urinary infection, ileus, and wound infection.

7.1.2.2 Wound Care

Wound condition is a very critical issue and must not be overlooked. Even if the operation was successful, the wound problem can cause limited ROM and it may progress to deep infection.

Dressing once every 3–4 days is enough unless any special conditions preexist. When performing wound dressing, any sign of infection, skin necrosis, or serous discharge from the incision or Hemovac insertion site should be carefully examined. *If there is a wound problem, active treatment should be started to prevent deep infection and to preserve the prosthesis*. Delayed management can cause limited ROM and pain even though the prosthesis is saved.

If there are any factors that may interfere with wound healing, they should be corrected; transfusion is needed if hemoglobin level drops below 10 g/dl and nutrition supply through an IV can be provided if there is hypoalbuminemia. If the blood sugar level is too high, it should be corrected and the patient should be asked to quit smoking as it can cause vasoconstriction and hamper wound healing.

Wound-related problems include serous discharge, tense hematoma, bullae, and superficial skin necrosis. These wound-related problems can cause full-thickness skin necrosis exposing the prosthesis and causing a deep infection.

If there is a *serous discharge* from the wound, a *wound swab should be taken for wound culture* and it should be checked whether the skin and subcutaneous sutures were done properly. *It is necessary to detect the source of the discharge*; if the discharge increases a lot during joint motion, it may be from inside of the joint. When discharge is noted, *sufficient gauze should be applied for compression dressing* so that the discharge is not exposed to the air, and *the ROM exercises such as CPM should be discontinued*. Prophylactic antibiotics can be continued. If the discharge persists for 4–5 days despite these managements or if it is assumed to be originating from inside of the joint, debridement can be considered in the operation room.

Hematoma develops in all patients in the early to midterm stage. Hence, the amount and the site of hematoma matter. *Tense excessive hematoma causes pain, compartment syndrome, and bullae formation, and it interferes with wound healing*. If bleeding or severe swelling persists, it becomes necessary to relieve it by all means. First, the joint exercises such as CPM should be restricted and discontinuation of anticoagulants should be carefully considered. It should be checked whether Hemovac is functioning properly if it has not yet been removed; resuming its function can help in reducing the hematoma. If Hemovac has already been removed, the total amount of bleeding from Hemovac is calculated in order to determine the method of management based on the amount of drained blood. If not much blood has drained, it is highly probable that Hemovac has not been functioning properly. In such a case, joint aspiration can be performed from the wound to reduce the pressure. Aspiration should be done carefully as it may cause persistent drainage from the aspiration site.

If the hematoma persists or if there is a risk of skin necrosis despite Hemovac has been functioning properly, it may be necessary to do angiography or to open the joint to identify the possible causes. However, this is not an easy decision to make. When the wound is opened, exploration should be focused on persistent bleeding from the lateral inferior genicular artery or middle genicular artery.

Sometimes, *bullae* develop due to swelling or poor venous circulation when the elastic bandage is too tight. If the bullae are peeled off, it can be painful and there is an increased risk of infection. Loosening the bandage, draining out the fluid with a syringe, and drying up the bullae is a more effective treatment method and is associated with less pain.

Since the wounds are likely to be accompanied with mild fever and swelling, it is recommended to apply an ice pack for about 20 min every 1–2 h. However, it should be avoided if there is any sign of skin necrosis as it may cause vasoconstriction.

7.1.2.3 Rehabilitation

After arthroplasty, *the purpose of rehabilitation is to maintain a healthy physical condition, improve the joint function, reduce complications, and extend the survival of the prosthesis*. Therefore, rehabilitation is essential for successful results. *Rehabilitation should be safe and effective and should progress gradually*.

Rehabilitation therapies should be individualized according to the patient's weight, activity, method of operation, and type of prosthesis used, and hence, there cannot be a standardized rehabilitation program. In particular, rehabilitation varies according to cementing or not, bone grafting, and ancillary procedures of the extensor mechanism. Also *the rehabilitation program should not be time bound. This means that if one goal is achieved earlier than expected, the next program can be started.*

Patient's muscular strength is decreased and the ROM is reduced postoperatively due to pain and muscle contracture. Postoperative rehabilitation includes ROM exercises, muscle-strengthening exercise, gait training, and recreation activities.

ROM Exercises

The range of motion is closely related to the function. *For performing activities of daily living, the flexion contracture should be less than 10° and flexion should be more than 95°.*

If a *rectus snip has been performed, the ROM exercises should be delayed by 2–3 weeks*. Even if other quadricepsplasty such as V–Y turndown has been performed, gentle limited ROM exercises should begin at 3–4 weeks as immobilization for 5–6 weeks significantly reduces the ROM. On the other hand, there is no need to delay the ROM exercises if a tibial tubercle osteotomy has been performed.

A preoperative flexion contracture has adverse effect on the postoperative ROM. If the patient has a flexion contracture of more than 20° preoperatively, further enhanced exercise program is needed postoperatively.

ROM exercises can be divided into active, passive, and continuous passive motion (CPM) exercises.

Active exercises are undertaken by the patients themselves and the rehabilitation program is focused on assisting the patient to perform the exercises. Active exercises include sitting on the edge of the bed, dropping and dangling the knee from the bed, bending the knee using a chair, and slowly squatting while holding a walker. Passive exercises are performed with assistance from the trained personnel according to the schedule. Passive exercises include bending the knee with a weight on the ankle while supporting the thigh with the patients' hands, bending the knee with the aid of a suspension sling, and passive manipulation by the physiotherapist. Those surgeons who prefer active exercises emphasize that there is no significant difference between active and passive exercises in terms of the final ROM. Repeated vigorous passive exercises aggravate the pain and causes arthrofibrosis resulting in a further limited ROM. Fox and Poss revealed that *repeated manipulation of the joint in patients with poor ROM improved the ROM initially, but the ROM was significantly decreased a year later.*

Whether or not to use CPM (continuous passive motion) and when to start CPM is also controversial. Surgeons who recommend CPM state that early ROM exercises play an important role in increasing the final range of motion. *With CPM, gradual and consistent ROM exercises can be performed in the early stage with less pain*, and it has the advantage of a shorter hospital stay. Johnson reported that CPM improved the range of motion at the long-term follow-up. However, Colwell and Morris stated that using CPM does not improve the range of motion, but reduces the pain and the duration of hospital stay. On the other hand, some surgeons *do not recommend CPM as it interferes with wound healing due to reduction in the oxygen tension of the tissues*, and it is an expensive treatment providing no significant ROM improvement. Pope et al. reported that CPM did not improve the range of motion, rather it *increased the use of pain killers and bleeding*. McInners et al. stated that there was no difference in the postoperative pain and the range of motion was same after 6 weeks with the use of CPM.

For several reasons, CPM is started not immediately after the operation but after removal of Hemovac. First, if CPM is started with Hemovac at the site, it can increase the amount of bleeding. Second, early CPM can affect wound healing. Third, CPM tends to aggravate the preexisting flexion contracture in the early stage of postoperative period. Finally, CPM can intensify the pain in the early postoperative stage.

When CPM is done, it is started from 30° and the angle is increased gradually till the pain is tolerable. It is recommended to increase the angle by 5–10° daily and continue

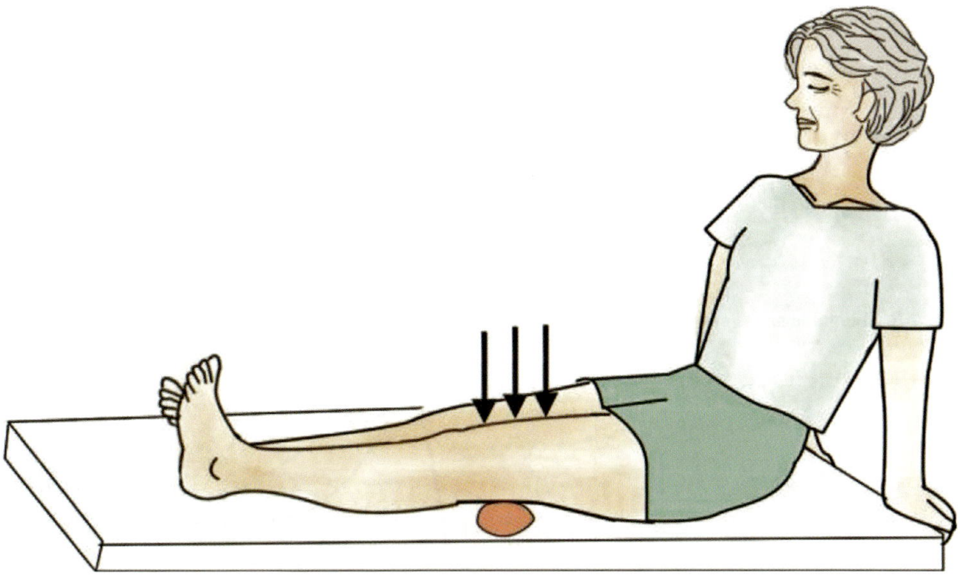

Fig. 7.1 Quadriceps setting exercise

CPM for more than 3 h a day. However, *it is advisable to discontinue the CPM if wound condition is poor or there is a risk of skin necrosis*. Colwell and Morris recommended that *the angle of CPM should not exceed 40° during the first 4 days as early CPM may result in decrease in the oxygen tension of the tissues*.

As the CPM angle does not coincide with the real knee joint motion, it should be remembered that the CPM angle is different from the real ROM.

If the *joint's ROM is seriously limited after the usual rehabilitation method, brisement can be performed under anesthesia. Brisement is most effective when performed within 3 weeks*; Yang et al reported good results by performing brisement under IV regional block in patients with flexion motion less than 90°.

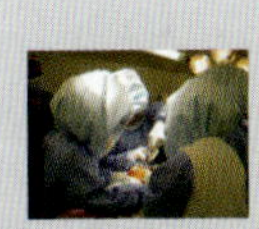

Author's Method

I believe that passive exercise would be needed if a certain degree of ROM is not achieved in the midterm stage. I have seen many patients who are fearful to undergo rehabilitation due to the pain during the early period and miss the appropriate time to improve the ROM.

The goal is to achieve a range of motion between 10° and 90° within the first week. Passive knee flexion is started if this goal is not achieved. Once 90° of flexion has been achieved, I allow the patients to select their exercise method.

Muscle-Strengthening Exercises

There are various muscle-strengthening exercises, and they should be performed consistently even after a few months.

Quadriceps Setting Exercise

Quadriceps setting exercise (QSE) is the most basic exercise and the patient should be trained preoperatively so that he/she can perform this exercise as soon as they wake up from the anesthesia.

For easy understanding of the patient, the patient is taught that this exercise is an "egg-breaking" exercise. It is performed as if an egg is placed under the knee joint and the patient has to break it with the knee extension motion. The patient is taught to extend the knee by performing quadriceps contraction for about 5 s and resting for 1 s (Fig. 7.1).

Ankle Pump Exercise

This exercise comprises of extending and flexing the ankle joint in supine position. It not only improves the muscular strength but also improves blood circulation of the lower limb (Fig. 7.2).

Straight Leg Raise Exercise

The operated leg is raised with the opposite knee bent (Fig. 7.3). Some patients cannot do the leg raising exercise due to the extension force rather than the flexion force of the hip joint. In such a case, phase conversion may be needed. The therapist supports the heel in the leg elevated position and the patient is asked to hold the leg up while the therapist removes his/her hand cautiously. Then hip extension power is converted into flexion power. In most of the cases, the patient is allowed to walk when the patient can raise the limb, but some patients gradually gain the strength to raise the leg as they start walking.

Fig. 7.2 Ankle pump exercise

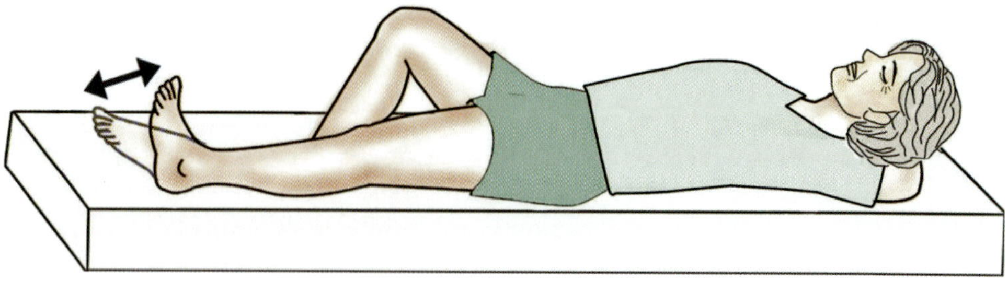

Fig. 7.3 Straight leg raise exercise

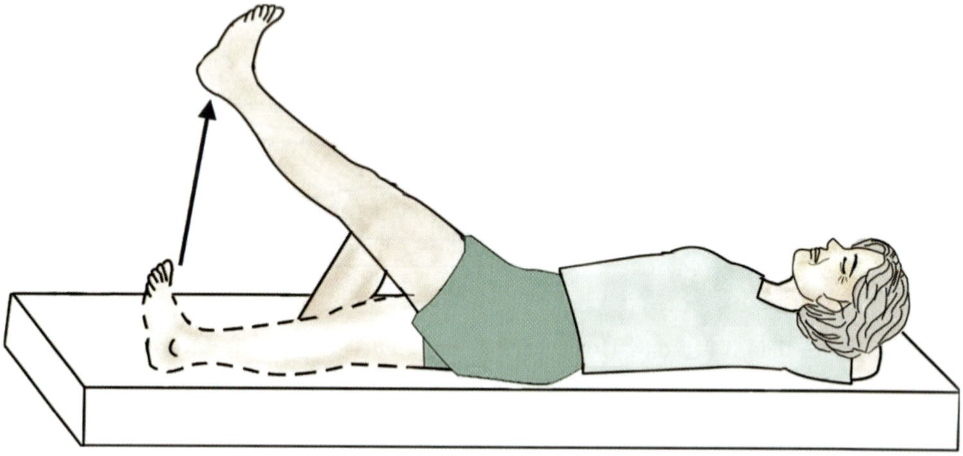

Other Exercises

The above-mentioned exercises are the most basic muscle-strengthening exercises. Other exercises include heel slide, knee press, and heel raise. Sometimes, Thera-Band with variable elasticity or electric stimulation can be used to improve the muscle power.

Modification of Exercises Program

These exercises are performed 2–3 times a day, and 30 repetitions are done at each time.

When performing these exercises, it is necessary to know their relationship with back pain. *Straight leg raise exercise is actually a provocative test for low back pain, and ankle pump exercise can also provoke back pain* in patients who do not have back pain, or it can *aggravate the preexisting back pain*. Since most of the elderly patients have back problems to a greater or lesser extent, this is not an infrequent occurrence. *If back pain occurs or worsens, it is necessary to discontinue the straight leg raise or ankle pump exercises* and perform the alternative exercises. Alternative exercises should also be discontinued if they cause back pain.

Gait Training

The initiation of gait training is determined based on whether the prosthesis is fixed with cement, whether bone grafting has been performed, whether or not a simultaneous operation has been performed and the level of muscular strength. If the patient cannot stand still due to dizziness, it is necessary to impart balance training before walking.

If the usual arthroplasty has been performed and the postoperative recovery has been uneventful, walking with a walker is allowed after postoperative 2–3 days as long as the patient can tolerate. In cementless fixation, weight bearing is not recommended until postoperative 4 weeks, and many surgeons recommend that full weight bearing should not be allowed earlier than postoperative 6–8 weeks. *In case of bone grafting, initial stability is important for the incorporation of grafted bone and weight bearing is allowed after 4–6 weeks*. However, toe touch gait for partial weight bearing with 10–15 kg may be tried earlier than 4–6 weeks.

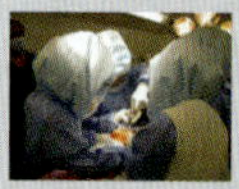

Author's Method

I allow every ordinary TKA patient to start walking with a walker on postoperative 3–4 days.

If the patient complains feeling of instability while walking, I always perform stress test on the knee joints. If there is no instability on stress test, the feeling comes from muscle weakness and I encourage the patient to strengthen the muscle power. If there is instability, I recommend brace fitting for 6 weeks until the ligaments that are responsible for the instability are scar bound.

7.1.3 Late Stage

After the stitches have been removed, the patients themselves should self-monitor their knee condition. Analgesics, anti-inflammatory drugs, and hypnotics are prescribed on discharge.

In this stage, the patient must continue the ROM and muscle-strengthening exercises so as to improve function. The patient is gradually weaned off the walker or crutches when the pain in the knee joint becomes tolerable and muscle power is improved.

As the patients should self-monitor, education regarding the warning signs of possible complications should be provided. The possible complications include wound problem, DVT, and infection.

If the patients develop any sign of the above complications, they should visit the hospital, and a careful checkup should be performed for their detection.

If the postoperative course is smooth, the patients are encouraged to increase their daily activities including stair walking, driving, and recreational activity. Light sports as well as occupational therapy can follow.

7.2 Education

Patients should be educated before discharge regarding "how to tackle" and "what to do" when something happens to the operated knee joint. Most of the patients would feel more pain after discharge and become anxious even after minor problems. *Explaining the progression of the postoperative course also helps to relieve the patients' anxiety and to increase their satisfaction*. It is necessary to explain regarding the pain, muscle weakness, motion limitation, loss of sensation on the lateral part of incision, crepitus sound, and heat sensation, which are noted in nearly every patient during the postoperative period.

One of the most common complaints is crepitus in the knee joint. Sharkey and Miller reported that about 63 % of patients experienced crepitus even after postoperative 6 months. The causes of crepitus are swelling, friction or fibrosis of the soft tissues, and impingement of the prosthesis. Crepitus not associated with pain is likely to disappear without the occurrence of any event. Many patients complain that the knee is heavy and feels somewhat unnatural, but these symptoms gradually disappear after 6 months. Also, hypoesthesia on the lateral side of the incision site is likely to improve to normal or near normal in 1 year.

Patients can take a shower or bath when the wound is completely healed. Close attention should be paid while applying the hot pack as the patients can experience burns due to the loss of sensation on the lateral side of the incision. The use of a cold pack is recommended more than that of a hot pack if there is heat sensation in the knee joint during exercise.

Muscle-strengthening exercises and ROM exercises must be continued at home.

Gait training is performed in a descending order of stability by the use of a walker, crutches, cane, and unsupported walking according to the patient's condition. *If possible, full weight bearing should be possible within 4–6 weeks*, and side step is allowed when the patient's walking improves.

Climbing up and down the stairs is also increased gradually according to the patient's condition. *When climbing up the stairs, the first step is taken with the healthy limb, followed by the operated limb and then the crutches or cane. When going down the stairs, the first step is taken with the crutches or cane, followed by the operated limb and then the healthy limb.*

The most important issue is the education about the prevention and management of infection. Patients should be instructed to visit the hospital if crust or skin necrosis develops on the wound, and local heat, general fever, or the pain tends to increase. *If possible, any major surgery that can last for more than 2 h should be delayed until at least postoperative 6 months*. In case an *invasive diagnostic method or tooth extraction* needs to be performed, it is necessary to let the physician prescribe *prophylactic antibiotics before performing these procedures*. However, some surgeons state that tooth extraction is not related to postoperative infection. What is most important is to get rid of infection source and not to delay the treatment of infectious disease. So, other infectious diseases such as common cold or urinary infection should be treated as early as possible. It is safer to perform any *major elective surgery* after at least postoperative 2 years; however, it is sometimes not very practical to wait for such a long time.

It is known that the knee joint returns to its normal condition *after postoperative 8 weeks* in order to be able to step on the brake pedal for *driving*. Therefore, it is safe for the patient to check his/her brake response time and *resume driving after 8 weeks*. However, Dalury et al. evaluated the brake response time and reported that the time to resume driving can be shortened to 4 weeks with the advancement of surgical technique, pain management, and rehabilitation.

Youm et al. surveyed 336 members of the American Academy of Hip and Knee Surgeons (AAHKS) and reported that full weight bearing was allowed at an average of 3.6 weeks, driving at an average of 5 weeks, and climbing up the ladder at 9 weeks in case of TKA with cementing. Fifty percent of responders answered that they allowed their patients to lift 50 lb after 14 weeks, but I believe that this weight is too heavy and is best avoided in the early period.

It is necessary to inform the patients that they are prohibited from *doing laborious work such as lifting heavy objects, squatting, walking for long hours, and going up and down the stairs frequently*.

The patient may be allowed to return to *sports* gradually as long as the joints are not stressed too much. If the operated joint is under excess loading or has undergone trauma, it can cause instability, loosening, or wear of the prosthesis. Therefore, *low-impact sports should be recommended.* Riding a bicycle on flat land, ballroom dancing, playing golf, skiing on gentle slopes, swimming, and walking may be allowed whenever possible, but some surgeons have different opinions regarding the activity of playing golf. Bowling, jazz dancing, bicycling, walking with quick steps, and table tennis can also be permitted, whereas skating, inline skating, and skiing should be allowed only in those patients who have a previous experience of these sports. Aerobics or tennis doubles may be allowed with the surgeon's permission. However, Rosenberg et al. advised that extra care is required for jogging and tennis as they impose excessive stress on the knee joint. *Higher impact sports that require techniques or competitive physical contact sports such as soccer, baseball, volleyball, handball, tennis singles, and hockey should be prohibited.*

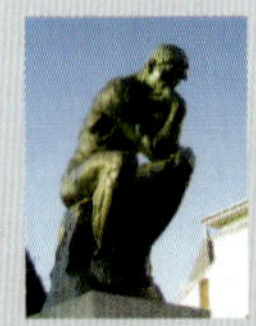

Author's Opinion

I allow swimming only in those patients who already know how to swim. When a person who cannot swim tries to learn swimming with an operated knee, the knee is likely to be exposed to excessive stress or injury.

Walking in the water is good for balance training, but it should be carefully done in the early postoperative period and it requires assistance. The buoyancy lightens the body in the water, but water resistance is much more than air resistance. Therefore even the healthy people, needs more strength while walking in the water.

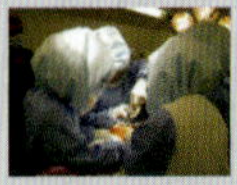

Author's Method

I personally hand over to the patients a booklet which they can take home after discharge and it has proved to be very useful. I have written the postoperative course in the booklet based on my experience. The brief summary is as follows.

There can be stinging pain along the incision scar for up to 6 weeks, and the pain may appear intermittently up to 3 months. I try to reassure the patient if there are no major problems on regular checkup. When the recovery is fast, the patients can walk without a walker or cane after 6 weeks. Walking distance should also be increased gradually. Simple calculation for determining the walking time is 10 multiplied by the postoperative period (months). For example, at postoperative 3 months, the patient is allowed to walk for 30 min, and at postoperative 6 months, the patient is allowed to walk for 60 min without resting. Walking for more than 1 h is allowed depending on the patient's condition.

The decreased sensation in the lateral part of the incision can persist for more than a year. I also emphasize that mild fever and swelling over the knee joint is normal during exercise or physiotherapy in the early postoperative period. Also, the crepitus may disappear spontaneously after a certain period of time and it is not a major problem even if the crepitus does not disappear.

I instruct the patients to do the ROM exercises until they can flex the knee by more than 90° by the first 2 weeks and then gradually increase flexion motion beyond 120°.

Since infection is the most serious complication, I inform the patients regarding the methods of prevention and what they should do when an infection is suspected. I do not allow invasive diagnostic procedure until postoperative 3 months and tooth extraction, vaccination, and major surgery until 6 months, if possible. I pay special attention for taking care of these patients so as not to miss the appropriate timing of management.

7.3 Follow-Up

Patients should be asked to follow up at postoperative 6 weeks, 3 months, 6 months, and 1 year and annually thereafter.

The most important goal of performing a regular checkup is to evaluate the pain and function. *Pain that aggravates over time or pain that cannot be tolerated should be evaluated considering its duration, severity, and causes so that appropriate treatment can be given.* The ROM and instability should also be checked for postoperative evaluation, and weight-bearing X-rays should be taken.

If the knee joint motion is limited, the causes should be identified. A flexion contracture of less than 10° is often corrected naturally in a year, and patients who achieved flexion of 95° or greater are encouraged to exercise without performing any additional procedure. If the patient can achieve flexion of less than 95°, more active ROM exercises are prescribed and frequent checkup is recommended. If flexion motion is less than 70°, brisement, arthroscopic surgery, or revision can be considered.

Major complications such as infection, wear, or loosening are treated according to their severity and progress. This is described in Chap. 8.

It is necessary to calculate the HSS score, KS score, and WOMAC score annually for the purpose of feedback and research.

Bibliography

Amin A, Watson A, Mangwani J, et al. A prospective randomised controlled trial of autologous retransfusion in total knee replacement. J Bone Joint Surg Br. 2008;90-B:451–4.

Busch CA, Shore BJ, Bhandari R, et al. Efficacy of periarticular multimodal drug injection in total knee arthroplasty. A randomized trial. J Bone Joint Surg Am. 2006;88-A:959–63.

Charoencholvanich K, Siriwattanasakul P. Tranexamic acid reduces blood loss and blood transfusion after TKA: a prospective randomized controlled trial. Clin Orthop. 2011;469:2874–80.

Cho WS, Kim JM, Ahn HS, et al. The effect of norepinephrine irrigation in primary total knee replacement arthroplasty. J Korean Orthop Assoc. 2004;39:247–51.

Cho WS, Youm YS, Yoon YS, et al. The effect of intraoperative regional analgesic injection in total knee arthroplasty. J Korean Orthop Assoc. 2006;41:989–93.

Clark CR, Spratt KF, Blondin M, et al. Perioperative autotransfusion in total hip and knee arthroplasty. J Arthroplasty. 2006;21: 23–35.

Colwell CW, Morris RN. The influence of continuous passive motion on the results of total knee arthroplasty. Clin Orthop. 1992;276:225–8.

Cushner FD. Preventing wound complication after total knee arthroplasty. In: Callaghan JJ, editor. The adult knee. 1st ed. Philadelphia, PA: Lippincott Williams & Wilkins; 2003. p. 1341–9.

Dalury DF, Lieberman JR, MacDonald SJ. Current and innovative pain management techniques in total knee arthroplasty. J Bone Joint Surg Am. 2011;93-A:1938–43.

Dalury DF, Tucker KK, Kelley TC. When can I drive?: brake response times after contemporary total knee arthroplasty. Clin Orthop. 2011;469:82–6.

D'Lima DD, Steklov N, Patil S, et al. The Mark Coventry Award: in vivo knee forces during recreation and exercise after knee arthroplasty. Clin Orthop. 2008;466:2605–11.

Denis M, Moffet H, Caron F, et al. Effectiveness of continuous passive motion and conventional physical therapy after total knee arthroplasty: a randomized clinical trial. Phys Ther. 2006;86: 174–85.

Deutsch A, Spaulding J, Marcus RE. Preoperative epoetin alfa vs autologous blood donation in primary total knee arthroplasty. J Arthroplasty. 2006;21:628–35.

Dorr LD, Raya J, Long WT, et al. Multimodal analgesia without parenteral narcotics for total knee arthroplasty. J Arthroplasty. 2008;23:502–8.

Ecker M, Lotke PA. Postoperative care of the total knee patient. Orthop Clin North Am. 1989;20:55–62.

Fox JL, Poss R. The role of manipulation following total knee replacement. J Bone Joint Surg Am. 1981;63-A:357–62.

Cushner F. Transfusion avoidance, blood loss, management, and total knee arthroplasty. In: Scott WN, editor. Surgery of the knee. 4th ed. Philadelphia, PA: Churchill Livingstone; 2006. p. 1828–36.

Gotlin RS. Rehabilitation. In: Scuderi GR, editor. Surgical techniques in total knee arthroplasty. 1st ed. New York, NY: Springer; 2002. p. 651–79.

Hartrick CT, Martin G, Kantor G, et al. Evaluation of a single-dose, extended-release epidural morphine formulation for pain after knee arthroplasty. J Bone Joint Surg Am. 2006;88-A:273–81.

Hatzidakis AM, Mendick RM, McKillip T, et al. Preoperative autologous donation for total knee arthroplasty: an analysis of risk factors for allogenic transfusion. J Bone Joint Surg Am. 2000;82-A:89–100.

Hunt KJ, Bourne MH, Mariani EM. Single-injection femoral and sciatic nerve blocks for pain control after total knee arthroplasty. J Arthroplasty. 2009;24:533–8.

Jensen CM, Pilegaard R, Hviid K, et al. Quality of reinfused blood drainage after total knee arthroplasty. J Arthroplasty. 1999;14: 312–8.

Johnson DP. The effect of continuous passive motion on wound healing and joint mobility after knee arthroplasty. J Bone Joint Surg. 1990;72-A:421–6.

Joo JH, Park JW, Kim JS, et al. Is intra-articular multimodal drug injection effective in pain management after total knee arthroplasty? A randomized, double-blinded, prospective study. J Arthroplasty. 2011;26:1095–9.

Keating EM, Meding JB. Perioperative blood management practices in elective orthopedic surgery. J Am Acad Orthop Surg. 2002;10: 393–400.

Keating EM, Ritter MA. Transfusion options in total joint arthroplasty. J Arthroplasty. 2002;17:125–8.

Kourtzis N, Pafilas D, Kasimatis G. Blood saving protocol in elective total knee arthroplasty. Am J Surg. 2004;187:261–7.

Lemos MJ, Healy WL. Blood transfusion in orthopaedic operations. J Bone Joint Surg Am. 1996;78-A:1260–70.

Lin PC, Hsu CH, Huang CC, et al. The blood-saving effect of tranexamic acid in minimally invasive total knee arthroplasty: is an additional pre-operative injection effective? J Bone Joint Surg Br. 2012;94-B:932–6.

McInners J, Larson MG, Daltroy LH, et al. A controlled evaluation of continuous passive motion in patients undergoing total knee arthroplasty. JAMA. 1992;268:1423–8.

McNair PJ, Marshall RN, Maguire K. Swelling of the knee joint: effects of exercise on quadriceps muscle strength. Arch Phys Med Rehabil. 1996;77:896–9.

Michelson JD, Lotke PA, Steinberg ME. Urinary-bladder management after total joint replacement surgery. N Engl J Med. 1988; 319:321–6.

Mizner RL, Petterson SC, Stevens JE, et al. Early quadriceps strength loss after total knee arthroplasty. The contributions of muscle atrophy and failure of voluntary muscle activation. J Bone Joint Surg Am. 2005;87-A:1047–53.

Mullaji A, Kanna R, Shetty GM, et al. Efficacy of periarticular injection of bupivacaine, fentanyl, and methylprednisolone in total knee arthroplasty: a prospective, randomized trial. J Arthroplasty. 2010;25:851–7.

Pang HN, Lo NN, Yang KY, et al. Peri-articular steroid injection improves the outcome after unicondylar knee replacement: a prospective, randomised controlled trial with a two-year follow-up. J Bone Joint Surg Br. 2008;90-B:738–44.

Park KK, Kim TK, Chang CB, et al. Normative temporal values of CRP and ESR in unilateral and staged bilateral TKA. Clin Orthop. 2008;466:179–88.

Parker MJ, Roberts CP, Hay D. Closed suction drainage for hip and knee arthroplasty. A metaanalysis. J Bone Joint Surg Am. 2004; 86-A:1146–52.

Peters CL, Shirley B, Erickson J. The effect of a new multimodal perioperative anesthetic regimen on postoperative pain, side effects, rehabilitation, and length of hospital stay after total joint arthroplasty. J Arthroplasty. 2006;21 Suppl 2:132–8.

Pope RO, Corcoran S, McCaul K, et al. Continuous passive motion after primary total knee arthroplasty. Does it offer any benefits? J Bone Joint Surg Br. 1997;79-B:914–7.

Ralley FE, Berta D, Binns V, et al. One intraoperative dose of tranexamic acid for patients having primary hip or knee arthroplasty. Clin Orthop. 2010;468:1905–11.

Rosenberg AG. Reducing blood loss in total joint surgery with a saline-coupled bipolar sealing technology. J Arthroplasty. 2007; 22:82–5.

Sculco TP. Global blood management in orthopaedic surgery. Clin Orthop. 1998;357:43–9.

Sharkey PF, Miller AJ. Noise, numbness, and kneeling difficulties after total knee arthroplasty: is the outcome affected? J Arthroplasty. 2011;26:1427–31.

Sharrock NE. Postoperative pain management. In: Scuderi GR, editor. Surgical techniques in total knee arthroplasty. 1st ed. New York, NY: Springer; 2002. p. 680–6.

Shen PC, Jou IM, Lin YT, et al. Comparison between 4-hour clamping drainage and nonclamping drainage after total knee arthroplasty. J Arthroplasty. 2005;20:909–13.

Slappendel R, Dirksen R. An algorithm to reduce allogenic red blood cell transfusion for major orthopedic surgery. Acta Orthop Scand. 2003;74:569–75.

Song MH, Kim BH, Kim TH. Is suction drainage necessary after total knee arthroplasty? J Korean Orthop Assoc. 2004;39:186–91.

Stålman A, Berglund L, Dungnerc E, et al. Temperature-sensitive release of prostaglandin E_2 and diminished energy requirements in synovial tissue with postoperative cryotherapy: a prospective randomized study after knee arthroscopy. J Bone Joint Surg Am. 2011;93-A:1961–8.

Stulberg BN, Zadzilka JD. Blood management issues using blood management strategies. J Arthroplasty. 2007;22:95–8.

Szczukowski Jr MJ, Hines JA, Snell JA, et al. Femoral nerve block for total knee arthroplasty patients: a method to control postoperative pain. J Arthroplasty. 2004;19:720–5.

Uckay I, Pittet D, Bernard L, et al. Antibiotic prophylaxis before invasive dental procedures in patients with arthroplasties of the hip and knee. J Bone Joint Surg Br. 2008;90-B:833–8.

Ulrich SD, Bhave A, Marker DR, et al. Focused rehabilitation treatment of poorly functioning total knee arthroplasties. Clin Orthop. 2007;464:138–45.

Underhill MA. Nursing care of a patient having a total knee arthroplasty. In: Scott WN, editor. The knee. 1st ed. St. Louise, MO: Mosby; 1994. p. 1229–38.

Vendittoli PA, Makinen P, Drolet P, et al. A multimodal analgesia protocol for total knee arthroplasty. A randomized, controlled study. J Bone Joint Surg Am. 2006;88-A:282–9.

Ververeli PA, Sutton DC, Hearn SL, et al. Continuous passive motion after total knee arthroplasty. Clin Orthop. 1995;321: 208–14.

Walker RH, Morris BA, Angulo DC, et al. Postoperative use of continuous passive motion, transcutaneous electrical nerve stimulation, and continuous cooling pad following total knee arthroplasty. J Arthroplasty. 1991;6:151–6.

Yang IH, Kim SH, Han CD. Early manipulation for flexion limitation after total knee arthroplasty. J Korean Knee Soc. 2004;16: 88–93.

Youm T, Maurer SG, Stuchin SA. Postoperative management after total hip and knee arthroplasty. J Arthroplasty. 2005;20: 322–4.

8 Complications

Since the purpose of arthroplasty is to reduce the pain and to maximize function for long term, the surgery cannot be considered successful if these goals are not achieved.

Although it is not clear as to what should be included under complications, it is a generally accepted concept to include all undesirable postoperative conditions under the heading of complications. These comprise of systemic complications and complications pertaining to the knee joint and may be caused due to the factors related to the patient, prosthesis, and/or the surgery.

8.1 Systemic Complications

Systemic complications are more common after TKA than after THA. These include myocardial infarction, pulmonary embolism, shock, cerebrovascular accident, renal failure, urinary retention, ileus, other organ infection, and deep vein thrombosis (DVT). Although not always possible, prevention of these complications is of utmost importance as they can lead to fatal results.

Once complications such as cerebrovascular accident, cardiopulmonary disease, or urinary retention occur, they are beyond the scope of management by an orthopedic surgeon. Although the help of a physician is required for management of complications such as deep vein thrombosis and fat embolism, I would like to describe them here since the orthopedic surgeons are required to diagnose and prevent these complications during the early postoperative period.

8.1.1 Deep Vein Thrombosis

Thrombosis occurs in the veins of the operated limb, and it interferes with the blood flow. *When the thrombus migrates into the cardiopulmonary system and causes a pulmonary embolism (PE), fatal results can occur*. Sometimes the term *VTE (venous thromboembolism) is often used pertaining to both DVT and PE*.

8.1.1.1 Etiology

The first stimulus that causes the formation of a thrombus develops during the perioperative period. It is assumed that it is caused by changes in coagulation factors due to the operation, vascular injury, use of tourniquet, and venous stasis due to long-term immobilization of the lower limbs. The use of tourniquet is controversial; Harvey et al. reported that the incidence of thrombosis was not related to the time of tourniquet inflation, but Aglietti et al. stated that the incidence of thrombosis increased when a tourniquet was not used.

8.1.1.2 Incidence

The incidence of thrombosis increases by about 20 times after a major operation. The incidence varies according to patients' risk factors, method of operation and anesthesia, ambulation period, and preventive anticoagulation therapy.

It is generally known that thrombosis is more common among patients who are *older, obese, have cancer, have a history of cardiopulmonary disease, have inherited coagulation disorder, have uncontrolled diabetes, or have been immobilized for long time*. Preoperative walking helps in the prevention of thrombosis; Pearse et al. reported that the incidence of thrombosis drops significantly when the patient is instructed to walk 24 h prior to the operation. The incidence of thrombosis after arthroplasty seems to vary among different races.

The incidence of thrombosis is known to decrease when continuous epidural anesthesia and regional anesthesia are used. Some authors reported an incidence of thrombosis of 58 % after simultaneous operation and of 75 % after two-stage operation when preventive measures were not taken. However, these incidences also vary according to the type of thrombosis. *Thrombosis can be classified into asymptomatic thrombosis which has no definite symptoms and gradually disappears, and symptomatic thrombosis*. The above incidences are those including asymptomatic thrombosis. The incidence of symptomatic thrombosis is 15–25 % and 0.1–2.0 % among them causes pulmonary embolism that can lead to death. Lotke and Lonner reported that *the incidence of*

W. Cho, *Knee Joint Arthroplasty*,
DOI 10.1007/978-3-642-39389-1_8,

fatal pulmonary embolism is very low and the correlation between pulmonary embolism and deep vein thrombosis is inconsistent.

The incidence of thrombosis after THA and after TKA is also different. Overall, thrombosis is less frequent after TKA than after THA. Symptomatic proximal vein thrombosis is common after THA. On the other hand, isolated proximal vein thrombosis rarely occurs after TKA, and the majority of thrombotic episodes are due to asymptomatic calf vein thrombosis. Also, 10–15 % of patients *experience thrombosis in the unoperated leg.*

The time of onset of thrombosis after THA and after TKA is different. The majority of thrombotic episodes occur during the first week after TKA, whereas the majority of thrombotic episodes occur during the first 3–4 weeks after THA.

8.1.1.3 Symptoms

Since most episodes of thrombosis are clinically silent, the only presentation could be in the form of unexpected death.

Post-thrombotic syndrome comprises of three or more of the following symptoms: swelling, skin induration, hyperpigmentation, venous ectasia, redness, pain on calf compression, and venous ulceration. The etiology of post-thrombotic syndrome is venous hypertension caused due to venous occlusion. The symptoms develop due to increased tissue pressure. However, many of these symptoms can occur postoperatively without the presence of thrombosis, so these cannot be considered as the pathognomonic symptoms of thrombosis. Some patients complain of persistent swelling over the calf at the regular follow-up, and I think the diagnosis in such cases would be post-thrombotic syndrome as a result of the development of microthrombi.

8.1.1.4 Diagnosis

Since many cases of thrombosis are asymptomatic, the diagnosis cannot be made based on the symptoms alone. *The D-dimer level, duplex sonography, and venography are the common diagnostic tools for DVT*, and these procedures should be performed when DVT is suspected.

Since checking the D-dimer level is simple, it is used as a screening test. Fibrin, the most important factor for coagulation, is broken down into fibrin degradation product (FDP) and D-dimer by plasmin, which is a fibrinolytic enzyme. Therefore, an increase in the D-dimer level indicates an increase of fibrin, which means that thrombus formation has occurred. However, the D-dimer level may be increased in inflammatory diseases and cancer. For the interpretation of the D-dimer level, if the level of D-dimer is normal, it suggests that there is no probability of DVT. However, if the D-dimer level is high, it does not always indicate DVT.

Duplex sonography is a good diagnostic method as it is noninvasive, relatively easy to perform and can detect the site and size of the thrombus along with the hemodynamic information of the thrombus. Brassard et al. stated that duplex sonography is very accurate when performed by an experienced examiner. However, it has low specificity and is used as a screening test.

Venography is accurate, but it is an invasive method and should be performed when there is any suspicion of thrombosis on the duplex sonography. In addition, magnetic resonance venography can be performed to confirm the presence of pelvic vein thrombus, and *lung perfusion scan or pulmonary angiogram can be performed when pulmonary embolism is suspected.*

8.1.1.5 Prevention

Prevention of thrombosis is more important than its treatment not only because it causes fatal complications, but it also leads to chronic pulmonary hypertension due to congestion, ulcers in the lower limbs due to swelling, recurrent thrombosis, and/or chronic venous stasis.

Thrombosis cannot be prevented in all cases with the preventive measures, but its incidence can be decreased according to the method of prevention. Wang et al. emphasized the use of antithrombotic agents in Asian patients, as thrombosis occurred in 71 % of patients who did not take antithrombotic agents and in 45 % of patients who took antithrombotic agents.

It is a general belief that antithrombotic agents cause problems related to bleeding, infection, and wound care. Therefore, *both the benefits and drawbacks of using antithrombotic agents should be considered.*

There are two basic treatment modalities: One is according to the recommendation of the American College of Chest Physicians (ACCP) and the other is according to the recommendation of the American Academy of Orthopedic Surgeons (AAOS). The basic differences between these two methods are whether to use an antithrombotic agent routinely and whether or not to use aspirin and mechanical devices for DVT prophylaxis.

The classic ACCP guideline recommended the routine use of antithrombotic agents whose effect has been established (excluding aspirin) in the patients who have undergone major orthopedic surgery. They recommended mechanical methods in only bleeding risk group. The ACCP considered all the patients who have undergone major orthopedic surgery as the risk group, and they disagreed on the effect of aspirin as an antithrombotic agent. Recently ACCP group agreed that orthopedic surgery is not as risky as before and modified the guidelines at ninth edition. In the current ninth edition, they still recommended routine use of antithrombotic agents in patients who have received major orthopedic surgery. Among the antithrombotic agents, low molecular weight heparin is more recommended. They recommend the use of IPCD (intermittent pneumatic compression device) in patients in whom bleeding risk is high and adding the IPCD to the pharmaceutical method during hospital stay.

The American Academy of Orthopedic Surgeons (AAOS) objected to the method suggested by the ACCP for the prevention of DVT based on the followings:

1. The method of arthroplasty that is being used now is different from that used 15 years ago in terms of techniques and operation time. This means that TKA is not a highly risky operation anymore. Hence, the method of prevention should not be based on the old concept of arthroplasty.
2. Cases reported in the literature after 1996 show that the incidence of symptomatic pulmonary embolism did not decrease with the use of low molecular weight heparin, warfarin, aspirin, or mechanical method.
3. There is not enough evidence to support the effectiveness of the ACCP recommendation, as the incidence of symptomatic or fatal embolism after arthroplasty is very low.
4. The risk of bleeding should be taken into consideration.

Novicoff et al. reported that the incidence of DVT did not drop and bleeding and hematoma increased significantly with the use of strict preventive measures as suggested by ACCP.

In fact, *the use of antithrombotic agents can reduce the incidence of asymptomatic thrombosis, but there is not enough evidence to support that this type of thrombosis progresses to symptomatic thrombosis.* In some cases, preventive methods are used only for legal defense. Therefore, the *AAOS largely categorized patients according to the risk of symptomatic pulmonary embolism (HD: high-risk DVT, SD: standard risk DVT) and the risk of bleeding (HB: high-risk bleeding, SB: standard risk bleeding). The patients were divided into four groups: HD and HB, HD and SB, SD and HB, and SD and SB. They suggested more reasonable mitigation guidelines than the ACCP guidelines according to patient grouping and added aspirin and mechanical intervention method targeting INR (International Normalized Ratio) below 2.0.* AAOA also modified the guideline recently by changing the DVT risk and bleeding risk criteria. The AAOA limits the high-risk group for DVT only to those patients who have a history of previous VTE and high-risk group for bleeding to those patients who have hepatic dysfunction or coagulation defect.

There are two methods of prevention: pharmaceutical and mechanical intervention.

Pharmaceutical agents should be effective, inexpensive, safe, and little, or no monitoring should be required. Most frequently used drugs include warfarin (Coumadin), low molecular weight heparin (LMWHs), other factor Xa inhibitors such as rivaroxaban and fondaparinux, ximelagatran and aspirin, etc.

Warfarin is the antagonist of vitamin K, and it is available for oral administration and can be used for about 3 months. Khatod et al. reported that only warfarin fared better than mechanical prophylaxis alone, whereas other forms of chemical prophylaxis revealed no significant differences. *Disadvantage of warfarin, however, is the narrow therapeutic window*; a little less dosage would not be effective and a little more dosage would increase the bleeding tendency. Another disadvantage is that the response to the drug varies significantly from patient to patient, and *continuous monitoring* is required for the drug interactions. Shorr et al. reported that using warfarin with NSAIDs increased the incidence of hemorrhagic peptic ulcer by 13 times. Also, *warfarin takes a longer time to become effective* (72–96 h), and *it is not as effective in patients of knee arthroplasty as it is in patients of hip arthroplasty.*

On the other hand, *low molecular weight heparin (LMWH) inhibits factor Xa by activation of antithrombin to prevent thrombosis.* Its molecular weight is 1,000–10,000 Da and it has a higher bioavailability and longer half-life than the regular heparin as it does not couple with plasma proteins and it does not attach to the internal walls of the vessels to a great extent. *Although LMWH has a drawback that a subcutaneous (SC) injection is required, it is much more effective than warfarin.* The risk of bleeding is decreased when it is used for preventive purpose since it does not increase the thromboplastin time. *Also, it is relatively safe and monitoring is not required.* Nevertheless, there is a higher risk of bleeding with LMWH as compared to warfarin.

Rivaroxaban and fondaparinux are the other factor Xa inhibitors. Rivaroxaban works directly on factor Xa to inhibit thrombin production and can be given orally without monitoring as it is highly specific and stable. However, it increases the risk of bleeding when given with aspirin, nonsteroid analgesics, or anti-inflammatory drugs. This agent should not be used in patients with severe hepatic and renal dysfunction. Jameson et al. compare the results of effects and side effects between LMWH and rivaroxaban and reported that the rivaroxaban had a higher wound complication rate and a lower DVT rate; however, there was no difference in the incidence of symptomatic PE or all cause of mortality. *Fondaparinux is an indirect factor Xa inhibitor that becomes effective by bonding with antithrombin. It should not be given within postoperative 6 h as it can increase the risk of bleeding, and monitoring is needed.* It is contraindicated in patients older than 75 years of age, weighing less than 50 kg, or who have poor renal function.

There is also a new drug called ximelagatran. It becomes active when it binds with thrombin and also works directly upon the thrombus. It is effective and relatively safe, and monitoring is not required. Colwell et al. reported that ximelagatran is more effective than warfarin in preventing thrombosis without any significant difference in bleeding tendency.

Aspirin inhibits platelet aggregation, thereby preventing thrombosis. It has an advantage of oral administration and low bleeding tendency, and it is cost effective. *However, there are different opinions regarding its effectiveness in prevention of thrombosis.*

There are controversies regarding the duration of VTE prophylaxis in TKA. *Some surgeons recommend the use of antithrombotic agents for about 7–10 days postoperatively as thrombosis mostly occurs between postoperative days 7 and 10 after TKA*, while others recommend its use for 4–5 weeks in patients who have a high risk of thrombosis.

Mechanical interventions include *graduated compression stockings (GCSs)*, *intermittent pneumatic compression (IPC)*, and *venous foot pumps (VFPs). These methods promote the circulation of venous blood to prevent thrombosis.*

The GCSs, in particular, are *not very effective* in TKA as they are in THA, and this is known to be related to the use of tourniquet. *The IPC* is effective in patients in whom preventive drugs are contraindicated. It should be applied for 17–20 h a day. The *benefit of this method is that there is no risk of bleeding*. The veins in the sole of the foot quickly fill and empty the venous blood during walking, and *VFPs mimic the effect of walking on the foot. These mechanical interventions can be more effective when used along with the pharmaceutical methods.*

Clinically, the methods of prevention can be used either according to the AAOS or AACP guidelines. On the other hand, patients can be simply divided into low-risk, moderate-risk, high-risk, and extremely high-risk groups, and prophylactic method is chosen according to the level of risk. Early gait training can be recommended in low-risk patients, pharmaceutical therapy with gradual addition of mechanical therapy in moderate- and high-risk patients, and heparinization with all other measures in extremely high-risk patients.

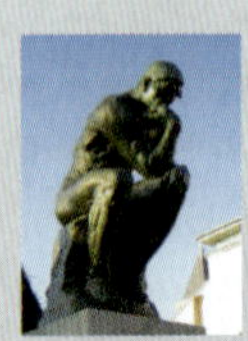

Author's Opinion

Patients who undergo arthroplasty are elderly, and hence, the risk of thrombosis is inevitably increased.

Although the incidence of thrombosis seems to vary among different races, prevention is necessary in order to ensure safety of the patients, to reduce the regional complications of thrombosis, and to protect the surgeon from legal issues.

As LMWHs and other factor Xa inhibitors are relatively safer drugs, they can be used for about 7–10 days after TKA, and the use of warfarin can be considered in high-risk patients even after discharge.

Among the mechanical methods, I do not recommend the use of GCSs as it is less effective. I prefer to use the IPC as it has no side effects and ensures a certain level of legal protection, and patients like to use it as it gives the feeling of a massage. Air cuff is fitted routinely from the operation room after wound closure and is kept for about a week.

Since I have used the IPC routinely, I have observed that the number of patients who complained of calf swelling and pain during hospital stay, and those who have post-thrombotic syndrome on outpatient care, was significantly decreased. I suppose that the IPC prevents the formation of microthrombi.

In high-risk patients, I recommend the use of a combination of pharmaceutical therapy and mechanical methods.

8.1.1.6 Treatment

Once thrombosis develops, it is important to prevent the formation of more thrombi, prevent pulmonary embolism, and treat the pulmonary embolism. *It is generally accepted concept that thrombi in the smaller veins can be ignored, but they can propagate in 5–23 % of cases, and 1.6 % of them can cause the symptomatic pulmonary embolism.*

When a thrombus is detected, thrombolytics such as heparin, warfarin, and low molecular weight dextran can be used considering the location of the thrombus, patient's age, and general condition.

The protocol for patients with documented thromboembolic disease by positive venography or ultrasound is that *patients with calf, popliteal or femoral thrombi, and asymptomatic pulmonary emboli should be treated with warfarin for 6 weeks. Symptomatic proximal vein thrombi and symptomatic pulmonary emboli should be treated with heparin until the effect of warfarin is established.* Physicians recommend the use of heparin injection through the IV route once thrombosis develops, but some orthopedic surgeons recommend the use of heparin injection through the IV route only in the extremely high-risk patient group. Kim et al. reported that it is acceptable not to give any drug unless symptomatic pulmonary embolism develops. The dosage of *heparin* is determined by the patient's general condition, and 5,000 U are given every 8–12 h for 1 week to 10 days through IV or IM injection. The problem is that heparin increases the amount of postoperative bleeding. Therefore, the PT (prothrombin time) should be between 15 and 17 s and the PT INR (International Normalized Ratio) should be maintained around 2.0. Careful monitoring throughout the injection period is required as it increases the bleeding tendency if the PT exceeds 20 s or the PTT (partial thromboplastin time) exceeds 50 s. To reduce the bleeding complication, direct infusion of thrombolytic agent into the thrombotic area through a catheter can be performed. But this method is associated with the risk of venous injury.

When pulmonary embolism occurs despite therapeutic warfarin, when warfarin is contraindicated in a high-risk patient, or *when complications develop as a result of anticoagulation, Mesh (Greenfield filter) is used as a radiological intervention to prevent the thrombus from propagating into the cardiopulmonary circulatory system.* Thrombectomy can be considered. However, this method is indicated in young patients in whom antithrombotic agents cannot be used, since this method can cause vascular injury.

8.1.2 Fat Embolism Syndrome

Fat embolism syndrome is caused due to an *increase in the intramedullary pressure* while using the intramedullary guide for osteotomy or while inserting the prosthesis with an extension stem.

The incidence of fat embolism syndrome is greater in the one-stage simultaneous operations, when intramedullary guide is used in femur and tibia concomitantly, when excessive reaming is done or the guide rod is inserted vigorously.

Fat emboli have a two-way adverse effect on the body. First, they block the blood supply, thereby burdening the heart (mechanical effect), which occurs mostly in the early stage. Second is the chemical effect that occurs after 48–72 h. The fat is degraded into free fatty acids by lipase, and the free fatty acid increases the capillary permeability and damages the alveolar tissues.

Symptoms include tachycardia, increased secretion, anxiety, drowsiness, and even unconsciousness. *The condition may often pass unrecognized* as a transient state of confusion after surgery.

There is no definite clinical diagnostic test, but hypoxia in the blood gas analysis and thrombocytopenia are generally observed.

For prevention of fat embolism syndrome, overdrilling of the femoral canal, gently placing the guide rod, copious irrigation, and the use of fluted guide rod are recommended.

Symptomatic management is done, and steroids can also be used when fat embolism has already developed.

8.2 Knee Joint Complications

8.2.1 Pain

Since pain relief is the main purpose of arthroplasty, the operation is considered unsuccessful if the patient suffers from postoperative pain. Pain is closely related to the time elapsed after the operation and is noted in almost all patients during the early stage. However, *it can be problematic if the pain is extremely severe even during the early stage, persists for a long time after the operation, or aggravates in comparison to preoperative state.*

8.2.1.1 Incidence

When Callahan et al. performed an analysis of 130 studies (9,879 patients) in 1994, 89.3 % of patients reported good or excellent results, 10.7 % of patients reported fair or poor results, and 3.7 % of patients eventually underwent revision arthroplasty at postoperative 4.1 years. With respect to the pain, 75 % of patients reported complete disappearance of pain, 20 % of patients reported mild pain, 3.7 % of patients reported moderate pain, and 1.3 % of patients reported severe pain. Cho et al. reported that 7 % of patients complained of pain to a greater or lesser extent at postoperative 1 year. Elson and Brenkel reported *a higher incidence of pain in the first knee of the two-stage operation, in patients who were younger than 60 years of age and who underwent lateral retinacular release, and in whom the posterior cruciate ligament had been sacrificed.*

8.2.1.2 Etiology

The causes of pain are largely classified into the intrinsic and extrinsic factors and unexplainable pain. Intrinsic factors are caused due to the problems within the knee joint, and they are further classified into inflammatory factors and mechanical factors. *Extrinsic factors are caused due to the problems outside of the knee joint.* They are mostly related to the disorders of the spine or the hip joints and are also related to the psychological factors. In some cases, however, the cause of pain is hard to identify clinically.

Intrinsic

Inflammatory

Bacterial infection and other inflammatory diseases or inflammatory reactions cause pain. In such cases, the patients *often complain of pain even when they are at rest.* Inflammatory disease is further subdivided into operation related and non-related. Operation non-related category includes rheumatoid arthritis, pigmented villonodular synovitis (PVNS), or Paget's disease. Inflammatory reactions are associated with joint swelling and pain. If there is fibrosis of the joint, it can limit the joint motion and can cause pain. Patients with allergies to metals also have similar symptoms as those in patients suffering from infection.

Mechanical

Mechanical causes of pain occur due to repeated stimulation of the knee joint, and excessive load or overuse of the knee joint. *This type of pain usually increases with activity.* The incidence of mechanical pain can vary according to the surgical procedures such as the method of fixation or patellar resurfacing etc.

The other causes of pain would be malalignment, instability, limited ROM, loosening and wear, and problems with the extensor mechanism, which are mostly due to *surgical failure*. Pes bursitis is also a type of inflammatory reaction caused due to irritation of the pes anserinus tendon by the prosthesis

Extrinsic

Extrinsic pain can be divided into operation related and non-related.

Some patients experience pain due to reflex sympathetic dystrophy. Reflex sympathetic dystrophy is one of the complex regional pain syndromes (CRPS). The possible etiology is conduction pathology of the sympathetic nerve due to trauma or surgery. Patients show hypersensitivity to pain even with minimal stimulation. The skin may be cold, discolored, and clammy due to sweating. Saphenous neuroma provokes pain by stimulus.

If the nature of pain is not very different from that before the operation, the cause of the pain is likely to be due to an extrinsic factor which is not related with operation. The patient may complain of persistent pain even though the operation has been successful in terms of alignment, ROM, and stability. In such a case, it is difficult to classify it as a complication of TKA. But persistent or recurring pain makes the patient feel that the operation was not successful. The evaluation of clinical results will show that the *knee function score is good, and yet the HSS score is poor.*

Elderly patients also have *back pain due to spinal stenosis* caused by degenerative spondylitis, and this is one of the most common operation non-related factors for knee joint pain. In particular, leg raising exercises after TKA can aggravate the back pain. In most of the patients, radiating pain is accompanied by back pain, while some patients have only mild or no back pain. Since the obturator nerve and the femoral nerve innervate both the hip and knee joints, there can be referred pain in the knee joint when there is *a lesion in the hip joint.*

Very high expectations, depression, other psychological problems, or secondary gain of the patients may also cause pain. Lundblad et al. reported that the patients with *severe preoperative pain are sensitive to the pain sensation* and experience more postoperative pain due to low pain threshold.

Mandalia et al. suggested the causes of pain according to the extrinsic and intrinsic factors. The table below is author's rearrangement of causes of pain based on Mandalia method (Table 8.1).

Unexplainable Pain

Some patients continue to complain of pain without any apparent causes for it. Khakharia et al. estimated the incidence of such cases to be approximately 1 in 300 arthroplasties. They presumed that unexplainable pain *is likely to occur in patients in whom the preoperative symptoms were worse than the pathologic condition of the knee joint.*

Infection, metal allergy, and reflex sympathetic dystrophy should be ruled out first. Overgrowth of the soft tissue, interposed meniscal fragment, lateral facet syndrome, irritation due to a retained osteophyte, extruded bone cement, popliteus tendon dysfunction, collateral ligament irritation caused by medial tibial displacement of the prosthesis, and even hypertrophic pulmonary osteoarthropathy can be the causes of unexplainable pain.

8.2.1.3 Diagnosis

The most important point in the diagnosis of pain is history taking. First, *the nature of pain* should be identified, followed by physical examination and the necessary tests. Infection should be ruled out first, and then the intrinsic factors should be studied. Extrinsic factors should be searched if no definite intrinsic factors are found. But, too much focus on the extrinsic factors may lead to missing an opportunity for making a timely diagnosis.

History Taking

The history relating to the intensity, site, timing, and provocating and relieving factors of pain should be taken. The first step in making a diagnosis is *to identify where and when the pain occurs.* The causes for pain are generally intrinsic when the pain is confined to the knee joint.

Neuroma or bursitis is associated with local pain and tenderness in the specific area, and it can be easily diagnosed by history taking. Reflex sympathetic dystrophy may be associated with severe pain and hypersensitivity of the skin in the operated limb. Rheumatoid arthritis may be suspected if the patient has polyarthralgia. If the pain is radiating to the lower limbs, focus should be on the extrinsic origin of pain.

The timing of the development of pain is also very indicative of its probable cause. Inflammation should be suspected if there is pain at rest. Persistent and extreme postoperative pain that does not disappear from postoperative day 1 (pain from day 1 onwards) is a strong sign of an infection. If there is instability or impingement of the soft tissues, pain is experienced from the early stage. On the other hand, delayed pain after a certain pain-free period is likely to be caused by inflammatory diseases, loosening or wear due to instability or malalignment, hematogenous infection, or stress fracture.

If the pain is aggravated by activity, it is likely to be of mechanical origin. Pain on weight bearing is mostly caused by instability and loosening. Pain while climbing up and down the stairs occurs when there are problems with the extensor mechanism such as patellar subluxation, patellar clunk syndrome, or impingement of the patella onto the PE. Pain in extension or flexion that limits the motion is caused by a narrow extension or flexion gap, swelling or hematoma, arthrofibrosis, insufficient removal of the spur, and impingement of the soft tissues.

Bizarre or unspecified pain may be of psychological origin.

Physical Examination

Firstly, it is necessary to observe *whether the joint is swollen and if there is a heat sensation.* If the joint is swollen, it is necessary to differentiate between swelling due to synovial

Table 8.1 Causes of pain according to author's rearrangement based on Mandalia et al. I. Intrinsic factors in the differential diagnosis of painful total knee replacement. II. Extrinsic factors in the differential diagnosis of painful total knee arthritis

I. Intrinsic factors	
Operation non-related	Operation related
I Rheumatoid arthritis	I Infection
II Pigmented villonodular synovitis	II Instability
III Paget's disease	III Malalignment
IV Overuse	IV Soft tissue impingement Fabellar impingement Popliteus impingement Component overhang
	V Arthrofibrosis
	VI Wear, osteolysis, and aseptic loosening
	VII Recurrent hemarthrosis
	VIII Pes anserinus bursitis
	IX Extensor mechanism problems Patellar maltracking Patellar clunk Extensor mechanism disruption (patellar fracture, patellar tendon rupture, quadriceps tendon rupture) Unresurfaced patella Undersized patellar button with lateral facet impingement Oversized patellar button with overstuffing Patella baja or alta
	X Metal allergy
II. Extrinsic factors	
Operation non-related	Operation related
I Hip pathology	
II Foot and ankle pathology	I Neurological Neuroma Complex regional pain syndrome
III Spinal disorders—stenosis/prolapsed disc	II Tendinopathy (patellar/quadriceps)
IV Vascular	
V Psychological condition	II Vascular—deep vein thrombosis
	III Heterotopic ossification
	IV Stress fracture and periprosthetic fracture
III. Unexplainable	

hypertrophy and simple effusion. Simple effusion is probably due to hemarthrosis or overactivity, while synovial hypertrophy is a manifestation of a chronic inflammatory lesion or chronic infection.

The easiest way to identify the site of the lesion is to palpate for tenderness. Tenderness on the medial side of the knee joint can be caused by overhang of the tibial prosthesis. If there is tenderness on the lateral side of the knee joint, there may be impingement of the popliteus tendon or a problem with the fabella regardless of snapping or clicking. Tendinitis or neuroma can be detected easily by the tender points.

Range of motion, muscle strength test, and instability of joint are also essential tests for making the diagnosis. Since malalignment and rotational deformity can be the cause of pain, they need to be examined as well.

The patella should be mobilized so as to check whether this causes pain. If there is pain along the lateral edge of the patella, it may be due to the lateral facet syndrome caused by the small patellar component in relation to the size of patella.

A lot of information can be obtained by observing the patient's gait.

If no intrinsic factors can be identified, extrinsic factors such as the spinal or hip lesions need to be examined.

Investigation

After physical examination, *X-rays should be taken first.* Simple X-rays can show the size and position of the prosthesis, its alignment, wear, and loosening along with patellofemoral alignment. If any abnormal findings are noted, it is important to *compare them with the previous X-rays* to know what has been changed.

If instability is suspected, stress or weight bearing X-ray should be taken to know the degree of joint laxity. If loosening or wear is suspected, an oblique view is needed in addition to the *A–P, lateral, and axial images, or fluoroscopy can be used for making a more accurate diagnosis.*

The next step is the study for differential diagnosis of the infection. Laboratory tests for *ESR and CRP* should be done routinely. If the results are abnormal, other chronic inflammatory diseases should be ruled out. If there are signs of inflammatory diseases, *joint fluid analysis* and *isotope test* can be performed based on the abnormal results. Bone scan, especially a WBC scan, is useful for making the diagnosis of infection, and it is clinically more significant when the scan is negative than when the scan is positive.

CT scan is useful for checking the rotational alignment of the prosthesis or when there is osteolysis. *MRI* is used occasionally to identify inflammatory disease or infection, but the metal interferes with imaging and much time is needed to get rid of metallic artifact. Murakami et al. reported that MRI is an effective modality in evaluating rotational alignment of component as well as extend of synovitis.

Reflex sympathetic dystrophy is diagnosed and tested by lumbar sympathetic ganglion block. Injection of local anesthetics is helpful for the diagnosis and treatment of bursitis or neuroma.

If allergy to the metal (metal sensitivity) is suspected, allergen testing is needed.

Arthroscopy can be performed *for obtaining the pathological specimen, removal of foreign body*, for adhesiolysis, and for treating the soft tissue impingement such as patellar clunk syndrome, but it is not used only for making a diagnosis.

X-ray, CT, or MRI of the spine or electromyogram can be performed for determining the causes of extrinsic pain.

As vascular diseases such as aneurysm, thrombosis, and atherosclerosis can be accompanied by pain, angiography may be needed if a vascular lesion is suspected.

If no causes can be detected after performing all these tests, consulting a neurologist or psychiatrist should be considered.

8.2.1.4 Treatment

The treatment of pain depends on its causes, intensity, and progression. If there is a definite cause of pain, it obviously requires treatment accordingly. However, the first step is to relieve the pain by medications and observe the progress unless there is an infection or rapid progression. Elson et al. stated that *telling the patients that the pain will get better helps to reduce the pain.*

Pain that is confined to a certain area such as bursitis or enthesopathy *can be treated by injecting local anesthetics and steroids*. If the cause originates from the synovial membrane, or if the pain is a result of mechanical block due to particles of PE debris or cement, *arthroscopy can be performed.*

In saphenous neuroma, simple resection of neuroma increases the possibility of a recurrence. Dellon et al. reported that they could reduce the incidence of recurrence of neuroma by intramuscular placement of the nerve ending or partially resecting a branch of the sensory nerve.

The treatment of reflex sympathetic dystrophy starts with administration of NSAIDs and muscle stimulation. Since reflex sympathetic dystrophy is accompanied by osteoporosis, weight bearing is encouraged and bisphosphonates can be administered. Psychiatric consultation may be helpful. If there is no response to the above methods, sympathetic block or sympathectomy may relieve the symptoms.

If infection, instability, wear, or loosening is the cause of pain and the speed of progression is fast, revision should be considered. Revision surgery is likely to fail if it is done without identifying the cause of pain. Mont et al. performed exploratory revision in patients with and without limited ROM and reported that it was successful in 60 % of patients with limited motion. Exploratory revision was successful in only 17 % of the patients who had pain without limited ROM, and the remaining patients complained of more pain. This means that revision surgery does not help in relieving the pain when its cause has not been identified.

8.2.2 Swelling

Swelling in the early postoperative period is considered normal. In patients who have undergone lateral retinacular release, the swelling would persist for a longer time. When the knee has been overused, it may be swollen even though there is no problem with the knee joint. Patients with rheumatoid arthritis may develop swelling as the disease progresses. *Abnormal extensor mechanism, problems with joint mechanics, instability, or arthrofibrosis may induce hypertrophy of the synovial tissue to cause persistent swelling.* When the PE is worn out, its particles cause synovitis which in turn causes swelling and pain. There have been some reports of recurrent hemarthrosis or swelling without definite etiology. Although there are numerous other causes that can give rise to swelling, the possibility of infection should be considered first. *Hence, the first step in making a diagnosis is to rule out infection*, and all tests for infection including arthrocentesis should be performed if there is persistent swelling and pain.

8.2.3 Motion Limitation

Motion limitation not only causes pain but also lowers patients' satisfaction due to functional disturbance. Motion limitation is the most common indication for revision surgery which does not exchange the implant. More flexion motion is better unless there is any problem with the knee mechanics. Normally, one can flex the knee up to 160°, but maximum flexion would probably be around 145° after TKA. Motion limitation can be classified into flexion contracture and limited flexion. Flexion of *at least 95° should be achieved in order to climb up and down the stairs without any handicap*, and full flexion is required for squatting. So more than 10° of flexion contracture and less than 95° of flexion can be included in motion limitation. *Flexion contracture causes more disability than that due to limited flexion*, and hence, flexion contracture should be corrected during the operation. However, in many cases, a flexion contracture of less than 10° during the early stage of the operation can be relieved with the passage of time.

8.2.3.1 Cause

After TKA, *the ROM is affected by the patient-related factors, surgical techniques, prosthesis design, and postoperative rehabilitation.*

Patient-Related Factors

One of the most important predisposing causes of limited ROM is the preoperative ROM. If the preoperative ROM was severely limited, the ROM would not be as much as that after ordinary arthroplasty due to quadriceps shortening and fibrosis of the soft tissues, even though the operation was successful. Also an extension lag may develop due to weakening of muscular strength when the quadriceps tendon or patellar tendon lengthening has been performed. If the preoperative ROM was less than 75°, the ROM may increase postoperatively, but in most of the cases, it is not more than 110°. Montgomery et al. reported that patients with ankylosed knee achieved an average flexion of 93° after TKA, and Naranja et al. reported that the average flexion achieved was only 62°.

It is believed that obesity affects the ROM, but this is because most patients cannot achieve enough flexion due to excessive subcutaneous fatty tissues on the thigh and calf. Otherwise, obesity does not affect the ROM to a great extent.

Other patient-related factors are preoperative diagnosis, body habits, and depressed patients with low threshold for pain. Patients who are prone to keloid formation may also be prone to develop arthrofibrosis.

Surgical Techniques

The range of motion is closely related to the surgical techniques. Most of the times, motion limitation is due to insufficient removal of spurs, flexion and extension gap imbalance, soft tissue impingement, and poor extensor mechanism.

If the *spurs on the posterior condyle of the femur* are not removed sufficiently, it causes extension or flexion motion limitation. *Gap balancing* is an important surgical technique for achieving a good ROM. When both the flexion and extension gaps decrease, flexion contracture and flexion limitation occur at the same time. Flexion contracture occurs when the extension gap is narrow and a narrow flexion gap decreases the angle of flexion. Reducing the *posterior slope of the tibia* narrows the flexion gap and decreases flexion motion. Excessive *joint line elevation* causes more tension on the soft tissues when the knee joint flexes by more than 90° and causes motion limitation. Also, *excessive tension on the posterior cruciate ligament in the CR type* can limit flexion and extension motion, and capsular contracture limits extension. *Problems with the extensor mechanism are also an important factor that limits motion*. Poor patellofemoral alignment causes the patients to avoid bending the knee joint due to anxiety and instability leading to limited motion. Correct component rotation is critical for patellar tracking, and internal rotation of the femoral and tibial components must be avoided. Bédard et al. suggested that internally rotated components compromised motion because of pain, patellar maltracking, a tight medial flexion gap, and limited femoral rollback on a high-conformity lateral tibial prosthesis. When the *prosthesis is too large*, it causes pain along with limited motion. Nicholls and Dorr stated that abnormal position of the prosthesis also causes limited motion.

Prosthetic Design

Prosthetic design can also affect the range of motion. Comparing the PS type with CR type, a better range of motion is achieved with the PS type than with the CR type, not only because it secures the rollback but also because it widens the flexion gap. Some surgeons emphasize that mobile-bearing prosthesis can increase the range of motion, while many surgeons report that it does not show any significant difference in the ROM. Constrained prosthesis not only interferes with the extension or flexion motion but also decreases the rotation and medial/lateral motion. There are some prostheses which increase the flexion motion, so-called high flexion knee. Many authors report that the use of "high flexion knee" increases the range of flexion motion, while others report no difference between conventional and "high flexion knee."

Postoperative Care

The ROM is also closely related to postoperative wound healing. If there is an *excessive hematoma or wound healing is delayed in the early postoperative period*, the pain limits the rehabilitation process and exercise is restricted during the treatment of the *wound*.

Swelling of the joint stimulates the mechanoreceptors in the joint capsule, thereby limiting the range of motion, and hence, persistent swelling results in limited ROM.

The ROM can be decreased if the patient is too anxious, lacks motivation, or is uncooperative with *rehabilitation* due to the abnormal response to pain and poorly controlled pain in *the early postoperative period.*

Miscellaneous

Other causes include infection, arthrofibrosis, and reflex sympathetic dystrophy. Arthrofibrosis, which develops as a result of combination of the aforementioned causes, is one of the common causes of stiffness following TKA. In cases in which *the ROM is good at first but becomes progressively limited later, we should suspect any of the following causes: infection, synovitis due to overuse, rheumatoid arthritis, wear debris, recurrent hemarthrosis, loosening or damaged prosthesis, etc.*

8.2.3.2 Treatment

Management is not very easy when the ROM is limited. The conservative treatment in the form of physiotherapy should be tried first and followed by graduated treatment protocol. When the desired ROM cannot be achieved, manipulation, brisement under anesthesia, arthroscopic adhesiolysis, open adhesiolysis, and revision TKA can be considered in that order.

Before revision arthroplasty is undertaken, the cause should be identified and the extrinsic factors should be ruled out.

If the range of motion is less than 95° until postoperative 4–6 weeks, more aggressive physiotherapy or manipulation can be considered. When this is done within postoperative 3 months, the results are promising. Numerous authors have reported successful results with manipulation. But manipulation is still a controversial issue. Brassard et al. and Maloney et al. stated that *manipulation can be attempted during the early stage of rehabilitation and brisement under anesthesia between postoperative 6 and 12 weeks achieved good results when flexion was less than 75°*. However, they advised that the procedure should be performed very carefully as it can cause a fracture or an avulsion fracture. The purpose of manipulation is to reduce intra-articular adhesions in order to normalize the early postoperative rehabilitation process and reduce the risk of developing a permanent limited ROM. Cates and Schmidt evaluated the stiff TKA and found that manipulation was most successful when it was performed within 8 weeks and in patients with full extension and at least 90° of flexion. Witvrouw et al. used computer-controlled motion technology (Antwerp, Belgium) device to provide static progressive stretch utilizing computer-controlled low-lead prolonged force so as to improve ROM. They reported that this device had equal or superior result than manipulation under anesthesia, especially in relieving flexion contracture.

Adhesiolysis using arthroscopy is another option. *Adequate timing of arthroscopic arthrolysis is 3–6 months after TKA*. Arthroscopy is done through 2–3 portals as in the usual arthroscopic surgery, but the prosthesis should not be damaged so as to avoid the development of scratches and wear particles. The joint is examined first without knee motion and is checked for adhesions. After this, it should be checked whether the soft tissues are impinging into the joint during knee motion. The impinging soft tissues should be removed, and any adhesions should be released using a trocar, basket forceps, or shaver. Diduch et al. demonstrated that adhesiolysis using arthroscopy increases the ROM by an average of 26°. Mont et al. also reported that *adhesiolysis using arthroscopy was successful in patients with limited motion without any apparent problem on the X-ray*.

In the case of severe ROM limitation with more than 20° of flexion contracture and less than 70° of flexion motion, arthroscopic treatment alone is less effective and open adhesiolysis is needed. It is desirable to perform adhesiolysis within 1 year of primary surgery. If such a *limited motion is caused due to patellofemoral malalignment or overstuffing of the extension and flexion gaps, there is no other option besides revision surgery. However, revision surgery is not always successful* if there is extensive scar formation due to arthrofibrosis or the *causes of limited ROM are unclear*. Revision surgery should include adhesiolysis and soft tissue balancing. Nelson et al. reported that revision of soft tissues improved the ROM in patients with an arc of motion between 15° and 75°, but the overall range of motion was improved up to a certain level. Bellemans et al. proposed a treatment method for flexion contracture. They divided the procedure into four steps, and the results were positive. The first step of the algorithm is removing the spur completely and increasing the resection of the distal femur by 2 mm and correcting the medial/lateral balance. The second step is gradually releasing the posterior capsule and gastrocnemius muscles. The third step is resecting the distal femur up to 4 mm, and the last step is performing hamstring tenotomy.

8.2.4 Instability and Dislocation

Instability is the second most common cause of revision surgery following infection, which is performed within 2 years after the index operation. The definition of instability is controversial, but it is accepted that instability is considered to exist when there is more than a 2 mm medial opening and a 3 mm lateral opening in extension and a 3 mm medial opening and a 4 mm lateral opening in flexion. A–P instability is defined if the tibia can be displaced by more than 5 mm or the joint can be dislocated. Also, the patella should not subluxate or disclocate.

Knee instability makes walking difficult and causes joint swelling and pain. When giving way on walking is accompanied with vague anterior knee pain, recurrent effusions, and soft tissue tenderness, instability should be suspected. In severe cases, it may cause joint dislocation. Also, *it worsens the prognosis as it causes wear or loosening from the early stage*. This is more prominently seen when the prosthesis has a flat articular surface.

8.2.4.1 Cause

Even if the operation was successful, *instability occurs if there is not enough muscular strength to support the joint.* Therefore, operation cannot be indicated in the patients with neuromuscular disorders. However, neuromuscular disorder may develop postoperatively and can cause instability of the operated joint.

Most of the times, instability is caused due to problems of the knee joint itself. Early instability may be a result of *surgical failure including malalignment, imbalance of flexion–extension gap, inadequate correction of the deformity, failure to achieve mediolateral balance, rupture of the PCL in the CR type, etc. Late instability is caused due to overuse of the joint and trauma, or it is secondary to complications such as infection, loosening, or wear.*

Instability is classified into anterior instability, instability in extension, instability in flexion, genu recurvatum, and global instability, and the causes and findings in each type of instability are different. In general, instability in extension manifests as mediolateral instability or genu recurvatum, while instability in flexion is manifested as A–P instability.

Anterior instability is associated with quadriceps weakness or subluxation or dislocation of the patella. In such a case, the patient shows quadriceps avoidance gait in which the patient is not willing to bend the knee and tends to lean forward while walking.

Instability in extension is further classified into symmetric instability and asymmetric instability, and *both types of instability tend to be worsened by malalignment and masked by good alignment. Symmetric instability is caused due to a wide extension gap. It occurs due to over-resection of the distal femur or by using a thinner PE to correct flexion and extension gap imbalance, and when incompletely released, collateral ligaments get detached during walking. Asymmetric instability is more common, and it is mostly due to inadequate release of the collateral ligaments on the contracted side*. In such a case, the contracted side is compressed and the other side is more opened (Fig. 8.1), leading to a seesaw effect. Insall stated that *valgus instability from over-release of the medial structures during correction of a fixed varus deformity is rare*. Koo and Choi reported that there was no significant difference between the MCL-preserved TKAs and the knees with an iatrogenic MCL injury. It may also occur due to *sinking down of the bone on one side when* the prosthesis is fixed to the weak bone or in case of valgus or varus tibial osteotomy.

Symmetric instability in flexion mostly occurs when the flexion gap widens or when the PCL is attenuated in TKA performed with the CR type. It also occurs when the flexion gap is excessively widened due to the use of a femoral prosthesis that is too small, the use of a thinner PE for correcting the flexion contracture, or when the posterior cruciate ligament is sacrificed. If it is severe, it can lead to posterior dislocation of the joint. Asymmetric instability in flexion occurs when soft tissues are released to a greater extent for correcting the varus–valgus deformity, and the rotation of the femoral prosthesis is incorrect.

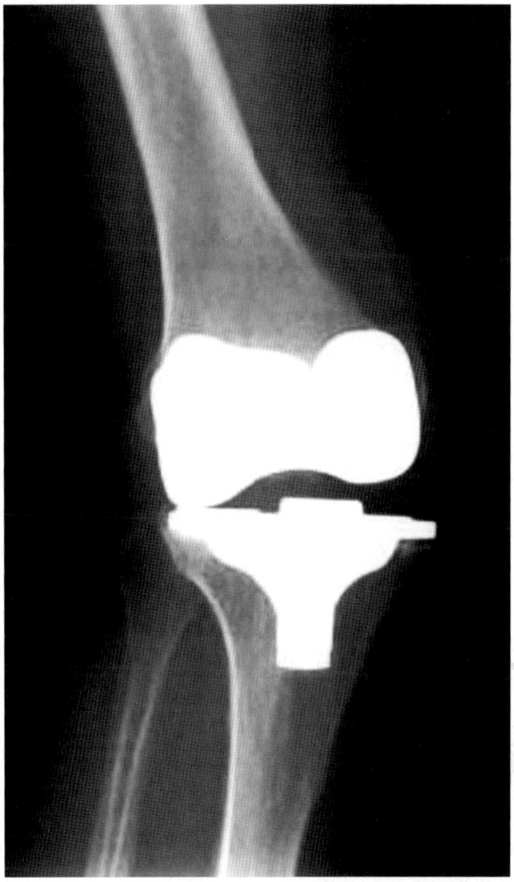

Fig. 8.1 Compression on one side leading to opening on the other side

The joint can be unstable in midflexion which makes it difficult to climb the stairs. This instability happens because balance is mostly tested in full extension or at 90° flexion during the operation. Midflexion instability leads to progressive stretching of secondary restraints, and accelerate PE wear. But it is often masked due to tightness of the posterior capsule in full extension. The joint line elevation affects the ligament tension at an intermediate angle to cause midflexion instability. The shift from a longer radius in extension to a shorter radius in flexion with a multi-radius design has been reported to cause instability between 30 and 45° of knee flexion.

Genu recurvatum can occur when the strength of hamstring muscles weakens or the extension gap is too wide. It can also develop with the use of the CR type of prosthesis when the posterior cruciate ligament gets absorbed in patients with RA or when the recessed posterior cruciate ligament gets ruptured.

Global instability occurs when one or more causes of instability occur in combination and when one-plane instability lasts longer.

Subluxation may occur with the use of the CR type of prosthesis, but subluxation is often overlooked because it

reduces spontaneously. Dislocation is the more aggravated form of instability. There are different opinions regarding the mechanism of knee dislocation. It is generally believed that dislocation occurs when a backward force is applied while the knee is slightly bent or when posterior and rotational forces are applied while the knee is in a flexed position. In patients with a valgus deformity, dislocation occurs when their legs are crossed. *The incidence of dislocation is higher in patients with a preoperative valgus deformity*. Lombardi et al. found that *the incidence of dislocation was higher in patients who had more flexion motion*.

Dislocation has been experienced more frequently with the use of the old PS type of prosthesis. Dislocation is related to location of the cam and height of the post, which is represented by the dislocation safety factor (DSF). Kocmond et al. defined the dislocation safety factor (DSF) as the vertical distance from the bottom of the femoral cam to the top of the tibial spine. The DSF increases as knee flexion increases, and it peaks at 70° of flexion and decreases thereafter, thereby increasing the risk of dislocation. The early PS type design had a lower post and the post was located on the posterior side, and hence, dislocation developed easily. Currently, improved prosthetic design with an increased jump distance has reduced the incidence of this complication. In a mobile-bearing joint, dislocation of the mobile-bearing prosthesis can occur along with instability when ligament balancing cannot be achieved.

8.2.4.2 Treatment

The method of treatment varies according to the type and degree of instability. If the instability is mild, the patients learn how to walk without difficulty. *Conservative treatment is recommended initially*. If the patient feels unstable during the first postoperative gait, the instability of the knee joint should be evaluated. If no problem is detected on the stress test, it is because of weak muscular strength, and more enhanced muscle strengthening exercises should be recommended. If muscular strength has been weakened due to a neurologic disorder, it needs to be addressed. If there is asymmetrical instability due to ligament or soft tissue imbalance in early stage, it is necessary to *fit a brace for approximately 6 weeks* for the soft tissues to become scar bound. If ligament instability is neglected at this time and the patient is allowed to walk without brace fitting, the ligament or soft tissues will heal in a relaxed state, and the instability will persist.

If moderate instability is not corrected by improving muscular strength or with the use of brace fitting, revision surgery is needed as it causes the knee to give way, and frequent subluxation or dislocation will cause early wear and loosening.

In symmetric instability in extension and genu recurvatum, exchange to the thicker PE and using a smaller femoral component is needed. In asymmetric extension instability, the contracted side should be released, and the use of a thicker PE is required. Pagnano et al. reported that replacing the CR type with the PS type of prosthesis showed good results.

Flexion instability can be managed by upsizing the femoral component following femoral posterior augmentation. Vince et al. described that it is important to align the limbs and balance the extension and flexion gaps. They concluded that when a *constrained prosthesis is used, good results can be expected even though the collateral ligaments are imbalanced. But in case the discrepancy between the flexion and extension gaps is marked, loosening developed eventually, even though the initial results were good*.

Acute dislocation can be reduced by pulling the tibia forward while the knee is fully bent, but revision is desirable according to the aforementioned principles of treatment since the possibility of recurrence of dislocation is high. In case of recurrent dislocation, it is required to perform revision and to insert a larger PE or perform component revision using a constrained type of prosthesis. Some authors reported that *arthrodesis was inevitable in severe cases*.

8.2.5 Vascular Complications

Direct injury to the vessels during arthroplasty is very rare. Popliteal arteries may be injured and aneurysm, pseudoaneurysm, or A–V fistula may develop during adhesiolysis in revision surgery, during posterior capsular stripping in patients with limited motion, or in limb salvage operation with the use of tumor prosthesis.

Yang et al. reported that the most dangerous zone of vascular injury during the operation is just lateral to the posterior center of the lateral condyle at the joint level, as the neurovascular structure is closest to the operation field at this area. Geertsema et al. experienced three cases of popliteal pseudoaneurysm. The most common mechanism for pseudoaneurysm formation is indirect trauma, which includes mechanical stretching, posterior capsule release, dislocating the knee, and thermal injury. They achieved successful revascularization by endovascular stenting.

Most of the times, the preoperative vascular disease is aggravated after the operation. Absolute vascular contraindications to TKA include the presence of confirmed vascular claudication on minimal or no activity, skin ulceration secondary to arterial insufficiency or venous stasis, and ischemia or necrosis of the toes.

If there is injury to the vessels during the operation or the vessels are occluded due to thrombosis, a vascular surgeon should be consulted emergently for seeking his/her help in treating these problems.

8.2.6 Nerve Palsy

Tibial nerve palsy can occur, but peroneal nerve palsy is the most common after TKA. Recently, some authors reported that tibial nerve palsy occurred in minimally invasive surgery when cement was pushed back to the posterior side.

Peroneal nerve palsy is caused due to *excessive stretching of the nerve while correcting a severe valgus deformity or flexion contracture*, injury during revision, fascial compression, disruption of vascular supply to the nerves, or external pressure, etc. Among them, *external pressure is the most common cause* of peroneal nerve palsy. Idusuyi and Morrey demonstrated that valgus deformity is the most common preoperative factor causing nerve palsy, and *the most common postoperative factor is incorrect position of the limb, while proprioception is lost with epidural block*. Other causes of nerve palsy could be the compression by bone or cement, improper use of tourniquet, or compartment syndrome due to excessive bleeding.

The method of treatment depends on the cause of nerve palsy. *Palsy caused by external pressure* in the early postoperative stage is temporary, and it gradually recovers with time when the elastic bandage is loosened and the knee is positioned at 30–60° flexion. *Early detection of palsy generally leads to a better prognosis. Tourniquet palsy requires observation. But palsy as a result of compartment syndrome needs active management such as surgical decompression.*

If nerve palsy persists for more than 3 weeks, electromyogram is necessary to identify the site and extent of nerve damage. *It is recommended to fit an ankle foot orthosis and perform passive ankle ROM exercises to prevent ankle contracture.*

Recovery starts from the motor function of the nerve, and most of the nerves recover without motor weakness; however, disorders of the sensory function often persist. Recovery may be delayed or impossible if there is excessive stretching of the peroneal nerve during the operation or if there is a complete palsy. Kim et al. reported that eight out of nine patients with peroneal palsy recovered, but one patient did not recover.

Krackow reported good results by performing exploration when palsy persisted for more than 2 months. Zywiel et al. also emphasized that nerve decompression improved the sensation and decreased the pain, and they recommended surgical decompression for patients who failed to improve with conventional conservative treatment. However, most of the surgeons agree that *exploration is not recommended in the early stage.*

8.2.7 Component Breakage

The causes of component breakage are multiple: design and material defects of the prosthesis, poor surgical techniques, and trauma. Most of the times, component breakage occurs when the hinge type or linked type of the constrained prosthesis is used for the young and active patients.

It is also closely related to the prosthesis design. It occurs when there is a groove or screw hole in the prosthesis; when there is no enhanced peripheral rim, with the use of porous coated prosthesis; or when a very thin cobalt chromium metal is used. The femoral component is broken when the femoral runner is thin; Whiteside et al. reported 32 cases of component breakage at the corner and the junction area out of 16,000 cases treated with Ortholoc II cementless prosthesis. The reduced thickness of the metal in these critical areas predisposed to the development of a fracture. Porous coating of the interface further weakened the prosthesis, and sintering process can degrade the quality of the base metal itself.

Some cases of tibial component breakage near the posterior cruciate ligament insertion site have been reported. Chatterji et al. analyzed 25 cases of tibial component breakage and reported that breakage occurred when the supporting bone showed an osteolytic defect, when the bone graft collapsed, or when avascular necrosis developed. In case of such bone defect, eccentric loading and condylar lift-off due to malalignment or PE wear impose an ongoing load causing a fatigue fracture.

The PS type of prosthesis occasionally shows wear and breakage of the post. The incidence of post fracture is higher in younger, obese, and male patients. It is caused due to the design defect, surgical failure, or both. Implants with a hole in the post for screw fixation, anteriorly placed post, and too closely located post and notch are predisposed to post wear and breakage. Hamai et al. and Akasaki et al. revealed that stress on the post is different in each implant and when stress exceeds the compressive yield strength of the post, it causes post wear and breakage. Surgical errors such as valgus malalignment, wide extension gap, instability, and excessive posterior slope predispose to a post fracture. *Among them, post wear and fracture occur most frequently when the post is under too much stress to block hyperextension during extension.*

When the prosthesis is broken, it causes instability, pain, or deformity, and revision is required.

8.2.8 Complications of the Extensor Mechanism

Complications of the extensor mechanism are the most common complications following TKA. Complications which are related to the extensor mechanism are anterior knee pain, extensor mechanism rupture, patellar fracture, malalignment or dislocation of the patella, patellar clunk syndrome, avascular necrosis of the patella, wear and loosening, etc.

The range of incidence is very wide from 5 to 60 %, because the scope for the complications differs according to the surgeon. Kim et al. reported an incidence of about 29 %, and subluxation of the patella was the most common complication. Meding et al. reported that patellar fracture and loosening of the patellar component were the most common complications excluding anterior knee pain and the risk of fracture was highest when lateral retinacular release had been performed in patients whose BMI was greater than 30. They also reported that the position of patellar component, thickness of the patella, and preoperative ROM and alignment are closely related to loosening. The incidence of these complications is decreasing with the improvement of the prosthesis and the evolution of surgical techniques, but there are still many unsolved problems. Non-resurfacing of the patella is preferred by some surgeons because of these complications, but non-resurfacing does not guarantee a reduction in the incidence of these complications.

Complications of the extensor mechanism not only cause pain and swelling, but they also alter the joint mechanics to aggravate the wear and loosening of other components and affect the survival of the prosthesis.

8.2.8.1 Anterior Knee Pain

Cause

Anterior knee pain is not always associated with the complications of the extensor mechanism itself, and its cause is often unclear. However, *it is mostly related to the problems with the extensor mechanism.*

Pain can occur if the stress imposed on the extensor mechanism exceeds the physiologic limit during squatting or climbing up and down the stairs. Also, overstuffing of the anterior knee joint or malalignment increases the diffuse or focal pressure, thereby causing anterior knee pain. Meftah et al. reported that the incidence of anterior knee pain at the 10-year follow-up was 22.2 % and that it was partly related to a specific implant used. Although it is controversial, pain is known to be more common among patients in whom the patella has not been resurfaced; Scott stated that pain is mostly due to the progression of the non-resurfaced lesion. Other causes of anterior knee pain are joint swelling, fibrosis of the anterior fat pad, neuroma, and tendonitis.

Treatment

Treatment varies according to the degree and cause of pain. *If the pain is not severe, observation is needed*; however, moderate pain requires conservative treatment such as medication or physiotherapy. In some cases, steroid injections can be used. *When the pain is severe, the patella can be resurfaced if it is thought that the pain is caused due to the unresurfaced patella. However, only patellar resurfacing may not solve this problem* in most of the cases. Hence, revision of all components may sometimes be necessary.

8.2.8.2 Rupture of the Extensor Mechanism

If there is rupture of the extensor mechanism, the extension function of the patella is lost, resulting in a very severe functional disturbance. The rupture of the extensor mechanism includes avulsion of the patellar tendon from the tibial tuberosity, patellar fracture, and quadriceps tendon rupture. Patellar fracture is further described in this chapter under Sect. 8.2.16.

Cause

General medical conditions leading to rupture of the extensor mechanism include rheumatoid arthritis, diabetes mellitus, chronic renal failure, hyperthyroidism, and steroid abuse.

Intraoperative rupture occurs when an excessive force is applied to improve the ROM in the patients with quadriceps contracture, ankylotic knee, osteoporosis, weak patella, or in revision cases.

Rupture may occur postoperatively when too much patellar osteotomy was done, too much fat pad was removed, lateral retinacular ligament was released, and transverse incision over the quadriceps tendon was made too close to the superior pole of the patella during paramedial arthrotomy. Malalignment of the extensor mechanism and severe global instability also provoke extensor tendon rupture. It also occurs when manipulation is applied to increase the ROM in the patients who have undergone a rectus snip or V–Y quadricepsplasty.

Infection and trauma are other causes of rupture *of the extensor mechanism.*

Diagnosis

Most of the patients complain of loss of extension even by a minor indirect trauma, and they may have no definite pain. Physically, dimpling is noted in the area of rupture. X-ray shows patella alta or patella baja. The site and degree of rupture can be detected on sonography or MRI.

Treatment

In case of partial tendon rupture, conservative treatment can yield good results. *In case of complete rupture, repair or reconstruction of the tendon should be performed. Excessive tension and circulatory disturbance interferes with the healing.* So, thoughtful planning should be estabilished before operation. In other words, medial incision used in the approach disrupts the vascular supply of the tendon from the medial side and the lateral inferior genicular arteries are often injured during meniscectomy or fat pad removal. If lateral retinacular release has been done, vascular supply is almost completely interrupted and *direct repair of the tendon is likely to fail.* Wilson and Venters performed primary repair of the patellar tendon rupture, and the operation failed in every case. *Therefore, semitendinosus tendon or gracilis tendon autograft can be used for augmentation while keeping the tibial insertion attached, or the tendon should be reconstructed with tendon allograft*. Cadambi and Engh performed autograft using semitendinosus tendon, Wilson et al. used plantaris autograft, and Jaureguito et al. used the medial head of the gastrocnemius with satisfying results. Emerson et al. recommended the use of allogeneic tendon graft, and I also obtained good results by performing allograft augmentation. A fresh-frozen allograft is a good candidate as an allogeneic tendon. The Achilles tendon is the most widely used. Zanotti et al. introduced the bone–patellar tendon–bone complex allograft and achieved a good success rate.

The tension is the key point during tendon reconstruction. Emerson et al. noted an average extension lag of 28° in 33 % of patients when the maximum tension was applied with the knee flexed at 60° under anesthesia. However, Nazarian et al. and Burnett and Bourne *recommended applying maximum possible tension while the knee is extended. This is because the allograft has a tendency to elongate and the ruptured portion of the tendon is likely to elongate as it is already shortened*. Lionberger and Correia recommended reinforcement with a dynamic and flexible leash to limit excursion of the patellar tendon while the repaired tendon heals.

For postoperative care, Nazarian et al. recommended the use of a plaster cast in extension for 6 weeks.

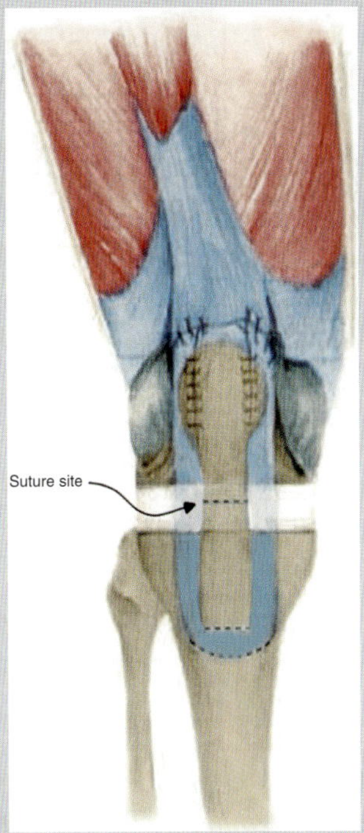

Fig. 8.2 Reconstruction of patellar tendon rupture using allograft. Proximal allograft is sutured to retinacular ligament and quadriceps tendon. Distal allograft is passed through the tibial bone

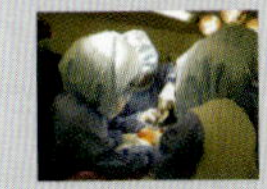

Author's Method

My method for allograft augmentation in case of patellar tendon rupture is to reinforce the repaired tendon using allogeneic hamstring tendon. First, I drill a hole distal to the tibial tuberosity, and the tendon is passed through this hole. The both ends of the allogeneic tendon are sutured to the soft tissues around the patella (Fig. 8.2). For quadriceps tendon rupture, I use Achilles tendon or iliotibial band to reinforce the repaired portion of quadriceps tendon.

I apply maximum tension during allograft augmentation while the knee is extended. After this, tension band suture technique is used to aid in postoperative rehabilitation.

For postoperative care, I identify the flexion angle that does not disrupt the sutures during the operation and start flexion exercises up to 20° less than this angle and avoid straight leg raising or active extension of the knee joint for the first 4–6 weeks.

8.2.8.3 Patellar Subluxation or Dislocation

Maltracking of the patella can cause anterior knee pain, limited ROM, and quadriceps weakness. The rate of wear and loosening and the incidence of patellar fracture can be accelerated due to the changes in the extensor mechanics (Fig. 8.3). However, Rand et al. *reported that only 1 % of patellar maltracking is actually associated with clinical symptoms*.

Cause

The *causes* of patellar subluxation or dislocation are largely divided into patient-related factors, prosthetic designs, and surgical techniques.

Chew et al. reported that there was an average of 5° postoperative patellar tilt even when patellar tracking was good during the operation, and this was *closely related to the patient's preoperative patellar tilt*. Preoperative valgus deformity is one of the predisposing factors of subluxation and dislocation. Patients who had *severe* preoperative *knee joint effusion* have a distended synovial membrane, and this

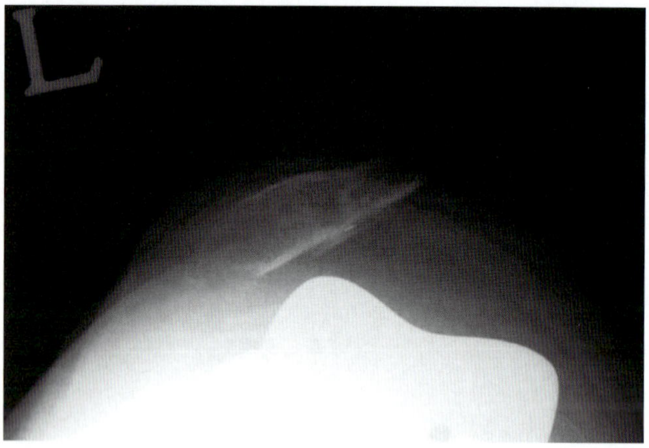

Fig. 8.3 Patellar dislocation

can be a cause of dynamic patellar instability during extension postoperatively, even though the tracking is good in the operation field.

Prosthetic design is closely related to patellar tracking. *Currently, patellar tracking has improved since the patella and the patellar groove have been modified into a patella-friendly shape.*

Surgical techniques are the most important factors for good patellar tracking. First, the tibiofemoral alignment should be correct. *Valgus deformity, if left uncorrected, causes maltracking. The position and rotation of the prosthesis are also important. Patellar tracking is improved by placing the tibial and femoral prosthesis laterally and the patella medially, and externally rotating the tibial and femoral components. Patellar instability also increases when the patella is resected asymmetrically or the resected patella is too thick.* The incidence of subluxation and dislocation also increases *when the femoral prosthesis is too large or the lateral retinacular ligament is too tight.* An anatomically shaped patella may aggravate maltracking if rotational alignment of the patellar component is not correct. Patellar instability can also occur when the arthrotomy site is disrupted due to excessive swelling, vigorous physiotherapy, or trauma.

Treatment

If there is no pain or if the subluxation is not severe, observation is needed and VMO (vastus medialis obliquus) strengthening exercises should be started.

In case of severe dislocation or if there is accompanying pain, the simplest method that can be performed is *lateral retinacular release and medial reinforcement* when the prosthesis is in its optimal position. Arthroscopic lateral retinacular release is performed occasionally. The next step, according to Grace and Rand, should be performing a *proximal realignment procedure* such as VMO advancement or V–Y quadricepsplasty for quadriceps balancing. Whiteside et al. suggested performing tibial tubercle osteotomy, but

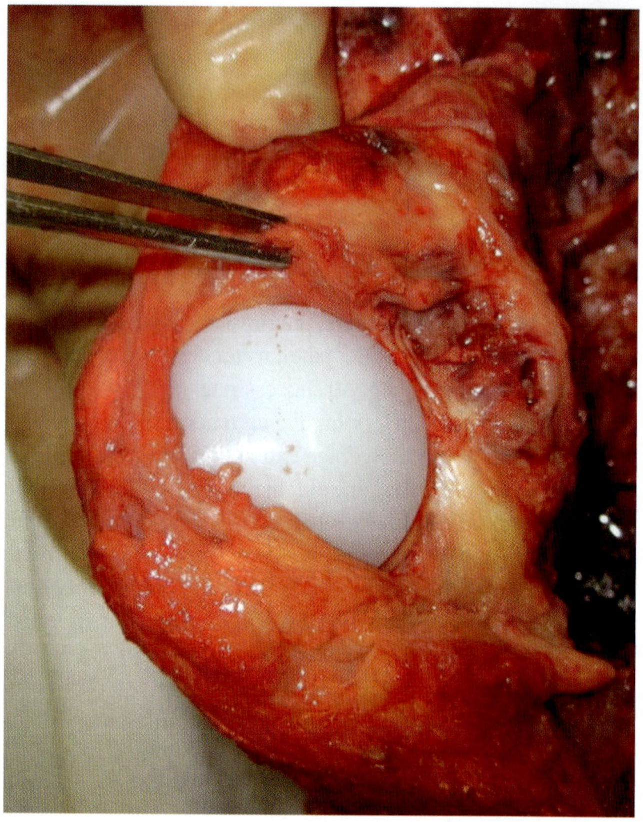

Fig. 8.4 Photography of patellar clunk syndrome. Fibrous nodule is picked up by forceps

Rand et al. are not in favor of performing this procedure because it causes many complications such as pain and nonunion. Nakajima et al. reported that Elmslie–Trillat operation and/or extensive lateral retinacular release showed good results.

If the prosthesis is not in its optimal position, lateral retinacular release can be tried first. If the problems are not solved after the lateral retinacular release, revision surgery should be performed to correct malposition and malrotation of the femoral, tibial, and patellar component.

8.2.8.4 Patellar Clunk Syndrome

Patellar clunk syndrome develops when the *scar tissues* located at the junction of the quadriceps tendon and patella, and causes irritation during flexion and extension motion. Such tissue growth is thought to originate from exposed cancellous bone at the margin of the components or due to chronic irritation of the synovium by the prosthetic prominences. Beight et al. noted that the causes of patellar clunk syndrome originated from the design problems of the femoral prosthesis, postoperative inflammatory reaction, and changes in the extensor mechanism.

Patella clunk syndrome occurs when the knee is *actively extended from 45 to 60° of flexion* (Fig. 8.4). *Catching occurs during the postoperative 6–12 months. This syndrome was more common with older PS type in which the femoral notch portion was extended proximally*. The current designs have a longer and deeper femoral sulcus which gradually adjusts to the shape of the femur and helps in reducing the incidence of patellar clunk syndrome significantly.

The results of treatment by removing the soft tissues using arthroscopy or open surgery *are good*. Diduch et al. demonstrated a success rate of 82 % by removal of the fibrous nodules using arthroscopy.

Synovial entrapment or hyperplasia is an entity similar to patellar clunk syndrome, but it is less well described. The location of the lesion is nearly the same as that in patellar clunk syndrome, but there are no discrete nodules. Rather than a clunk or catch, the patient experiences pain and crepitus, typically when the knee is extended actively from 90° of flexion. Treatment of synovial entrapment or hyperplasia depends on the degree of symptoms. If the symptoms (pain and/or crepitus sound) are mild, assurance of the patient is enough. If the symptoms are severe, arthroscopic examination followed by synovectomy is needed.

Patellar crepitus is defined as a palpable, continuous grinding sensation, and the symptoms of patellar crepitus are secondary to those of peripatellar fibrosynovial hyperplasia which develops at the junction of the superior pole of the patella and the distal quadriceps tendon. Dennis et al. reported that the causes of patellar crepitus are multifactorial including previous knee surgeries, decreased component size and composite thickness, shorter patella tendon length, and increased femoral condylar offset. Crepitus which is not related with pain needs observation. If the crepitus is accompanied with pain, the causes of pain should be searched and corrected.

8.2.8.5 Avascular Necrosis of the Patella

The incidence of avascular necrosis of the patella increases when the superior lateral genicular arteries are injured during lateral retinacular release. *Avascular necrosis of the patella has the tendency for revascularization in 6 months to 1 year.*

It is unclear as to whether or not avascular necrosis of the patella causes anterior knee pain, and there are also various theories regarding its contribution to patellar complications such as loosening and fracture. Theoretically, it is believed that it contributes to the incidence of patellar fracture.

8.2.8.6 Wear and Loosening

When the patellar prosthesis is under excessive load, the incidence of wear and loosening is increased. Meding et al. reported that *obesity* predisposes to patellar component loosening up to 6.3 times. Loosening can develop due to repeated squatting and when the bone quality is not good due to bone necrosis. The incidence of wear appears to increase with the patient's weight, postoperative range of motion, and the duration of implantation. *The surgical factors that increase the wear are malalignment of the extensor mechanism, joint line elevation, and lateral retinacular release*. Vanbiervliet et al. demonstrated via an in vitro study that patellar maltracking due to an internally rotated femoral component may lead to an increased patellar component wear. *Prosthetic design also plays an important role; metal-backed patella causes wear more rapidly due to thin PE*. The current all-poly patellar component has a significantly reduced incidence of wear.

When wear or loosening develops, the prosthesis should be removed and the condition of the remaining patella should be checked to decide whether or not to re-resurface the patella. In low-demand patients, simple patellar component removal and patelloplasty using an arthroscopic burr may suffice. However, early wear and loosening in young patients might need revision of the femoral or tibial component according to its cause.

8.2.9 Hematoma and Wound Drainage

It is not surprising that a postoperative hematoma can occur as the TKA procedure involves numerous bone cuts, intramedullary canal violation, and soft tissue release.

There are multimodal approaches for minimizing the intraoperative bleeding. *Plugging the intramedullary canal, not performing the lateral retinacular release by accurate patellofemoral balancing, and meticulous hemostasis can decrease the initial blood loss*. However, to deflate the tourniquet and intraoperative hemostasis is a controversial issue.

The incidence of infection is increased due to prolonged wound drainage. Patel et al. stated that the serous discharge may persist for a long time in patients who are morbidly obese, take anticoagulants, or have excessive drainage.

When a postoperative wound drainage occurs, the first step is to take a wound swab, and a period of immobilization and observation is needed. If the discharge is profuse and if it increases with joint motion, the discharge may be coming from inside of the joint. If the bleeding continues and is suspected to be originated from inside of the joint, the knee can be reopened and the source of bleeding should be identified. *Indications for surgical evacuation of a hematoma include wound dehiscence, impending skin necrosis, persistent sanguineous leakage from the incision site, and severe pain. Probing and squeezing the wound to evacuate the hematoma are not recommended* because these could lead to retrograde contamination.

8.2.10 Superficial Infection and Skin Necrosis

When wound healing is not satisfactory, there may be a serous discharge from the wound, crust formation, or skin

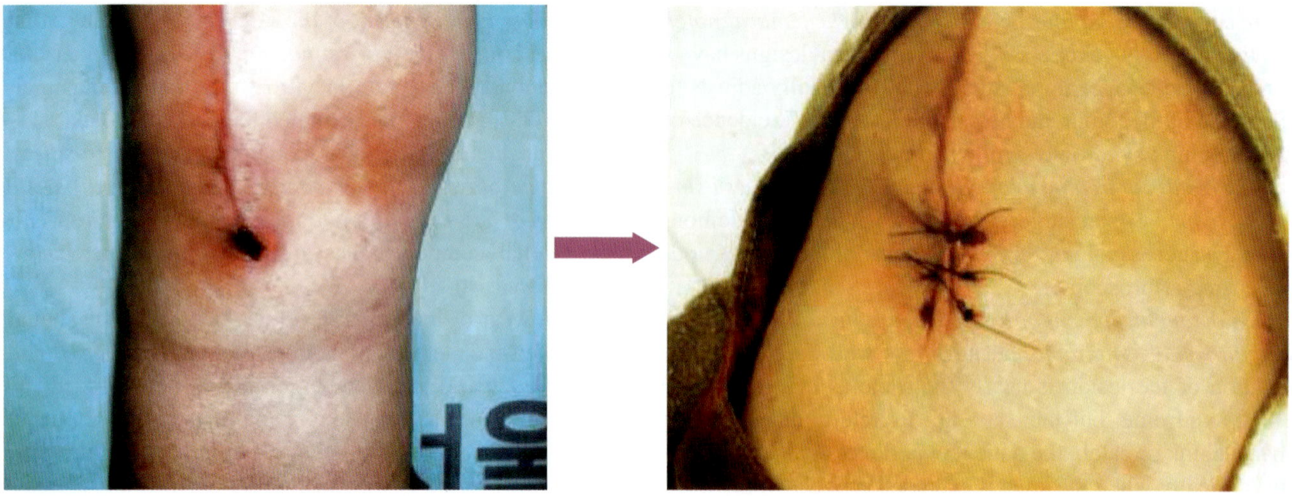

Fig. 8.5 Treatment of the crust

necrosis and superficial infection. When skin necrosis develops, it should be regarded as superficial infection.

A superficial infection is confined to the skin and subcutaneous tissues and does not extend to the fascia, but *active management* is required from the beginning *as it can progress to skin necrosis and deep infection if it is not treated adequately*.

Systemic factors which have an adverse effect on wound healing include obesity, malnutrition, prolonged corticosteroid or nonsteroidal anti-inflammatory drug use, DM, an immunocompromised state, and a history of smoking. Wilson et al. reported that *the incidence of superficial infection is high* when the patient is *obese* because it is difficult to perform an adequate approach and there is excessive discharge after surgery. However, Stern and Insall have an opposite opinion, and they state that superficial infection is not related to obesity. *Smoking* can also be a very important cause of skin necrosis due to constriction of the capillary vessels. *Steroid therapy* interferes with wound healing by decreasing the immunity and inhibiting fibroblast proliferation.

Local factors are vascular insufficiency of the lower limbs, when an improper skin incision and approach was utilized in the patients with poor skin condition due to a previous surgery, patient who had infectious disease that affected the knee joint, patients with a severe deformity, the incision was exposed to air for a long time, and closure was done improperly. *Since lateral retinacular release also increases the incidence of superficial infection*, Johnson et al. suggested preserving the superior lateral genicular arteries as much as possible. The incidence of *superficial infection* would further increase if CPM is started early or if the wound is not treated adequately. It is most common in the area just proximal to the patella and around the tibial tuberosity. The tibial tuberosity area, in particular, has a thinner soft tissue envelope, and this causes an easier spread of the superficial infection to the bone.

If purulence or erythema is not severe, the initial management should include careful dressing, immobilization, and observation. It is necessary to isolate the organism before starting the antibiotics and to delay the rehabilitation program such as CPM until the wound condition improves.

When superficial epidermal loss occurs in an area smaller than 2–3 cm^2, several modified dressing protocols can be used and the surgeon waits until the granulation tissue appears. If the wound is small and yet the skin condition is poor, marginal debridement and resuturing of the wound is recommended.

The crust formation at the incision site is essentially different from the crust of an abrasion wound, and hence, it is not recommended to wait until the crust peels off. Instead, *wound revision should be performed as soon as possible when the demarcation becomes definite* (Fig. 8.5).

There are several reasons for performing wound revision. First, the crust formed on an abrasion wound heals faster due to abundant blood supply, but the crust formed on a surgical incision has a poor blood supply and hence takes a longer time to heal. Second, crust formed on an abrasion wound is not deep, and there exists a defense mechanism of penetration into the deeper tissues, and it does not cause many problems even if the wound gets deeper. On the other hand, the crust formed on a surgical scar masks the wound penetration, and it is likely to be connected to the joint through the incision site. As a result, deep wound infection can develop. Third, motion restriction is needed for a certain period of time for crust healing, and this could delay rehabilitation, thereby causing problems such as soft tissue adhesion or limited motion. *In widespread skin necrosis, however, overaggressive debridement can lead to deep infection*. It is sometimes needed to wait until the eschar demarcates.

The most difficult judgement to make is to determine whether the necrosis is confined to the subcutaneous layer or it is connected to a deeper part. If the duration of necrosis is short, it can be considered to be confined to the superficial layer.

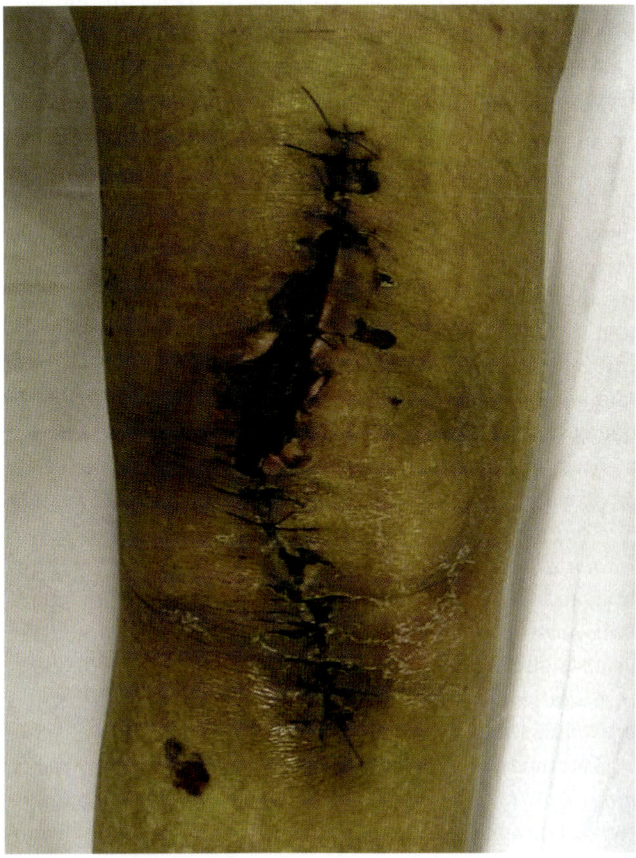

Fig. 8.6 Skin necrosis after arthroplasty

Skin grafting is preferred if the area of skin necrosis is too large for performing simple skin closure and there is a risk of skin necrosis after wound revision. In some cases, Hallock recommended the use of local fasciocutaneous flap. If the necrosis has extended to the muscle layer, the prosthesis can be seen through the wound, there is persistent drainage, or the amount of discharge increases with joint motion, these can be regarded as the signs of joint involvement (Fig. 8.6). In such a case, a plastic surgeon should be consulted for flap surgery, and the next step of treatment should be planned carefully.

The most frequently used flap material is the medial head of gastrocnemius; it is detached from the Achilles tendon insertion area and turned to the proximal part (Fig. 8.7). The medial head is better than the lateral head because it gives a good coverage, has a wide range of movement for treating the defects in both the patella and the tibial tuberosity, and has less postoperative motion limitation. Gerwin et al. reported that all their cases were successfully treated with this method when the prosthesis was removed and about 83 % of cases were successfully treated with this method when the prosthesis was retained. Another tissue available is the soleus flap. If other materials are unavailable, free muscle flaps such as latissimus dorsi or rectus abdominis should be used.

8.2.11 Deep Infection

Deep infection could be the most awful complication after arthroplasty. The *prognosis of deep infection is worst among all complications once it develops, and the joint almost never returns to the previous condition*. It usually requires revision, and there is no guarantee that one revision would be enough. In addition, long-term use of antibiotics is physically and financially burdening, and it is stressful to both the patient and the surgeon.

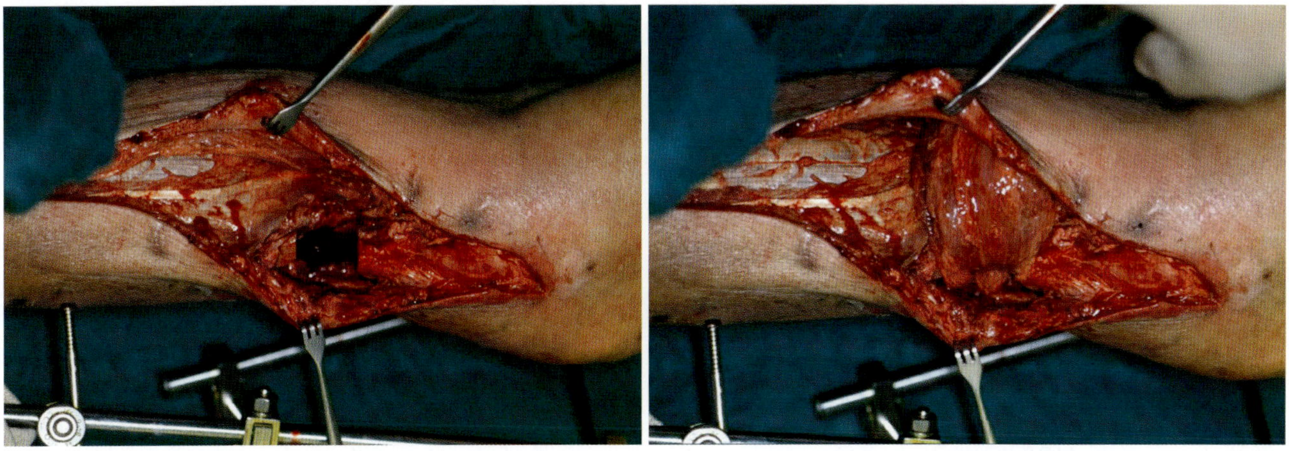

Fig. 8.7 Medial head gastrocnemius muscle flap (Courtesy JP Hong). *Left*: soft tissue defect before flap surgery. *Right*: after flap surgery

8.2.11.1 Classification

Deep infection is classified into *four types according to the time of onset. Type I is an acute infection that occurs within postoperative 4 weeks, type II is a chronic infection that persists for more than 4 weeks, type III is an acute hematogenous infection* that develops suddenly in a well-functioning artificial joint, and *type IV includes a positive culture from the specimen taken during revision* for probable aseptic failure. Segawa et al. defined the type IV deep *infection* as type I deep *infection* and the type I deep *infection* as type IV *deep infection*.

8.2.11.2 Incidence

The incidence of infection after primary TKA continues to increase. The incidence of infection varies from surgeon to surgeon. Most surgeons reported the range of incidence of infection between 0.5 and 2.0 %; Hanssen et al. reported an incidence of 2.0 % among 16,035 cases of primary arthroplasty and 5.6 % among 2,714 cases of revision performed between 1969 and 1996 at the Mayo Clinic. Teeny et al. reported that about half of the deep infections are caused due to superficial infection, persistent serous discharge, skin dehiscence, and skin necrosis, and joint swelling increases the incidence of deep infection.

Deep infections are known to be *more common after TKA than after THA*, because the knee joint is a relatively superficial joint and the surgical approach leads to vascular interruption to the skin when the subcutaneous tissues are stripped off.

The infection rate is also higher *in the one-stage simultaneous operation*.

8.2.11.3 Cause

It is believed that the patient's general condition, surgical techniques, surgical environment, and postoperative care affect the occurrence of infection.

It is assumed that acute infection is related to the surgical environment and procedures in patients with various risk factors, whereas acute hematogenous infection is caused due to the patient's poor general condition or in patients with mechanically or biomechanically unstable knee joint.

Patient-related risk factors are the general and local factors. In terms of *the general factors*, infection rate is thought to be related with *poor nutrition* (albumin 3.5 g/dl↓) and comorbidities such as *chronic exhaustive diseases, sexually transmitted diseases, diabetes mellitus, cardiopulmonary diseases, and urethritis, etc.* Wilson et al. found that the patients with *rheumatoid arthritis* have decreased immune function leading to poor wound healing, which doubles the infection rate. Other risk factors include *long-term use of steroid therapy, chronic alcohol addiction, AIDS, history of smoking, organ transplantation, and malignant tumor. Morbid obesity* may also cause an increase in the incidence of infection. Jämsen et al. reported that diabetes and morbid obesity increased the risk of periprosthetic infection.

Local factors are prior open knee surgery, periarticular open fracture, and prior history of septic arthritis or adjacent osteomyelitis.

Operation time seems to play an important role in the occurrence of infection. Longer operation time means longer exposure to the air and longer nonphysiologic state of the tissues. Peersman et al. stated that the incidence of infection is significantly increased if the operation time exceeds 2.5 h.

Surgical environment is theoretically a very convincing factor, but in fact, there is no definite evidence for development of infection based on the quality of surgical environment alone. It is very hard to clarify the relationship between the incidence of infection and surgical environment, because the incidence of infection is very low and is related to various factors. Strict surgical asepsis is critical for everyone attending the operation. When it comes to preparing for the operation, appropriate attire such as body exhaust suit, access restriction of persons to the operating room, installation of laminar flow, and meticulous surgical drape are thought to decrease the incidence of infection. Under any circumstances, the rate of infection caused due to the surgical or environmental factors should not be greater than 0.5 %.

Long-term insertion of the Hemovac and being in a bedridden state for a long time are also the risk factors for infection, and the patient becomes susceptible to infection due to *long-term hospitalization*. When patients have pneumonia or urinary infection, it may be a source of prosthetic infection.

Malalignment and instability worsen the condition of the prosthesis and increase the risk of infection.

The type of the prosthesis used is also important; when a *hinged prosthesis is used*, macrophage-linked membrane is formed around the stem, and this tissue reduces the phagocytic activity, which in turn increases the risk of infection.

8.2.11.4 Diagnosis

Rapid and expedient diagnosis is essential so as not to delay the treatment. Diagnostic tests include blood test, X-rays, arthrocentesis, bone scan, and biopsy based on the medical history and physical examination.

In acute infection, there is persistent *pain*, and it is noted even when the *patient is resting*. The pain that does not disappear from postoperative day 1 (day 1 onward pain) strongly suggests the presence of an acute infection. However, in chronic infection, the pain may not be definite, and it may sometimes be difficult to differentiate a chronic infection from the other complications because there may not be any specific symptoms except for mild pain and swelling.

On physical examination, the joint is swollen and warm and the joint motion is limited, but these symptoms are also commonly found during the early postoperative stage even though there is no infection. Persistent drainage, of course, can be associated with deep infection.

Therefore, the diagnosis mostly relies on the laboratory studies for infection, which includes WBC, ESR, and CRP. The *ESR and CRP are the more commonly used* in the orthopedic field. CRP is more sensitive than ESR in patients with infection, and hence, it is very reliable unless the patient has inflammation in the other region of the body. The CRP level is the highest on postoperative 2–3 days and drops down to normal in about 3 weeks. In my experience, however, there were a considerable number of patients whose CRP level did not drop down to normal after 3 weeks, and in most of them, it eventually returned to normal without any treatment for infection. I am not certain as to whether or not this feature is related with simultaneous operation. So, *the pattern of the CRP curve is more important than the numerical values. It requires close observation if the CRP level rises again after it had dropped or if it remains persistently high.* Parvizi et al. believed that synovial CRP assay holds great promise as a diagnostic marker for periprosthetic infection. The ESR level is the highest at about 1 week after the operation and gradually returns to normal in about 3 months. However, it can be higher than normal for up to 1 year. Di Cesare et al. found that the interleukin-6 (IL-6) level, which was produced by macrophages, was a more accurate marker than either the ESR or the CRP level.

X-ray may not show abnormal findings at first, but bone destruction, loosening of the prosthesis and periosteal new bone formation can be seen as the infection progresses. The *bone destruction* shows some irregular borders around the prosthesis, which is a little different from that in osteolysis (Fig. 8.8). In some cases, gas forms in the soft tissues. It is not easy to differentiate between aseptic loosening and infectious loosening on the X-ray, but *if loosening occurs around all components, it is a strong sign of infectious loosening*. In other words, *aseptic loosening generally affects only one component, but infection affects all the components*.

Arthrocentesis is essential for making the diagnosis of infection. The joint fluid should be checked for its color and viscosity along with chemical analysis and cell counts. There is a possibility of infection if the WBC count is greater than 50,000 cells/μL and the proportion of polymorphonuclear cells (PMN) is more than 65 % in the non-replaced joint. However, after TKA, an infection should be *suspected if the WBC count is more than 1,500–2,000 cells/μL and the proportion of PMN cells is more than 65 %, and there certainly is an infection if the WBC count is more than 3,000 cells/μL.* But these counts can vary according to the timing of arthrocentesis from the index operation or from the onset of symptoms. In patients with infection which developed within 3 months, the synovial fluid cell count and proportion of PMN cells can be much higher (approximately 20,000 cells/μL and 89 %, respectively). In this respect, Bedair et al. stated that the optimal synovial fluid white blood cell cutoff value was 27,800 and the use of standard cutoff value (3,000) would have led to unnecessary reoperation. Barrack et al. noted that in contrast to aspiration of hip joints after THA, the false-positive results are more common after TKA and the false-negative is more likely after THA.

In the chemical analysis, it is important to check whether the protein level has increased and sugar level has dropped. However, this may not be applicable when there is a chronic infection.

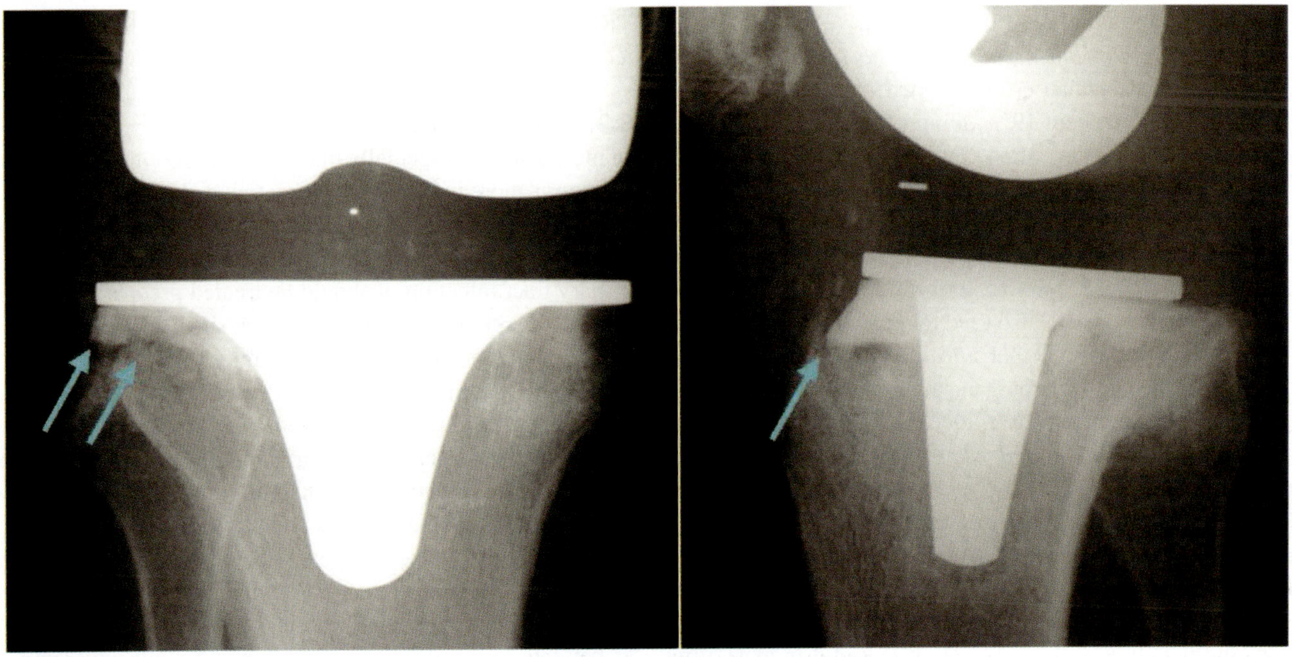

Fig. 8.8 X-ray showing a deep infection. There is bone destruction with periprosthetic loosening

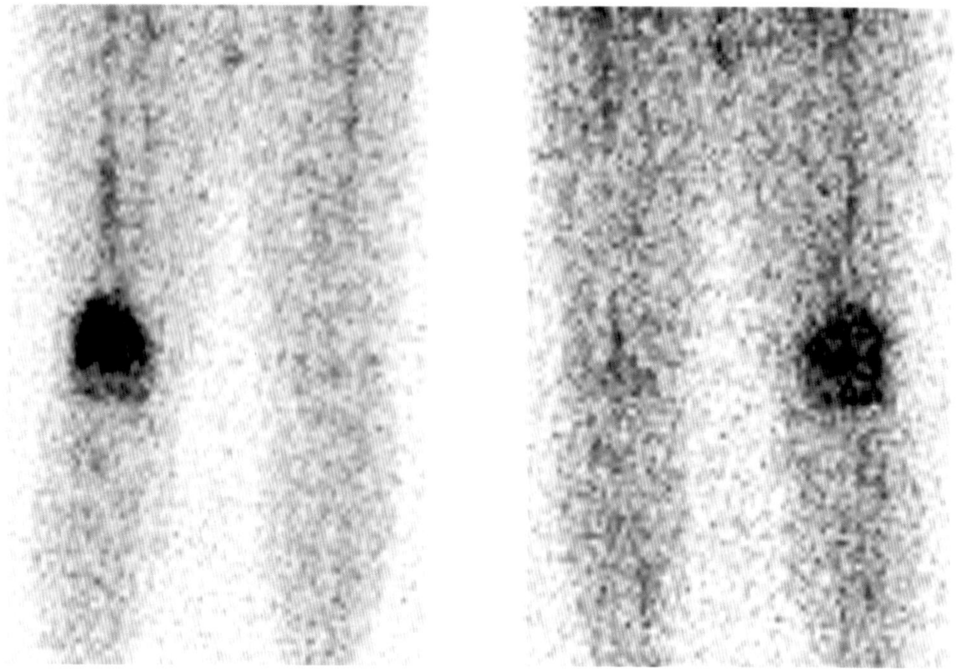

Fig. 8.9 WBC scan for deep infection. Hot uptake is observed around the prosthesis in the right knee joint

Smear and culture should be performed to detect the causative organism and to determine its sensitivity to antibiotics. The smear helps to identify whether the organism is gram-positive or gram-negative so as to choose the antibiotics to be administered before the antibiotic sensitivity results are obtained. However, gram staining may show high false-positive results. *The most common organism is Staphylococcus aureus (50–65 %), and MRSA is the most troublesome among them.* Sometimes, it presents as a mixed infection, and it is likely to occur when there is a wound problem. Other organisms including Streptococcus, *Escherichia coli*, and tuberculous bacilli, and fungi may also be found.

Failure to isolate the organism does not mean that there is no infection. Peersman et al. reported that organism could not be isolated in about 19 % of infected TKAs. Isolation of organism often fails when antibiotics have been used; Barrack et al. reported that the organism can be isolated when antibiotics are stopped for about 4 weeks. *AAOS recommends that antibiotic therapy should be stopped for a minimum of 2 weeks* prior to performing intra-articular culture. Other methods are also used for detecting the organism. Kobayashi et al. found that *ultrasonication* breaks up the biofilm formed by microorganism on the implant surface, thereby increasing the possibility of isolation of the microorganism. *Amplification and sequencing of 16S ribosomal deoxyribonucleic acid* by polymerase chain reaction improved the diagnosis of prosthetic infection. This is based on the theory that all pathogenic bacteria have 16S RNA. Detection of 16S RNA can be done by amplification of DNA. Although this technique is not widely available in most centers and is only used for research, it is useful in expediting the identification of slow-growing bacteria and the detection of bacteria that cannot be cultured. *On the other hand, it does not necessarily mean that the isolated organism is the causative organism for the infection.*

Bone scan is very useful for making the diagnosis of infected arthroplasty. The technetium (Tc) scan, 3-phase scan, and WBC scan are available. As the technetium scan is nonspecific, the 3-phase scan or WBC scan is recommended, but the results of these scans may be difficult to interpret. The results of both the technetium scan and WBC scan performed simultaneously are more accurate (Fig. 8.9).

For an even more accurate diagnosis, the specimen is taken for *biopsy* during arthroscopic examination or revision TKA. The specimen is examined histologically and subjected to culture for microorganism.

8.2.11.5 Prevention

In most diseases, especially in infection following TKA, prevention is more important than treatment. *If the general factors can be improved before the operation*, all possible methods should be used to improve them. If the patient has urinary tract infection, it should be treated preoperatively. If patient has skin ulcers at the operation site, it is ideal to wait for at least 3 months before performing a TKA. In order to reduce the local risk factors, it is recommended to ask the patient to quit smoking for at least 3 weeks before surgery.

It is controversial whether the *preoperative prophylactic antibiotics* are effective. AlBuhairan et al. reviewed 11,343 patients through meta-analysis and reported that *the prophylactic antibiotics* helped to prevent the infection. AAOS suggested that the preoperative prophylactic antibiotics should not be withheld in patients with a probability of infection or in patients with established infection who are undergoing reoperation. *The first-generation cephalosporin is used* as a prophylactic antibiotic. *However, the AAOS recommended the use of vancomycin in the hospital or institute where the occurrence of MRSA has been previously reported.* Smith et al. reported that the use of vancomycin as the perioperative prophylactic antibiotics for primary TKA appeared to be effective in decreasing the rate of periprosthetic infection.

There are different opinions regarding the timing and duration of prophylactic antibiotics. Many reports have suggested the use of antibiotics for just 24 h. Classen et al. recommended administrating antibiotics once 30–40 min before the operation and they should not be given for more than 48 h postoperatively to reduce the risk of urinary tract infection. However, I am of the opinion that antibiotics can be given for 3–4 days or for a longer period in patients in whom the operation time was longer, who had undergone knee surgery previously, who had poor skin condition, who had received steroid injection into the joint, who had rheumatoid arthritis, or who were at high risk of infection for other reasons.

The operation should be precise and accurate and should not last for a very long time.

Some surgeons recommend the use of antibiotic-loaded bone cement (ALBC). Josefsson and Kolemrt emphasized *the use of antibiotic-loaded cement routinely*, which leads to an increase in the concentration of antibiotics at the operation site and promote the delivery of the antibiotics to the area where antibiotics cannot reach due to poor blood supply. Chiu et al. expressed the same opinion that the use of ALBC reduces the incidence of infection. However, Masini et al. did not recommend the use of antibiotic-loaded cement routinely since some patients are allergic to antibiotics, resistant strains can develop, and the cement may be weakened. Instead, they suggested its use in revision surgeries and in patients with high risk of infection. Namba et al. reported that ALBC does not help in preventing infection.

To prevent hematogenous infection, an invasive procedure should not be performed within 2 years of TKA. Durack reported that when 2 years had not elapsed after TKA, the incidence of infection was particularly high in case operation was done for dental or genitourinary system. *Practically, invasive procedures that potentially cause bacteremia should simply be avoided at least in the first 3–6 months after TKA. Durack suggested the use of prophylactic antibiotics 1 h before the invasive procedure of the genitourinary system or oral surgery* in patients with diabetes, rheumatoid arthritis, or in high-risk patients and if the operation time is expected to be longer than 75 min. However, some authors state that the use of prophylactic antibiotics before dental treatment is meaningless. Uckay et al. stated that oral bacteria are anaerobic bacteria or streptococci which are different from those found in the artificial joint infection and temporary asymptomatic bacteremia occurs after dental treatment and disappears quickly. They concluded that it is more dangerous to have an oral infection than it is to treat the dental problem. Despite of this theory, many surgeons recommend prophylactic antibiotics during dental treatment because if an infection develops, it can cause serious problems.

8.2.11.6 Treatment

The goal of treatment is to eradicate the infection first and restore the knee function to the preinfection state as much as possible.

As patients may require antibiotic administration for a long time and they may undergo several operations, their general condition, their life expectancy, and quality of life should be taken into consideration.

The method of treatment is decided based on the antibiotic sensitivity of the organism, duration of infection, skin and soft tissue conditions, integrity of the extensor mechanism, fixation state of the prosthesis, and bone defect. Surgeon's ability and patient's expectations should also be taken into consideration. Segawa et al. stated that the *factors which have a negative impact on the treatment of infection include immunocompromised conditions, bone necrosis and loss, and poor soft tissues surrounding the joint.*

According to Segawa et al., *successful treatment* of the infected arthroplasty is defined as *no clinical evidence of infection for 2 years and restoration of adequate function after arthroplasty*. The definition of adequate function here is the ability to walk with minimal pain and no radiological loosening of the prosthesis. *The results of treatment depend mainly on the condition of the patient and causative organism.* Mortazavi et al. observed that negative culture or MRSA infection increased the risk of failure by more than fourfold and twofold, respectively. Hence, the evaluation of results according to the method of treatment is less reliable if these conditions are not considered. Mcpherson et al. suggested a grading system for a better clarification of the infection eradication rate of each treatment method. Since the infection eradication rate varies significantly according to the type of infection, the patient's general condition, and the condition of the knee joints, they emphasized that *the results of treatment should be judged* based on three factors, (1) *the type of infection* (acute postoperative, acute hematogenous, late chronic), (2) *systemic host grade according to the medical and immune state condition (uncompromised, compromised, significantly compromised)*, and (3) *the local extremity grade (uncompromised, compromised, significantly compromised).* Therefore, evaluating the success rate of infection eradication without applying the Mcpherson's grading system may be inaccurate.

Since the Mcpherson's method was introduced recently, it must be understood that the previously reported success rates were the general success rates without considering the patient's condition or infection type.

Antibiotics should be used regardless of the method of treatment. They must be *bactericidal* based on the antibiotic sensitivity test and should be continued for *at least 4–6 weeks. Antibiotic therapy differs greatly from surgeon to surgeon, but there are some general principles which need to be followed.* Vancomycin is started from the beginning if the smear shows gram-positive cocci as it indicates the possibility of occurrence of MRSA. Even if *MRSA is sensitive to cephalosporin, vancomycin is the most effective* and cephalosporin derivatives are not recommended. *Quinolone is also not recommended as many strains of staphylococcus become resistant to it.* Vancomycin is also the first choice for patients who are allergic to cephalosporin or penicillin derivatives.

After analyzing 146 patients with deep infection, Fulkerson et al. recommended the general guidelines for antibiotic use. Vancomycin is used when the acute or chronic postoperative infection is due to gram-positive cocci or when gram staining fails to detect the organism. Combination of cefazolin and gentamicin is used for acute hematologic infections. For gram-negative organisms, third- or fourth-generation cephalosporin or combined therapy with aminoglycoside and penicillin, ampicillin, or quinolone derivatives can be used. Mixed infection with gram-positive and gram-negative organisms needs vancomycin in combination with third- or fourth-generation cephalosporin. When the organism cannot be isolated, vancomycin and gentamicin should be administered.

Zimmerli et al. found that many organisms form a mucopolysaccharide biofilm when the prosthesis becomes infected, and this *biofilm increases the bacterial resistance to the antibiotics*. Since *rifampin facilitates the penetration of antibiotics into the biofilm*, they recommended addition of rifampin in cases with long-standing infections to achieve synergistic effects.

At times, *long-term oral antibiotic therapy* is used, but it is *not recommended* as this promotes development of resistant strains and causes bone loss accompanied by various side effects.

Guidelines for administrating antibiotics are summarized in Table 8.2.

Treatment options include antibiotic suppression only, drainage and debridement, one-stage revision, two-stage revision, arthrodesis, resection arthroplasty, and amputation.

The use of suppressive antibiotic therapy yields a success rate of less than 20 %. It can be selectively used in the acute streptococcal infection in the patient who is healthy with no wound problems or when the patient's general condition is too poor to undergo an operation. If type IV infection has been found, it is a general principle to use only suppressive antibiotics. Segawa et al. reported that type IV infection was treated only with an antibiotic injection in all five of his cases without recurrence. *But antibiotic suppression prolongs the duration of treatment and often makes the subsequent treatment difficult due to delay of definite treatment. The prerequisites for this therapy are that the microorganism should be susceptible to an oral antibiotic, the antibiotics should be tolerated by the patient without serious toxicity, and prosthesis should be stable.* Prognosis of antibiotic suppression therapy is worse with staphylococcus or gram-negative organisms. The presence of other joint arthroplasties or presence of cardiac valvular disease is a relative contraindication. *Use of a combined regimen of rifampin with quinolone has been reported to be more successful.*

If it is a tuberculous infection, it can be treated by antituberculous chemotherapy. Marmor et al. experienced good results by providing antituberculous chemotherapy for 6–18 months with the prosthesis retained while observing changes in the CRP.

Debridement or drainage with prosthesis retention can be attempted in acute stage of type I and type III infection when the prosthesis being stable and the organism is sensitive to antibiotics. The success rate was reported to be 20–30 %. Arthroscopic surgery can be used as a means to irrigate the joint, but it shows a low success rate. Sherrell et al. experienced high failure rates of subsequent two-stage reimplantation.

The most common method of treating infection is *revision TKA*. *Prosthesis needs to be removed in cases with deep infection due to a resistant strain, long-standing infection and when loosening of the prosthesis is noted.* Revision TKA can be performed in one stage or in two stages. This is further described in Chap. 9. Surgical treatment modality of infected TKA is summarized in Table 8.3.

Arthrodesis can be performed when the patient is a young active laborer, the extensor mechanism is lost, the infection is with a resistant strain, the patient cannot endure several operations due to poor general condition, the infection has recurred after revision TKA, or *there is the risk of reinfection due to poor skin or soft tissue conditions*. After arthrodesis, the patients cannot mobilize the joint, but it has the advantage of *reducing the reinfection rate and provides stable and pain-free knee joint*. Methods of achieving arthrodesis include external fixation, internal fixation, and intramedullary (IM) nailing. Among these, IM nailing is the most preferred method. Arthrodesis can also be done in two

Table 8.2 Brief summary for guidelines of administrating antibiotics according to the organism of infected arthroplasty

	Gram (+)			Gram(−)	Mixed	MDR	Undetermined
	Streptococcus	Staphylococcus	MRSA				
First-generation cephalosporin	+						
Third- or fourth-generation cephalosporin	+			+	②		
Penicillin or ampicillin				②			
Aminoglycoside				①			②
Quinolone				②			
Vancomycin		+	+		①	+	①
Rifampin		③	③		③	③	③

MRSA methicillin-resistant staphylococcus aureus, *MDR* multi-drug resistant organism
+: single use, ①: first-line antibiotics, ②: combination therapy with first-line antibiotics, ③: combination therapy is recommended

Table 8.3 Surgical treatment strategy according to the type of infected arthroplasty

	Streptococcus Sensitive drug (+)	MRSA MDR
Type I<2 weeks (acute)	Debridement and PR One-stage revision	Two-stage revision
>2 weeks	One-stage revision or Two-stage revision	
Type II>4 weeks (chronic)	Two-stage revision	
Type III (acute hematogenous)	Same with acute infection	
Type IV (intraoperative culture (+))	Antibiotic suppression and observation	

MRSA methicillin-resistant staphylococcus, *MDR* multi-drug resistant organism, *PR* prosthesis retention

stages; the first stage includes prosthesis removal, extensive debridement, and insertion of antibiotic-loaded cement, while the second stage includes performing arthrodesis after removal of antibiotic-loaded cement. The success rate of arthrodesis varies from surgeon to surgeon and from method to method. *Factors causing nonunion include a huge bone defect, poor condition of the remaining bones, inadequate fixation, and persistent infection.* Some surgeons report a success rate of 95–100 %, but Rand et al. reported a success rate of 70–81 % in infection of an ordinary prosthesis and 56 % in infection of a hinged prosthesis. Broderson et al. and Rand et al. also agreed that the incidence of nonunion is higher with the use of the hinged prosthesis due to a huge bone defect.

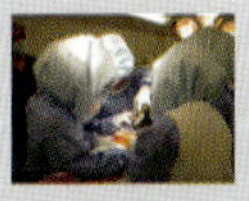

Author's Method

I suggest arthrodesis in case of recurrence of infection after revision TKA. Re-revision TKA yields an even lower success rate, and it is uncertain as to how many operations would be needed. Also, the patient's general condition can worsen, pain may persist, and function can decrease due to poor soft tissues and bone quality. Considering the social and financial circumstances, it is practically difficult to persuade the patient to undergo one more operation if re-revision fails.

Arthrodesis can be performed in one stage or in two stages according to the degree of infection. However, it is very difficult to achieve bone union, and it takes a long time in a severe bone defect.

If there is a severe bone defect or the condition of the bone is not good, I perform debridement and curettage of the bone marrow cavity and fix the femur and tibia with a flexible nail and fill cement into the gap. This method is not for achieving real bony union, but it allows early mobilization, and I have achieved good results in many patients (Fig. 8.10).

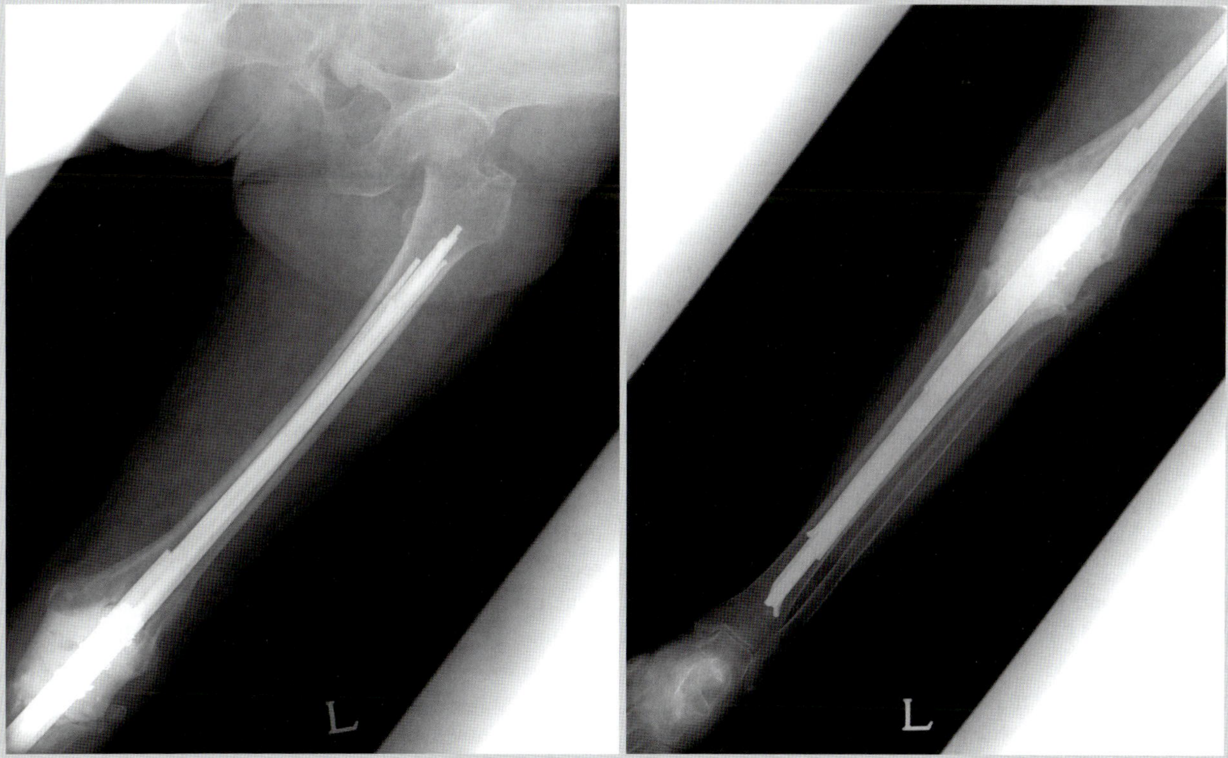

Fig. 8.10 Arthrodesis using a flexible nail

Resection arthroplasty can be performed when the patient has a severe bone defect and has difficulty in movement due to rheumatoid arthritis, *when the infection may threaten the patient's life, when the patient cannot undergo revision TKA*, or when performing TKA is meaningless. Patient may be able to move the knee in the 30° arc of motion and needs brace fittings for ambulation. It is easier for the patient to sit down than that after arthrodesis, but the joint becomes unstable for walking and the pain may persist. If the patient is not satisfied with the results of resection arthroplasty, arthrodesis can be performed later. The knee joint sometimes undergoes spontaneous fusion.

Amputation can be considered when the organisms are not sensitive to any antibiotics, infection threatens the patient's life, several operations have failed, the joint function cannot be maintained by any method, the bone defect is too severe to use tumor prosthesis or APC (allograft prosthetic composite), etc.

8.2.12 Aseptic Loosening

Loosening means the separation of the artificial prosthesis from the bone causing instability of the prosthesis. Loosening can occur between the cement and the bone or between the prosthesis and the cement.

The loosening caused due to the long-term use of prosthesis is inevitable; however, early loosening has specific causes including patient-related factors, implant design, and surgical failure.

The distinction between osteolysis and loosening is sometimes ambiguous, and both the terms can sometimes be used interchangeably. Some surgeons take them into account as different presentations of one phenomenon, but it is necessary to differentiate between these two conditions since the prosthesis can be separated from the cement without osteolysis.

Miller et al. explained that the mechanism causing loosening is initiated by micromotion between the components and the bone. The other possible mechanisms are component subsidence and periprosthetic osteolysis. If the prosthesis has sunk by more than 5°, the cancellous bone surrounding the prosthesis loses its trabecular network and forms a shell to cause a bone defect, which leads to an increase in the PE wear as a result of the deformity. The worn PE particles are resorbed by the macrophages provoking an inflammatory reaction, which predisposes to further bone destruction.

8.2.12.1 Cause

Patient-Related Factors

Loosening increases when the *knee joint is overused or patients are engaged in prohibited activities*. The incidence of loosening increases when the *bone is weak or osteopenia is severe* since the supporting strength of the prosthesis is decreased. According to Lombardi et al., there are some patient-related factors including obesity, knee motion over 115°, and very active male patients that may lead to loosening.

Implant Design

Implant design is the most common cause of loosening. Articular conformity, motion constraint, fixation method, modularity, and stem shape and length are the implant design factors related to loosening. *The incidence of loosening of cementless type of prosthesis, high-flex designs, the prosthesis with high conformity, and the constrained prosthesis is high.* This is because of the greater shear stress between the bone and the prosthesis. The incidence of loosening of modern prostheses has markedly decreased compared to that of the past through the modification of component design.

Surgical Factors

Malalignment and Instability

One of the most important predisposing surgical factors is *malalignment*. The incidence of loosening is bound to increase if malalignment imposes too much load on one side. Lotke and Lonner and Dorr et al. stated that *malalignment is the most important factor in aseptic loosening*, and Lee et al. reported that loosening increases when the tibial prosthesis is shifted to the medial side by 4 mm or when there is a varus deformity of more than 2°. However, Hsu et al. and Smith et al. stated that malalignment does not always causes loosening. There is increased patellar component loosening when the bone is resected asymmetrically or aligned poorly. *Instability* also causes loosening as a result of failure to distribute the load evenly.

Cement Fixation Technique

It is obvious that poor fixation leads to increased loosening. If cementing is done *without proper treatment of the sclerotic bone or repeated joint motion is allowed before the cement is fully set during cement fixation, the rate of loosening increases. The time and method of cement fixation* is also important; Dorr recommended cementing the patella within 2 min, the tibia in 3–4 min, and the femur in 6–7 min. He also recommended removing the extruded cement and then pressing the component while extending the knee until the cement is fully set. *The depth of cement penetration into the bone affects the rate of loosening*. Walker et al. stated that the ideal depth of penetration is 3–4 mm. While Brassard et al. recommended the depth of 2–3 mm, and 5 mm or a deeper penetration caused thermal necrosis and bone weakening leading to increased loosening. Long-term follow-up studies of TKA using old cementing techniques without using pulsatile lavage reported adequate bone penetration of the cement and have shown an extremely good survival rate with minimal loosening.

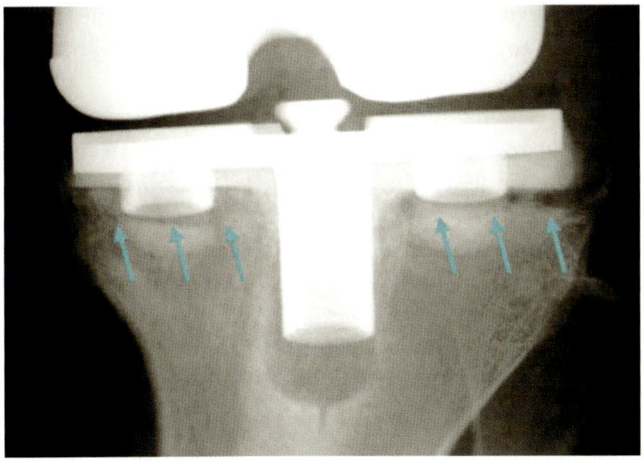

Fig. 8.11 Aseptic loosening. *Arrows* indicate separation the prosthesis from bone

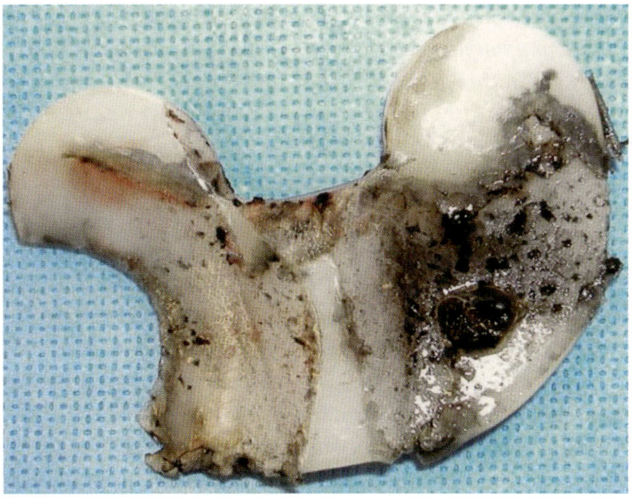

Fig. 8.12 Wear of the polyethylene

8.2.12.2 Diagnosis

In the early stage, a radiolucent line is seen along the boundary of the component on X-ray, and this is followed by tilting and subsidence of the prosthesis with progression of loosening. Although theoretically there should be no gap between the cement and the prosthesis, a *gap of up to 2 mm between the cement and the bone is considered to be clinically acceptable.*

Loosening is more common around the tibial component (Fig. 8.11). However, this is because loosening is not easily detected on the femoral side due to incorrect projection of the X-ray beam. If the angle of radiological projection is oblique, loosening on the femoral side can be masked due to overlapping on the X-rays. Therefore, X-rays need to be taken accurately to diagnose loosening appropriately. Fehring et al. recommended fluoroscopy-aided X-rays which are taken during weight bearing. It is beneficial to diagnose loosening that cannot be detected on simple X-rays.

The American Knee Society adopted a scoring system at the site of radiolucency to determine the loosening. The *roentgenographic evaluation and scoring system* assigns 1 point for every millimeter based on the radiolucency in each zone (Fig. 3.2). *Loosening can be diagnosed if the score is more than 4 points, in case of implant subsidence or migration, cement fracture, hot uptake in delayed phase of the three-phase bone scan*, and *asymmetric wear associated with osteolysis* on simple A–P X-rays. *However, radiolucency in the cementless type means that there is no bony ingrowth. Therefore, loosening of the cementless type may progress when a radiolucent line is seen.* It is also *necessary to compare with previous X-rays* in order to determine the stability of prosthesis or the progression of loosening.

It is important to differentiate this condition from septic loosening. Even though it is very difficult to differentiate between both these conditions clinically or radiologically, *the diagnosis is likely to be septic loosening when loosening is found around all the components.*

8.2.12.3 Treatment

Loosening does not always cause serious symptoms, and hence, the treatment is done according to the symptoms and progression of loosening. *Revision TKA is needed if pain is associated with instability and the aforementioned X-ray findings are seen. Once the decision is made, it is recommended to perform revision TKA as soon as possible in order to preserve more bone.* The method of revision is further described in Chap. 9.

8.2.13 Wear

Wear is a very common and serious complication, which accounts for about 25 % of all revision TKAs and is known to be more common after TKA than after THA. Wear of the patellar component due to the use of a metal-backed patella was more common in the past, but the wear of the tibial PE is common nowadays.

When wear occurs, the vicious cycle of osteolysis starts leading to loosening which in turn increases the wear. Wear can occur uniformly, but early wear tends to be the eccentric wear on the medial or posteromedial side (Fig. 8.12). Initial wear is confined to the PE; however, the wear progressively extends to the metal.

Wear is largely classified into abrasive/adhesive wear, fatigue wear, scratching, and corrosive wear.

Abrasive wear is simple grinding and adhesive wear is defined as grinding with a compressive force, but these two types of wear have been combined into one type of wear as they actually occur concurrently. Burnishing is the most common finding *in abrasive/adhesive wear. It is the wear of the surface due to constant repeated contact, and hence, it is significantly influenced by the material of the counter part of the PE. The hip joint is a ball and socket joint, and it is mostly affected by the abrasive/adhesive wear and is more influenced by properties of the femoral head.*

Delamination, crack, and pitting are fatigue type of wear due to repeated trauma rather than due to repeated grinding on the surface and occur when the shape of the PE changes. This type of wear develops from the inside of the PE, and hence, it is influenced mainly by the nature of the PE itself. Delamination wear is common in the knee joint due to its complex kinematics, but undersurface wear in mobile-bearing knee is actually the abrasive/adhesive wear.

Scratching occurs on the surface mostly due to third-body wear as a result of impingement of the cement or bony particles. Corrosive wear is the chemical wear.

8.2.13.1 Cause

Wear, just as loosening, is closely related to the time elapsed after TKA. *Wear which is caused due to the long-term use of the prosthesis cannot be avoided, but early wear is mostly caused due to overuse, surgical failure, and PE defect.*

Patient's Activity

It is obvious that *vigorous and incautious activity* increases the wear. Since the wear is proportionate to the amount and duration of loading, it increases due to overactivity, squatting, in obese patients, etc.

Surgical Techniques

Incorrect operation can cause *malalignment and instability*. Any form of malalignment, regardless of the direction (mediolateral, anterior–posterior, or rotational) and site (tibiofemoral or patellofemoral), leads to focal concentration of stress on the PE. Instability also imposes stress on the PE, thereby accelerating the wear.

When the *joint space is overstuffed*, stress increases during the joint motion, thereby increasing the wear rapidly. If the extension gap is wide, hyperextension of the knee joint increases the contact stress on the anterior aspect of the post, and this can increase the wear rate of the post in PS type of prosthesis. Callaghan et al. noticed that the post is severely worn when the knee is hyperextended.

If cement around the notch area in PS open box type of the prosthesis is not removed completely and when the cement or the bone debris is caught between the components, it causes a third-body wear.

Prosthesis Defect

Design

The design and nature of PE material can affect wear rate of prosthesis. This is described in more details in Chap. 2, and hence, I will briefly describe it here.

In terms of the design, *low conformity or flat design increases the stress* on the PE, thereby increasing the wear rate, and excessive conformity restricts the rotational movement, thereby increasing the stress on the PE during rotation to cause loosening and wear.

Since sliding motion compared to rolling contributes more to the wear, the design that leads to *too much roll back increases the wear. Loose fixation between the tibial tray and the PE increases the PE motion, and an uneven surface treatment of the tibial component increases an undersurface abrasive/adhesive wear.*

For the patella, metal backing of the patellar component leads to an increased wear due to a decrease in the PE thickness. The sombrero type of patellar component that fits into the shape of the femoral trochlea is known to have a low wear rate, whereas the dome type of patellar component increases the contact stress.

Materials

When titanium articulates with PE, i.e., when the femoral component is made of titanium, the wear rate increases. On the other hand, ceramic has a lower wear rate.

Various attempts have been made to increase the strength of the PE in order to reduce the wear, but only the abrasive wear could be decreased and not the delamination wear. Most of the wear of the knee joint is the delamination wear, and the advantage of using a cross-linked PE in the knee joint is doubtful.

It is reported that the wear increases significantly when the PE is thinner than 6 mm. Wear also increases *when there is a fusion defect in PE or heat press is applied for surface treatment* as in the earlier type of PCA Knee (Porous Coated Anatomic Knee, Howmedica, Rutherford, NJ).

Sterilization and Storage

Wear varies according to the amount of gamma radiation and the presence of oxygen during sterilization; the most desirable type of sterilization is the EO gas sterilization. *The location and duration of storage* is also related to the wear; *3–4 years of shelf storage increases the wear as a result of oxidative degradation.*

8.2.13.2 Symptoms and Diagnosis

When wear develops, there is no particular clinical symptom initially. *As wear progresses, however, the patient experiences instability, pain, crepitus, swelling, and difficulty in walking, and joint subluxation may finally occur. Development of a popliteal cyst may be an indirect sign of wear.*

The joint space looks narrower as compared to that in the previous X-ray, and stress X-ray is useful (Fig. 8.13). *When the wear progresses to the metal, a metal line can be seen on the X-ray* (Fig. 8.14). *Ultrasonography* has been shown to be helpful in evaluating the PE thickness accurately. Teeter et al. proposed a micro-CT technique by which volumetric and surface scanning can be obtained.

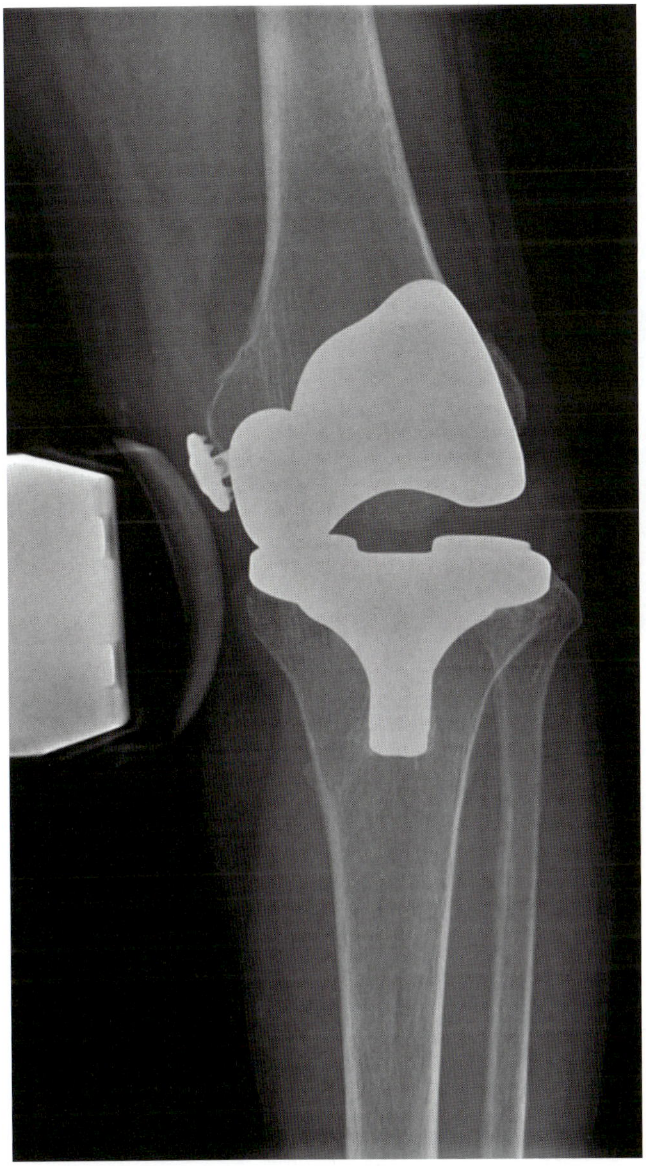

Fig. 8.13 X-ray findings of the wear. The medial side is narrower and the lateral side is wider on varus stress image

8.2.13.3 Treatment

If wear is noted, its management depends on the amount of wear and duration of usage of the prosthesis. *If the wear is confined to the PE which has been used for long duration, the PE can simply be changed.* If the wear has extended to the metal, performing a revision TKA is inevitable. Hence, it is important to diagnose the wear before metal involvement. This is one of the reasons why an annual follow-up is required in arthroplasty patients.

If early wear is found, it is likely to recur in cases when only the PE has been changed without any correction of the causative factor. If the wear is caused due to asymmetric instability, ligament balancing should be done and a thicker PE can be used. *Otherwise, it is necessary to perform revision for replacing all the components.*

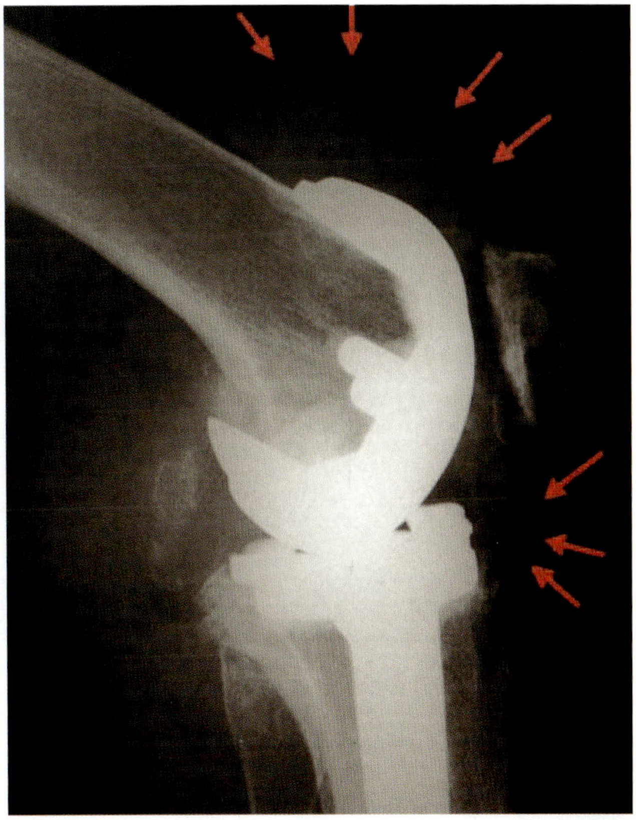

Fig. 8.14 Metal line due to metal wear (*arrows*)

8.2.14 Osteolysis

8.2.14.1 Cause

Osteolysis generally *occurs when the PE wear particles cause inflammatory reactions* and when there is an infection (Fig. 8.15). With the current improvement in PE materials, the incidence of wear and its resultant osteolysis have decreased. Metal particles also cause osteolysis; titanium is known to cause more amount of osteolysis than cobalt chrome.

Histologically, there is formation of hypercellular membrane containing histiocytes and giant cells which are activated by wear particles. Therefore, the particle size of the wear debris is important. According to Song et al., the particle size varies from 1 to 100 μm when observed under scanning electron microscopy (SEM). Large particles do not cause osteolysis, but *any particle smaller than 3 μm is absorbed by giant cells, thereby causing inflammatory reactions. If these particles do not penetrate into the cancellous bone, osteolysis does not occur. Hence, when the cancellous bone is properly sealed with cement, the incidence of osteolysis is decreased.* On the other hand, the incidence of osteolysis increases if the prosthesis is press fitted, when screw fixation is done without cement, or when the cement is broken.

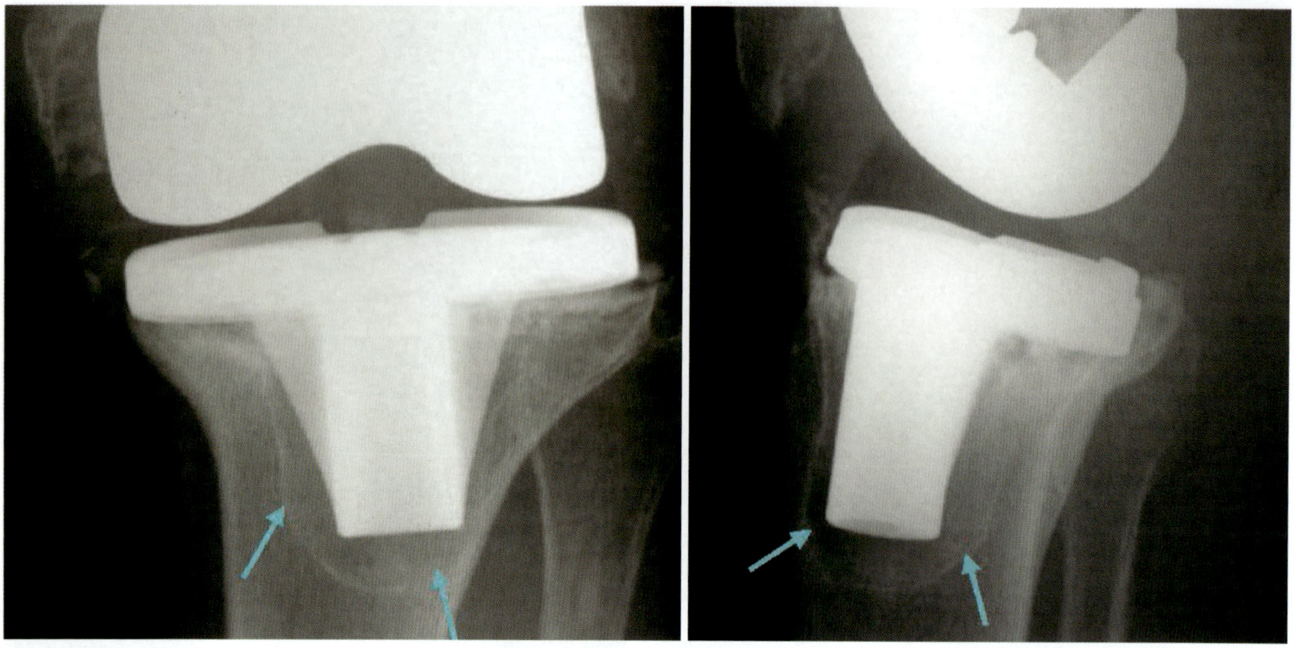

Fig. 8.15 X-ray showing osteolysis (*arrows*)

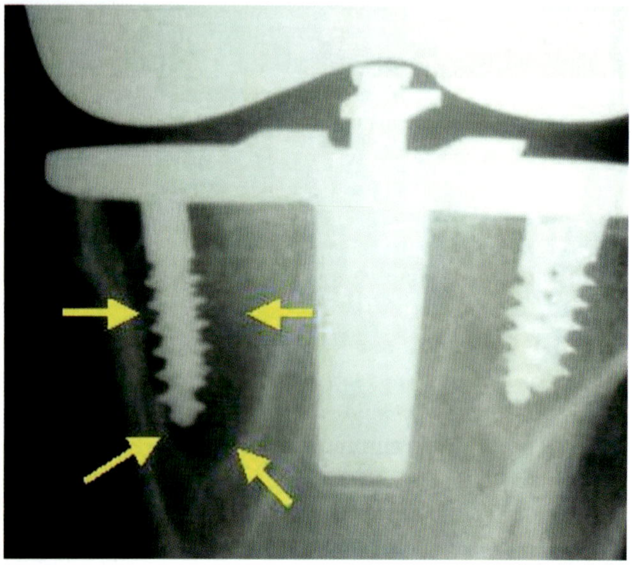

Fig. 8.16 Osteolysis around the screw (*arrows*)

Therefore, osteolysis is very closely related to the prosthetic design; Brassard et al. reported that *about 16 % of patients* suffered from *osteolysis when the tibia was fixed with screws*. And among them the PS type of prosthesis was used in 65 % of the cases (Fig. 8.16).

8.2.14.2 Incidence

Osteolysis is also closely related with the time elapsed after TKA, and it generally does not occur within 2 years. Robinson et al. reported that it occurs at an average of 56 months. *The progression of osteolysis differs according to the age, gender, tissue reaction, activity, alignment, and stability*.

Wear is more common after TKA than after THA, but *osteolysis is less common after TKA than after THA*. According to Engh et al., there are several *reasons* for this. The first reason is the *size of particles produced*. In the knee joint, the particle size is large due to delamination wear. The second reason is that the *synovial cavity of the knee joint is more extensive to absorb the wear particles easily*. The third reason is that *the knee joint is sealed better with cement on the surface of the bone*. The fourth reason is that *the knee joint experiences less shear and tensile forces* than the hip joint, and hence, *cement breakage occurs less frequently in the knee joint*.

Osteolysis mostly occurs in the tibia; Peters et al. explained that *this is because the particles tend to precipitate due to weight bearing and gravity, osteolysis may not be seen on the X-ray of the femoral side, and screw fixation has been used on the tibial side*.

8.2.14.3 Diagnosis

The symptoms of patients with osteolysis vary. Most patients with a well-fixed component are asymptomatic. But osteolysis eventually causes synovitis which provokes pain and swelling and leads to instability of the joint.

Diagnosis is made primarily on simple X-rays. *Radiolucency may be increased and partial or focal bone destruction may be seen on the X-ray*. Absence of trabeculae in the cancellous bone and geographic demarcation by a shell of bone can be seen. Diagnosis can be more accurate when the latest X-ray is compared to the previous X-ray. *Osteolysis on the X-ray tends to be much smaller than the real size of the osteolytic lesion. CT is of great help* in detecting the site and extent of osteolysis. Vessely et al. suggested that osteolysis can be diagnosed more accurately by an MRI using the metal suppression method.

8.2.14.4 Treatment

While treating osteolysis, observation is required when the prosthesis is stable, the lesion is small, and there are no apparent symptoms. Medical management with bisphosphonates and calcium supplementation can be initiated during the observation period.

If there is swelling and/or pain and the *prosthesis becomes unstable, there are two options. One option is the debridement, changing the PE and curettage followed by impaction of the defect with a morcellized bone graft. The other option is revision of components*. Callaghan et al. reported durable midterm results with extensive graft incorporation after PE exchange.

8.2.15 Heterotopic Ossification

Heterotopic ossification is a very rare complication following TKA, and it is not as common as that following THA.

Risk factors include male gender, obesity, history of heterotopic ossification, and patient with ankylotic spondylitis. Surgical factors include excessive injury to the periosteum, quadriceps muscle injury, hematoma formation due to inadequate hemostasis, anterior notching, and bony fragments remaining within the muscle.

The symptoms include pain and limited motion, but they vary according to the extent of ossification.

Heterotopic ossification is easy to diagnose on the X-ray, but bone scan or alkaline phosphatase level is useful for making an early diagnosis and for anticipating the prognosis.

Conservative treatments including *radiation therapy and administration of indomethacin are known to be effective*. Continuous passive exercise prevents adhesion and scar formation, but vigorous rehabilitation can aggravate the symptoms. Cho et al. reported that conservative treatment achieved good results in patients with heterotopic ossification.

8.2.16 Periprosthetic Fracture

The definition of a periprosthetic fracture differs from surgeon to surgeon, for example, fracture occurring within 15 cm of the prosthesis, within 9 cm from the joint line, or within 5 cm of the medullary stem. However, periprosthetic fracture may be defined as *all the cases in which the fracture treatment and its method have a direct influence on the prognosis of arthroplasty*.

It is difficult to decide the best treatment modality for periprosthetic fracture because it is mostly accompanied by osteopenia; there are many factors that influence the prognosis including fixation state of the prosthesis, displacement and comminution of the fracture fragment, and patients' general condition and knee joint condition before/after fracture.

The incidence of nonunion is high since the patients are older in age and have various medical comorbidities, vascularity may be poor due to arthroplasty, and the prosthesis and cement are placed around the fracture site. The incidence of *periprosthetic fracture* is about 0.6–2.5 % after TKA, which is not as high as that after THA. The incidence of *periprosthetic fracture* is higher when the old type of prosthesis is used.

8.2.16.1 Cause

General factors include *osteopenia* or any condition that can cause osteopenia such as rheumatoid arthritis, long-term steroid therapy, and neurologic deficiency. Local factors can be divided into intraoperative and postoperative factors.

Intraoperative Factors

Femoral fracture can occur during the operation when the guide rod is improperly inserted into the medullary canal, the femoral *component of the PS type is implanted without enough box cutting, or box cutting is too large, thereby weakening the bone*. It is known that a fracture is more common at the medial femoral condyle because the bone mass of the medial condyle decreases dramatically in the metaphyseal area and less bone is left after box cutting (Fig. 8.17).

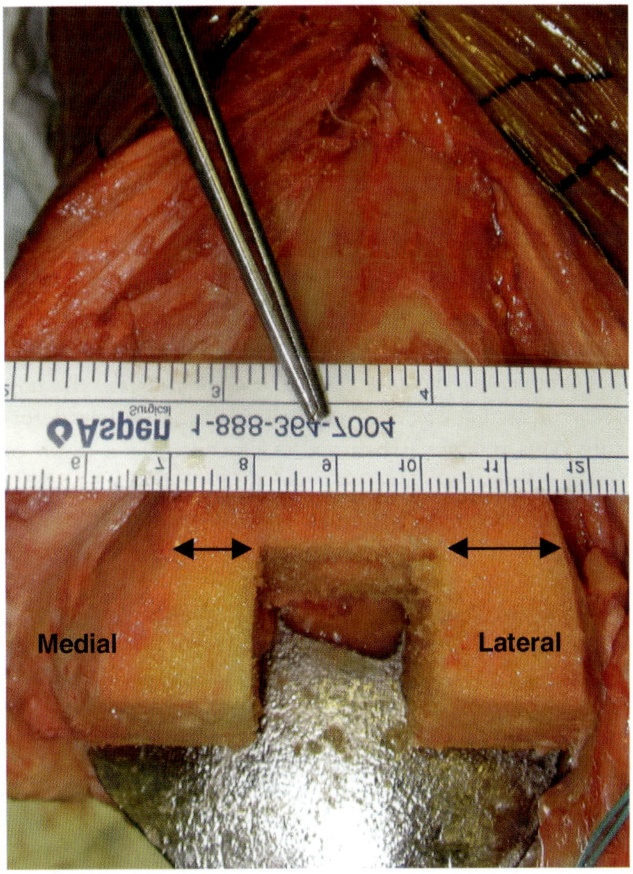

Fig. 8.17 The reason why fracture of the medial condyle using the PS type occurs more frequently than that of the lateral condyle during notch osteotomy

However, I have experienced more fractures of the lateral condyle than medial condyle. I think this is because the lateral condyle is less stronger due to a weak cortical buttress than the medial condyle.

Tibial fracture is caused due to excessive traction of soft tissues in patients with osteopenia, when the stem hole is made too small on the plateau, and when a forceful keeling procedure is done to fix the stem. When the prosthesis is implanted in patients with a flexion contracture, forceful extension of the knee joint causes compression of the anterior part of the tibial plateau, causing a fracture in osteoporotic patients.

In revision TKA, fracture may develop during removal of the implant and reaming or insertion of the extension stem. Fracture of the patella occurs most commonly during revision.

Postoperative Factors

Postoperatively, fracture can occur due to *trauma* such as fall or traffic accidents, or as a result of *repeated stress and fatigue* without definite trauma.

In femoral fractures, there are different theories regarding whether anterior notching of the femur is a predisposing factor for fracture. *Notching generally refers to an anterior resection more than 3 mm deeper than normal.* Ritter et al. reported that *anterior notching* is not related to periprosthetic fracture, but Scott et al. and most of the other surgeons believe that anterior notching acts as *stress riser as fracture tends to occur from the notching area in the early postoperative period in patients with osteopenia.* Lesh et al. revealed that notching decreases the bending strength by 18 % and the torsional strength by 39 %. Zalzal et al. also reported that notching more than 3 mm with sharp corners starting from the end of the femoral prosthesis often leads to a fracture due to stress concentration.

There are reports that *the pin used in the navigation system causes a fracture in patients with osteopenia.*

Sometimes, a fracture similar to a compression fracture occurs in the lateral condyle, thereby causing a valgus deformity. This fracture is believed to be caused as a result of osteonecrosis due to excessive soft tissue stripping in valgus deformity, or preexisting valgus malalignment increases the eccentric load on the lateral condyle in patients with osteopenia (Fig. 8.18).

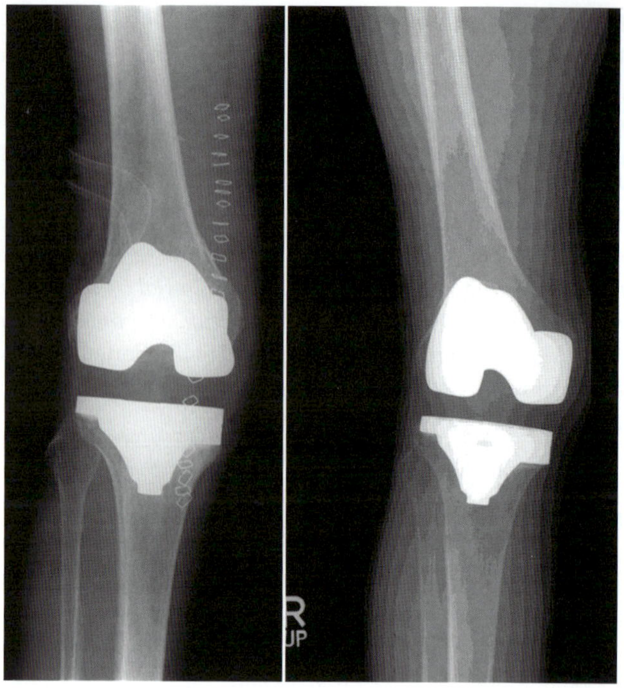

Fig. 8.18 Valgus deformity due to fracture of the lateral condyle. *Left*: X-ray taken immediately postoperatively shows good alignment. *Right*: X-ray at postoperative 2 months shows valgus deformity due to lateral condylar fracture

When an extension stem is used, a too thick stem causes endosteal thinning during reaming and the site of the stem ends increases the possibility of a fracture.

A tibial fracture can be caused due to incorrect positioning of the prosthesis, when cement is not used, tibial tubercle osteotomy has been done, or osteolysis develops.

Patellar fracture can be caused due to trauma, but it is mostly a fatigue fracture (Fig. 8.19). *Patellar fracture may not have definite pain* and may be associated with sudden loss of extension power causing difficulty in walking and climbing up and down the stairs. Men are at a higher risk for fracture than women, and about half of the fractures occur in the first year. The incidence is reported to be between 0.15 and 3.7 %.

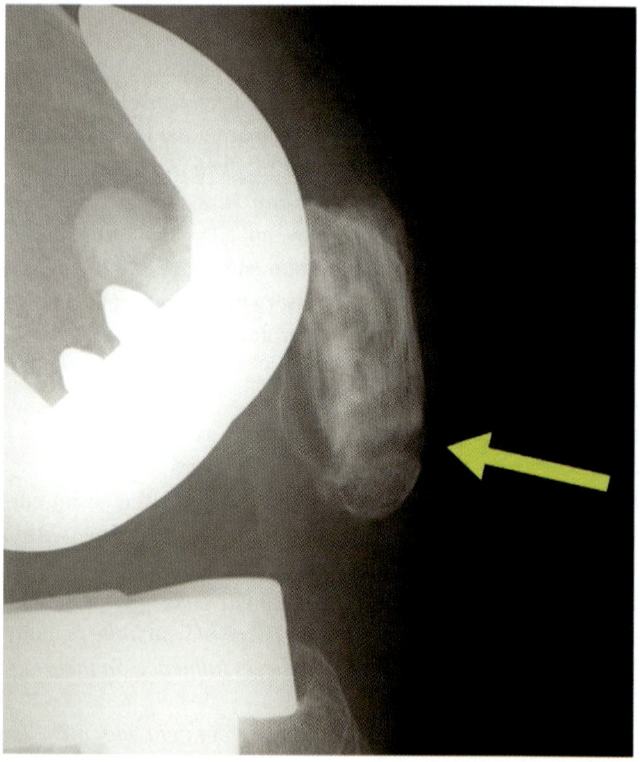

Fig. 8.19 Patellar fracture

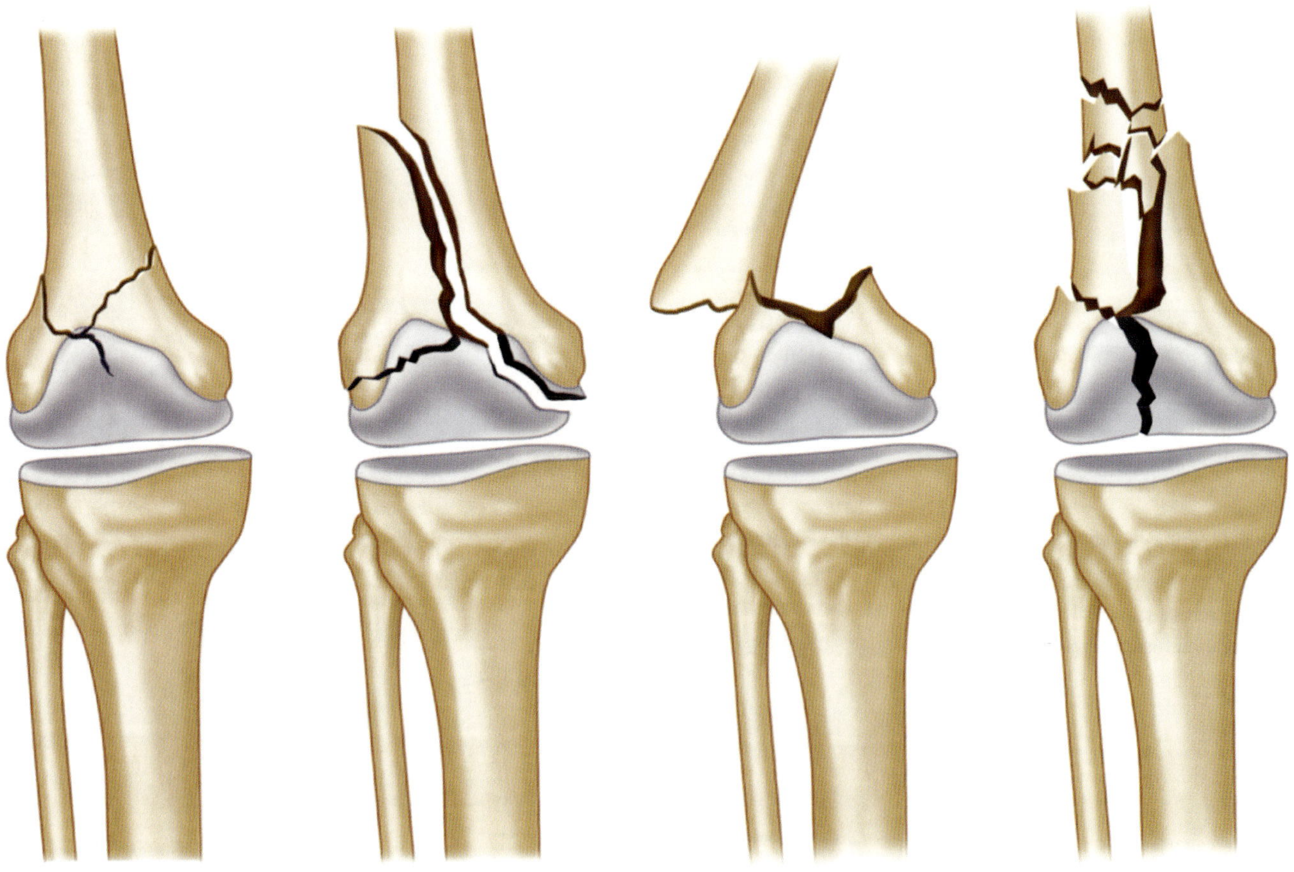

Fig. 8.20 The Neer classification

Possible causes include patellar maltracking, too much or too little patellar bone resection, avascular necrosis due to lateral retinacular release, and revision surgery. Tria et al. reported that avascular necrosis of the patella is the common cause of fracture and the incidence is increased among patients who had undergone lateral retinacular release. Figgie et al. reported that patellar alignment is closely related to the severity of fracture. *Prosthetic design* is also a causative factor; fracture is *more common when there is one fixation hole in the center*. Insall–Burstein PS type often causes fatigue fracture of the patella because the shape and A–P length of the femoral prosthesis increase the stress on the patella.

8.2.16.2 Classification

Femur

The Neer classification has been used for periprosthetic fractures of the femur. He classified the fractures according to the displacement of fracture and the degree of comminution (Fig. 8.20). Type I refers to a fracture without displacement, and type II is a fracture with displacement, among which type IIa indicates medial displacement and type IIb indicates lateral displacement. Type III refers to a fracture of the femoral condyle and shaft. Here, displacement indicates more than 5 cm of displacement of fracture fragments or more than 5° of angulation. However, this classification is not specific for a periprosthetic fracture but for a general supracondylar fracture of the femur, and the stability of prosthesis which is the most important prognostic factor for a periprosthetic fracture has not been taken into consideration.

Rorabeck and Taylor developed a modified form of the Neer classification for periprosthetic fractures of femur. *Type I is a fracture without displacement, and type II is a fracture with displacement, but the prosthesis is stable. Type II fracture is further classified into IIA (without comminution) and IIB (comminuted). Type III fracture has an unstable prosthesis regardless of the displacement*. This method is more practical for deciding the method of treatment because the prosthesis stability is the most decisive factor for periprosthetic fracture treatment.

Su et al. suggested a new classification method for surgical treatment, because an operation is required in most of fracture cases. Operative method varies mainly according to the level of fracture and stability of the prosthesis. I am of the opinion that the Su classification is simple and very practical.

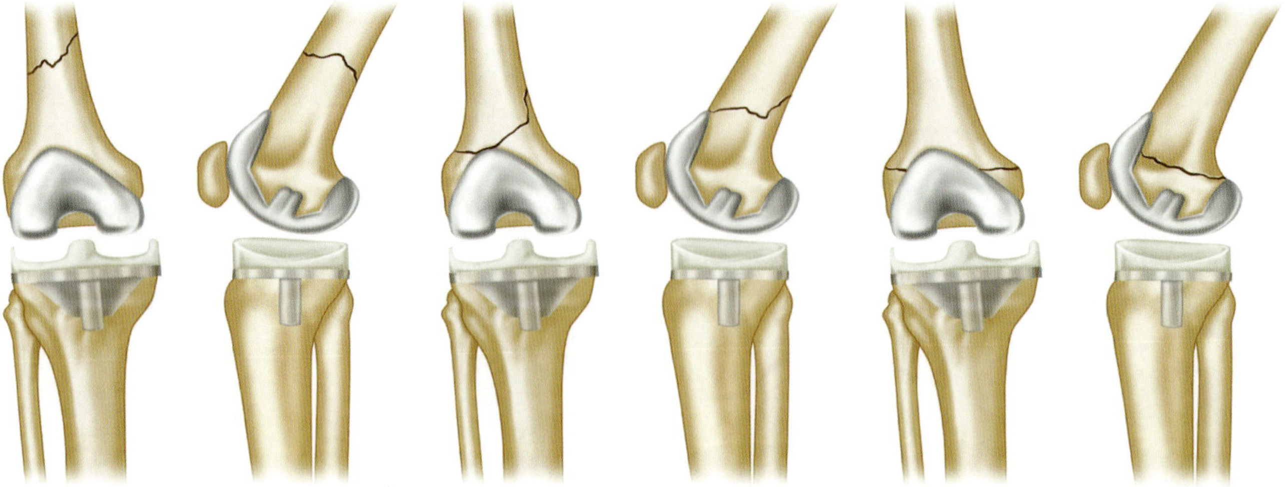

Fig. 8.21 Su's classification for fractures around the femoral prosthesis

Fig. 8.22 The Felix classification for tibial fractures

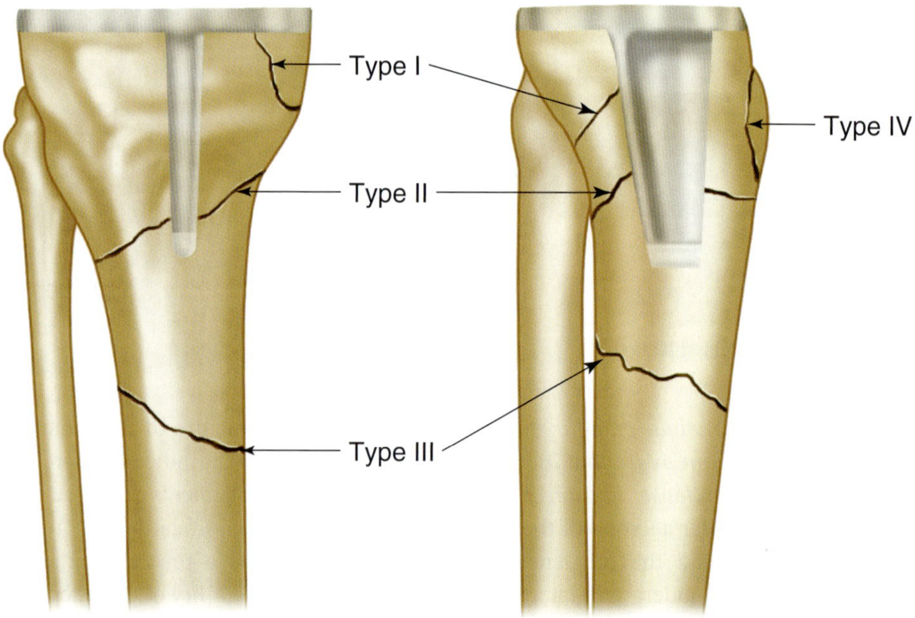

They have classified the fractures according to the level of fracture. *Type I is when the fracture is proximal to the prosthesis, type II is when the fracture starts near the prosthesis, and type III is when the fracture is located within the prosthesis* (Fig. 8.21). They suggested IM nailing for type I fracture, IM nailing or plate fixation for type II fracture, and internal fixation using plate or revision TKA with the use of a stem for type III fracture according to the prosthesis stability.

Tibia

Tibial fracture is very rare, and the most popular classification for tibial periprosthetic fracture is the *Felix classification*, in which the fracture is classified according to the level of fracture, timing of occurrence of fracture, and stability of the prosthesis (Fig. 8.22).

In this method, *fractures are classified according to the fracture site into type I plateau fracture, type II fracture adjacent to the prosthetic stem, type III fracture distal to the stem, and type IV tibial tubercle fracture. It is also classified into type A (fracture with a stable prosthesis) and type B (fracture with an unstable prosthesis) according to the prosthesis stability and type C (intraoperative fracture) according to the timing of fracture*. However, this method is based on the frequency of occurrence, and it is a little complicated to be standardized for deciding the treatment method.

Patella

The most popular classification method for a patellar fracture is *Goldberg's classification*, which classifies patellar

Fig. 8.23 Goldberg's classification of patellar fractures

TYPE	DESCRIPTION
I	Fractures not involving the implant/composite or quadriceps mechanism (marginal fractures)
II	Fractures disrupting the quadriceps mechanism or the fixation of the implant
IIIA	Non-displaced inferior pole fractures with intact patellar ligament
IIIB	Inferior pole fractures with patellar ligament rupture (displaced avulsions)
IV	Fracture-dislocation of the patella (shear fractures)

EXAMPLE/DIAGRAM

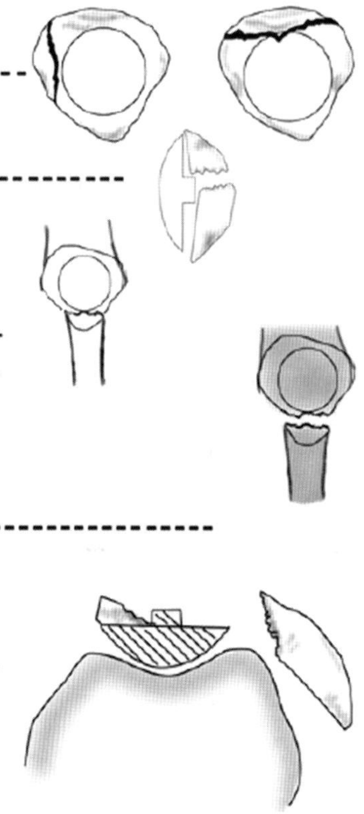

fractures into five types. *Type I* patellar fracture is the fracture which is *not associated with disruption of the extensor mechanism or prosthesis fixation*, *type II* patellar fracture is the fracture in which the *extensor mechanism or prosthesis fixation is disrupted*, *type IIIA* patellar fracture is the fracture at the *inferior pole of the patella without disruption of the extensor mechanism*, *type IIIB* patellar fracture *is the fracture at the inferior pole of the patella with disruption of the extensor mechanism*, and *type IV* patellar fracture *is the fracture with dislocation of the patella* (Fig. 8.23). The drawback of this classification system is that the severity of fracture does not increase gradually and there may be confusion regarding the severity of some fractures. For example, type IIIA patellar fracture is similar to type I patellar fracture and type IIIA patellar fracture has a better prognosis than type II patellar fracture.

Ortiguera and Berry proposed a new classification method focusing on three main factors: integrity of the extension mechanism, fixation state of the implants, and the remaining bone stock. This classification is simple and systematic. In this classification, type I is intact extensor mechanism with well-fixed patella, type II is extensor mechanism disruption, type III is loose patellar component and bone stock for revision is adequate, and type IV is loose patellar component and bone stock for revision is poor.

8.2.16.3 Treatment

Goal

The goal of treatment is to restore the knee function to the level as before the fracture. The prosthesis should be stable and well aligned, and the knee should flex more than 90°.

Principle

To determine the treatment method, fracture is first classified into intraoperative and postoperative fracture because intraoperative fracture mostly has minimal displacement and can be managed during the operation.

Intraoperative Fracture

Tibial or femoral fracture that occurs during the operation is mostly a split fracture or a burst fracture, and any special management other than screw fixation may not be required. If stability of the fracture cannot be secured with this treatment, buttress plate or extension stem may be used. No particular postoperative management may be needed except for brace fitting and delayed weight bearing.

However, patellar fracture usually occurs during revision surgery, and the method of treatment is not simple because there is inadequate bone stock and the patella is mostly avascular. Tension band wiring is one option, although it is not the ideal method. After reduction and fixation, ligament augmentation is needed in special situation. Non-resurfacing of the patella or patellectomy is another option.

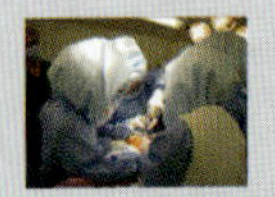

Author's Method

In the event of a patellar fracture during operation, I perform encirclage suture technique to address this problem.

In this technique, I pass a nonabsorbable suture (Ethibond) through the tendons and retinacular ligaments along the entire periphery of the patella and tighten it with the knee completely extended position. With this technique, the fracture usually gets anatomically approximated, and the results are satisfying (Fig. 8.24).

The advantage of this technique is that satisfactory reduction and fixation of the fracture can be achieved, vascularity is better preserved than tension band technique using K-wire, and cerclage wire and hardware is not seen radiologically.

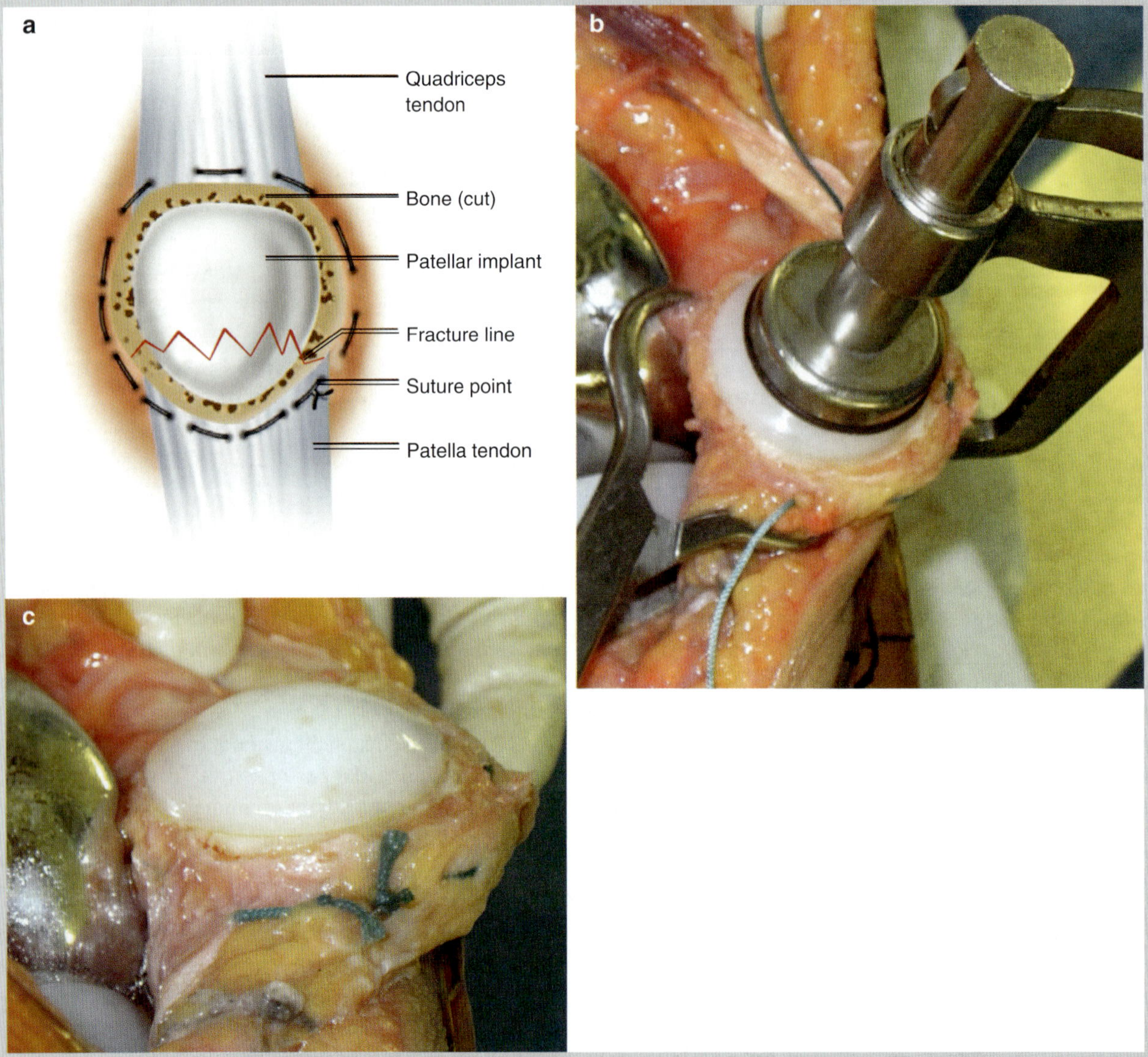

Fig. 8.24 Treatment of intraoperative patellar fracture. (**a**) Schematic drawing, (**b**) encirclage suture technique, (**c**) after reduction

Postoperative Fracture

When the prosthesis is stable, the fracture can be treated with the conservative or operative method. Although this is controversial, *open reduction is preferred so as to reduce the incidence of complications and maintain the function, unless there is a non-displaced fracture or patella fracture.*

The surgeons who prefer the conservative treatment state that the operation is difficult to perform in osteopenic patients and there is a high risk of complications such as nonunion and infection. Hence, they state that an operation should be the last resort for fracture treatment. Some surgeons state that revision can be performed after union depending on the patient's condition.

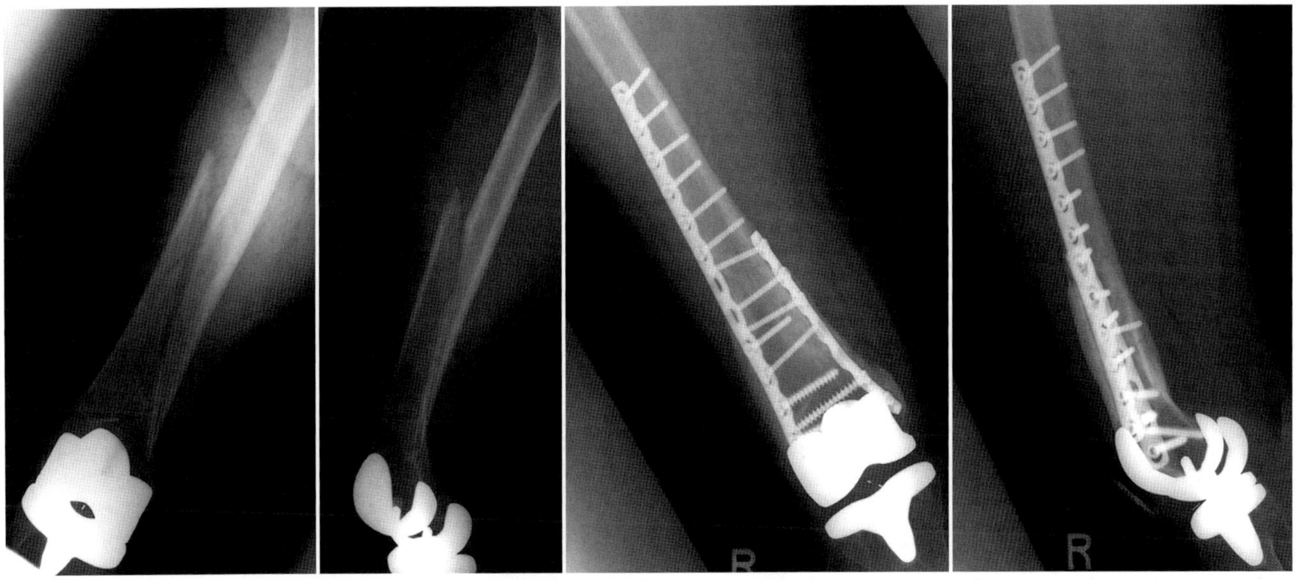

Fig. 8.25 Open reduction in a femoral periprosthetic fracture

On the other hand, the surgeons who are in favor of the operative treatment state that several complications such as bedsores and pneumonia are likely to develop due to prolonged immobilization and the results of the operative treatment are better than those of the conservative treatment. Operative procedure reduces, the incidence of third-body wear caused by bony fragment, and achieves more ROM and better alignment.

If the prosthesis is not stable, revision TKA is needed. Theoretically, open reduction is performed at the fracture site and a long stem can be used for revision TKA in case of an unstable prosthesis. However, the surgical procedure is technically demanding as it is difficult to fix the plate due to osteopenia, and screw should be inserted so as not to interfere with the stem insertion.

In some cases, bone grafting or cementing is needed.

Treatment Method for Each Bone

Femur

In Rorabeck type I fracture, wherein there is a linear fracture or there is almost no displacement, *cast immobilization can be done. The acceptable alignment* for conservative treatment, although it varies from surgeon to surgeon, *is less than 10° of angulation in all directions and less than 5 mm of displacement. In type II fracture, close reduction or traction can be performed first. If the fracture is reduced to achieve an acceptable alignment, conservative treatment can be performed. Open reduction is needed if the fracture cannot be reduced or it is difficult to maintain the reduction. However, many surgeons recommend open reduction and internal fixation in this type of fracture regardless of displacement. Type III fracture, wherein the prosthesis is unstable, requires revision TKA using medullary stem after open reduction and internal fixation. Tumor prosthesis* can be used primarily in cases with severe comminution.

Surgical treatment options include open reduction and internal fixation, external fixation, or revision TKA. Internal fixtures that can be used are the blade plate, T or condylar buttress plate, simple plate, or LCP (locking compression plate) according to the level of fracture or the degree of comminution. The blade plate is stable, but it may be impossible to insert it as the blade is located too distally and special surgical techniques are required for its insertion. *LCP is very useful in fractures with accompanying osteopenia* as this plate provides better stability than the other plates (Fig. 8.25). IM nailing may also be performed, but there is more probability of *malunion or nonunion* than that with the use of other internal fixtures. There are several types of IM nails including the Rush nail, supracondylar nail, or modified Huckstep nail. It is difficult to insert Rush nails in a fracture at a very distal level, and their use can also aggravate the preexisting fracture. Supracondylar nail cannot be used with the close box type of PS prosthesis and is known to cause nonunion more often as the thinner nail should be used. However, Jabczenski and Crawford reported good results with the use of a supracondylar nail.

When internal fixation with plate and screws is done, loss of fixation may occur, while IM nailing can cause migration, shortening, nonunion, or infection.

Bone grafting is often needed for fracture healing, and bone cement may be added if screw fixation is not secure. In such a case, special techniques are needed so that the cement does not leak out to the cortex or gets interposed between the fracture fragments. Healy et al. recommend creating a window in the supracondylar area for bone grafting or cementing in order to reinforce the fixation (Fig. 8.26).

Kumar et al. experienced good results by inserting allogeneic fibular graft into the medullary canal and buttress plate fixation, and Lee et al. introduced a method of fixation after allogeneic bone impaction.

External fixation can be another option, but it is associated with high risk of infection, and it is likely to fail in patients with osteopenia.

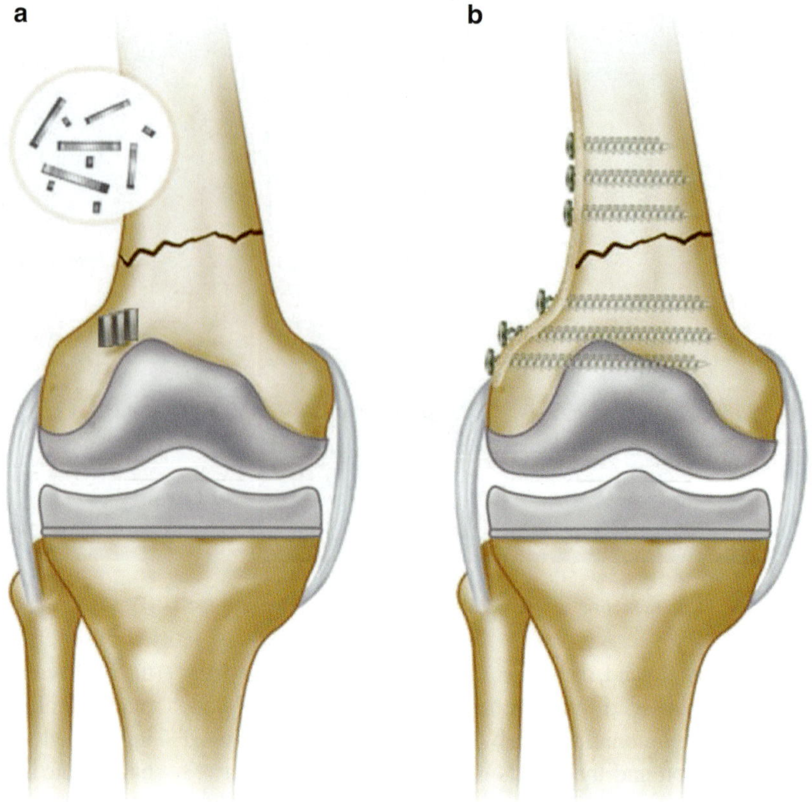

Fig. 8.26 Healy's method to reinforce fracture with a bone graft. (**a**) A window is made for allograft reinforcement the periprosthetic fracture, (**b**) after plate and screw fixation

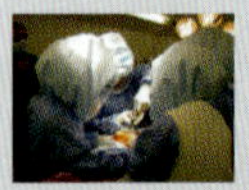

Author's Method

There may be a valgus deformity due to compression fracture of the lateral femoral condyle.

I perform impaction of compression fracture and reinforce the defect with a metal augment and cementing rather than reduction and bone grafting, and this is followed by buttress screw fixation at the proximal part of fracture in order to improve the stability (Fig. 8.27).

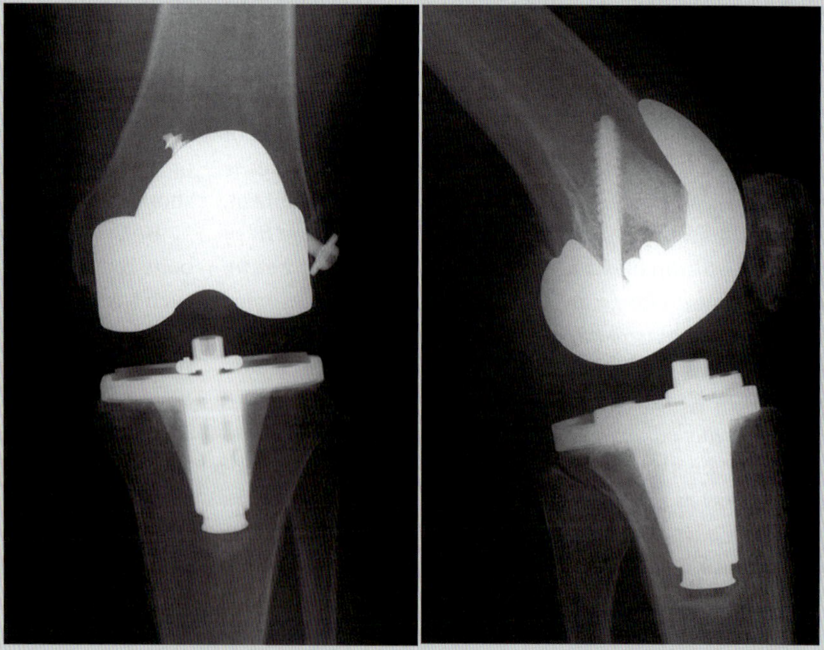

Fig. 8.27 X-ray of a lateral femoral periprosthetic fracture. Metal augment is used for compression fracture of the lateral femoral condyle, and buttress screw is inserted. Good alignment and stability are obtained

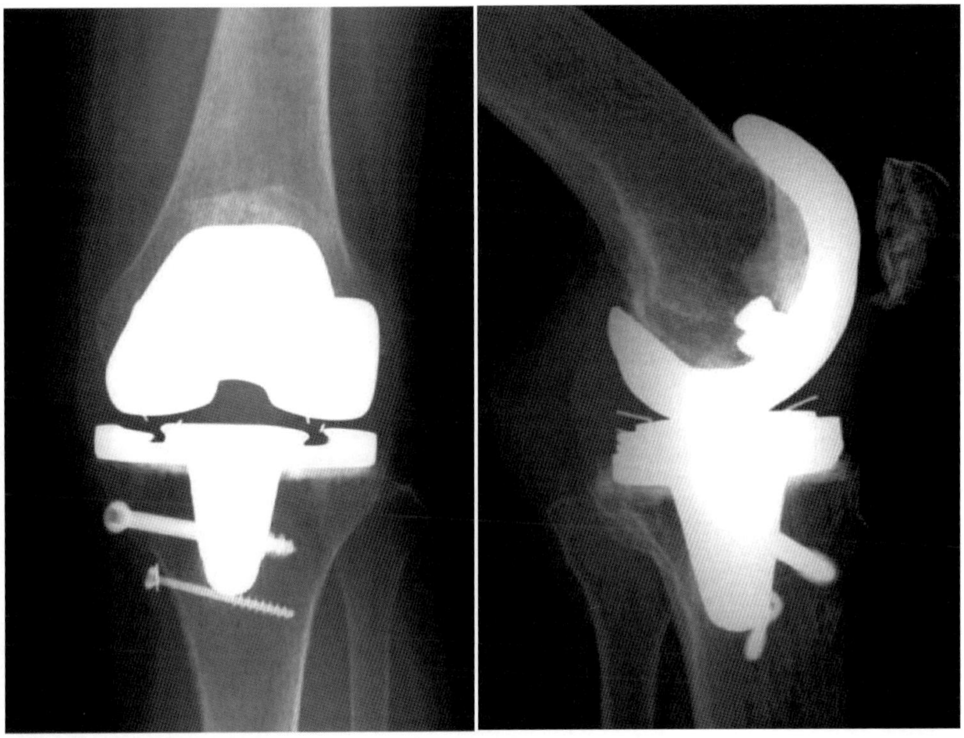

Fig. 8.28 Screws are inserted into the intraoperative tibial fracture

Revision TKA is performed with an extension stem when the prosthesis is unstable. The length of the stem should extend proximally more than two times the diameter from the fracture line. If an extension stem is not available, APC (allograft prosthesis composite) or tumor prosthesis can be used. Appleton et al. stated that the hinge type of constrained prosthesis is recommended in patients who are older and have limited mobility, although it is associated with the high risk of loosening.

Tibia

Tibial periprosthetic fractures can be treated based on the Felix classification. The treatment principles are not very different from those applied to the femur. *Treatment differs according to the time, the level of fracture, and prosthesis stability. A fracture that occurs during the operation is mostly a vertical fracture with minimal displacement, so it is enough to perform a lag screw fixation* (Fig. 8.28). However, some surgeons state that *a vertical fracture* does not need any special management. *If there is displacement, an extension stem can be used and the fragments are fixed with screws.*

A postoperative fracture with a stable prosthesis requires open reduction and internal fixation, and a bone graft is needed depending on the degree of comminution and the degree of displacement. Revision TKA is required if the prosthesis is unstable. In type IV fracture which is the fracture of the tibial tuberosity, conservative treatment can be sufficient in cases with minimal displacement and surgical treatment is required in cases with marked displacement.

In case of fracture due to a high-velocity injury, there may be an accompanying neurovascular injury which needs an emergent vascular surgery (Fig. 8.29).

Patella

The principles of treatment of patellar fractures vary according to the degree of comminution, component loosening, and maintenance of the extensor mechanism. The goal of treatment is the restoration of extensor function. When there is no component loosening with minimal displacement and the extensor power is maintained, conservative methods such as knee immobilizer or cylinder cast are recommended.

When there is more than 2 cm of displacement, a severe extensor defect, or patellar component loosening, surgical intervention is needed. However, surgical methods are not recommended even in cases with rupture of the extensor mechanism if the patient is too old with a mobility problem, has poor skin condition, or is generally weak due to the other physical conditions. *Despite a widely displaced patellar fracture, some patients may have reasonable extensor power and little extensor lag because of intact medial and lateral retinacular soft tissues.*

Surgical methods include tension band wiring, removal of only the loosened patellar component, partial or total resection of the patella with autogenous or allogeneic ligament augmentation, or whole extensor mechanism allograft. *Tension band wiring can be performed when the bony fragment is large, there is good quality of the bone, and the prosthesis is stable.* However, Vince et al. stated that tension

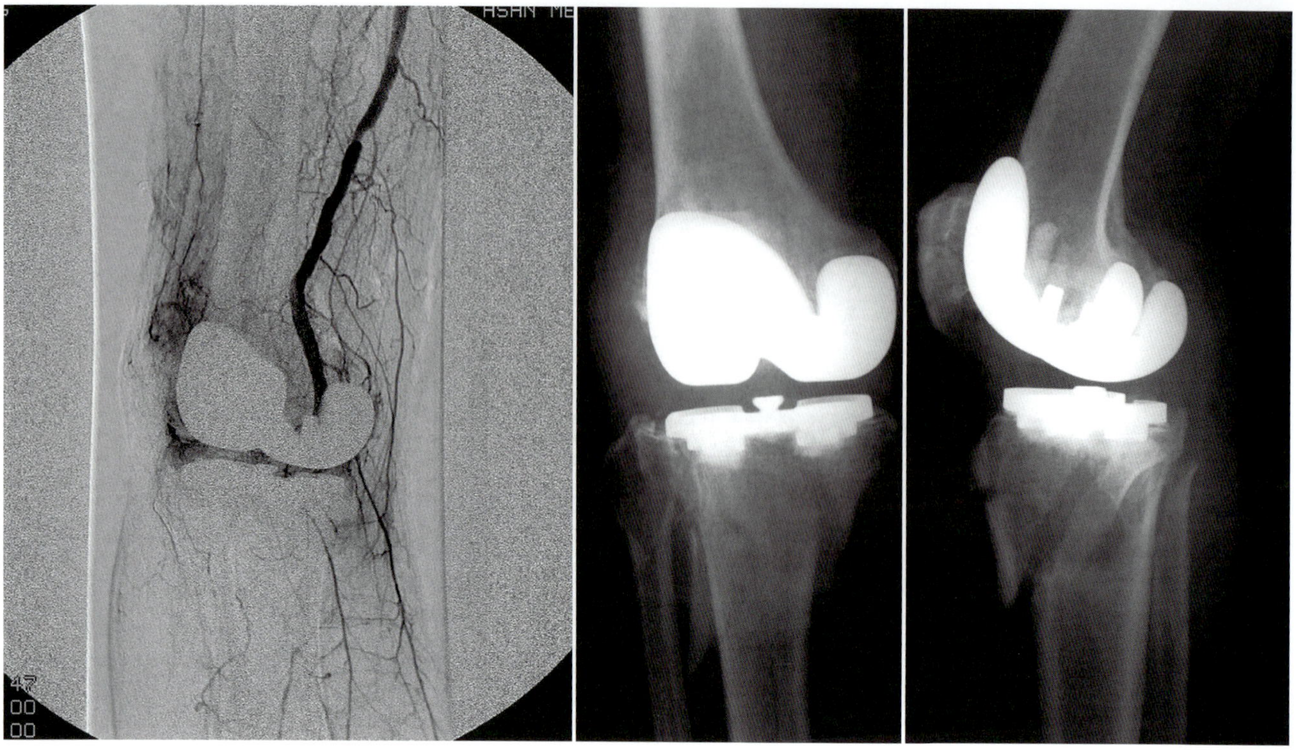

Fig. 8.29 Fracture around the tibial prosthesis accompanied by a vascular injury

band wiring is not recommended since it disrupts the blood supply which is already poor due to the TKA operation and fracture. Hence, some surgeons prefer *allograft augmentation rather than internal fixation of the fracture fragment.*

If the prosthesis has loosened due to a comminuted fracture or the fracture is associated with avascular necrosis of the patella, removal of only the patellar component or partial or total resection of the patella can be performed and the fracture site can be augmented using the Achilles tendon allograft. Whole extensor mechanism allograft reconstruction with patella and patellar tendon augmentation technique has also been introduced.

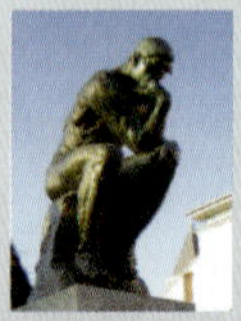

Author's Opinion

My principles for treatment of periprosthetic fractures are based on the degree of osteopenia, site and degree of comminution, and stability of the prosthesis.

I usually perform the operation whenever possible, provided the patient's general condition permits. The difficulties related to the morbidity of an operation may be one of the reasons for choosing conservative treatment. Even though the displacement is within the acceptable range of conservative treatment, cast immobilization in the elderly patients increases the chances of general complications, and there is a high possibility of limited range of motion and malunion.

The level of fracture and the degree of osteopenia are the key decision-making factors for operative method rather than the degree of comminution or displacement. I prefer plate and screw fixation except when it is very difficult to reduce the fracture in the area proximal to the prosthesis. In that case, I do IM nailing. I sometimes use the Cho plate which I have designed for internal fixation of the periprosthetic fracture. The Cho plate has transverse wiring holes through the horizontal plane of the plate for augmenting the fixation with wires at the site where screws cannot be inserted (Fig. 8.30).

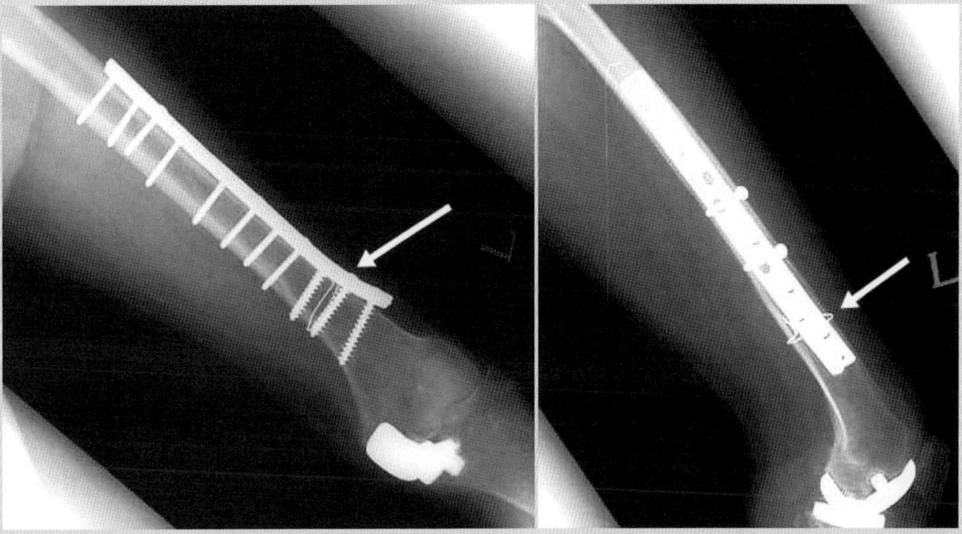

Fig. 8.30 Treatment of a periprosthetic fracture using the Cho plate. Wires are passed through the transverse holes in order to reinforce the plate fixation

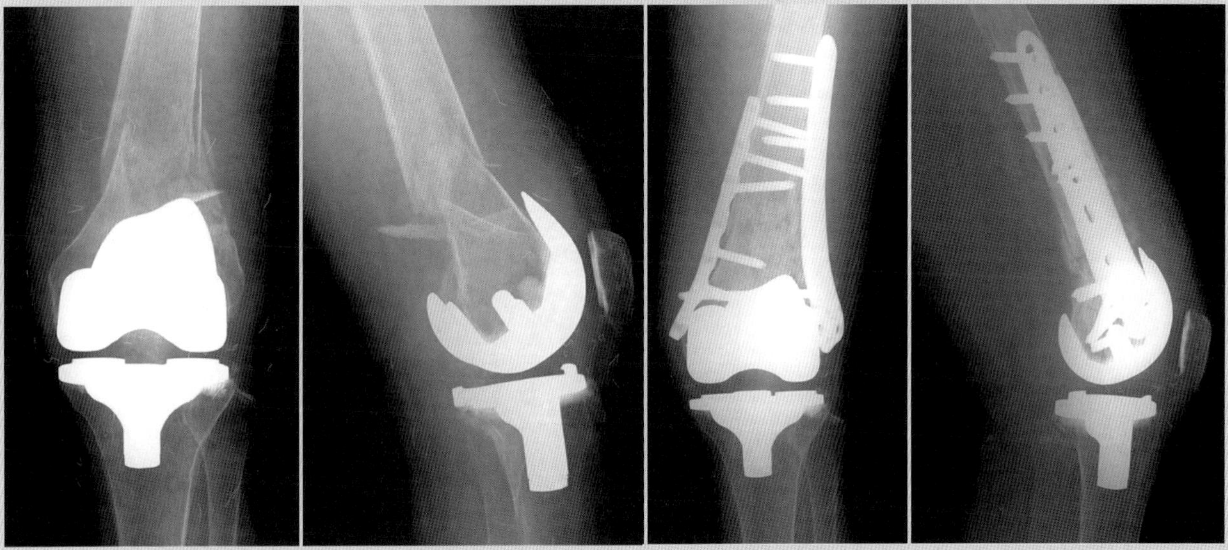

Fig. 8.31 X-ray of internal fixation of a periprosthetic fracture using the LCP and buttress plate plate

If osteopenia is not very severe and the metaphyseal fracture is comminuted to a lesser extent, I perform internal fixation regardless of the degree of displacement and do bone grafting if needed. Mostly I use the LCP for internal fixation as it is compatible with the anatomy of this site. LCP is not bulky and hence can be handled easily and ensures a relatively stable fixation in the osteoporotic bone. I sometimes use dual buttress plates (Fig. 8.31).

In severe comminution, an internal fixator can still be used. Biologic fixation method is applied wherein the bony fragments are reduced by indirect method.

In a severe osteoporotic fracture that cannot be fixed, cementing technique may help in the fixation of plate and screws (Fig. 8.32). In other words, stability of the fracture site should be primarily established by internal fixation and the cement can be used for additional fixation. However, special surgical techniques are required for cementing.

When the fracture is within the confines of the prosthesis and shows severe comminution, it is generally associated with loosening of the prosthesis. I consider using the tumor prosthesis in such a case rather than performing internal fixation and revision TKA (Fig. 8.33).

If there is loosening between the prosthesis and the fragments, and comminution is not severe, I try internal fixation and revise the TKA with the use of a long extension stem.

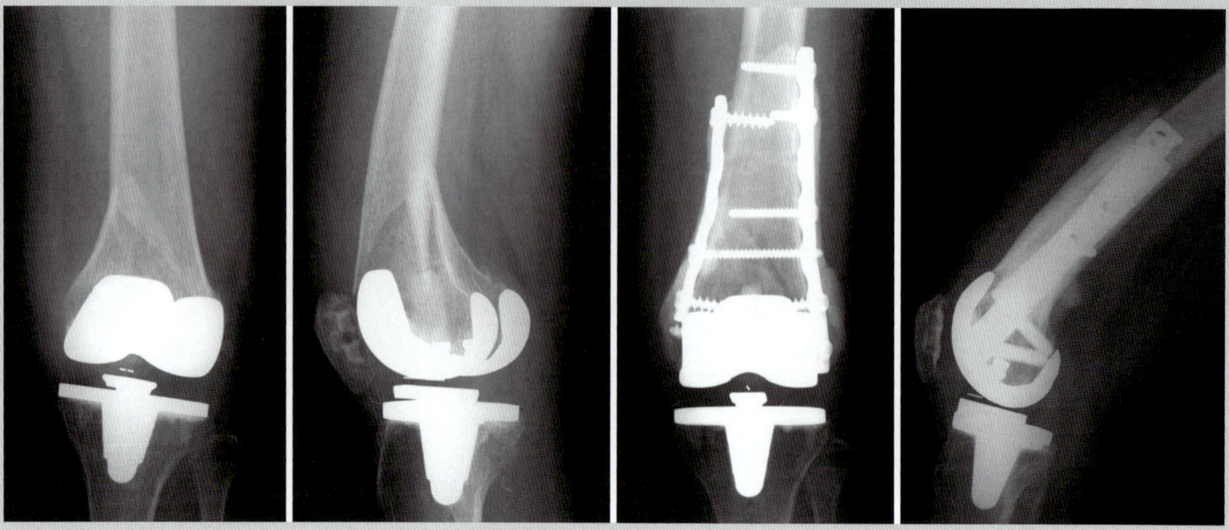

Fig. 8.32 Treatment of a periprosthetic fracture with cement augmentation

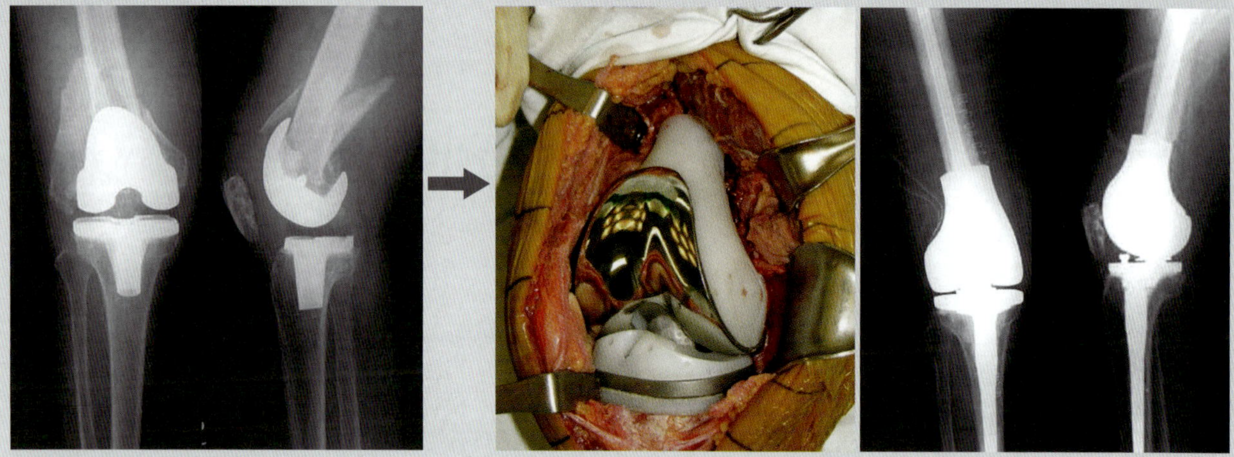

Fig. 8.33 Treatment of a periprosthetic fracture using tumor prosthesis

8.3 Results

There are many reports of good results for the treatment of femoral or tibial periprosthetic fractures; however, the treatment is not simple and the complication rate is reported to be between 25 and 75 %.

Conservative treatment takes a long time and is associated with an increased possibility of general complications due to long-term immobilization and malunion. Healy et al. and Culp et al. reported good results with open reduction and internal fixation, but it was difficult to achieve fixation in patients with osteopenia and was often accompanied by nonunion.

It takes about 5–6 months to achieve bony union regardless of the method used. Kraay et al. and McLaren et al. reported good results with revision TKA. However, good results mean only acceptable results when considering the limited situations.

Bibliography

Aaron RK, Scott R. Supracondylar fracture of the femur after total knee arthroplasty. Clin Orthop. 1987;219:136–9.

Aglietti P, Baldini A, Vena LM, et al. Effect of tourniquet use on activation of coagulation in total knee replacement. Clin Orthop. 2000;371:169–77.

Ahmad R, Kumar GS, Katam K, et al. Significance of "hot patella" in total knee replacement without primary patellar resurfacing. Knee. 2009;16:337–40.

Akasaki Y, Matsuda S, Shimoto T, et al. Contact stress analysis on the conforming post-cam Mechanism in posterior-stabilized total knee arthroplasty. J Arthroplasty. 2008;23:736–43.

AlBuhairan B, Hind D, Hutchinson A. Antibiotic prophylaxis for wound infections in total joint arthroplasty: a systematic review. J Bone Joint Surg. 2008;90-B:915–9.

Appleton P, Moran M, Houshian S, et al. Distal femoral fracture treated by hinged total knee Replacement in elderly patients. J Bone Joint Surg. 2006;88-B:1065–70.

Asp JPL, Rand JA. Peroneal nerve palsy after total knee arthroplasty. Clin Orthop. 1990;261:233–7.

Austin MS, Parvizi J, Grossman S, et al. The inferior vena cava filter is effective in preventing fatal pulmonary embolus after hip and knee arthroplasties. J Arthroplasty. 2007;22:343–8.

Ayers DC. Evaluation of the symptomatic total knee replacement. In: Callaghan JJ, editor. The adult knee. 1st ed. Philadelphia: Lippincott Williams & Wilkins; 2003. p. 1405–12.

Backstein D, Safir O, Gross A. Periprosthetic fractures of the knee. J Arthroplasty. 2007;22:45–9.

Barrack RL, Jennings R, Wolfe M, et al. The value of preoperative aspiration prior to total knee revision. Clin Orthop. 1997;345:8–16.

Barrack RL, Schrader T, Bertot AJ, et al. Component rotation and anterior knee pain after total knee arthroplasty. Clin Orthop. 2001;392:46–55.

Bedair H, Ting N, Jacovides C, et al. The Mark Coventry Award: diagnosis of early postoperative TKA infection using synovial fluid analysis. Clin Orthop. 2011;469:34–40.

Bédard M, Vince KG, Redfern J, et al. Internal rotation of the tibial component is frequent in stiff total knee arthroplasty. Clin Orthop. 2011;469:2346–55.

Beight JL, Yao B, Hozack WJ, et al. The patellar "clunk" syndrome after posterior stabilized total knee arthroplasty. Clin Orthop. 1994;299:139–42.

Bellemans J, Vandenneucker H, Victor J, et al. Flexion contracture in total knee arthroplasty. Clin Orthop. 2006;452:78–82.

Berry DJ. Patellar fractures in total knee arthroplasty. In: Scott WN, editor. Surgery of the knee. 5th ed. Philadelphia: Churchill Livingstone; 2011. p. 1381–5.

Berger RA, Della Valle CJ, Rabash HE. Patellofemoral problems in total knee arthroplasty. In: Callaghan JJ, editor. The adult knee. 1st ed. Philadelphia: Lippincott Williams & Wilkins; 2003. p. 1245–58.

Bert JM. Dislocation/subluxation of meniscal bearing elements after New Jersey low-contact stress total knee arthroplasty. Clin Orthop. 1990;254:211–5.

Bhutta MA, Doorgakant A, Marynissen H. Tibial nerve impingement secondary to posterior cement extrusion after unicompartmental knee arthroplasty. J Arthroplasty. 2010;25:1168.e17–8.

Bindelglass DF, Cohen JL, Dorr LD. Patellar tilt and subluxation in total knee arthroplasty: relationship to pain, fixation, and design. Clin Orthop. 1993;286:103–9.

Bloebaum RD, Nelsonk K, Dorr LD, et al. Investigation of early surface delamination observed in retrieved heat-pressed tibial inserts. Clin Orthop. 1991;269:120–7.

Board TN, Karva A, Board RE, et al. The prophylaxis and treatment of heterotopic ossification following lower limb arthroplasty. J Bone Joint Surg. 2007;89-B:434–40.

Bocell JR, Thorpe CC, Tullos JH. Arthroscopic treatment of symptomatic total knee arthroplasty. Clin Orthop. 1991;271:125–34.

Brassard MF, Insall JN, Scuderi GR, et al. Complication of total knee arthroplasty. In: Insall JN, Scott WN, editors. Surgery of the knee. 4th ed. New York: Churchill Livingstone; 2006. p. 1716–60.

Briard JL, Hungerford DS. Patellofemoral instability in total knee arthroplasty. J Arthroplasty. 1989;4:87–97.

Broderson MP, Fitzerald RH, Deterson LFA, et al. Arthrodesis of the knee following failed total knee arthroplasty. J Bone Joint Surg. 1979;61-A:181–5.

Brooks MK, Palestro CJ, Weissman BN. Imaging of total knee arthroplasty. In: Scott WN, editor. Surgery of the knee. 5th ed. Philadelphia: Churchill Livingstone; 2011. p. 125–39.

Brown GA. Venous thromboembolism prophylaxis after major orthopaedic surgery: a pooled analysis of randomized controlled trials. J Arthroplasty. 2009;24:77–83.

Brown GA, Parratte S, Pagnano MW. Instability in total knee arthroplasty. In: Scott WN, editor. Surgery of the knee. 5th ed. Philadelphia: Churchill Livingstone; 2011. p. 1359–66.

Burnett RS, Berger RA, Paprosky WG, et al. Extensor mechanism allograft reconstruction after total knee arthroplasty. A comparison of two techniques. J Bone Joint Surg. 2004;86-A:2694–9.

Burnett RS, Bourne RB. Periprosthetic fractures of the tibia and patella in total knee arthroplasty. Instr Course Lect. 2004;53:217–35.

Burnett RS, Butler RA, Barrack RL. Extensor mechanism allograft reconstruction in TKA at a mean of 56 months. Clin Orthop. 2006;452:159–65.

Cadambi A, Engh GA. Use of a semitendinosus tendon autogenous graft for rupture of the patellar ligament after total knee arthroplasty: a report of seven cases. J Bone Joint Surg. 1992;74-A:974–9.

Callaghan JJ, O'Rourke MR, Goetz DD, et al. Tibial post impingement in posterior stabilized total knee arthroplasty. Clin Orthop. 2002;404:83–8.

Callaghan JJ, Reynolds ER, Ting NT, et al. Liner exchange and bone grafting: rare option to treat wear and lysis of stable TKAs. Clin Orthop. 2011;469:154–9.

Callahan CM, Drake BG, Heck DA, et al. Patient outcomes following tricompartmental total knee. Replacement. A meta-analysis. JAMA. 1994;271:1349–457.

Cates HE, Schmidt JM. Closed manipulation after total knee arthroplasty: outcome and affecting variables. Orthopedics. 2009;32:398.

Chatterji U, Ashworth MJ, Smith AL, et al. Retrieval study of tibial baseplate fracture after total knee arthroplasty. J Arthroplasty. 2005;20:101–7.

Chew JT, Stewart NJ, Hanssen AD, et al. Differences in patellar tracking and knee kinematics among three different total knee designs. Clin Orthop. 1997;345:87–98.

Chiba J, Schwedeman LJ, Booth RE, et al. A biomechanical histologic and immunohistologic analysis of membranes obtained from cemented and cementless total knee arthroplasty. Clin Orthop. 1994;299:114–24.

Chiu YS, Chen WM, Huang CK, et al. Fracture of the polyethylene tibial post in a NexGen posterior stabilized knee prosthesis. J Arthroplasty. 2004;19:1045–9.

Chmell MJ, Moran MC, Scott RD. Periarticular fractures after total knee arthroplasty: principles of management. J Am Acad Orthop Surg. 1996;4:109–16.

Cho SD, Park KW, Lee CC. Heterotopic ossification after total knee arthroplasty. J Korean Knee Soc. 2002;14:126–30.

Cho WS, Ahn HS, Kim MY, et al. Pain after total knee arthroplasty. J Korean Orthop Assoc. 2006;41:129–33.

Clarke HD, Math KR, Scuderi GR. Polyethylene post failure in posterior stabilized total knee arthroplasty. J Arthroplasty. 2004;19:652–7.

Classen C, Evans RS, Pestotnik SL, et al. Timing of prophylactic administration of antibiotics and the risk of surgical-wound infection. N Engl J Med. 1992;326:281–6.

Collier JP, Mayor MD, McNamara JL, et al. Analysis of the failure of 122 polyethylene inserts from uncemented tibial knee components. Clin Orthop. 1991;273:232–42.

Colman WW, Ries MD. Miscellaneous complication. In: Callaghan JJ, editor. The adult knee. 1st ed. Philadelphia: Lippincott Williams & Wilkins; 2003. p. 1389–404.

Colwell Jr CW, Berkowitz SD, Lieberman JR, et al. Oral direct thrombin inhibitor ximelagatran compared with warfarin for the prevention of venous thromboembolism after total knee arthroplasty. J Bone Joint Surg. 2005;87-A:2169–77.

Colwell Jr CW, Hardwick ME. Rationale for low-molecular-weight heparin prophylaxis after total knee arthroplasty. Clin Orthop. 2006;452:181–5.

Cowell GW, Boom SJ, Ablett MJ. Thrombosis of popliteal artery pseudoaneurysm by deployment of angioplasty balloon after total knee arthroplasty. J Arthroplasty. 2009;24:825.e11–3.

Craig SM. Soft tissue considerations in the failed total knee arthroplasty. In: Scott WN, editor. The knee. 1st ed. St. Louis: Mosby; 1994. p. 1279–95.

Cuckler JM. The infected total knee: management options. J Arthroplasty. 2005;20 Suppl 2:33–6.

Culp RW, Schmidt RG, Hanks G, et al. Supracondylar fracture of the femur following. Prosthetic knee arthroplasty. Clin Orthop. 1987;222:212–22.

Cushner FD. Preventing wound complications after total knee arthroplasty. In: Callaghan JJ, editor. The adult knee. 1st ed. Philadelphia: Lippincott Williams & Wilkins; 2003. p. 1341–50.

Dalury DF, Jiranek WA. The incidence of heterotopic ossification after total knee arthroplasty. J Arthroplasty. 2004;19:447–52.

Della Valle CJ, Sporer SM, Jacobs JJ, et al. Preoperative testing for sepsis before revision total knee arthroplasty. J Arthroplasty. 2007;22:90–3.

Della Valle CJ, Parvizi J, Bauer TW, et al. American Academy of Orthopaedic Surgeons clinical practice guideline on: the diagnosis of periprosthetic joint infections of the hip and knee. J Bone Joint Surg. 2011;93-A:1355–7.

Dellon AL, Mackinnon SE, Pestron KA. Implantation of sensory nerve into muscle. Ann Plast Surg. 1984;12:30–40.

Dennis DA. Periprosthetic fractures following total knee arthroplasty. Instr Course Lect. 2001;50:379–89.

Dennis DA. Arthrodesis and resection arthroplasty for the failed total knee arthroplasty. In: Scott WN, editor. The knee. 1st ed. St. Louis: Mosby; 1994. p. 1345–51.

Dennis DA, Kim RH, Johnson DR, et al. The John Insall Award: control-matched evaluation of painful patellar crepitus after total knee arthroplasty. Clin Orthop. 2011;469:10–7.

Di Cesare PE, Chang E, Preston CF, et al. Serum interleukin-6 as a marker of periprosthetic infection following total hip and knee arthroplasty. J Bone Joint Surg. 2005;87-A:1921–7.

Diduch DR, Scuderi GR, Scott WN, et al. The efficacy of arthroscopy following total knee replacement. Arthroscopy. 1997;13:166–71.

Dolan MM, Kelly NH, Nguyen JT, et al. Implant design influences tibial post wear damage in posterior-stabilized knees. Clin Orthop. 2011;469:160–7.

Dorr LD, Boiardo RA. Technical considerations in total knee arthroplasty. Clin Orthop. 1986;205:5–11.

Dorr LD, Serocki JH. Mechanism of failure of total knee arthroplasty. In: Scott WN, editor. The knee. 1st ed. St. Louis: Mosby; 1994. p. 1239–49.

Drancourt M, Stein A, Argenson JN, et al. Oral treatment of Staphylococcus spp. infected orthopaedic implants with fusidic acid or ofloxacin in combination with rifampicin. J Antimicrob Chemother. 1997;39:235–40.

Durack DT. Prevention of infective endocarditis. N Engl J Med. 1995;332:38–44.

Elson DW, Brenkel IJ. A conservative approach is feasible in unexplained pain after knee replacement: a selected cohort study. J Bone Joint Surg. 2007;89-B:1042–5.

Elson DW, Brenkel IJ. Predicting pain after total knee arthroplasty. J Arthroplasty. 2006;21:1047–53.

Emerson Jr RH, Head WC, Malinin TI. Reconstruction of patellar tendon rupture after total knee arthroplasty with an extensor mechanism allograft. Clin Orthop. 1990;260:154–61.

Engh GA, Ammeen DJ. Periprosthetic fractures adjacent to total knee implants: treatment and clinical results. J Bone Joint Surg. 1997;79-A:1100–13.

Engh GA, Parks NL, Ammeen DJ. Tibial osteolysis in cementless total knee arthroplasty. A review of 25 cases treated with and without tibial component revision. Clin Orthop. 1994;309:33–43.

Falck-Ytter Y, Francis CW, Johanson NA. Prevention of VTE in orthopedic surgery patient: antithrombotic therapy and prevention of thrombosis, 9th ed.: American College of Chest Physicians evidence-based clinical practice guidelines. Chest. 2012;141(S): 278–325.

Fehring TK, McAvoy G. Fluoroscopic evaluation of the painful total knee arthroplasty. Clin Orthop. 1996;331:226–33.

Felix III NA, Stuart MJ, Hanssen AD. Periprosthetic fractures of the tibia associated with total knee arthroplasty. Clin Orthop. 1997; 345:113–24.

Figgie III HE, Brody GA, Inglis AE, et al. Knee arthrodesis following total knee arthroplasty in rheumatoid arthritis. Clin Orthop. 1987;224:237–43.

Figgie III HE, Goldberg VM, Figgie MP, et al. The effect of alignment of the implant on fractures of the patella after condylar total knee arthroplasty. J Bone Joint Surg. 1989;71-A:1031–9.

Freedman KB, Brookendal KR, Fitzgerald H, et al. A meta-analysis of thromboembolic prophylaxis following elective total hip arthroplasty. J Bone Joint Surg. 2000;82-A:929–38.

Freeman MA, Bradley GW, Revell PA. Observations upon the interface between bone and polymethylmethacrylate cement. J Bone Joint Surg. 1982;64-B:489–93.

Friedman RJ. Prevention of thrombophlebitis in total knee arthroplasty. In: Scott WN, editor. Surgery of the knee. 4th ed. Philadelphia: Churchill Livingstone; 2006. p. 1837–47.

Fulkerson E, Valle CJ, Wise B, et al. Antibiotic susceptibility of bacteria infecting total joint arthroplasty sites. J Bone Joint Surg. 2006;88-A:1231–7.

Gallagher J, Rorabeck C, Bourne R. Patella resurfacing in total knee arthroplasty. In: Scott WN, editor. Surgery of the knee. 4th ed. Philadelphia: Churchill Livingstone; 2006. p. 1574–91.

Garvin KL, Konigsberg BS. Infection following total knee arthroplasty: prevention and management. J Bone Joint Surg. 2011;93-A: 1167–75.

Geertsema D, Defoort KC, van Helemondt GG. Popliteal pseudoaneurysm after total knee arthroplasty: a report of 3 cases. J Arthroplasty. 2012;27:1581.

Gerwin M, Rothaus KU, Windsor RE, et al. Gastrocnemius muscle flap coverage of exposed or infected knee prosthesis. Clin Orthop. 1993;286:64–70.

Goldberg VM, Figgie HE, Inglis AE, et al. Patellar fracture type and prognosis in condylar total knee arthroplasty. Clin Orthop. 1988;236:115–22.

Grace JN, Rand JA. Patellar instability after total knee arthroplasty. Clin Orthop. 1988;237:184–9.

Gupta SK, Chu A, Ranawat AS, et al. Osteolysis after total knee arthroplasty. J Arthroplasty. 2007;22:787–99.

Halket A, Stratford PW, Kennedy DM, et al. Using hierarchical linear modeling to explore predictors of pain after total hip and knee arthroplasty as a consequence of osteoarthritis. J Arthroplasty. 2010;25:254–62.

Hallock GG. Salvage of total knee arthroplasty with local fasciocutaneous flaps. J Bone Joint Surg. 1990;72-B:1236–9.

Hamai S, Miura H, Matsuda S, et al. Contact stress at the anterior aspect of the tibial post in posterior-stabilized total knee replacement. J Bone Joint Surg. 2010;92-A:1765–73.

Han HS, Kang SB, Yoon KS. High incidence of loosening of the femoral component in legacy posterior stabilised-flex total knee replacement. J Bone Joint Surg. 2007;89-B:1457–61.

Han Z, Burnham CA, Clohisy J, et al. Mycoplasma pneumoniae periprosthetic joint infection identified by 16S ribosomal RNA gene amplification and sequencing: a case report. J Bone Joint Surg. 2011;93-A:e103.

Hanssen AD, Osmon DR, Nelson CL. Prevention of deep prosthetic joint infection. J Bone Joint Surg. 1996;78-A:458–71.

Harvey EJ, Leclerc J, Brooks CE, et al. Effect of tourniquet use on blood loss and incidence of deep vein thrombosis in total knee arthroplasty. J Arthroplasty. 1997;12:291–6.

Healy WL, Siliski JM, Incavo SJ. Operative treatment of distal femoral fractures proximal to total knee replacements. J Bone Joint Surg. 1993;75-A:27–34.

Hooker JA, Lachiewicz PF, Kelly SC. Efficacy of prophylaxis against thromboembolism with intermittent pneumatic compression after primary and revision total hip arthroplasty. J Bone Joint Surg. 1999;81-A:690–6.

Hsu HP, Garg A, Walker PS, et al. Effect of knee component alignment on tibial load distribution with clinical correlation. Clin Orthop. 1989;248:135–44.

Hsu RW, Himeno S, Coventry MB, et al. Normal axial alignment of the lower extremity and load bearing distribution at the knee. Clin Orthop. 1990;255:215–27.

Idusuyi OB, Morrey BF. Peroneal nerve palsy after total knee arthroplasty. J Bone Joint Surg. 1996;78-A:177–84.

Insall JN, Binazzi R, Soudry M, et al. Total knee arthroplasty. Clin Orthop. 1985;192:13–22.

Jabczenski FF, Crawford M. Retrograde intramedullary nailing of supracondylar femur fracture above total knee arthroplasty: a preliminary report of four cases. J Arthroplasty. 1995;10: 95–101.

Jameson SS, Rymaszewska M, Hui AC, et al. Wound complications following rivaroxaban administration: a multicenter comparison with low-molecular-weight heparins for thromboprophylaxis in lower limb arthroplasty. J Bone Joint Surg. 2012;94-A:1554–8.

Jämsen E, Nevalainen P, Eskelinen A, et al. Obesity, diabetes, and preoperative hyperglycemia as predictors of periprosthetic joint infection: a single-center analysis of 7181 primary hip and knee replacement for osteoarthritis. J Bone Joint Surg. 2012;94-A:e101.

Jaureguito JW, Dubois CM, Smith SR, et al. Medial gastrocnemius transposition flap for the treatment of disruption of the extensor mechanism after total knee arthroplasty. J Bone Joint Surg. 1997;79-A:866–73.

Johanson NA. Extensor mechanism failure: treatment of patella fracture, dislocation, and ligament rupture. In: Lotke PA, editor. Master techniques in orthopedic surgery. Knee arthroplasty. 1st ed. New York: Raven; 1995. p. 219–40.

Johanson NA, Lachiewicz PF, Lieberman JR, et al. American academy of orthopaedic surgeons clinical practice guideline on prevention of symptomatic pulmonary embolism in patients undergoing total hip or knee arthroplasty. J Bone Joint Surg. 2009;91-A:1756–7.

Johnson DP, Eastwood DM. Lateral patellar release in knee arthroplasty: effect on wound healing. J Arthroplasty. 1992; 7(Suppl):427–31.

Johnson DR, Friedman RJ, McGinty JB, et al. The role of arthroscopy in the problem total knee replacement. Arthroscopy. 1990; 6:30–2.

Josefsson G, Kolemrt L. Prophylaxis with systemic antibiotics versus gentamicin bone cement in total hip arthroplasty. A ten year survey of 1,688 hips. Clin Orthop. 1993;292:210–4.

Kathod M, Inacio MC, Bini SA, et al. Pulmonary embolism prophylaxis in more than 30,000 total knee arthroplasty patients: is there a best choice? J Arthroplasty. 2012;27:167–72.

Katz MM, Hungerford DS, Krackow KA, et al. Reflex sympathetic dystrophy as a cause of poor results after total knee arthroplasty. J Arthroplasty. 1986;1:117–24.

Keating EM, Ritter MA, Harty LD, et al. Manipulation after total knee arthroplasty. J Bone Joint Surg. 2007;89-A:282–6.

Kevin RM, Syed FZ, Catherine P. Imaging of the painful total knee arthroplasty. In: Scott WN, editor. Surgery of the knee. 4th ed. Philadelphia: Churchill Livingstone; 200. p. 193–200.

Khakharia S, Nett MP, Hajnik CA, et al. Complications of total knee arthroplasty. In: Scott WN, editor. Surgery of the knee. 5th ed. Philadelphia: Churchill Livingstone; 2011. p. 1293–319.

Kilgus DJ, Howe DJ, Strang A. Results of periprosthetic hip and knee infections caused by resistant bacteria. Clin Orthop. 2003;404:116–24.

Kim KY, Cho WS, Lee SH, et al. Study on the incidence of pulmonary embolism before and after hip and knee replacement arthroplasties. J Korean Orthop Assoc. 1994;29:816–24.

Kim YH, Yoo JH, Kim JS. Factors leading to decreased rates of deep vein thrombosis and pulmonary embolism after total knee arthroplasty. J Arthroplasty. 2007;22:974–80.

Kobayashi N, Bauer TW, Tuohy MJ, et al. Brief ultrasonication improves detection of biofilm-formative bacteria around a metal implant. Clin Orthop. 2007;457:210–3.

Kocmond JH, Delp SL, Stern SH. Stability and range of motion of Insall-Burstein condylar prosthesis. A computer simulation study. J Arthroplasty. 1995;10:383–8.

Koo MH, Choi CH. Conservative treatment for the intraoperative detachment of medial collateral ligament from the tibial attachment site during primary total knee arthroplasty. J Arthroplasty. 2009;24:1249–53.

Kosy JD, Eyres KS, Toms AD. The value of magnetic resonance imaging in investigating a painful total knee arthroplasty. J Arthroplasty. 2011;26:977.e9–12.

Kraay MJ, Goldberg VM, Figgie MP, et al. Distal femoral replacement with allograft/prosthetic reconstruction for treatment of supracondylar fracture in patients with total knee arthroplasty. J Arthroplasty. 1992;7:7–16.

Krackow KA, Maar DC, Mont MA, et al. Surgical decompression for peroneal nerve palsy after total knee arthroplasty. Clin Orthop. 1993;292:223–8.

Kumar A, Chambers I, Maistrelli G, et al. Management of periprosthetic fracture above total knee arthroplasty using intramedullary fibular allograft and plate fixation. J Arthroplasty. 2008;23: 554–8.

Lachiewicz PF. How to treat a tibial post fracture in total knee arthroplasty? A systematic review. Clin Orthop. 2011;469: 1709–15.

Lachiewicz PF, Kelly SS, Haden LR. Two mechanical devices for prophylaxis of thromboembolism after total knee arthroplasty. J Bone Joint Surg. 2004;86-B:1137–41.

Lachiewicz PF, Soileau ES. The rates of osteolysis and loosening associated with a modular posterior stabilized knee replacement. J Bone Joint Surg. 2004;86-A:525–30.

Landy MM, Walker PS. Wear of ultra-high molecular-weight polyethylene components of 90 retrieved knee prostheses. J Arthroplasty. 1988;3(Suppl):73–85.

Large TM, Kellam JF, Bosse MJ, et al. Locked plating of supracondylar periprosthetic femur fractures. J Arthroplasty. 2008;23: 115–20.

Laskin RS. The painful knee. Orthopedics. 1999;22:869–70.
Laskin RS, Beksac B. Stiffness after total knee arthroplasty. J Arthroplasty. 2004;19 Suppl 1:41–6.
Laskin RS, O'Flynn HM. The Insall Award. Total knee replacement with posterior cruciate retention in rheumatoid arthritis. Problems and complications. Clin Orthop. 1997;345:24–8.
Lee GC, Nelson CL, Virmani S, et al. Management of periprosthetic femur fractures with severe bone loss using impaction bone grafting technique. J Arthroplasty. 2010;25:405–9.
Leone JM, Hanssen AD. Management of infection at the site of a total knee arthroplasty. J Bone Joint Surg. 2005;87-A:2335–48.
Lesh ML, Schneider DJ, Deol G, et al. The consequences of anterior femoral notching in total knee arthroplasty. A biomechanical study. J Bone Joint Surg. 2000;82-A:1096–101.
Li S, Scuderi GR, Furman BD, et al. Assessment of backside wear from the analysis of 55 retrieved tibial inserts. Clin Orthop. 2002;404:75–82.
Lieberman JR, Baker J. Prevention of deep venous thromboembolism after total knee arthroplasty. In: Callaghan JJ, editor. The adult knee. 1st ed. Philadelphia: Lippincott Williams & Wilkins; 2003. p. 1291–305.
Lieberman JR, Hsu WK. Prevention of venous thromboembolic disease after total hip and knee arthroplasty. J Bone Joint Surg. 2005;87-A:2097–112.
Lintner DM, Bocell JR, Tullos HS. Arthroscopic treatment of intra-articular fibrous bands after total knee arthroplasty. Clin Orthop. 1994;309:230–3.
Lionberger DR, Correia N. Protection of repaired patellar tendons a surgical technique. J Arthroplasty. 2011;26:969–71.
Lombardi AV, Engh GA, Volz RG, et al. Fracture/dislocation of the polyethylene in metal backed patellar components in total knee arthroplasty. J Bone Joint Surg. 1988;70-A:675–9.
Lotke PA, Lonner JH. Deep venous thrombosis prophylaxis: better living through chemistry-in opposition. J Arthroplasty. 2005;20 Suppl 2:15–7.
Lundblad H, Kreicbergs A, Jansson KA. Prediction of persistent pain after total knee replacement for osteoarthritis. J Bone Joint Surg. 2008;90-B:166–71.
Maheshwer CB, Mitchell E, Kraay M, et al. Revision of the patella with deficient bone using a biconvex component. Clin Orthop. 2005;440:126–30.
Maloney WJ. The stiff total knee arthroplasty. J Arthroplasty. 2002;17:71–3.
Mandalia V, Eyres K, Schranz P, et al. Evaluation of patients with a painful total knee replacement. J Bone Joint Surg. 2008;90-B: 265–71.
Marculescu CE, Cantey JR. Polymicrobial prosthetic joint infections: risk factors and outcome. Clin Orthop. 2008;466:1397–404.
Mariani BD, Martin DS, Levine MJ, et al. The Coventry Award. Polymerase chain reaction detection of bacterial infection in total knee arthroplasty. Clin Orthop. 1996;331:11–22.
Markel DC, York S, Liston MJ Jr, et al. Venous thromboembolism: management by American Association of Hip and Knee Surgeons. J Arthroplasty. 2010;25:3–9.e1–2.
Masini MA, Maguire JH, Thornhil TS. Infected total knee arthroplasty. In: Scott WN, editor. The knee. 1st ed. St. Louis: Mosby; 1994. p. 1261–78.
Marmor M, Parnes N, Dekel S. Tuberculosis infection complicating total knee arthroplasty: report of 3 cases and review of the literature. J Arthroplasty. 2004;19:397–400.
Mauerhan DR. Fracture of the polyethylene tibial post in a posterior cruciate-substituting total knee arthroplasty mimicking patellar clunk syndrome. J Arthroplasty. 2003;18:942–5.
McAndrew CM, Fitzgerald SJ, Kraay MJ, et al. Incidence of post-thrombotic syndrome in patients undergoing primary total knee arthroplasty for osteoarthritis. Clin Orthop. 2010;468:178–81.
McGrath MS, Mont MA, Siddiqui JA, et al. Evaluation of a custom device for the treatment of flexion contractures after total knee arthroplasty. Clin Orthop. 2009;467:1485–92.
McLaren AC, Dupont JA, Schroeber CD. Open reduction internal fixation of supracondylar fractures above total knee arthroplasties using the intramedullary supracondylar rod. Clin Orthop. 1994;302:194–8.
McPherson EJ, Tontz Jr W, Patzakis M, et al. Outcome of infected total knee utilizing a staging system for prosthetic joint infection. Am J Orthop. 1999;28:161–5.
Meding JB, Fish MD, Berend ME, et al. Predicting patellar failure after total knee arthroplasty. Clin Orthop. 2008;466: 2769–74.
Meehan J, Jamali AA, Nguyen H. Prophylactic antibiotics in hip and knee arthroplasty. J Bone Joint Surg. 2009;91-A:2480–90.
Meftah M, Ranawat AS, Ranawat CS. The natural history of anterior knee pain in 2 posterior-stabilized, modular total knee arthroplasty designs. J Arthroplasty. 2011;26:1145–8.
Meneghini R, Hanssen AD. The infected total knee replacement. In: Scott WN, editor. Surgery of the knee. 4th ed. Philadelphia: Churchill Livingstone; 2006. p. 1782–98.
Merkow RL, Soudry M, Insall JN. Patellar dislocation following total knee replacement. J Bone Joint Surg. 1985;67-A:1321–7.
Miller J. Improved fixation in total hip arthroplasty using L.V.C. surgical technique (brochure). Warsaw, IN: Zimmer; 1980.
Mont MA, Serna FK, Krackow KA, et al. Exploration of radiographically normal total knee replacements for unexplained pain. Clin Orthop. 1996;331:216–20.
Mont MA, Seyler TM, Marulanda GA, et al. Surgical treatment and customized rehabilitation for stiff knee arthroplasties. Clin Orthop. 2006;446:193–200.
Mont MA, Waldman B, Banerjee C, et al. Multiple irrigation, debridement, and retention of components in infected total knee arthroplasty. J Arthroplasty. 1997;12:426–33.
Montgomery WH, Insall JN, Haas SB, et al. Primary total knee arthroplasty in stiff and ankylosed knees. Am J Knee Surg. 1998;11:20–3.
Monto RR, Garcia J, Callaghan JJ. Fatal fat embolism following total condylar knee arthroplasty. J Arthroplasty. 1990;5:291–9.
Mortazavi SM, Vegari D, Ho A, et al. Two-stage exchange arthroplasty for infected total knee arthroplasty: predictors of failure. Clin Orthop. 2011;469:3049–54.
Mraovic B, Hipszer BR, Epstein RH, et al. Preadmission hyperglycemia is an independent risk factor for in-hospital symptomatic pulmonary embolism after major orthopedic surgery. J Arthroplasty. 2010;25:64–70.
Murakami AM, Hash TW, Hepinstall MS, et al. MRI evaluation of rotational alignment and synovitis in patients with pain after total knee replacement. J Bone Joint Surg. 2012;94-B:1209–15.
Nakajima A, Watanabe H, Rokkaku T, et al. The Elmslie-Trillat procedure for recurrent patellar subluxation after total knee arthroplasty. J Arthroplasty. 2010;25:1170.e1–5.
Namba RS, Chen Y, Paxton EW, et al. Outcomes of routine use of antibiotic-loaded cement in primary total knee arthroplasty. J Arthroplasty. 2009;24(6 Suppl):44–7.
Naranja RJ, Lotke PA, Pognano MW, et al. Total knee arthroplasty in previously ankylosed or arthrodesed knee. Clin Orthop. 1996;331:234–7.
Nazarian DG, Booth Jr RE. Extensor mechanism allografts in total knee arthroplasty. Clin Orthop. 1999;367:123–9.
Neer II CS, Grantham SA, Shelton ML. Supracondylar fracture of the adult femur: a study of one hundred and ten cases. J Bone Joint Surg. 1967;49-A:591–613.
Nelson CL, Green TG, Poster RA, et al. One day versus seven days of preventive antibiotic therapy in orthopedic surgery. Clin Orthop. 1983;176:258–63.

Nelson CL, Kim J, Lotke PA. Stiffness after total knee arthroplasty. J Bone Joint Surg. 2005;87-A Suppl 1:264–70.

Nercessian OA, Ugwonali OF, Park S. Peroneal nerve palsy after total knee arthroplasty. J Arthroplasty. 2005;20:1068–73.

Nett MP, Scuderi GR. Revision of aseptic failed total knee arthroplasty. In: Scott WN, editor. Surgery of the knee. 5th ed. Philadelphia: Churchill Livingstone; 2011. p. 1327–45.

Nicholls DW, Dorr LD. Revision surgery for stiff total knee arthroplasty. J Arthroplasty. 1990;5:73–7.

Novicoff WM, Brown TE, Cui Q, Mihalko WM, et al. Mandated venous thromboembolism prophylaxis: possible adverse outcomes. J Arthroplasty. 2008;23:15–9.

O'Rourke MR, Callaghan JJ, Goetz DD, et al. Osteolysis associated with a cemented modular posterior cruciate substituting total knee design. Five to eight-year follow-up. J Bone Joint Surg. 2002;84-A:1362–71.

Oethinger M, Warner DK, Schindler SA, et al. Diagnosing periprosthetic infection: false-positive intraoperative gram stains. Clin Orthop. 2011;469:954–60.

Ortiguera CJ, Berry DJ. Patellar fracture after total knee arthroplasty. J Bone Joint Surg. 2002;84-A:532–40.

Pagnano MW, Hanssen AD, Lewallen DG. Flexion instability after primary posterior cruciate retaining total knee arthroplasty. Clin Orthop. 1998;356:38–46.

Pandher DS, Boparai RS, Kapila R. Biceps tendinitis as a cause of acute painful knee after total knee arthroplasty. J Arthroplasty. 2009;24:1292.e15–8.

Parks NL, Engh GA, Topoleski LD, et al. Modular tibial insert micromotion. Clin Orthop. 1998;356:10–5.

Parvizi J, Ghanem E, Sharkey P, et al. Diagnosis of infected total knee: findings of a multicenter database. Clin Orthop Relat Res. 2008;466:2628–33.

Parvizi J, Han SB, Tarity TD, et al. Postoperative ileus after total joint arthroplasty. J Arthroplasty. 2008;23:360–5.

Parvizi J, Zmistowski B, Berbari EF, et al. New definition for periprosthetic joint infection. J Arthroplasty. 2011;26:1136–8.

Parvizi J, Mckenzie JC, Cashman JP. Diagnosis of periprosthetic joint infection using synovial C-reactive protein. J Arthroplasty. 2012;27 Suppl 8:12–6.

Patel VP, Walsh M, Sehgal B, et al. Factors associated with prolonged wound drainage after primary total hip and knee arthroplasty. J Bone Joint Surg Am. 2007;89:33–8.

Pearse EO, Caldwell BF, Lockwood RJ, et al. Early mobilisation after conventional knee replacement may reduce the risk of postoperative venous thromboembolism. J Bone Joint Surg Br. 2007;89:316–22.

Peersman G, Laskin R, Davis J, et al. Infection in total knee replacement: a retrospective review of 6,489 total knee replacements. Clin Orthop. 2001;392:15–23.

Peters Jr PC, Engh GA, Dwyer KA, et al. Osteolysis after total knee arthroplasty without cement. J Bone Joint Surg. 1992;74-A:864–76.

Puloski SK, McCalden RW, MacDonald SJ, et al. Tibial post wear in posterior stabilized total knee arthroplasty. An unrecognized source of polyethylene debris J Bone Joint Surg. 2001;83-A:390–7.

Rand JA. Neurovascular complications of total knee arthroplasty. In: Rand JA, editor. Total knee arthroplasty. 1st ed. New York: Raven; 1993. p. 417–22.

Rand JA, Morrey BF, Bryan RS. Patellar tendon rupture after total knee arthroplasty. Clin Orthop. 1989;244:233–8.

Rao AR, Engh GA, Collier MB, et al. Tibial interface wear in retrieved total knee components and correlations with modular insert motion. J Bone Joint Surg. 2002;84-A:1849–55.

Riddle DL, Wade JB, Jiranek WA, et al. Preoperative pain catastrophizing predicts pain outcome after knee arthroplasty. Clin Orthop. 2010;468:798–806.

Ries MD, Badalamente M. Arthrofibrosis after total knee arthroplasty. Clin Orthop. 2000;380:177–83.

Rimnac CM, Wright TM. Retrieval analysis of knee replacement. In: Scott WN, editor. The knee. 1st ed. St. Louis: Mosby; 1994. p. 1251–60.

Ritter MA, Campbell ED. Postoperative patellar complications with or without lateral release during total knee arthroplasty. Clin Orthop. 1987;219:163–8.

Ritter MA, Faris PM, Keating EM. Anterior femoral notching and ipsilateral supracondylar femur fracture in total knee arthroplasty. J Arthroplasty. 1988;3:185–7.

Robinson EJ, Mulliken BD, Bourne RB, et al. Catastrophic osteolysis in total knee replacement. Clin Orthop. 1995;321:98–105.

Rorabeck CH, Taylor JW. Periprosthetic fractures of the femur complicating total knee arthroplasty. Orthop Clin North Am. 1999; 30:265–77.

Rosenberg AG, Berger RA. Alternative procedures for the management of an infected total knee. In: Scuderi GR, editor. Surgical techniques in total knee arthroplasty. 1st ed. New York: Springer; 2002. p. 491–9.

Sachs RA, Smith JH, Kuney M, et al. Does anticoagulation do more harm than good?: a comparison of patients treated without prophylaxis and patients treated with low-dose warfarin after total knee arthroplasty. J Arthroplasty. 2003;18:389–95.

Schindler OS. Patellar resurfacing in total knee arthroplasty. In: Scott WN, editor. Surgery of the knee. 5th ed. Philadelphia: Churchill Livingstone; 2011. p. 1161–90.

Schroer WC, Calvert GT, Diesfeld PJ, et al. Effects of increased surgical volume on total knee arthroplasty complications. J Arthroplasty. 2008;23:61–7.

Scott RD. Anterior femoral notching and ipsilateral supracondylar femur fracture in total knee arthroplasty. J Arthroplasty. 1988;3:381.

Scott RD. Patellofemoral complications associated with total knee arthroplasty. In: Scott RD, editor. Total knee arthroplasty. 1st ed. Philadelphia: Saunders; 2006. p. 54–62.

Scott RD. Sepsis and total knee arthroplasty. In: Scott RD, editor. Total knee arthroplasty. 1st ed. Philadelphia: Saunders; 2006. p. 103–9.

Scott RD. Staying out and getting out of trouble during total knee arthroplasty. In: Scott RD, editor. Total knee arthroplasty. 1st ed. Philadelphia: Saunders; 2006. p. 110–6.

Scuderi GR. Complications after total knee arthroplasty: how to manage patients with osteolysis. J Bone Joint Surg. 2011;93-A: 2127–35.

Scuderi GR. The stiff total knee arthroplasty: causality and solution. J Arthroplasty. 2005;20 Suppl 2:23–6.

Segawa H, Tsukayama DT, Kyle RF, et al. Infection after total knee arthroplasty. A retrospective study of the treatment of eighty-one infections. J Bone Joint Surg. 1999;81-A:1434–45.

Severson EP, Hanssen AD. The infected total knee arthroplasty. In: Scott WN, editor. Surgery of the knee. 5th ed. Philadelphia: Churchill Livingstone; 2011. p. 1346–58.

Sharkey PF, Hozack WJ, Rothman RH, et al. Insall Award paper. Why are total knee arthroplasties failing today? Clin Orthop. 2002;404:7–13.

Sherrell JC, Fehring TK, Odum S, et al. The Chitranjan Ranawat Award: fate of two-stage reimplantation after failed irrigation and débridement for periprosthetic knee infection. Clin Orthop. 2011;469:18–25.

Shorr RI, Ray WA, Danghorty JR, et al. Concurrent use of nonsteroidal anti-inflammatory drugs and oral anticoagulants places elderly persons at high risk for hemorrhagic peptic ulcer disease. Arch Intern Med. 1993;153:1665–70.

Silva M, Kabbash CA, Tiberi III JV, et al. Surface damage on open box posterior-stabilized polyethylene tibial inserts. Clin Orthop. 2003;416:135–44.

Sinha RK, Rubash HE. Extensor mechanism rupture. In: Callaghan JJ, editor. The adult knee. 1st ed. Philadelphia: Lippincott Williams & Wilkins; 2003. p. 1351–8.
Smith JL, Tullos HS, Davidson JP. Alignment of total knee arthroplasty. J Arthroplasty. 1989;4 Suppl 1:55–61.
Song EK, Yoon TR, Joo DC. Analysis of wear particle in association with aseptic loosening in cementless total knee arthroplasty. J Korean Knee Soc. 1999;11:143–8.
Stern SH, Insall JN. Total knee arthroplasty in obese patients. J Bone Joint Surg. 1990;72-A:1400–4.
Su ET, Kubiak EN, Dewal H, et al. A proposed classification of supracondylar femur fractures above total knee arthroplasties. J Arthroplasty. 2006;21:405–8.
Surface MF, Berzins A, Orban RM, et al. Backsurface wear and deformation in polyethylene tibial inserts retrieved postmortem. Clin Orthop. 2002;404:14–23.
Teeny SM, Dorr L, Murato G, et al. Treatment of infected total knee arthroplasty: irrigation and debridement versus two-stage reimplantation. J Arthroplasty. 1990;5:35–9.
Teeter MG, Naudie DD, McErlain DD, et al. In vitro quantification of wear in tibial inserts using microcomputed tomography. Clin Orthop. 2011;469:107–12.
Trampuz A, Hanssen AD, Osmon DR, et al. Synovial fluid leukocyte count and differential for the diagnosis of prosthetic knee infection. Am J Med. 2004;117:556–62.
Tria AJ, Harwood DA, Alicea JA, et al. Patellar fractures in posterior stabilized knee arthroplasties. Clin Orthop. 1994;299:131–8.
Uçkay I, Hoffmeyer P, Trampuz A, et al. Antibiotic prophylaxis before dental procedures in arthroplasty patients. Rev Med Suisse. 2010;6:727–30.
Vanbiervliet J, Bellemans J, Verlinden C, et al. The influence of malrotation and femoral component material on patellofemoral wear during gait. J Bone Joint Surg. 2011;93-B:1348–54.
Vaughn BK, Knezevich S, Lombardi AV, et al. Use of the Greenfield filter to prevent fatal pulmonary embolism associated with total hip and knee arthroplasty. J Bone Joint Surg. 1989;71-A:1542–8.
Vessely MB, Frick MA, Oakes D, et al. Magnetic resonance imaging with metal suppression for evaluation of periprosthetic osteolysis after total knee arthroplasty. J Arthroplasty. 2006;21:826–31.
Vince KG, Abdeen A, Sugimori T. The unstable total knee arthroplasty: causes and cures. J Arthroplasty. 2006;21 Suppl 1:44–9.
Vince KG, Nakasone C. Extensor mechanism disruption after total knee arthroplasty. In: Scott WN, editor. Surgery of the knee. 4th ed. Philadelphia: Churchill Livingstone; 2006. p. 1814–27.
Vince KG, Bédard M. Extensor mechanism disruption after total knee arthroplasty. In: Scott WN, editor. Surgery of the knee. 5th ed. Philadelphia: Churchill Livingstone; 2011. p. 1386–410.
Waldman BJ, Mont MA, Hungerford DS. Total knee arthroplasty infections associated with dental procedures. Clin Orthop. 1997;343:164–72.
Walker PS, Soudry M, Ewald FC, et al. Control of cement penetration in total knee arthroplasty. Clin Orthop. 1984;185:155–64.
Wang CJ, Wang JW, Weng LH, et al. Prevention of deep-vein thrombosis after total knee arthroplasty in Asian patients. Comparison of low-molecular-weight heparin and indomethacin. J Bone Joint Surg. 2004;86-A:136–40.
Wang H, Simpson KJ, Chamnongkich S, et al. Biomechanical influence of TKA designs with varying radii on bilateral TKA patients during sit-to-stand. Dyn Med. 2008;7:12.
Warren JP, Olanokun TK, Cobb AG, et al. Laxity and function in knee replacements: a comparative study of three prosthetic designs. Clin Orthop. 1994;305:200–8.
Wasilewski RC, Barden RM, Rosenberg AG. Results of different surgical procedures on total knee arthroplasty infections. J Arthroplasty. 1996;11:931–8.
Wasilewski SA, Frankl U. Arthroscopy of the painful dysfunctional total knee replacement. Arthroscopy. 1989;5:294–7.
White RH, Henderson MC. Risk factors for venous thromboembolism after total hip and knee replacement surgery. Curr Opin Pulm Med. 2002;8:365–71.
Whiteside LA. Cementless total knee design. In: Scott WN, editor. Surgery of the knee. 5th ed. Philadelphia: Churchill Livingstone; 2011. p. 1112–24.
Whiteside LA. Clinical results of the Whitesides Ortholoc total knee replacement. Orthop Clin North Am. 1987;20:113–24.
Whiteside LA, Fosco DR, Brooks JG. Fracture of the femoral components in cementless total knee arthroplasty. Clin Orthop. 1993;286:71–7.
Wilson FC, Venters GC. Results of knee replacement with the Wallidus prosthesis: an interim report. Clin Orthop. 1976;120:39–46.
Wilson MG, Kelley K, Thornhill TS. Infection as a complication of total knee-replacement arthroplasty. Risk factors and treatment in sixty-seven cases. J Bone Joint Surg. 1990;94-A:58–64.
Witvrouw E, Bellemans J, Victor J. Manipulation under anaesthesia versus low stretch device in poor range of motion after TKA. Knee Surg Sports Traumatol Arthrosc. 2012.
Wong P, Gross AE. The use of structural allografts for treating periprosthetic fractures about the hip and knee. Orthop Clin North Am. 1999;30:259–64.
Woolson ST, Pottorff G. Venous ultrasonography in the detection of proximal vein thrombosis after total knee arthroplasty. Clin Orthop. 1991;273:131–5.
Yang D, Zhou Y, Tang Q, et al. Anatomical relationship between the proximal tibia and posterior neurovascular structures: a safe zone for surgeries involving the proximal tibia. J Arthroplasty. 2011;26:1123–7.
Zalzal P, Backstein D, Gross AE, et al. Notching of the anterior femoral cortex during total knee arthroplasty characteristics that increase local stresses. J Arthroplasty. 2006;21:737–43.
Zanotti RM, Freiberg AA, Matthews LS. Use of patellar allograft to reconstruct a patellar tendon-deficient knee after total joint arthroplasty. J Arthroplasty. 1995;10:271–4.
Zimmeri W, Widmer AF, Blatter M, et al. Role of rifampin for treatment of orthopedic implant-related staphylococcal infections: a randomized controlled trial. Foreign-body infection (FBI) study group. JAMA. 1998;279:1537–41.
Zmistowski B, Restrepo C, Kahl LK, et al. Incidence and reasons for nonrevision reoperation after total knee arthroplasty. Clin Orthop. 2011;469:138–45.
Zywiel MG, Mont MA, McGrath MS, et al. Peroneal nerve dysfunction after total knee arthroplasty: characterization and treatment. J Arthroplasty. 2011;26:379–85.

Revision Arthroplasty

9

Artificial joints do not assimilate into the human body and are not as durable as the human joints. Hence, artificial joints require a revision surgery after a certain period of time. Even though the artificial joint has not been used for a long time, revision arthroplasty may be needed in cases of severe pain and significant functional loss or when complications develop.

Operative procedures for revision arthroplasty are generally more difficult than those for primary TKA and their prognosis is not as good as that of primary TKA. The operation may fail in the absence of thoughtful planning.

I would like to describe aseptic and septic revision arthroplasty separately as there are several differences between the two operations.

9.1 Introduction

The number of patients requiring revision arthroplasty is increasing. There are many reasons for this. First, the number of primary TKAs has increased significantly. Second, the indication for primary TKA has extended to young active patients. Third, the life span has prolonged and the patients now live longer than the expected TKA survival.

The need for revision before the average survival time of the artificial joint is considered to be a failure of the artificial joint under any circumstance. *The most common indications of revision TKA are infection, followed by wear and loosening. Other causes are osteolysis, instability, stiffness, extensor mechanism dysfunction, and fracture.*

The outcomes of revision TKA are not as good as those of primary TKA, but the results vary from surgeon to surgeon. Ritter et al. reported that the survival rate of revision TKA was 97 % at 6 years, while Haas and Dennis reported a survival rate of 83 % at 8 years. Sheng et al. analyzed 2,637 cases of revision TKA performed in Finland and reported that the 2-year survival rate was 96 %, 5-year survival rate was 89 %, and 10-year survival rate was 79 %. *Prognosis was better when the patients were older than 70 years of age, when 5 years had elapsed from the time of primary TKA, and when the patellofemoral alignment was good.* Singh et al. reported that *activity is often restricted after revision TKA in case the patient is a woman, is over 80 years of age, and/or is exceedingly overweight (BMI > 40).* Suarez et al. reported that 46 % of cases of failed revision TKA were due to infections.

Similar to primary TKA, *the goal of revision TKA is to reduce pain, to improve function, and to provide a mechanically stable joint.* For this purpose, it is necessary to reconstruct the bone defect, to establish mediolateral and extension–flexion gap balance, and to restore the extensor mechanism.

There are several factors to be considered while performing a revision TKA. First, it is necessary to know the causes of a failed TKA. Wear and loosening which has developed after 15 years of use is considered to be natural, whereas early wear and loosening is caused due to surgical failure, prosthesis defect, or overactivity of the patient. Revision TKA should be done to correct the causative factors. *The probability of failure is high when revision TKA is performed simply to relieve pain without identifying the causes of failure.* Revision TKA should be performed only when it is certain that the cause of pain is not reflex sympathetic dystrophy or the pain is not due to extrinsic causes. *Second, the necessity and timing of the operation should be considered.* Revision TKA should be performed when the pain is very severe, the patient cannot walk, or the lesion is progressing rapidly. It is not appropriate to perform revision simply because there are complications and the clinical manifestations are progressing. Patient's general condition, activity, and life expectancy should also be considered. Just as there are indications for primary TKA, there also are indications for revision TKA. *Indications for revision TKA should be decided more carefully* as revision TKA is technically more demanding and has a poorer prognosis. *However, once the decision has been made to perform revision TKA, it should be done as soon as possible* in order to reduce the bone defect caused by osteolysis and instability and to prevent the

W. Cho, *Knee Joint Arthroplasty*,
DOI 10.1007/978-3-642-39389-1_9, © Springer-Verlag Berlin Heidelberg 2014

progression of synovitis. *Third, surgeons* should be humble when evaluating their experiences or level of skills since an *operation beyond their abilities can worsen the results of revision TKA*.

9.2 Revision for Aseptic Failure

If there is no infection, revision TKA can be largely classified into *partial replacement and total replacement of the component*. If the wear is confined to the PE or loosening has developed in only one component despite of the long-term use, it may not be necessary to replace all the components. Engh et al. reported that isolated PE exchange for wear or osteolysis showed similar result with full revision when the component are well aligned and well fixed. However, *many surgeons report that when partial replacement is done, the results are not good*. Hence, it is increasingly recommended to replace all the components even when the problems are confined to one component. In cases of early wear and loosening, replacing all the components is required as it is likely to be caused due to surgical failure or implant defect.

9.2.1 Preoperative Checkup

9.2.1.1 General Condition

As revision surgery takes a long time and considerable bleeding is expected, patient's general conditions including cardiopulmonary function and compromised immune system should be carefully evaluated. Also, infections in the other organs and diabetes mellitus should be treated or controlled before the revision TKA since the risk of infection is high.

9.2.1.2 Analysis of the Causes

The causes of failure of primary TKA should be identified before revision TKA based on the patient's medical history, physical examination, and X-rays.

Loosening of the tibial or femoral component was the most common cause of revision TKA when the first-generation prosthesis and constrained type prosthesis were used, while patellar component loosening occurred mostly with the use of the second-generation prosthesis due to improper selection of implant or maltracking. The causes of loosening include an obese patient, overactivity, malalignment, instability, osteoporotic bone, and constrained type of prosthesis. Most of the times, it is necessary to *establish a method for reconstructing the bone defect and for ensuring stable fixation*. Currently, *wear* is one of the major reasons for performing revision TKA. This may be related to the patient, implant, and surgical factors. *The method of treatment varies according to the causes, period from primary TKA, and extent of wear*. If *motion limitation* is simply due to adhesions, enhanced rehabilitation program should be started first, and brisement and simple adhesiolysis with arthroscopy can be followed in order to increase the ROM. *If the ROM is limited due to the flexion/extension gap discrepancy or other surgical faults, revision TKA should be performed to correct the gap discrepancy. The incidence of revision TKA due to instability is not high, but surgical correction is needed in severe cases.* The cause of instability is mostly surgical failure to achieve the balance, which includes flexion/extension gap imbalance, inadequate release of the ligament, and patellar maltracking in addition to wear and loosening. Muscle weakness or trauma is another cause of instability.

An extrinsic lesion can affect the results of primary TKA and it should be evaluated before revision surgery. The hip and ankle joint pathology and the deformity of the femur and tibia are another cause of failure of primary TKA.

9.2.1.3 Preoperative Knee Joint Assessment

Physical Examination

The first step in preoperative assessment is to *check the skin condition*. The site and condition of the incision scar, the elasticity of skin, and vascularity are the important elements that affect the prognosis of revision. Second, the treatment method for revision TKA can differ according to the *condition of the knee joint and its function*. This includes the degree of instability, deformity, limited ROM, and muscle strength. It is necessary to determine the degree, site, direction of deformity and whether it is a fixed or flexible deformity in order to plan the revision. The *degree of limited motion* and its causes are very important factors for deciding the revision and for choosing the method of revision. The methods of revision can be different according to the causes of limited motion such as adhesions of soft tissues or gap discrepancy due to surgical failure. Dorr stated that soft tissues often need special management when the preoperative flexion motion is less than 90° or the flexion contracture is greater than 15°. *The quadriceps muscle power* also has a significant impact on the prognosis of revision TKA, and hence its tension and extensor lag should be evaluated before surgery.

Radiological Examination

The degree of deformity, bone defect, instability, and patellar tracking should be examined on the plain X-ray. Loosening may only be seen when the projection is accurate and its accuracy increases with the use of fluoroscopy. *On X-ray, bone defect appears much smaller than its actual size. Stress X-ray also helps in checking the instability* whether it is due to PE wear, relaxation of ligaments, or prosthesis instability. *X-ray of the contralateral knee* is necessary in order to compare both sides and to check the prosthesis size.

In some cases, CT scan can be of great help to assess the degree of osteolysis, rotational deformity, and the position of the prosthesis.

Miscellaneous

Before revision TKA, the possibility of an infection should always be ruled out and any suspicious factor should be thoroughly examined. Barrack et al. and Duff et al. suggested performing a routine arthrocentesis before revision TKA.

Finally, the size and *brand of the primary prosthesis* should be checked to determine whether that product had any material or design defect, whether it is appropriate for revision and which options are available.

9.2.2 Surgical Procedure

The surgical procedures that can be considered based on the preoperative analysis include *which type of prosthesis is to be used, which approach will be better, how the prosthesis can be removed, how to perform osteotomy and bone reconstruction, how the soft tissue treatment can be done to achieve balancing, and how to fix the prosthesis.*

9.2.2.1 Implant selection

Implant selection is usually done before the operation, and it is desirable to select an implant that offers all the options since the surgical procedure may change during the operation. Since the current prostheses have a modular system, all sizes of each component need to be kept ready. *Metal augment and an extended stem with an offset stem, should be available.* Also, it is desirable to use the prosthesis which has an instrument for easy removal of the implant.

Factors that affect implant selection include range of motion, instability of the joint, amount and type of bone defect, alignment of lower limbs, patellar tracking, and type and shape of the prosthesis used in the primary TKA.

The most important factor is the motion constraint of the implant. Less constraint is better for long-term survival of the implant, but constrained prosthesis may be required in some cases of revision TKA. *The CR type of prosthesis can be used when only the PE needs to be replaced in patients in whom this type of prosthesis has been used before and in whom the PCL is sound.* The benefit of using this type of prosthesis is that it minimizes the bone loss. However, there are a few problems when revision is to be done; it is not easy to correct the deformity and it is difficult to achieve the balance. If the PCL is not normal, it might be difficult to achieve stability in flexion or the ROM may be limited. Clinically, this type of prosthesis can be used by experienced surgeons only when there is little deformity, instability, and bone loss.

The PS type of prosthesis is the most appropriate implant when the flexion and extension gaps have been restored, the joint line is retained, and the collateral ligament has been balanced. The benefit of using this type of prosthesis is that it provides reliable substitution when the PCL is missing or incomplete, it makes it easy to correct the deformity, it is stable in flexion, and the patient can achieve a good range of motion. The drawbacks of PS type of prosthesis is that posterior dislocation may occur if the collateral ligaments are not balanced or when there is flexion and extension gap discrepancy. Gustke reported that 82 % of cases of revision TKA can be done with semiconstrained implants.

Constrained type of prosthesis is used when there is marked instability due to severe collateral ligament deficiency or when there is moderate to severe flexion/extension gap discrepancy. In other words, a constrained prosthesis is used when there is mediolateral instability in extension or dislocation of the prosthesis occurs in flexion. There are *two types of constrained prosthesis, VVC (varus–valgus control) type and linked type*, and some of the linked types allow for rotation. The appropriate type of *constrained prosthesis* should be selected according to the degree of instability. In general, the linked type can correct the instability in a more strict sense than the VVC type, but the motion constraint is increased. The linked type can be used in *severe instability, severe bone defect, or hyperextension as it constrains motion more than the VVC* type. As a result, the linked type is associated with a higher rate of loosening.

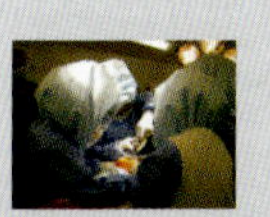

Author's Method

I recommend the PS type in most revision cases, and the constrained type is used only if it is absolutely indicated. The decision for using of constrained type is determined by the balance of extension and flexion gaps and the status of the collateral ligament before or during the operation. When an infection and severe instability have persisted for a long time, when AORI Type III bone defect exists or when joint dislocation has occurred, I use the constrained type for revision TKA. In such cases, the collateral ligaments are unreliable even though they appear sound in the operation field. Also, the constrained type is used if dislocation in flexion develops with an adequate extension gap state during the operation.

I decide to use the constrained type by increasing the PE thickness step by step. I start with a PE that seems to fit the flexion/extension gap and followed by inserting a one-size thicker PE in flexion state. In most cases, the flexion gap adapts to this thickness, but flexion contracture occurs because the extension gap becomes narrow. I extend the knee forcefully. If the flexion contracture is corrected with the one-size thicker PE, I try the same procedure again with a two-size thicker PE. If the flexion contracture disappears with a two-size thicker PE, a constrained prosthesis is used since these findings indicate that the joint capsule or ligament tissues are unreliable for stability.

Custom-made prosthesis has fallen out of favor since the modular type component has been introduced. *APC* (allograft prosthesis composite) can be used when there is a severe bone defect, but the junction with the host bone site may not be well united, and infection may occur more frequently. Therefore, it would be more convenient and safer to *use the tumor prosthesis rather than the APC in the patient with a severe bone defect.*

In patellar revision, biconvex prosthesis, inset patella, or trabecular metal augment can be considered when there is a severe cavitary defect.

9.2.2.2 Approach

The most important surgical step in revision TKA is the approach. Wound edge necrosis and extensor mechanism rupture are the most critical complications that can adversely affect the outcome of revision TKA. If the *approach is insufficient and lateral traction or eversion of the patella cannot be achieved, revision TKA cannot be performed properly and it is highly likely to fail.* Harwin recommended brisement before skin incision in patients with ankylosed knee. Approach varies based on the previously used approach, soft tissue coverage, deformity, and joint motion, but *it is recommended to use the same approach as that used in primary TKA*. However, the subvastus approach should be avoided even though it has been used before. If problems with the skin and/or soft tissues are suspected, a plastic surgeon should be consulted in advance. If excessive tension in the skin is expected, tissue expanders may be used before revision TKA. Arthrotomy is done along the previous incision line if there is remaining suture material.

If the patient has good preoperative range of motion, a routine medial release allows the tibia to be rotated externally and subluxated anteriorly, which is usually sufficient for exposure. If there is contracture of the ligamentous tissues, it is necessary to release the tissues en bloc. The medial contracture may require release up to the whole superficial MCL, pes anserinus, and semimembranosus tendon, thereby allowing anterior translation and external rotation of the tibia so that the tibia can be exposed as much as possible. If there is a lateral contracture, the iliotibial band, joint capsule, and popliteus tendon may be released step by step.

If exposure is not enough for revision arthroplasty using the above methods, ancillary procedures for the quadriceps mechanism such as rectus snip, V–Y quadricepsplasty, tibial tubercle osteotomy, or subperiosteal peel can be performed subsequently.

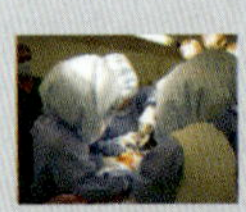

Author's Method

I believe that the approach is the most important factor in revision TKA. If the patella is not everted or laterally retracted during revision TKA, the exposure will be limited and the surgical procedure will be restricted.

In order to do patellar eversion, hypertrophic fibrous tissues on the lateral side of the quadriceps and patella tendon is removed completely and adhesiolysis is done as well in advance. On careful observation, I can easily define the junction between tendinous and fibrous tissue. Once this is done, the patella can be everted or laterally retracted in most of the cases (Fig. 9.1). *During eversion of the patella, the patellar tendon* may be stripped off or an avulsion fracture may develop. I use a protector or mini plate to prevent this occurrence. I had used the rectus snip approach to ensure an adequate operation field until I developed this technique. But I have not needed any ancillary procedures to the quadriceps tendon ever since I used this technique.

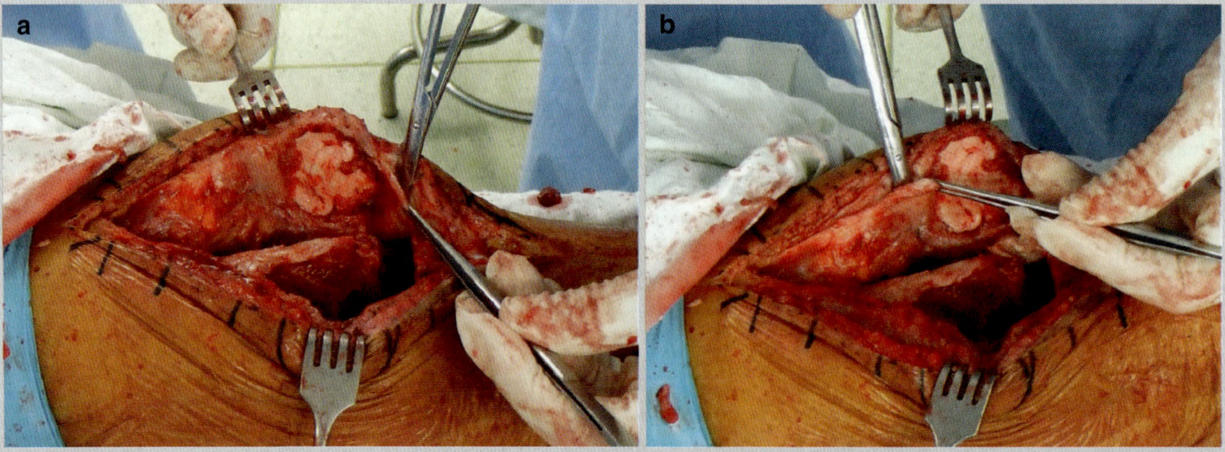

Fig. 9.1 Removing the hypertrophic fibrous tissues from patella tendon (**a**) and quadriceps tendon (**b**) Thick fibrous tissue should be removed

9.2.2.3 Implant Removal

Implant removal is an even more critical procedure during revision TKA. If it is done with less amount of bone loss, the subsequent procedure becomes easier and the operation has good prognosis. Hence, implant removal should be done carefully in order to minimize the bone loss.

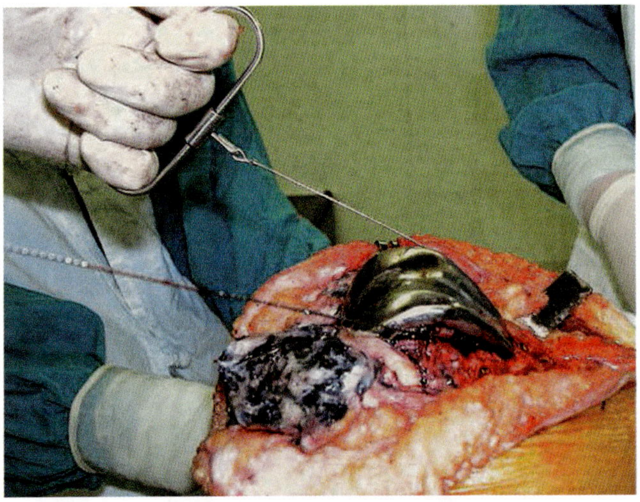

Fig. 9.2 Separating the prosthesis using a Gigli saw

For easy removal of the implant, sliding hammer, microsaw, Gigli saw, diamond-tipped drill, etc., should be kept ready. At first the PE is removed. There is usually no problem while removing the snap-fitted PE, but it is sometimes necessary to cut the PE which was fixed with screws or metal rod. After removal of the PE, the femoral, tibial, and patellar prostheses are removed in that order. It is technically more difficult to remove the tibial prosthesis first and the tibial bone might be injured while removing the femoral prosthesis. Patellar component is removed lastly because removing the patellar component first may weaken the patella and a patellar fracture may occur during the subsequent surgical procedures.

Microsaw is more recommended than Gigli saw for separating the prosthesis from the bone. Gigli saw can separate only the anterior portion of the femur, it can cause too much bone loss at the chamfer area and may cause contamination as the handle portion of the Gigli saw can get easily slipped off (Fig. 9.2). On the other hand, *microsaw can reach almost all areas except for the posterior portion of the prosthesis. So, the use of microsaw can minimize the bone loss and it is also convenient to use* (Fig. 9.3).

Finally, an extractor is used to remove the prosthesis. If the *stem does not come out, a window can be made in the anterior cortex of the femur. In the tibia, a window can be made in relation to the tibial tubercle osteotomy.*

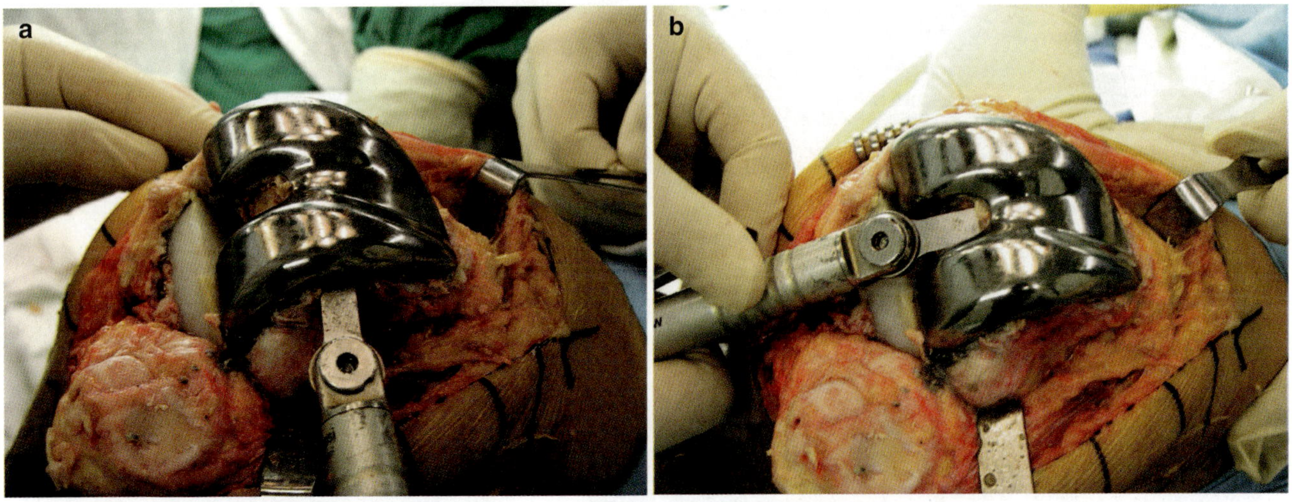

Fig. 9.3 Separating the prosthesis from the bone using a microsaw. The distal (**a**) and notch area (**b**) is separated

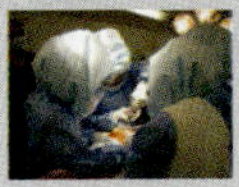

Author's Method

My method of implant removal is different from the others. It is a very simple and effective technique and it reduces the amount of bone loss. First, I *drill a hole to make a mark* at around 5–6 cm proximal to the joint line on the lateral side of the femoral metaphysis *before removing the femoral prosthesis* and measure its distance from the joint line. Even in revision TKA, the height of the femoral prosthesis is usually maintained. So this hole is *used as the index of the joint line* which is one of the most important points of the surgical technique for revision TKA (Fig. 9.4). After making a mark, *I remove the fibrous tissues around the femoral prosthesis* using a knife or a thin osteotome to define the boundaries.

I use a microsaw to separate the prosthesis from the bone, and then instead of using an extractor, I tap the medial and lateral sides alternately with a hammer. The seesaw effect helps to separate the prosthesis from the bone. Then, I use an impactor to tap the anterior flange of the femoral prosthesis. This makes it easy to remove the prosthesis as it has already been separated. In this manner, the prosthesis can be removed with almost no bone loss (Fig. 9.5).

While removing the tibial component, the anterior and medial sides are separated using a microsaw, while the lateral and posterior sides are separated using a Gigli saw. Again, the mediolateral and anteroposterior sides are tapped alternately with a hammer and impactor (Fig. 9.6). While removing the prosthesis, the tibial plateau can get compressed if the osteotome is used as a lever. Hence, I use the extractor or impactor in the reverse direction. In the modular type, it is sometimes easier to separate the tibial plate and the stem first. After removal of the tibial plate, the stem is separated from the bone with a gouge and is removed.

Removal of the patellar component is done in the end. The patella is removed by stripping off the fibrous tissues and bony overgrowth from margins of the prosthesis and followed by separating the prosthesis from the bone using a microsaw. And then I remove the patellar component using an osteotome and the instrument that I have designed (Fig. 9.7). In a metal-backed patella, I remove the PE first to see the outline of the metallic component. I sometimes cut the lugs using Midas Rex (Medtronic, Minneapolis) and then dig them out. Since the removal of the patellar component is likely to cause a fracture due to excessive bone loss, I take special care to prevent this occurrence.

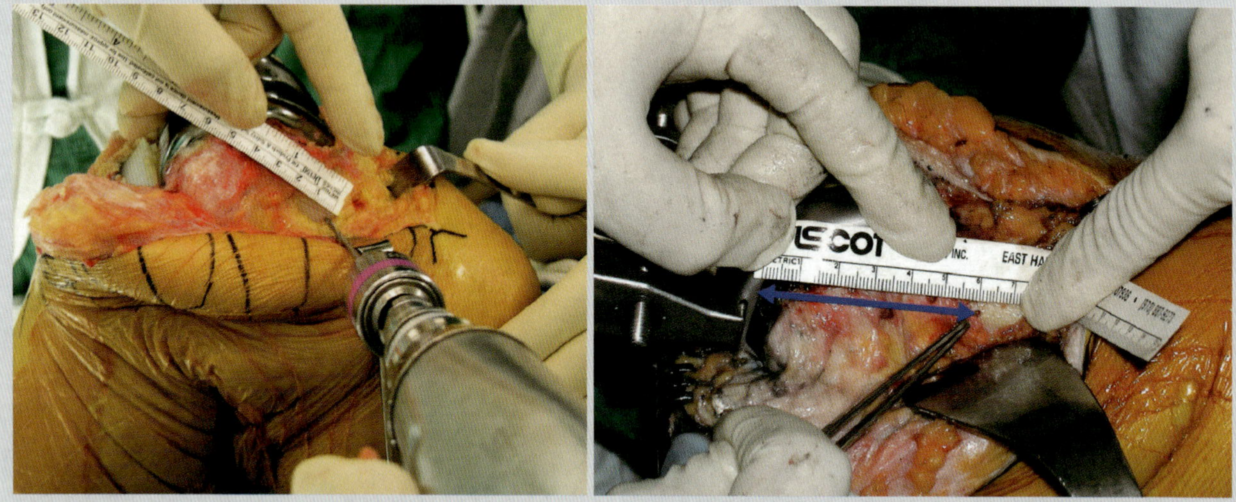

Fig. 9.4 The method to maintain the joint line. The *left* image shows a marking about 5–6 cm proximal to the joint line before removing the prosthesis. The *right* image shows the technique of measuring the size of bone defect after inserting a trial implant up to the marked level

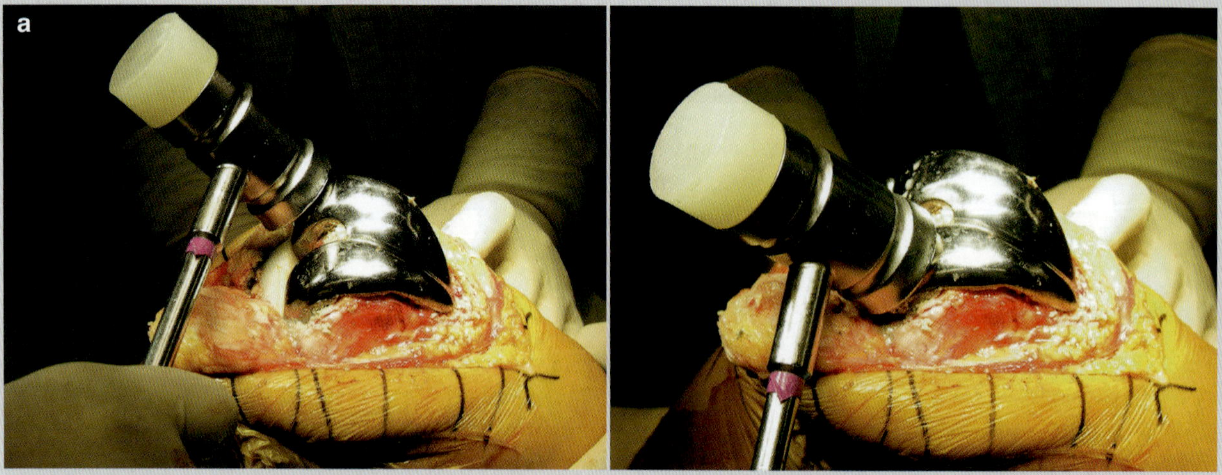

Fig. 9.5 Method of removing the femoral prosthesis. (**a**) Separating the femoral prosthesis from the bone by tapping the medial and lateral sides alternately with a hammer. (**b**) Removing the prosthesis with an impactor. (**c**) After removal of the prosthesis using my technique (There is almost no bone loss after removal of the prosthesis.)

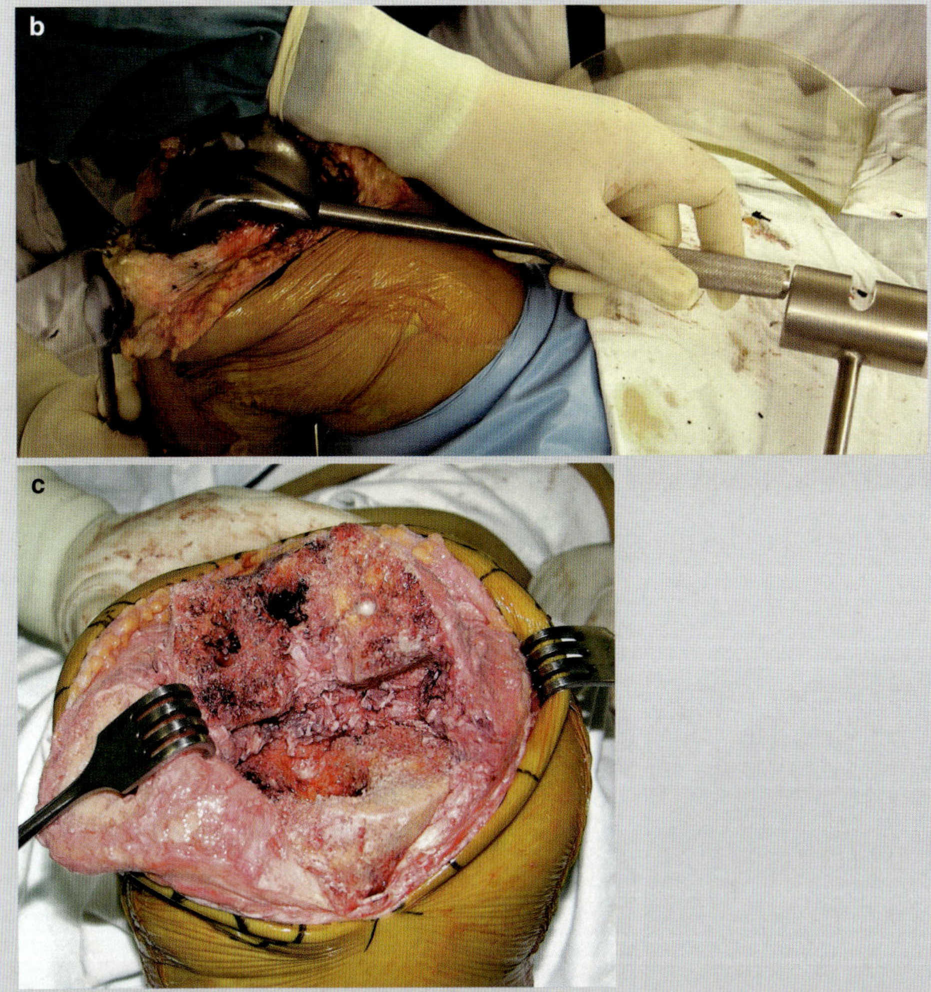

Fig. 9.5 (continued)

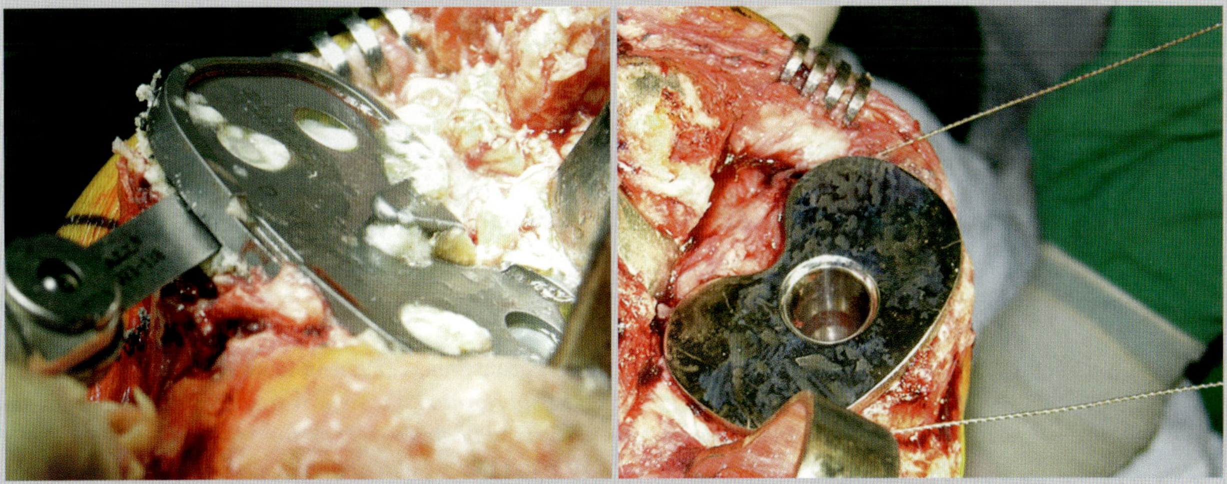

Fig. 9.6 Method of removing of tibial component. *Left*: Anterior portion is separated using microsaw. *Right*: Posterior portion is separated by Gigli saw. Next procedure is same with removal of femoral prosthesis

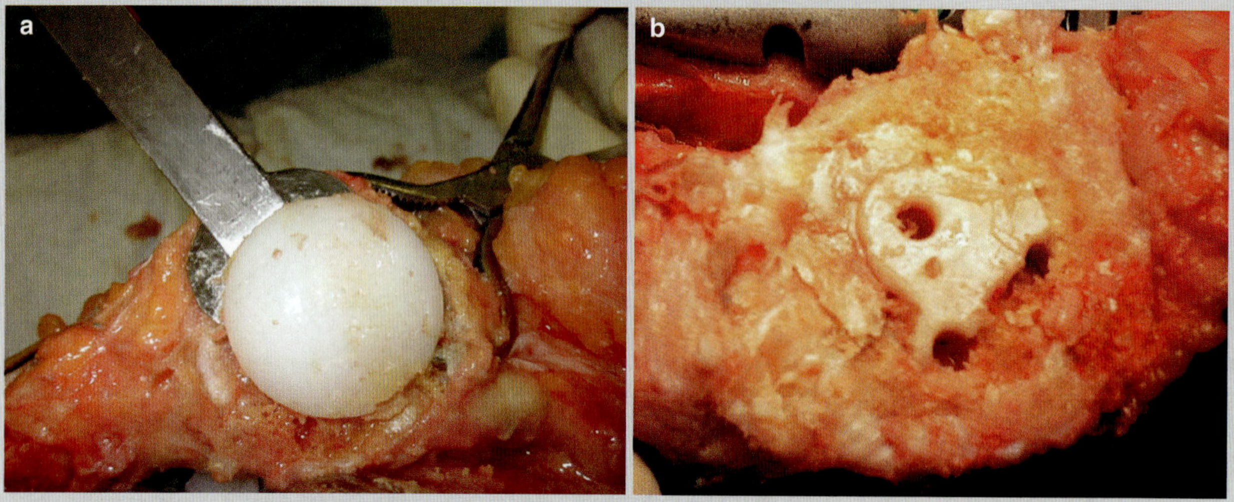

Fig. 9.7 Method of removing the patellar prosthesis using patella remover (**a**) and after its removal (**b**)

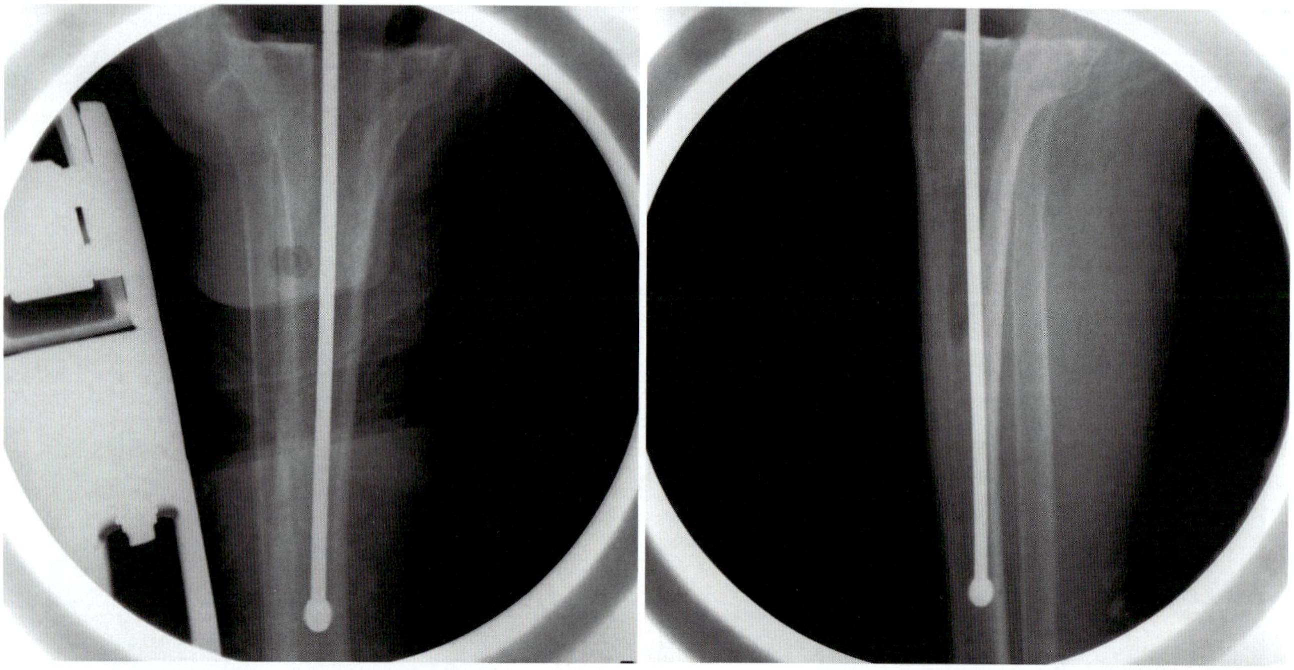

Fig. 9.8 Use a C-arm to check whether the medullary reamer is in its correct position or not. The reamer is located in the medullary canal

After removal of the prosthesis, it is recommended to remove the remaining bone cement. *In aseptic revision TKA, cement may not be removed if its removal causes a large bone defect.* But in septic revision, all the cement should be removed as the cement may be the source of infection. The reamer can be used to remove the cement from the medullary canal. *While reaming, care should be taken so that the reamer does not perforate the cortex of the tibia* instead of reaming the cement. This happens sometimes because the cement is too hard. *If the cortex of the tibia is perforated, the neurovascular structures in the calf are likely to be injured. Therefore, it is recommended to use C-arm to check whether reaming is done correctly* (Fig. 9.8).

After removal of the cement from the medullary canal, the fibrous membrane on the inner surface of the bone and intramedullary canal should be curetted completely until the healthy bone is exposed in order to improve fixation of the prosthesis.

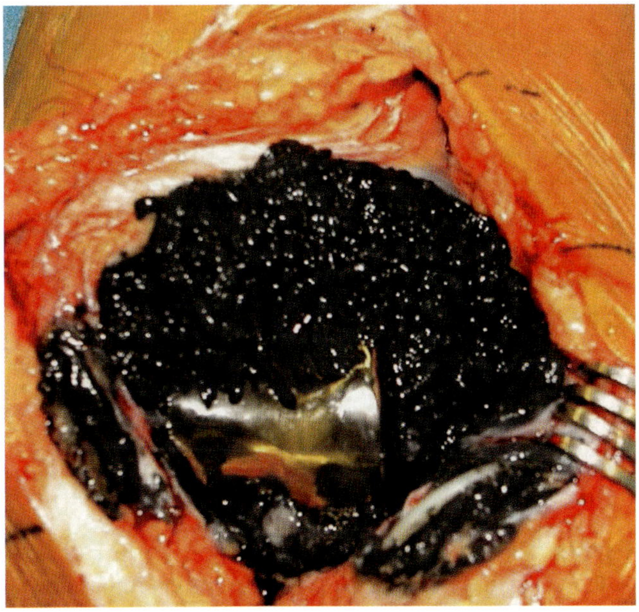

Fig. 9.9 Black colored soft tissue and synovium due to metallosis

9.2.2.4 Soft Tissue Treatment

If wear has extended to the metal, synovium and soft tissues are stained black due to metallosis (Fig. 9.9). Even a small amount of metal debris can stain the bone, and hence it needs to be excised meticulously. In most cases, however, such meticulous excision is impossible as it is dangerous to the neurovascular system and it can be found outside of the joint. In revision for loosening or osteolysis, the color of the synovium may have changed to a grayish shade. This is the osteolysis phenomenon caused due to the PE particles rather than metallosis and these particles must be removed meticulously. As the synovial membrane is adhered to the surrounding soft tissues and the joint capsule is weak, *caution is needed to prevent a neurovascular injury while performing debridement of the posterior synovial membrane and the capsule.*

After synovectomy, *the hypertrophic fibrous tissues in the supracondylar area of the femur should be removed. If these tissues are not removed, they will worsen the patellar alignment, restrict flexion motion, and interfere with skin closure.* Therefore, fibrous tissues in the supracondylar area must be *removed without any hesitation* not only for improving the extensor mechanism but also for achieving a better ROM.

9.2.2.5 Osteotomy and Bone Reconstruction

Removal of the prosthesis is followed by bone reconstruction and soft tissue balancing. *The basic principle of revision arthroplasty involves maintaining the joint line and performing a kinematically stable arthroplasty that is well fixed and well aligned.*

The causes of bone defect noted during revision TKA are infection, loosening, osteolysis, stress shielding, instability, etc. The bone defect becomes larger during removal of the implant.

Bone defect should be reconstructed by any method which achieves stability of the prosthesis and balancing of the knee joint. In the femur, maintenance of the joint line is strongly related to the amount of reconstruction. If the extension gap is narrow in an adequate flexion gap state, the joint line can be elevated by 4–5 mm using the PS type of prosthesis. Vince stated that *it is much more important to establish the extension and flexion gap balance, ligament balance, and prosthesis fixation rather than retaining the joint line in revision TKA. An excessive tibial osteotomy weakens the bone that supports the prosthesis and a smaller prosthesis with a thicker PE may be required.* Therefore, the bone defect should be reconstructed as much as possible. General principles of bone reconstruction are described in Sect. 5.1, and hence, surgical techniques for each part are briefly described here.

Tibia

The tibial bone reconstruction is the foundation of revision arthroplasty because the level of tibial osteotomy affects both the extension and flexion gaps. Hence, I will describe the tibial procedure first. *Intramedullary method is strongly recommended for alignment and reconstruction of the tibia* because an extension stem needs to be inserted in many cases, and the amount of resection increases when bone resection is performed by using the extramedullary method since additional bone cutting is needed more frequently. *As the tibial component is usually perpendicular to the extension stem, the posterior slope of the tibia should be 0°.* If the posterior slope is between 3 and 5° just like in primary TKA, the posterior portion of the tibial prosthesis does not make any contact with the bone when an extension stem is used. The size of the prosthesis and the length and diameter of the extension stem are chosen, and the medullary canal is reamed. After osteotomy, the center of rotation is determined. *A little more external rotation is preferable for better patellar tracking.* When bone grafting has been performed, the tibial prosthesis tends to be inserted in an internally rotated state if the rotation has been matched with the shape of the bone graft. To prevent this occurrence, *the rotation should be checked with the tibial tuberosity as a landmark.*

Femur

In femoral reconstruction, the first step is to determine the size of the femoral prosthesis. Since bone loss has occurred in the anterior or posterior portion of the femur while removing the prosthesis, many surgeons *tend to make a mistake of choosing a smaller prosthesis. With respect to the prosthesis size, the A–P length is more important than the width.* The size of the prosthesis that is removed, the contralateral

X-rays, and the flexion gap may be helpful to determine the prosthesis size. A larger prosthesis is chosen if the flexion gap is wide and a smaller prosthesis is chosen if it is narrow.

Correct rotation of the femoral component is utmost important. If the rotation of the remaining bone is not aligned with the epicondylar axis, one side of the posterior condyle can be resected more and the other side may need metal augmentation for achieving correct external rotation. As there are many incidences of bone loss at the epicondylar area, it is convenient and reasonable to use the gap technique for determining the femoral rotation.

The next step is *reaming* the medullary canal and osteotomy is done as per the manual for each prosthesis. *As most of cases have anterior bony defect*, there is a tendency to set the reaming point on the posterior side. In such a case, *the prosthesis is inadvertently inserted with anterior angulation* when an extension stem is used. On the other hand, *too little reaming of the posterior portion increase the size of prosthesis and the anterior gap between the prosthesis and the bone*. In such a situation, it is not recommended to use a prosthesis that is too large, and hence, it needs to be decided whether to lower down the reaming point, whether to use an offset stem, or to insert the prosthesis at a slight anterior angulation. *When the extension stem is already attached, the axis of distal osteotomy should be same with the stem axis of the prosthesis which is fixed between 5 and 7° in the coronal plane.*

To check the amount of the distal bone defect, a trial implant is inserted up to the level of the joint line. The guideline for the joint line is 1 cm inferior to the patella, 1 cm superior to the fibular head, 2.5 cm inferior to the lateral epicondyle, or 3.0 m inferior to the medial epicondyle.

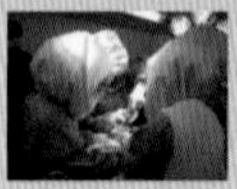

Author's Method

I start with the tibial preparation when performing a revision TKA, because the exposure is much better, it is more convenient to balance the joint gap, and it is easier to determine external rotation of femoral component and balance the soft tissues.

When performing a revision TKA, there is no reliable index for osteotomy. Therefore, I do not use any instrument for bone resection. Instead, I insert the trial implant first up to the adequate level and check the bone defect. In the tibia, I use the tibial tuberosity or fibular head as a landmark. In the femur, I use the point which has been marked before removal of the femoral prosthesis as the landmark for the joint line.

I insert a trial implant up to this point and check the flexion and extension gaps. And then, I choose the method of reconstruction. According to the gap balance, I decide whether to do bone grafting or to use a metal augment. If osteotomy is needed, minimal bone resection is preferred. I just trim the host bone rather than doing osteotomy so that the bone graft or metal augment fits well. As a result, stability of the prosthesis can be achieved with minimal bone resection.

Rotational alignment is adjusted by patellar tracking and a metal augment on femoral posterior condyle is used when needed.

Patella

Although management of the patella has an enormous impact on the results of revision TKA, it is often not discussed in detail. *The method of management of the patella is determined based on whether or not patellar resurfacing has been performed during primary TKA, the state of patellar component, the type of prosthesis used, patellofemoral alignment, and the amount of the remaining bone.*

When treating the patella, rupture of the extensor mechanism should be avoided. In order to do so, the adhesions in the gutter area should be released before eversion or retraction of the patella. It is also recommended to protect the patellar tendon from being stripped off or perform a rectus snip, V–Y quadricepsplasty, or tibial tubercle osteotomy in advance.

Patella baja is a common finding during revision TKA. The patellar tendon can be lengthened or tibial tubercle osteotomy can be performed, but it is not recommended due to rupture of the tendon or nonunion, respectively. An alternative option would be to downsize the patella, not to resurface the patella or to use a beveled form of tibial PE.

In revision TKA, *management of the patella includes re-resurfacing of the patella only to treat complications confined to the patella, reimplantation of other components and not of the patella, reimplantation of all components, and removal of the patella followed by patelloplasty.* Berry and Rand reported that patient satisfaction was lower *when only re-resurfacing of the patella was done as opposed to whole component reimplantation* and about 53 % of patients were dissatisfied with patellar re-resurfacing only. Burke et al. observed that in isolated revision of metal-backed patella, the re-resurfaced patella was in a good condition, but 15 % of patients *needed a revision TKA due to the other component-related problems* within an average period of 78 months. This manifests that complications of the patella can be associated with problems of other components. However, Ko et al. *recommended re-resurfacing of the patella only when the patient was old and the activity level was lower with a relatively good patellar tracking*.

There are a few benefits when the patella is not re-resurfaced during revision TKA. First, there is a low risk of patellar fracture; second, patellar bone stock is retained; third, operation can be performed faster; and fourth, it is more economical. *The prerequisites for not re-resurfacing the patella are; first, prosthesis fixation should be stable; second, there should be no infection; third, there should be minimal surface damage and the type of prosthesis should be dome-shaped and not metal-backed patella; and finally, proper patellar tracking is maintained.* Barrack stated that the metal-backed type should be removed and re-resurfaced if it can be anticipated that there would be more than 12 mm of remaining bone after removal of the patellar component. If the remaining bone is expected to be less than 12 mm and the aforementioned conditions are fulfilled, the patella can be retained. In other words, non-resurfacing the patella is recommended when the patellar bone stock is insufficient or the bone quality of the patella is extremely poor. Lonner et al. obtained good results by retaining the PE, provided that the PE has not oxidized and emphasized the importance of sterilization method. They also insisted that manufacturing mismatch is acceptable with most contemporary designs.

If the patella is loosened, damaged, or not positioned correctly, it should be re-resurfaced or treated with the other methods. If re-resurfacing is planned, there should be more than 12 mm of the remaining bone for achieving stable fixation and more than half of the surface should be even in thickness after bone resection. *If there is 10–12 mm of the remaining patella, a biconvex patella or inset patella can be used.*

If the thickness is less than 10 mm and if there is a cavitary defect like the shape of crab shell, just trimming the margin without resurfacing, patelloplasty which involves covering with soft tissues after bone grafting, trabecular metal augmentation, resection arthroplasty, gull wing osteotomy, or subsynovial iliac grafting can be performed. Dalury and Adams reported that patelloplasty appeared to be a satisfactory option in the management of the patella in revision TKA. This is described in more details in Sect. 5.1.

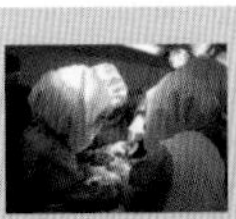

Author's Method

I do not re-resurface the patella only for isolated patellar problem. This is because the causes of patellar problems are complex. I remove the patella if patellar wear is severe, loosening has developed, there is a metal-backed patella, or if the patellar component is incompatible with revised femoral component.

If the remaining bone is more than 10 mm, I try to re-resurface the patella. In case the remaining bone is less than 10 mm, I have tried several methods including trimming the margin and non-resurfacing the patella, patelloplasty with bone graft, gull wing osteotomy, and using the trabecular system. Among them, trabecular augmentation showed better results.

9.2.2.6 Balancing

In revision TKA, bone reconstruction and balancing are interrelated procedures and cannot be performed separately. After bone reconstruction, extension, and flexion gap, balance should be achieved. The gapper or tensioner can be used for checking the balance, but checking with the trial implant is more recommended during this procedure.

Since balancing in revision TKA is basically similar to balancing in primary TKA, refer to Sect. 4.5. In summary, *the extension and flexion gaps are balanced according to the size of the femoral prosthesis and management of the distal femur*. Mihalko and Krackow stated that these principles are very convenient for achieving gap balancing in revision TKA. They used a distal femoral augment to adjust the extension gap and used different sizes of the femoral prosthesis to adjust the flexion gap (Fig. 9.10). If the extension gap is wider, the distal femur is augmented. The offset stem can be used to adjust the sagittal position of the femoral component more anteriorly or a smaller femoral prosthesis can be used to widen the flexion gap. If the flexion gap is wider, more bone resection may be performed in the distal femur to widen the extension gap or a larger prosthesis can be used and the posterior bone defect is filled with posterior metal augment so as to decrease the flexion gap. The size of the prosthesis and distal femoral resection must be within the permissible range.

Vince suggested three steps for bone reconstruction and soft tissue balancing. The first step is tibial platform reconstruction. The second step is stabilization of the knee in flexion by appropriate femoral rotation, femoral component size, and establishing the joint line. The third step is stabilization in extension by flexion and extension gap balance.

Mediolateral balance is achieved by releasing the ligament on the contracted side as much as the loosened ligament. However, in revision TKA, a thicker PE or constrained prosthesis may be needed in certain cases when all the ligaments have weakened or it is difficult to achieve sufficient reconstruction of the bone defect.

Patellofemoral malalignment needs to be readjusted since the primary femoral or tibial implant might have been inserted in internal rotation. The external rotation based on the epicondylar axis on the femoral side and the tibial

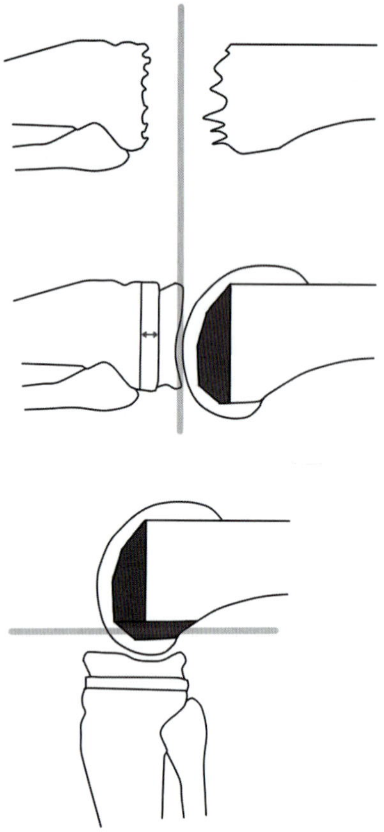

Fig. 9.10 A model for balancing the extension and flexion gaps using a distal augment and a larger size of the femoral prosthesis

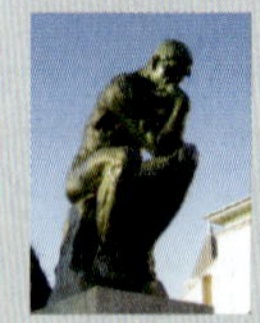

Author's Opinion

I have the experience of performing a revision TKA for patellar dislocation. I removed the femoral and tibial prosthesis and reinserted them in externally rotated position and performed lateral retinacular release. But I could not achieve satisfying results because the positioning of the femoral and the tibial component in external rotation was limited. In such a case, derotational osteotomy on the femoral side can be considered as the axis of the external rotation can be adjusted without implant removal.

tuberosity on the tibial side or by checking the patella tracking is needed and corrected if it is malrotated.

In a revision TKA, there is a high risk of patellofemoral malalignment and the incidence of lateral retinacular release is also high. Tibial tubercle osteotomy can be performed in revision for achieving patellofemoral alignment, but it is not easy to decide considering nonunion due to vascular disturbance and pain after osteotomy. If the management of the patella cannot be done by any of the method, patellectomy can be an option that can be considered.

9.2.2.7 Fixation

If the revised prosthesis is thought to be unstable, it is recommended to use an extension stem. In some cases, an offset stem may be needed according to the position of prosthesis. Conditt et al. stated that in case of a bone defect in the proximal tibia, it is recommended to fill the medullary canal (medullary canal filling by the stem) rather than improving bone coverage so as to ensure stability and emphasized using the extension stem.

There are controversies regarding the application of cement to the stem. Many surgeons do not recommend the use of cement if the stem is fixed according to the press-fit concept, but Engh et al. reported that *cementing the stem* after allogeneic graft *showed good results*. Vince et al. recommended cementing when a constrained prosthesis is used and when there is osteopenia. Fehring et al. reported that cementing the stem resulted in a stable fixation in about 93 % of patients, while only 71 % of patients showed stable fixation when cementing was not done. Peters et al. stated that the risk of infection is high when cementing of the stem is not done. On the contrary, Sah et al. revealed that modified hybrid stem fixation (metaphyseal cementing and cementless diaphyseal engaging stem) is durable at a mean 5-year follow-up. *In general, shorter extension stem (25 to 30 mm) which do not engage into the diaphysis or long and small diameter stems which do not fill the canal should be cemented.*

When cementing is done after bone grafting, two-stage cementing is recommended: first stage is done in the tibia and the patella and coating on the morcellized bone graft on the femoral side, and second stage is done in the femoral side. Internal rotation should be avoided when inserting the tibial and femoral components, and femoral component should be inserted with extension force to prevent insertion of prosthesis in anterior angulation of the femoral component (Fig. 9.11).

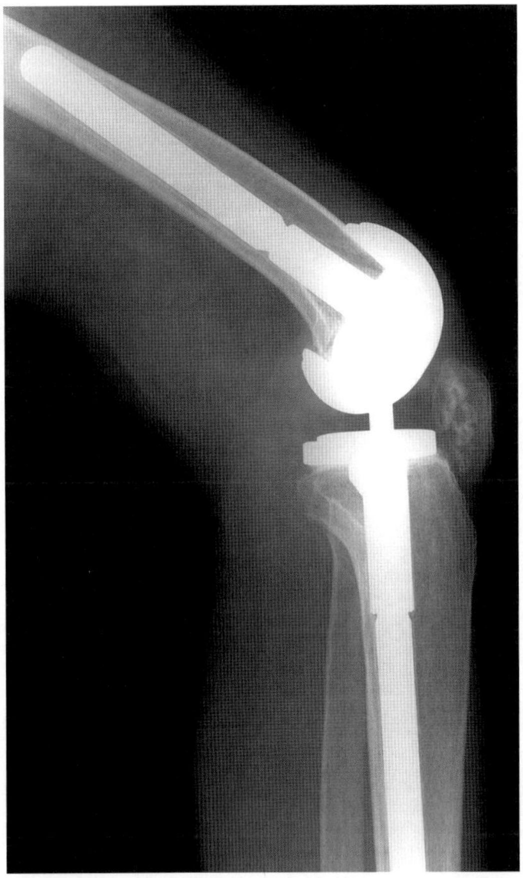

Fig. 9.11 Anterior angulation of the femoral prosthesis which is a common pitfall in revision TKA

9.3 Revision of Unicompartmental Knee Arthroplasty (UK)

In general, the survival rate of UK is inferior to that of TKA, and hence the revision rate of UK is higher than that of TKA. There are different opinions about revision of UK. Some surgeons insist that revision of UK is more difficult than that of TKA, while others have an opposite opinion. Since the current UK prosthesis has the concept of surface replacement, revision of UK is not more difficult than that of TKA if implant removal is done carefully.

The surgical methods vary according to the causes of failure. It is not recommended to perform revision to UK again except for exchanging the PE, since the supporting bone is weak and is accompanied by degenerative changes in the other parts of the joint and soft tissues. In case instability develops as a result of PE wear and over-release of the medial collateral ligament, the PE can be replaced with a thicker one after ligament balancing. PE dislocation may occur in mobile-bearing UK. This is mostly due to flexion and extension gap imbalance, which needs balancing of ligaments and exchange with a thicker PE (Fig. 9.12). However, PE exchange should be done carefully by an experienced surgeon. So revision TKA is more recommended.

Pain and limited motion also causes a problem in UK, just like in primary of TKA. The revision of UK is also likely to fail if the causes for failure remain undetected. In case of loosening, there is always an accompanying bone defect. Hence, it is very important to remove the prosthesis with minimal bone loss as in revision TKA. If this is done well, the revision procedure is much easier with the use of an only metal augment on the tibial side (Fig. 9.13).

Osteotomy is performed in a manner similar to that in conventional TKA. However, care should be taken while performing distal osteotomy of the femur since there are bone defects on the medial condyle which can make the osteotomy inaccurate. Also, the use of the ligament tension technique is recommended to determine the external rotation due to a bone defect on the posterior side of the medial femoral condyle.

In conclusion, *extension of the skin incision from the pre-existing scar, careful removal of the prosthesis, correct osteotomy, and more meticulous ligament balancing enable revision of UK to TKA easily.*

9.4 Revision of Infected TKA

Infection following arthroplasty *requires a revision TKA in almost all cases*. Other methods except for revision are described in Chap. 8.

Revision TKA is the best treatment method for an infected TKA. However, it must be planned very carefully since it has one more goal that is to eradicate the infection, and several operations may be needed in order to achieve this goal.

Contraindications for revision TKA are persistent infections and when the patient cannot undergo several operations due to the general condition. If the extensor mechanism has been disrupted and/or skin condition is poor, knee fusion is more recommended than revision TKA. Revision can be done in one stage or in two stages.

Revision TKA can be performed in one stage if the causative organism is sensitive to antibiotics in an acute infection, but the success rate is not as good as that of the two-stage revision. *The two-stage revision has a higher success rate, and hence, it is considered to be the principle*

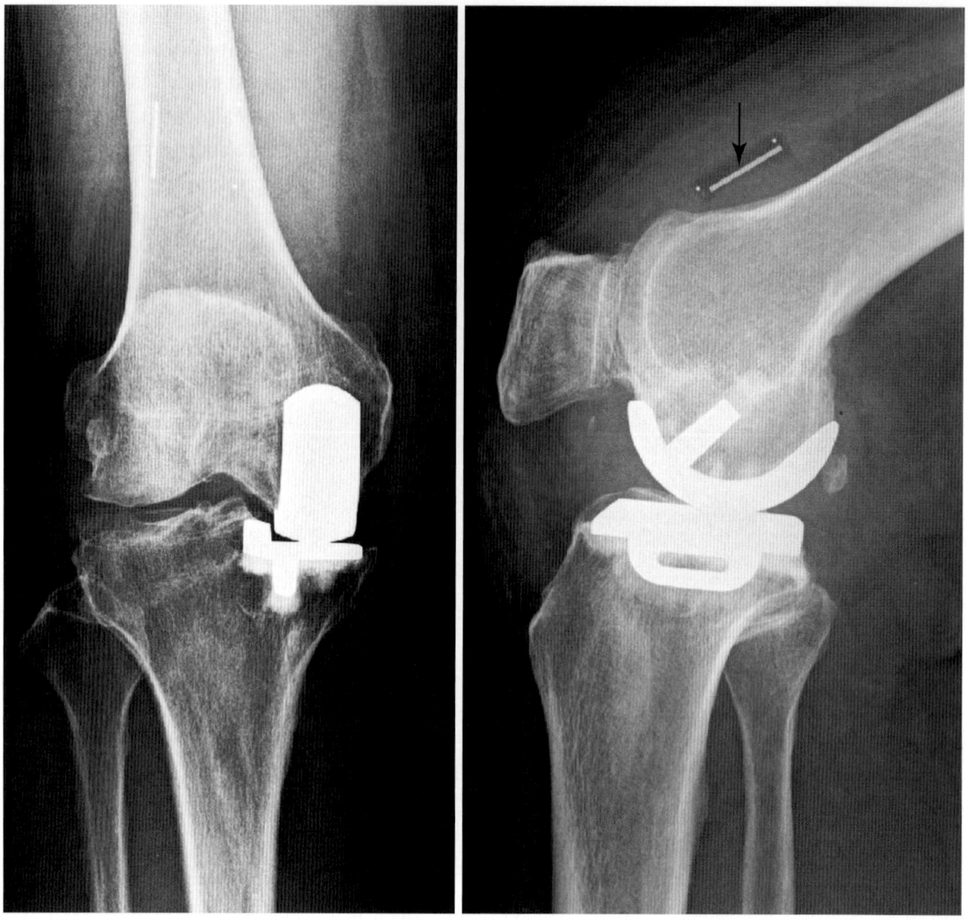

Fig. 9.12 PE dislocation in UK. Polyethylene metal marker is located in the supracondylar area (*arrow*)

method of treatment for an infected TKA. Teeny et al. reported that in 71 % of patients who had an infection for more than 2 weeks, the infection could not be eradicated with debridement and drainage, but all 9 cases who underwent the two-staged revision TKA were successful without recurrence of infection. Hofmann et al., Windsor et al., Goldman et al., and Cho et al. reported that more than 90 % of two-stage revision TKAs were successful. Hanssen and Rand compared the results through the meta-analysis and reported that 74 % of cases were successful when one-stage revision TKA using antibiotic-loaded cement was performed, 72 % of cases were successful when two-stage revision TKA was performed within 3 weeks after removal of the prosthesis and antibiotics were not used in the cement, 88 % of cases were successful when two-stage revision TKA was performed at an interval of more than 6 weeks without the use of antibiotics in the cement, and 91 % of cases were successful when two-stage operation was performed at an interval of more than 6 weeks and antibiotic-loaded cement was used.

Although, some surgeons suggest that the functional results of revision of an infected TKA are not very different from those of aseptic revision, in reality, this seems not to be true.

9.4.1 One-Stage Revision TKA

Revision TKA can be performed in one stage in case of an acute infection with antibiotic-sensitive organism in aged and in patients with restricted activity. The benefit of this method is that it reduces the duration and cost of treatment. However, *it has a critical drawback of a higher recurrence rate of infection than that of two-stage revision*.

Factors related to the success rates include an infection of not more than 4-week duration, gram-positive cocci which are sensitive to antibiotics, absence of osteomyelitis, and younger and healthier patients.

Although one-stage revision shows a higher recurrence rate of infection than that of two-stage revision, the success rate of one-stage revision can be as high as 70–80 % if patient selection is done properly and debridement is performed meticulously.

In case of the one-stage revision TKA, intravenous antibiotics should be used for at least 6 weeks. Zimmerli stated that one-stage revision can be done in patients who do not show any signs of a systemic infection, and he recommended antibiotic therapy for 2–3 weeks before performing one-stage revision if the organisms have been identified preoperatively. Whiteside et al. introduced one-stage uncemented

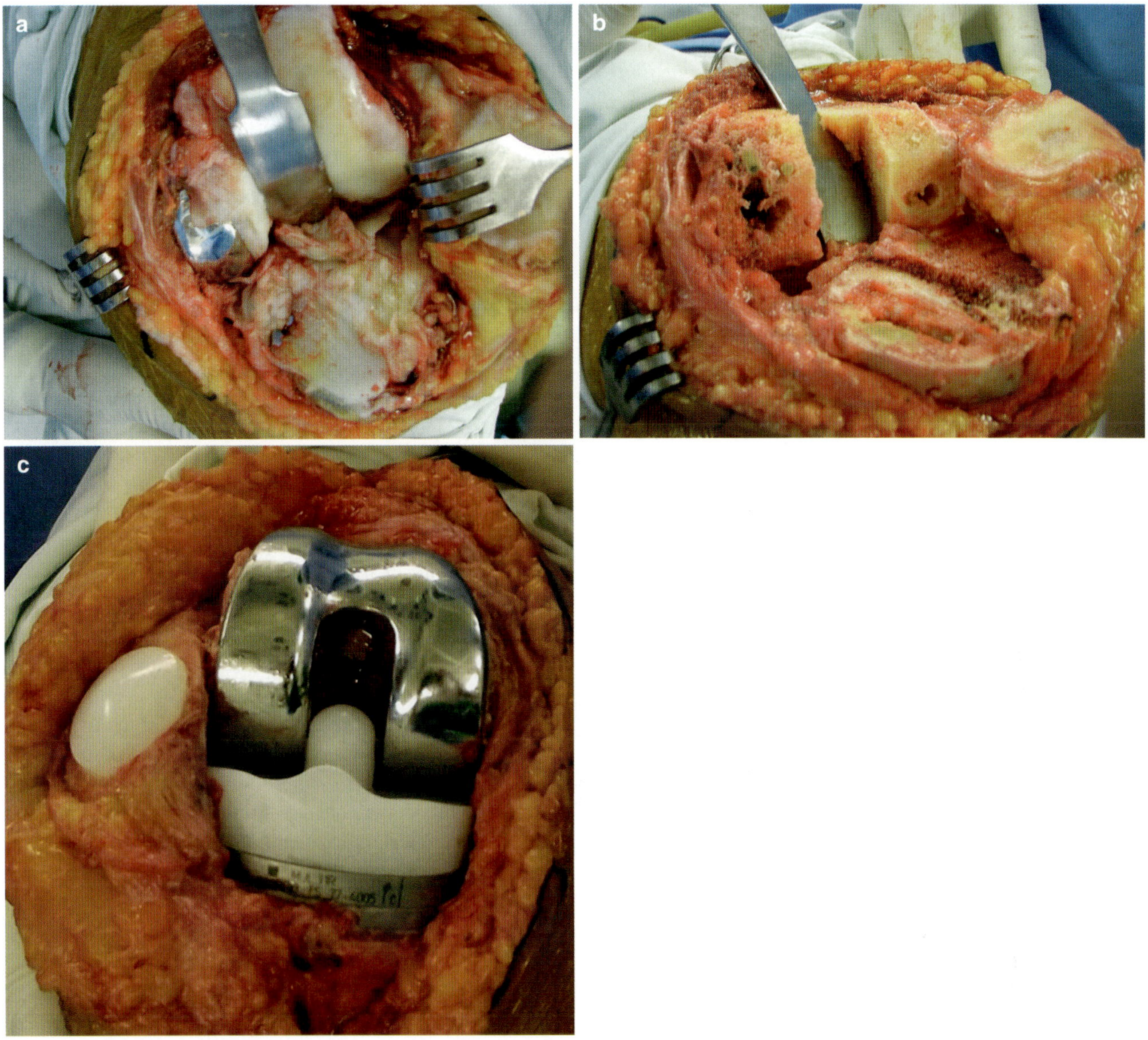

Fig. 9.13 Revision of UK. (**a**) Before removal of the implant. Degenerative changes are seen in the other parts of the joint. (**b**) After osteotomy. Only the tibial portion needs metal augmentation. (**c**) Revision TKA with metal augment on the tibial bone defect

revision and direct intra-articular infusion of vancomycin. They achieved an eradication rate of 94 % in MRSA infection. Buechel introduced another method; the operation field is soaked in povidone iodine for 30 min and the wound is closed after releasing the tourniquet while antibiotics are administered through an intravenous injection.

The surgical procedure of one-stage revision TKA is basically the same as that of aseptic revision TKA except for meticulous debridement of the infected tissues. Remaining cement should be removed and bone graft is used after immersion in antibiotic solution to reduce the recurrence of infection. When cementing is done, antibiotic-loaded cement is used and cementing on the stem is recommended in order to obliterate the dead space within the medullary canal.

9.4.2 Two-Stage Revision TKA

Since Insall et al. introduced two-stage revision in 1983, it *has been the gold standard for the treatment of infected arthroplasty.*

9.4.2.1 First Operation

In the first operation, implant removal, debridement, and insertion of antibiotic-loaded cement are done.

Skin is incised along the scar of the primary TKA. In case there is a draining sinus, the skin is removed in an elliptical shape and all scar tissues should be excised completely for easier skin suturing and for preventing reinfection. After arthrotomy, it is necessary to take the specimen from 4 to 5 sites for isolation of organisms and biopsy.

In case of long-standing or chronic infection, *the fibrosis of the soft tissues and granulation tissues often make the eversion of the patella difficult, and hence, debridement is performed on the lateral side first. If the patella cannot be everted or laterally retracted, lateral retinacular release can be performed at the beginning*. If exposure is not adequate despite of lateral retinacular release or *a limited ROM is expected due to shortening of the quadriceps tendon, rectus snip can be done primarily*. V–Y quadriceps turndown is not recommended since it causes vascular disruption and there is a marked functional loss and tibial tubercle osteotomy is neither recommended as it requires internal fixation. Removal of the prosthesis is easier when the duration of infection is longer, but removal of the prosthesis may not be easy when it is accompanied by weakening and destruction of the bone. Therefore, it is important to take special care in order to minimize the bone loss. For prosthesis removal, refer to the methods described under Sect. 9.2.2.3. Infected soft tissues as well as cement or necrotic tissues should be removed meticulously again after implant removal.

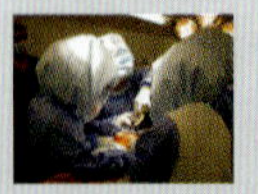

Author's Method

When performing synovectomy, I try to peel off the synovium en bloc. I do meticulous debridement around the posterior capsule, gutter, medullary canal, and lug hole. I try to remove all the fibrous tissue on the supracondylar area and lateral to the quadriceps and patella tendon. This procedure helps to retract or evert the patella easily, to reduce the skin tension during closure, and to improve postoperative ROM. After medullary cavity curettage is completed, it is packed with a gauze so as to prevent contamination. I mix 1 g cefazolin or 1 g vancomycin in 10 cc normal saline, and the skin, subcutaneous tissues, joint cavity, and the medullary canal are soaked in this solution. In this state, I proceed with debridement and curettage for about 10 min without irrigation and then irrigate the joint. This procedure is done repetitively for about 2–3 times. When debridement is not done adequately, the color of saline is opaque, and hence I repeat this procedure until the saline becomes transparent. Some surgeons have an opposite opinion about the local application of concentrated antibiotics and they state that the antibiotics have high toxicity and higher concentration is not always more effective. They state that this method may increase the resistance of organisms, cause allergic reactions, and it is not theoretically supported. However, based on my experience, I have achieved good results with a recurrence rate of infection of less than 5 %, although it is unclear whether this result is attributable to the use of this method.

In most of the cases, antibiotic-loaded cement is left in situ for 6–8 weeks before reimplantation. Antibiotic-loaded cement has been popular in infected arthroplasty since Buchholz et al. mixed gentamicin in Palacos bone cement to increase the local concentration of antibiotics. *The antibiotics mixed with cement should be heat stable and water soluble*; the most widely used antibiotics are *gentamicin, cefazolin, tobramycin, and vancomycin*.

Sensitive antibiotics should be used, but other antibiotics can also be mixed together because the organisms cannot always be clearly identified and there is a risk of mixed infections. Azzam et al. suggested mixing the bone cement with vancomycin or tobramycin to prevent mixed infections. Streptomycin can be used when arthroplasty is infected with tuberculous bacillus. Marra et al. mixed 750 mg of amphotericin B into four packs of Palacos bone cement to manage fungal infection.

Kurd et al. recommended 3–4 times even up to eight times of antibiotic concentration than ordinary amount of antibiotics. This means that up to 3.0–4.0 g of vancomycin or 3.6 g of tobramycin can be used for one 40 g pack of cement. *The rationale for using highly concentrated antibiotics is that the strength of cement is not very important as the purpose of using antibiotic-loaded cement is not to achieve fixation of the prosthesis but to act as a source of local antibiotics temporarily*. The adverse effect of highly concentrated antibiotics on the body is not very considerable. Springer et al. reported that 36 cases of infection were managed with high concentration of antibiotic-loaded cement and only one case showed temporary increase in the creatinine level with no major side effects.

The factors that affect the release of antibiotics include the type of antibiotics, amount of antibiotics, type of cement, and surface area of cement. In terms of the concentration of antibiotics, Penner et al. reported that CMW1 and CMW3 released about 30–40 % less antibiotics compared to Palacos in an in vitro study. It is known that antibiotics are released to a lesser extent when they are hand-mixed. *Antibiotic releasing times differ from 1 to 80 days according to the type of cement, concentration, and amount of antibiotics*. Goss et al. reported that antibiotics are mostly released during the first 24 h and are not released after 1 week. *Palacos is known to release*

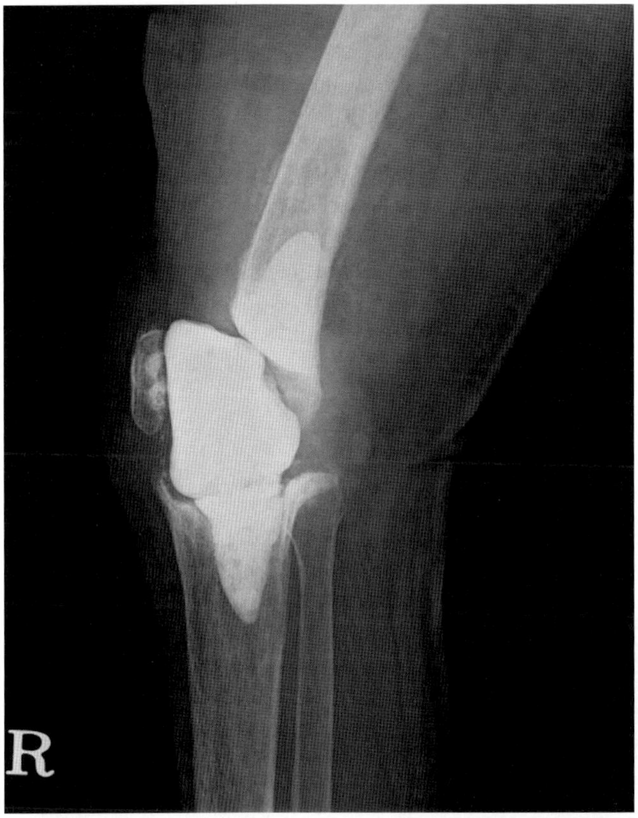

Fig. 9.14 X-rays of dislocated block type of cement

antibiotics for a longer time than the other types of cement, and hence Palacos is recommended when high concentration and longer duration of antibiotic release is required. An experiment demonstrated that the release time of antibiotics is prolonged without altering the strength of cement when bacterial cellulose is mixed with antibiotics before mixing with cement.

Antibiotic-loaded cement can be used in the form of cement beads, blocks (fixed), or articulating cement spacer. Cement beads are mostly used to fill the dead space; however, it takes time to make them during the operation and it often induces fibrosis. *In a joint cavity, blocks or articulating cement spacers are used. Whether to use blocks or articulating cement spacers depends on the amount of bone loss, condition of soft tissues, necessity of joint motion, market availability, and preference of the surgeon.*

The block type is cheap and it is easy to prepare. It consistently releases antibiotics, reduces the dead space, retains the joint gap until the subsequent operation, and allows for walking with brace fitting by *ensuring a certain level of stability*.

What needs to be taken into consideration is that *the cement block should be larger than the bone*; otherwise, it becomes unstable leading to an increased risk of dislocation while walking and causes bone loss (Fig. 9.14). Most of the times, the block is prepared during the operation, but a product of flat-molded arthrodesis block (antibiotic-loaded bone cement spacer: ALBCS) is also available.

Antibiotic-loaded *articulating cement spacer* (mobile articulating spacer or PROSTALAC (prosthesis of antibiotic-loaded acrylic cement)) can also be used. This type is thought to *have the benefit of joint motion and stability*, and about 75° of flexion can be achieved. Ha introduced a method for molding a similar shape from the prosthesis that has been removed.

When articulating cement spacer is used, it is easier to perform a revision TKA as it reduces the stiffness and the range of motion is improved more after revision than with the use of the block type.

Anderson et al. reported that a 3–115° of joint motion was achieved with the use of articulating cement spacer and the average HSS score was 91 after revision TKA. Hoffman et al. reported 4–104° of joint motion and HSS score of 89 points. Emerson et al. reported the comparative analysis which suggested that the range of motion was significantly improved to 108° with the articulating cement spacer, while it was 94° with the block type. Hsu et al., Fehring et al., Jones et al., Incavo et al., and Gooding et al. also reported that articulating cement spacer showed better clinical results than the block type.

According to Lombardi et al., *the drawbacks of articulating cement spacer are that the cement particles can cause problems when used for a long time and joint motion may delay the healing of soft tissues and may cause recurrence of infection*. Huang et al. stated that when articulating cement spacer was used, abrasion caused cement debris and this was associated with extensive scar formation. Adhesions in the suprapatellar pouch area often required an additional procedure for patellar exposure and the range of motion was not any better than that with the block type at the last follow-up. Haddad et al. emphasized that articulating cement spacer could cause instability of the patellofemoral joint and collateral ligaments, and increased the risk of dislocation. However, Johnson et al. reported that reinfection rate, Knee Society scores, and ROM were comparable between the static and dynamic spacer groups.

Considering that it takes 6–8 weeks to perform a revision surgery, some surgeons state that it is not absolutely necessary to use articulating cement spacer unless revision TKA is being performed simultaneously in both knee joints due to infection in both knee joints.

Regardless of whether the block type or articulating cement spacer is used, insertion of antibiotic-impregnated medullary dowels is strongly recommended.

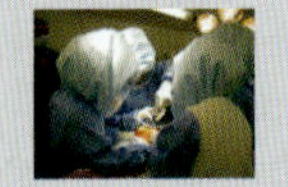

Author's Method

I make the cement block in two steps. The ratio of cement and antibiotics is 1:3. In the first step, I use one pack to fill the medullary cavity. When the cement is in the dough stage, I make intramedullary dowels for inserting into the femoral and tibial canals, and for filling into the patellar or femoral lug site. I can minimize the dead space in this manner. I do not allow the cement to get firmly attached to the bone by repeatedly mobilizing the cement dowels when the cement is setting so that it becomes easier to remove them during the 2nd stage of operation.

And then, I use two packs of cement to make a block for inserting into the gap between the femur and the tibia. I knead the cement to increase the surface area from where the antibiotics are released. As this cement is being used temporarily, its strength does not matter. At the end of the dough stage, I make the cement into a flat disk shape for easier insertion and make it as large as possible for providing the stability of the joint. When heat is generated, I perform saline irrigation for cooling so as to protect the neurovascular structures from thermal injury. When the cement has almost cured, I repetitively flex and extend the knee so that the cement is not fixed on the bones (Fig. 9.15).

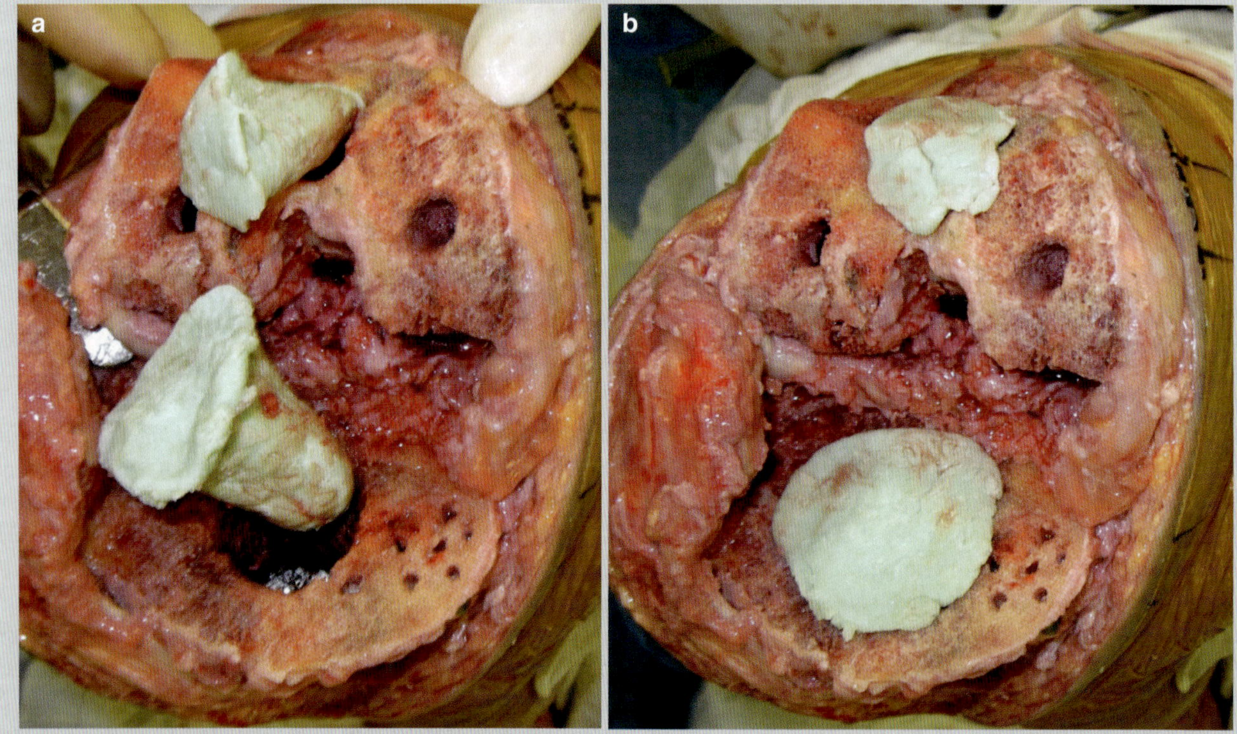

Fig. 9.15 The use of cement to decrease the dead space after removal of the prosthesis. The medullary canals of the femur and tibia are filled with the cement in the shape of a column or dowel (**a, b**). The femoro-tibial joint gap is filled with block-shaped antibiotic cement (**c**)

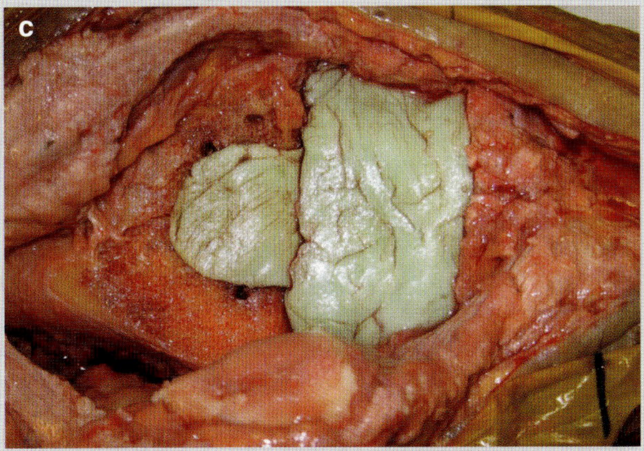

Fig. 9.15 (continued)

Antibiotics should be administered continuously through the IV route until reimplantation of prosthesis. When block type articulating cement is used, knee immobilizer is fitted for walking and weight bearing is permitted when the patient tolerates.

The timing for reimplantation is determined according to the clinical symptoms along with the ESR and CRP levels. Prosthesis can be inserted after 4 weeks of the 1st stage of the operation, but most surgeons wait until at least 6–8 weeks. Scott stated that the white blood cell count and its differential count in the joint fluid analysis are very important while making the decision of performing reimplantation of the prosthesis. When more than 10 weeks have elapsed after antibiotic cement insertion, fibrosis and foreign body reaction occur thereby making the reimplantation of the prosthesis difficult. If the clinical symptoms and laboratory results do not return to normal until this time, re-debridement or arthrodesis can be considered after a careful review.

9.4.2.2 Second Operation

Reimplantation of the prosthesis can be performed once it is confirmed that the infection has resolved based on the clinical symptoms and laboratory tests. *Generally, it is considered that the infection has resolved if the patient has no generalized fever, the incision scar has healed, there is no local warmth or erythema near the incision site, and the CRP level has returned to normal.* Insall et al. stated that the soft tissues should be in a good condition and there should be no signs of infection in the joint fluid analysis in order to perform a revision TKA, while Mont et al. emphasized the need to perform an organism culture and sensitivity test using the specimen obtained through the biopsy or joint fluid analysis before the revision TKA. They reported better results by using the following protocol: administer the antibiotics for 4–6 weeks and discontinue the antibiotics for 4–6 weeks, and this is to be followed by performing a culture. If the culture is negative, perform reimplantation of the prosthesis. If the culture is positive, readminister the antibiotics. Whiteside stated that the ESR must show a decreasing pattern and the CRP level should be within the normal range.

In the operation field, the *Mirra criteria* is most widely used to determine whether or not the infection is still persisting; *a frozen section showing the presence of more than 5 WBCs per high power field indicates the possibility that the infection still exists.* In such a case, revision TKA should be cancelled and performing re-debridement or arthrodesis should be considered.

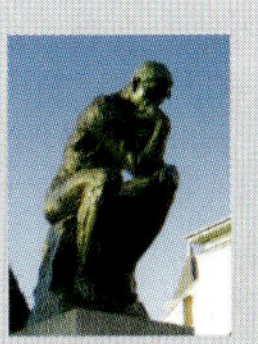

Author's Opinion

It is doubtful whether the Mirra criteria is the absolute criteria for reimplantation of the prosthesis.

In case of a type IV infection, when an infection has been detected postoperatively in the specimen obtained from revision surgery, many surgeons reported that the reinfection rate is not very high with the use of antibiotic suppression or even with no special management. I think that this type IV infection is not quite different from the situation wherein the clinical findings and CRP show no signs of infection and only the WBC count on frozen section is more than 5. I believe that the operative findings are more decisive than the Mirra criteria. Of course, if the operation field is unclean, the number of WBCs is markedly elevated.

For frozen section, I adopt a numbering system for the specimen: No 1, from the supracondylar area; No 2, from the interspace between the femur and the tibia; No 3, from the femoral intramedullary canal; No 4, from the tibial medullary canal; and No 5, from the most unclean tissues. In the area wherein the WBC count is more than 5, I perform more meticulous debridement.

I have performed revision TKA when the WBC count was more than 5 and less than 20 per high power field but the operation field was clean. The reinfection rate was below 5 %.

The procedure of revision TKA is the same as that described in "Aseptic revision." A marginal difference between the two operations is that *antibiotic-loaded cementing is strongly recommended around extension stem in septic revision cases.* While performing bone grafting, it is recommended that the bone graft is immersed in a saline solution containing antibiotics.

Bibliography

Anderson SP, Sculco PK, Heitkemper S, et al. An articulating spacer to treat and mobilize patients with infected total knee arthroplasty. J Arthroplasty. 2009;24:631–5.

Azzam K, McHale K, Austin M, Purtill JJ, Parvizi J. Outcome of a second two-stage reimplantation for periprosthetic knee infection. Clin Orthop. 2009;467:1706–14.

Bare J, MacDonald SJ, Bourne RB. Preoperative evaluations in revision total knee arthroplasty. Clin Orthop. 2006;446:40–4.

Barrack RL. Specialized surgical exposure for revision total knee arthroplasty: quadriceps snip and patellar turndown. Instr Course Lect. 1999;48:149–52.

Barrack RL. Managing the patella in revision total knee arthroplasty. In: Callaghan JJ, editor. The adult knee. 1st ed. Philadelphia, PA: Lippincott Williams & Wilkins; 2003. p. 1473–83.

Barrack RL, Ingraham R, Matzkin E, et al. Revision knee arthroplasty with patella replacement versus bony shell. Clin Orthop. 1988;356:139–43.

Barrack RL, Jennings RW, Wolfe MW, et al. The Coventry Award. The value of preoperative aspiration before total knee revision. Clin Orthop. 1997;345:8–16.

Berry DJ. Preoperative planning for revision total knee arthroplasty. In: Callaghan JJ, editor. The adult knee. 1st ed. Philadelphia, PA: Lippincott Williams & Wilkins; 2003. p. 1413–9.

Berry DJ, Rand JA. Isolated patellar component revision of total knee arthroplasty. Clin Orthop. 1993;286:110–5.

Bertin KC, Freeman MAR, Samuelson KM. Stemmed revision arthroplasty for aseptic loosening of total knee replacement. J Bone Joint Surg Br. 1985;67-B:242–8.

Bozic KJ, Kurtz SM, Lau E, et al. The epidemiology of revision total knee arthroplasty in the United States. Clin Orthop. 2010;468:45–51.

Brassard MF, Insall JN, Scuderi GR. Revision of aseptic failed total knee arthroplasty. In: Scott WN, editor. Surgery of the knee. 4th ed. Philadelphia, PA: Churchill Livingstone; 2006. p. 1761–81.

Buchholz GW, Elson RA, Heinert K. Antibiotic-loaded acrylic cement: current concepts. Clin Orthop. 1984;190:96–108.

Buechel FF. Primary exchange revision arthroplasty using antibiotic-impregnated cement for infected total knee replacement. Orthop Rev. 1990;19:83–8.

Burke WV, Ammeen DJ, Engh GA. Isolated revision of failed metal-backed patellar components: outcome with minimum 4-year follow-up. J Arthroplasty. 2005;20:998–1001.

Cadambi A, Jones RE, Maale GE. A protocol for staged revision of infected total hip and knee arthroplasties: the use of antibiotic-cement-implant composites. Int Orthop. 1995;3:133–45.

Calton TF, Fehring TK, Griffin WL. Bone loss associated with the use of spacer blocks in infected total knee arthroplasty. Clin Orthop. 1997;345:148–54.

Cho WS, Jeong YG, Park JH, et al. Treatment of infected total knee arthroplasty. J Korean Orthop Assoc. 2001;36:561–7.

Conditt MA, Parsley BS, Alexander JW, et al. The optimal strategy for stable tibial fixation in revision total knee arthroplasty. J Arthroplasty. 2004;19 Suppl 2:113–8.

Dalury DF, Adams MJ. Minimum 6-year follow-up of revision total knee arthroplasty without Patella reimplantation. J Arthroplasty. 2012;27 Suppl 8:91–4.

Della Valle CJ, Bogner E, Desai P, et al. Analysis of frozen sections of intraoperative specimens obtained at the time of reoperation after hip or knee resection arthroplasty for the treatment of infection. J Bone Joint Surg Am. 1999;81-A:684–9.

Dennis DA. Revision knee arthroplasty: How I do it. In: Insall JN, Scott WN, editors. Surgery of the knee. 3rd ed. New York, NY: Churchill Livingstone; 2001. p. 1934–41.

Dorr LD. Revision knee arthroplasty. How I do it. In: Insall JN, Scott WN, editors. Surgery of the knee. 3rd ed. New York, NY: Churchill Livingstone; 2001. p. 1925–33.

Duff G, Lachiewicz PF, Kelley S. Aspiration of the knee joint before revision arthroplasty. Clin Orthop. 1996;331:132–9.

Emerson Jr RH, Muncie M, Tarbox TR, et al. Comparison of a static with a mobile spacer in Total knee infection. Clin Orthop. 2002;404:130–8.

Engh GA, Herzwurm PJ, Parks NL. Treatment of major defects of bone with bulk allografts and stemmed components during total knee arthroplasty. J Bone Joint Surg Am. 1997;79-A:1030–9.

Engh Jr CA, Parks NL, Engh GA. Polyethylene quality affects revision knee liner exchange survivorship. Clin Orthop. 2012;470:193–8.

Fehring TK, Griffin WL. Revision of failed cementless total knee implants with cement. Clin Orthop. 1998;356:34–8.

Fehring TK, Odum S, Olekson C, et al. Stem fixation in revision total knee arthroplasty. A comparative analysis. Clin Orthop. 2003;416: 217–24.

Friedman RJ, Hirst P, Pose R, et al. Results of revision total knee arthroplasty performed for aseptic loosening. Clin Orthop. 1990;255:235–41.

Gallagher J, Rorabeck C, Bourne R. Patella resurfacing in total knee arthroplasty. In: Scott WN, editor. Surgery of the knee. 4th ed. Philadelphia, PA: Churchill Livingstone; 2006. p. 1574–91.

Ghanem E, Ketonis C, Restrepo C, et al. Periprosthetic infection: where do we stand with regard to gram stain? Acta Orthop. 2009;80:37–40.

Gioe TJ, Killeen KK, Grimm K, et al. Why are total knee replacements revised? : analysis of early revision in a community knee implant registry. Clin Orthop. 2004;428:100–6.

Goldman RT, Scuderi GR, Insall JN. Two-stage reimplantation for infected total knee replacement. Clin Orthop. 1996;331:118–24.

Gooding CR, Masri BA, Duncan CP, et al. Durable infection control and function with the PROSTALAC spacer in two-stage revision for infected knee arthroplasty. Clin Orthop. 2011;469:985–93.

Goss B, Lutton C, Weinrauch P, et al. Elution and mechanical properties of antifungal bone cement. J Arthroplasty. 2007;22:902–8.

Gustke KA. Preoperative planning for revision total knee arthroplasty: avoiding chaos. J Arthroplasty. 2005;20 Suppl 2:37–40.

Ha CW. A technique for intraoperative construction of antibiotic spacers. Clin Orthop. 2006;445:204–9.

Haas BD, Dennis DA. Implant selection in revision total knee arthroplasty. In: Callaghan JJ, editor. The adult knee. 1st ed. Philadelphia, PA: Lippincott Williams & Wilkins; 2003. p. 1447–53.

Haddad FS, Masri BA, Campbell D, et al. The PROSTALAC functional spacer in two-stage revision for infected knee replacement. Prosthesis of antibiotic-loaded acrylic cement. J Bone Joint Surg Br. 2000;82-B:807–12.

Hanssen AD. Reimplantation for infection after total knee arthroplasty. In: Callaghan JJ, editor. The adult knee. 1st ed. Philadelphia, PA: Lippincott Williams & Wilkins; 2003. p. 1509–17.

Hanssen AD, Rand JA. Evaluation and treatment of infection at the site of a total hip or knee arthroplasty. J Bone Joint Surg Am. 1998;80-A:910–22.

Harwin SF. Revision arthroplasty. How I do it. In: Insall JN, Scott WN, editors. Surgery of the knee. 3rd ed. New York, NY: Churchill Livingstone; 2001. p. 1967–74.

Hofmann AA, Kane KR, Tkach TK, et al. Treatment of infected total knee arthroplasty using an articulating spacer. Clin Orthop. 1995;321:45–54.

Huang HT, Su JY, Chen SK. The results of articulating spacer technique for infected total knee arthroplasty. J Arthroplasty. 2006;21: 1163–8.

Incavo SJ, Wild JJ, Coughlin KM, et al. Early revision for component malrotation in total knee arthroplasty. Clin Orthop. 2007;458: 131–6.

Insall JN, Thompson FM, Brause BD. Two-stage reimplantation for the salvage of infected total knee arthroplasty. J Bone Joint Surg Am. 1983;65-A:1087–98.

Johnson AJ, Sayeed SA, Naziri Q, et al. Minimizing dynamic knee spacer complications in infected revision arthroplasty. Clin Orthop. 2012;470:220–7.

Ko PS, Ip D, Chow KP, et al. The role of intraoperative frozen section in decision making in revision hip and knee arthroplasties in a local community hospital. J Arthroplasty. 2005;20:189–95.

Koh JS, Yeo SJ, Lo NN, et al. Isolated patellar revisions for failed metal-backed components: 2- to 9-year follow-up. J Arthroplasty. 2004;19:880–6.

Kurd MF, Ghanem E, Steinbrecher J, et al. Two- stage exchange knee arthroplasty: does resistance of the infecting organism influence the outcome? Clin Orthop. 2010;468:2060–6.

Laskin RS. Management of the patella during revision total knee replacement arthroplasty. Orthop Clin North Am. 1998;29: 355–60.

Lombardi Jr AV, Berend KR, Adams JB, et al. Articulating antibiotic spacers: the standard of care for an infected total knee arthroplasty. Orthopedics. 2007;30:782. 786–7.

Lonner JH, Mont MA, Sharkey PF, et al. Fate of unrevised all-polyethylene patellar component in revision total knee arthroplasty. J Bone Joint Surg Am. 2012;85-A:56–9.

Marra F, Robbins GM, Masri BA, et al. Amphotericin-B loaded bone cement to treat osteomyelitis caused by Candida albicans. Can J Surg. 2001;44:383–6.

Mihalko WM, Krackow KA. Flexion and extension gap balancing in revision total knee arthroplasty. Clin Orthop. 2006;446:121–6.

Mirra JH, Marder RA, Amstutz HC. The pathology of failed total joint arthroplasty. Clin Orthop. 1982;170:175–83.

Mont MA, Waldman BJ, Hungerford DS. Evaluation of preoperative cultures before second-stage reimplantation of a total knee prosthesis complicated by infection. A comparison-group study. J Bone Joint Surg Am. 2000;82-A:1552–7.

Mori R, Nakai T, Enomoto K, et al. Increased antibiotic release from a bone cement containing bacterial cellulose. Clin Orthop. 2011;469:600–6.

Nett MP, Scuderi GR. Revision of aseptic failed total knee arthroplasty. In: Scott WN, editor. Surgery of the knee. 5th ed. Philadelphia, PA: Churchill Livingstone; 2011. p. 1327–45.

Parsley B, Sugano N, Bertolusso R, et al. Mechanical alignment of tibial stems in revision total knee arthroplasty. J Arthroplasty. 2003;18 Suppl 1:33–6.

Penner MJ, Duncan CP, Masri BA. The in vitro elution characteristics of antibiotic-loaded CMW and Palacos-R bone cements. J Arthroplasty. 1999;14:209–14.

Peters CL, Erickson J, Kloepper RG, et al. Revision total knee arthroplasty with modular components inserted with metaphyseal cement and stems without cement. J Arthroplasty. 2005;20:302–8.

Peters CL, Erickson JA, Gililland JM. Clinical and radiographic results of 184 consecutive revision total knee arthroplasties placed with modular cementless stems. J Arthroplasty. 2009;24:48–53.

Ranawat CS, Flynn Jr WF. Principles of planning and prosthetic selection for revision total knee replacement. In: Scott WN, editor. The knee. 1st ed. St. Louis, MO: Mosby; 1994. p. 1297–303.

Rand JA, Bryan RS. Reimplantation for salvage of an infected total knee arthroplasty. J Bone Joint Surg Am. 1983;65-A:1081–6.

Ries MD, Haas SB, Windsor RE. Soft-tissue balance in revision total knee arthroplasty. Surgical technique. J Bone Joint Surg Am. 2004;86-A Suppl 1:81–6.

Ritter MA, Eizemler LE, Fechtman RW, et al. Revision total knee arthroplasty: a survival analysis. J Arthroplasty. 1991;6:351–6.

Rorabeck CH, Taylor J. Revision knee arthroplasty. How I do it. In: Insall JN, Scott MN, editors. Surgery of the knee. 3rd ed. New York, NY: Churchill Livingstone; 2001. p. 1949–57.

Sah AP, Shukla S, Della Valle CJ, et al. Modified hybrid stem fixation in revision TKA is durable at 2 to 10 years. Clin Orthop. 2011;469:839–46.

Sanchez F. Revision knee arthroplasty. How I do it. In: Insall JN, Scott WN, editors. Surgery of the knee. 3rd ed. New York, NY: Churchill Livingstone; 2001. p. 1942–8.

Scott G, Freeman MAR. Single-stage revision of infected total knee replacement. In: Scuderi GR, editor. Surgical techniques in total knee arthroplasty. 1st ed. New York, NY: Springer; 2002. p. 465–70.

Scott RD. Reoperation after total knee arthroplasty. In: Scott RD, editor. Total knee arthroplasty. 1st ed. Philadelphia, PA: Saunders; 2006. p. 117–22.

Scuderi GR, Clarke HD. Two-stage reimplantation. In: Scuderi GR, editor. Surgical techniques in total knee arthroplasty. 1st ed. New York, NY: Springer; 2002. p. 471–2.

Seel MJ, Hanssen AD, Berry DJ, et al. Patellar component resection arthroplasty for the severely compromised patella during revision total knee arthroplasty. Orthop Trans. 1995;19:338–9.

Severson EP, Hanssen AD. The infected total knee arthroplasty. In: Scott WN, editor. Surgery of the knee. 5th ed. Philadelphia, PA: Churchill Livingstone; 2011. p. 1346–58.

Sheng PY, Konttinen L, Lehto M, et al. Revision total knee arthroplasty: 1990 through 2002.A review of the Finnish arthroplasty registry. J Bone Joint Surg Am. 2006;88-A:1425–30.

Singh JA, O'Byrne MM, Harmsen WS, et al. Predictors of moderate-severe functional limitation 2 and 5 years after revision total knee arthroplasty. J Arthroplasty. 2010;25:1091–5.

Smith PN, Rorabeck CH. Component removal. In: Scuderi GR, editor. Surgical techniques in total knee arthroplasty. 1st ed. New York, NY: Springer; 2002. p. 377–89.

Springer BD, Lee GC, Osmon D, et al. Systemic safety of high-dose antibiotic-loaded cement spacers after resection of an infected total knee arthroplasty. Clin Orthop. 2004;427:47–51.

St John TA, Hozack WJ, Sharkey PF. Implant removal in revision total knee arthroplasty. In: Callaghan JJ, editor. The adult knee. 1st ed. Philadelphia, PA: Lippincott Williams & Wilkins; 2003. p. 1431–6.

Suarez J, Griffin W, Springer B, et al. Why do revision knee arthroplasties fail? J Arthroplasty. 2008;23:99–103.

Teeny SM, Dorr L, Murata G, et al. Treatment of infected total knee arthroplasty. Irrigation and debridement versus two-stage reimplantation. J Arthroplasty. 1990;5:35–9.

Vail TP, Lang JE. Surgical techniques and instrumentation in total knee replacement arthroplasty. In: Scott WN, editor. Surgery of the knee. 4th ed. Philadelphia, PA: Churchill Livingstone; 2006. p. 1455–521.

Vince KG. Revision knee arthroplasty. How I do it. In: Insall JN, Scott WN, editors. Surgery of the knee. 3rd ed. New York, NY: Churchill Livingstone; 2001. p. 1958–66.

Vince KG, Blackburn DC, Ortaaslan SG, et al. "Gull wing" osteotomy of the patella in total knee arthroplasty. J Arthroplasty. 2000;15: 254–9.

Vince KG, Long W. Revision knee arthroplasty. The limits of press fit medullary fixation. Clin Orthop. 1995;317:172–7.

Whiteside LA. Treatment of infected total knee arthroplasty. Clin Orthop. 1994;299:169–72.

Whiteside LA, Peppers M, Nayfeh TA, et al. Methicillin-resistant Staphylococcus aureus in TKA treated with revision and direct intra-articular antibiotic infusion. Clin Orthop. 2011;469:26–33.

Willson SE, Munro ML, Sandwell JC, et al. Isolated tibial polyethylene insert exchange outcomes after total knee arthroplasty. Clin Orthop. 2010;468:96–101.

Windsor RE, Insall JN, Urs WK, et al. Two-stage reimplantation for the salvage of total knee arthroplasty Complicated by infection: further follow-up and refinement of indications. J Bone Joint Surg Am. 1990;72-A:272–8.

Zimmerli W. Prosthetic joint infection: Diagnosis and treatment. Curr Infect Dis Rep. 2000;2:377–9.

10 Optional Techniques

10.1 Introduction

The development of surgical tools and technology has extended its territory to newer surgical fields. Good examples include computer assisted surgery and arthroscopic surgery.

The introduction of computers in arthroplasty has improved the accuracy of the operation and the use of robots has made it possible to reach the lesions where human hands cannot reach. Also, attempts have been made to reduce morbidity and to allow early mobilization by minimizing the length of the incision. Minimal incision and computer assisted surgeries have become the optional techniques of arthroplasty.

In this chapter, I would like to describe Computer Assisted Orthopedic Surgery (CAOS) and Minimally Invasive Surgery (MIS).

10.2 Computer Assisted Orthopedic Surgery

10.2.1 Overview

The prognosis of arthroplasty is affected by the patient-related factors, implant-related factors, surgical techniques and postoperative management. Among all these factors, the most important factor is the surgical techniques.

The surgical procedures that affect the prognosis include the approach, osteotomy, ligament balancing and fixation. In terms of alignment, the failure rate significantly increases if there is more than 3–4° varus or valgus malalignment and the ROM decreases by 20° even if there is just 2.5 mm of difference in the A–P position of the femoral component. Teter et al. reported that 8 % of cases showed malalignment of more than 4° when an extramedullary guide was used for the tibial osteotomy. However, this is based only on the two dimensional X-rays and a higher incidence of malalignment may be noted in the three dimensional plane. Such an error is detected in about 10 % of cases performed even by the experienced surgeons, since the performance of an operation largely depends on the judgment of the eye and experience of the surgeon. *Computer assisted surgical techniques were developed in order to minimize the errors that can develop with the conventional techniques*. Of course, even with the use of computers, surgical errors can occur during the placement of cutting blocks, the actual performance of osteotomy or fixation of prosthesis, etc. Although the occurrence of errors varies according to the type of computer system, computer assisted surgery aims to achieve malalignment of less than 1° and malpositioning of less than 1 mm through the use of a navigation system for osteotomy and balancing.

Currently, it is believed that alignment in the coronal plane is accurate when the navigation system is used. In the sagittal plane, however it is difficult to assess the accuracy as there is still no definite theory regarding the sagittal axis. CAOS tends to cause slight hyperextension compared to that with the conventional technique because the center of motion does not coincide with the center of mechanical axis in sagittal plane. There are still problems to be solved with respect to the rotational alignment. *Currently, computer assisted surgical techniques are used not only for osteotomy but also for soft tissue balancing using a tensioner or distractor.*

The benefit of computer assisted surgery in the artificial joint is that *it is accurate and highly reproducible*. As the medullary guide is not needed, *bleeding and the risk of embolism are reduced* and there is an improvement in the documentation that *helps in the research*.

The drawbacks of this technique are that a longer operation time is required and it is expensive. Computer assisted systems *can also give rise to errors. The causes of errors include registration errors (error in, error out), and problems not related to the computer system but related to the surgical techniques*, e.g., change of position of the cutting block during drilling, incorrect use of ligament alignment jig, incorrect osteotomy due to a wide slot or flexible cutting blade, or improper cementing for fixation, etc. Also, *a learning curve* is involved for using this technique, and the *surgeons who have a poor understanding with the conventional techniques are likely to make errors*.

W. Cho, *Knee Joint Arthroplasty*,
DOI 10.1007/978-3-642-39389-1_10, © Springer-Verlag Berlin Heidelberg 2014

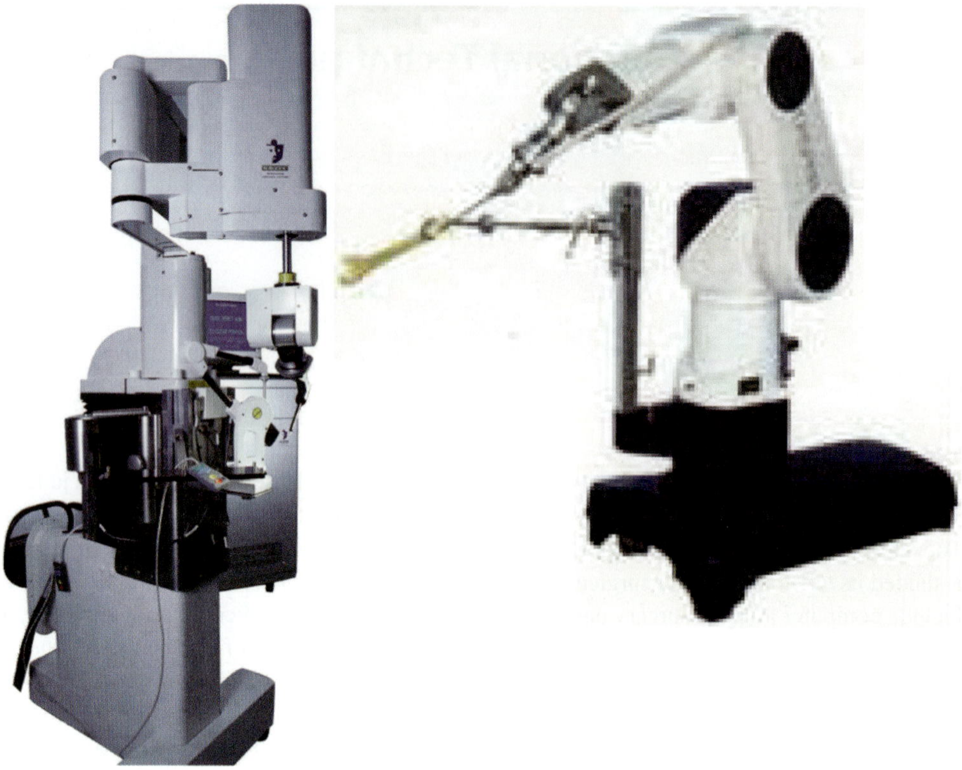

Fig. 10.1 ROBODOC (Integraged surgical systems, Davis, CA) and CASPAR systems (U.R.S.-ortho GmbH & Co. KG, Rastatt, Germany)

10.2.2 History

Computer assisted surgery was first used in a neurosurgical operation for the brain and spine in the 1980s for determining the accurate location at which the operation was to be performed.

In orthopedic surgery, it was first used by Kaiura in 1986 to determine the center of the femoral head with the robot by applying the kinematic registration technique through the preoperative CT scan. In the 1990s, it was introduced in TKA after accurate pointing of the important landmarks was possible. Soon afterwards, fluoroscopy was used to obtain images during the operation until Saragaglia et al. developed a navigation system using the OrthoPilot for imageless surgery in 1997.

10.2.3 Type

There are various types of computer assisted surgery systems produced by different manufacturers, but Picard classified them according to the performance and the method used to obtain the image. *In terms of performance, there are active, semi-active, and passive types* of computer assisted surgery systems, *and in terms of the method used to obtain the images, there are image-free, preoperative image-based, and intraoperative image-based types*. When all these systems are taken into account in combination, theoretically there can be nine types (3 × 3), but not all these combinations do actually exist.

10.2.3.1 Classification According to the Performance

Active System

Active type uses computer systems in all or part of the preparation and operative procedure and the robot system is included in this type. In the robot system, the robot performs the surgery instead of the surgeon and the accuracy is very high. It was used limitedly in the early stage of computer assisted surgery, but it has been transformed into the modern robot assisted surgery since the development of the navigation system.

The robot can perform osteotomy and soft tissue release without any injury to the ligaments, nerves or vessels. Robot systems include the Robodoc and Caspar systems, and these systems perform concise, clear, accurate and effective three-dimensional operations (Fig. 10.1). Also, some of the surgical procedures such as intramedullary drilling can be avoided just like in the navigation surgery. It helps in cementless prosthesis due to an accurate osteotomy as it mills the surface without sawing.

Robot assisted surgery comprises of the pin type or the pinless type and preoperative CT is required for both types. In the pin type, a stab wound is made under local anesthesia before the operation and a self-tapping screw is fixed onto the pelvic bone, femur and tibia. These screws act as indicators of spatial orientation of the patient's real bone for three dimensional verification. In the more recently developed pinless type, the process of inserting the pins before surgery is bypassed. Patient information based on the CT images including the position of the joint, size of the tibia and femur, and degree of deformity is stored in the computer, which enables to perform cyber surgery and to plan the operation. During the operation, the robot and the knee should be securely fixed to prevent micro-motion. The actual shape of the patient's joint and bone is matched *with the information already stored in the computer using a probe attached to the robotic system. This process of registration and verification is the most important step in robotic surgery*. Once the registration is completed, the robot mills the bone finely and accurately with an error of less than 0.25 mm as planned during the preoperative cyber surgery, and then the pre-selected prosthesis is inserted to complete the operation (Fig. 10.2).

However, the robot system requires preoperative imaging and registration, it is bulky, it may hinder the normal operation process, and it is too time-consuming and expensive. A learning curve is also needed for using the robot system.

Saragaglia et al. reported that accuracy with less than 3° outliers can be achieved in 75 % of patients when the computer was not used, in 84 % of patients when the computer was used and in more than 95 % of patients when the robot system was used. Park and Lee reported the comparison between the robot system and the conventional method, which suggested that the robot system was clearly useful in terms of preoperative planning, accuracy and postoperative alignment, but the incidence of complications such as fracture or peroneal nerve palsy was higher in the early period of this technique.

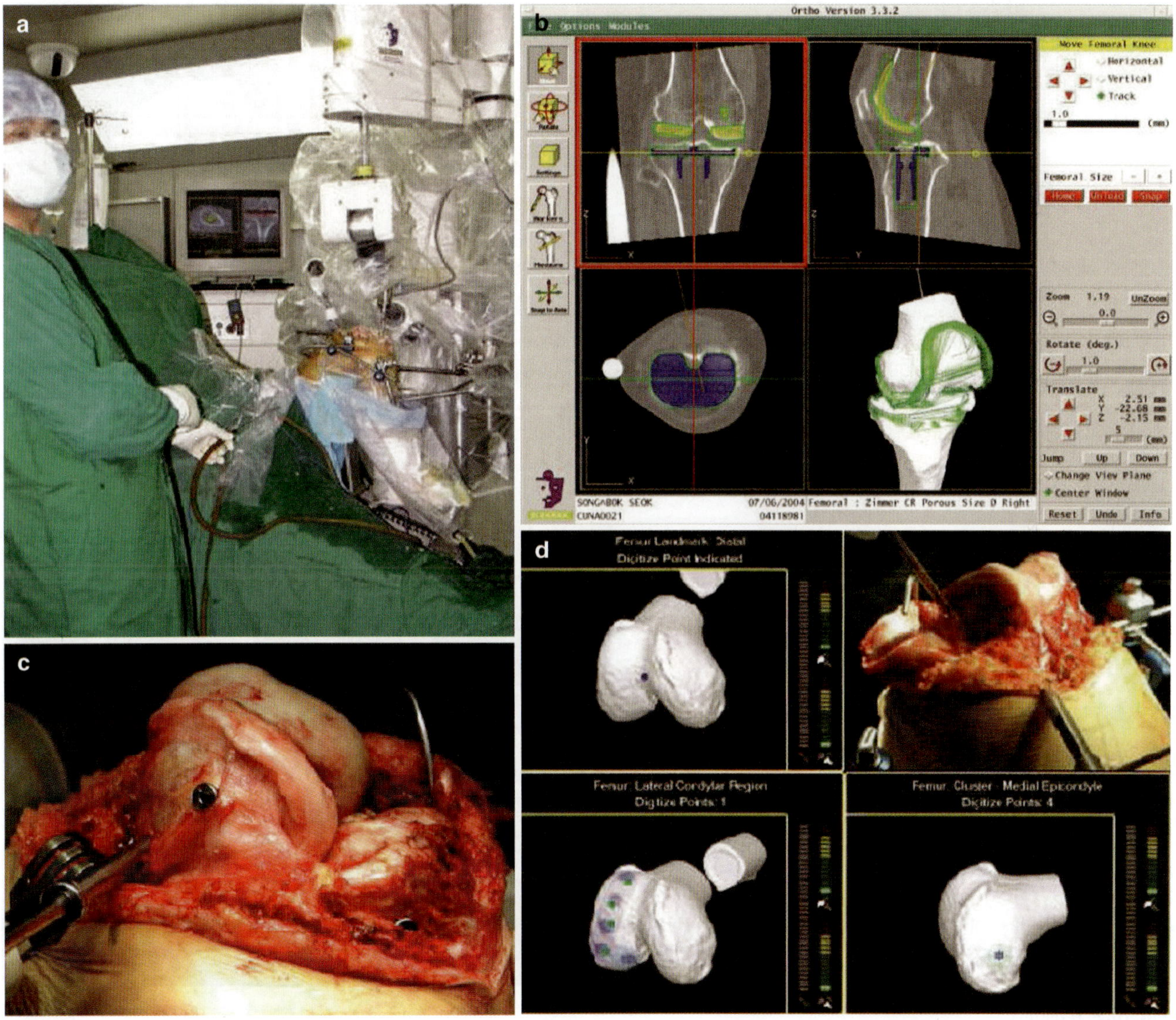

Fig. 10.2 Operative procedures of pinless Robodoc system. (**a**) Robodoc system, (**b**) planning through the preoperative cyber surgery, (**c**) exposing the joint and inserting the screw into the femur, (**d**) registration process, (**e**) verification process, (**f**) immediately before milling the bone, (**g**) milling process, (**h**) after milling the bone, (**i**) after inserting the prosthesis

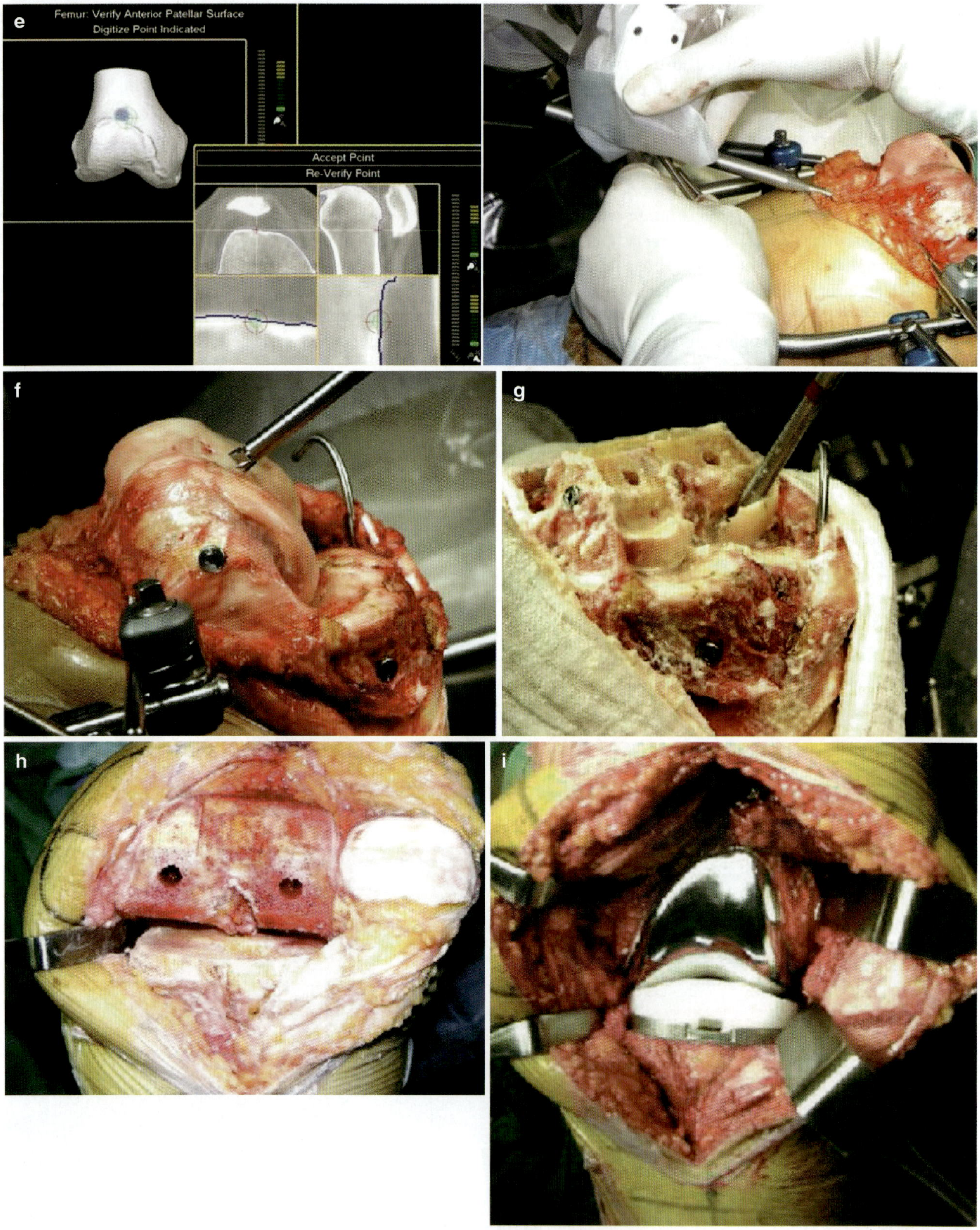

Fig. 10.2 (continued)

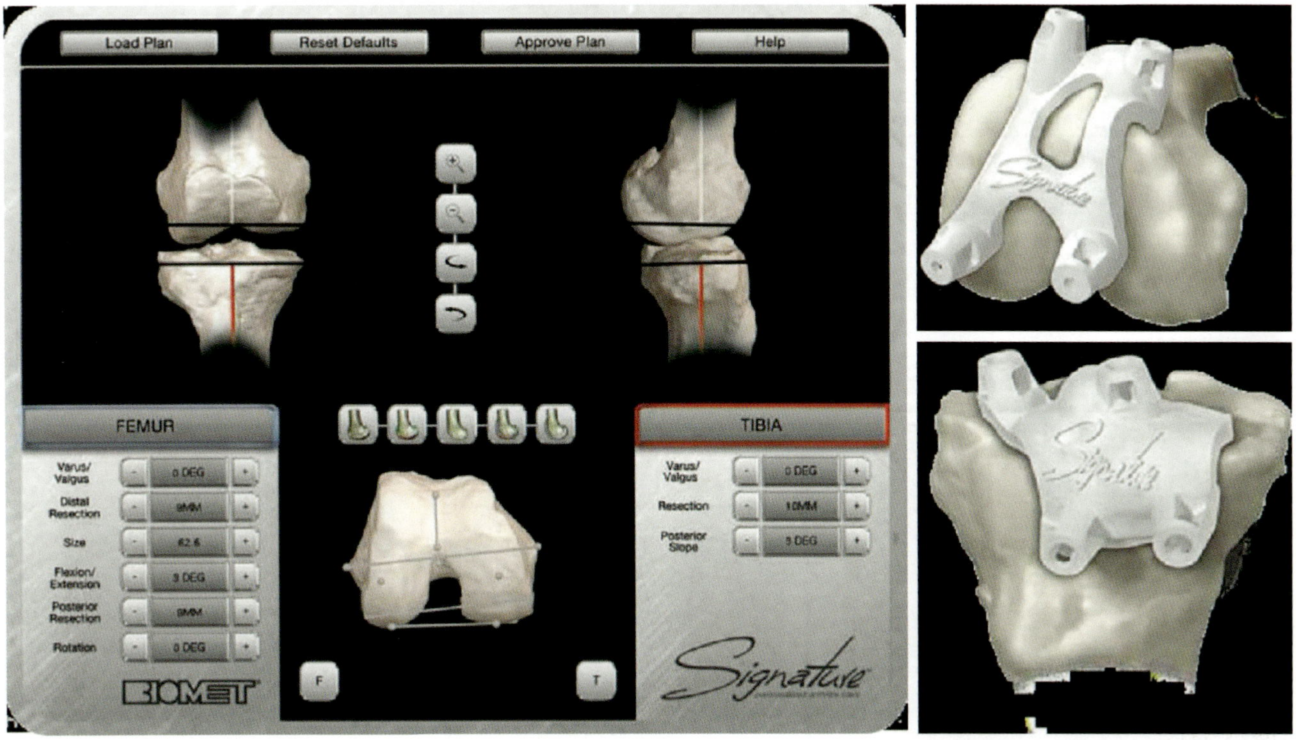

Fig. 10.3 Patient-specific templating system (Biomet, Warsaw IN)

Semi-active System

Surgery is performed by both the surgeon and the robot; the robot guides the surgeon and controls the surgeon when osteotomy exceeds the normal range, or the surgeon can move the robot's arms. The Acrobot can be classified into the active system or the semi-active system and it also requires preoperative imaging and registration during surgery.

Passive System

Surgery is performed solely by the surgeon. The passive system includes the *navigation system and the patient specific instrument (PSI) or the patient-specific templating system. The navigation system is used to guide the operation and it is more recommended by the US FDA*.

In arthroplasty, *navigation* refers to registering the patient information in the computer in order to guide the performance of an accurate operation. *Kinematic registration by joint motion detects the center of the joint and a probe is used for surface registration of the size and shape of the bone*. This process simulates the real shape of the patient's bone based on the registered information in order to secure *accurate positioning of surgical instruments for osteotomy*.

The patient-specific templating system, which is still in its toddler stage, uses preoperative CT or MRI. MRI has the theoretical advantages of detecting the cartilage and of being a radiation free imaging modality. However, MRI images have more segmentation difficulties than CT images, which may be the cause of malpositioning of the template. There are two methods of patient-specific templating system: one is the pin placement technique and the other is the cutting guide technique. *In the pin placement technique, a preoperative CT or MRI is used to create the positioning guide in order to locate the position of the pin for osteotomy and the same conventional cutting jig is used (Fig. 10.3). In the cutting guide technique, the surgeon uses the custom made guides to perform the osteotomy without using the conventional cutting guide*. There are two aligning method in PSI system: one is kinematic alignment and the other is mechanical alignment method. Mechanical alignment method needs detecting the center of hip, knee and ankle joint on CT or MRI to restore mechanical alignment. The MRI or CT of the joint is needed and release of collateral ligaments and retinacular ligament are not performed in kinematic alignment system. The concept of kinematic alignment, is quite different from that of conventional mechanical alignment. The purpose of kinematic alignment is to restore pre-arthritic state to improve clinical result. In case of mechanical alignment method, just similar to conventional instrument method, Nunley et al. experienced more varus outliers than the kinematic alignment method. During the operation, osteophytes should not be removed because they may be used as a reference for positioning the cutting guides. The femoral guides are usually used first to make more space for the tibial cutting guide. So, aligning the joint along the mechanical axis is just a reference. This is described in details under Sect. 4.4.

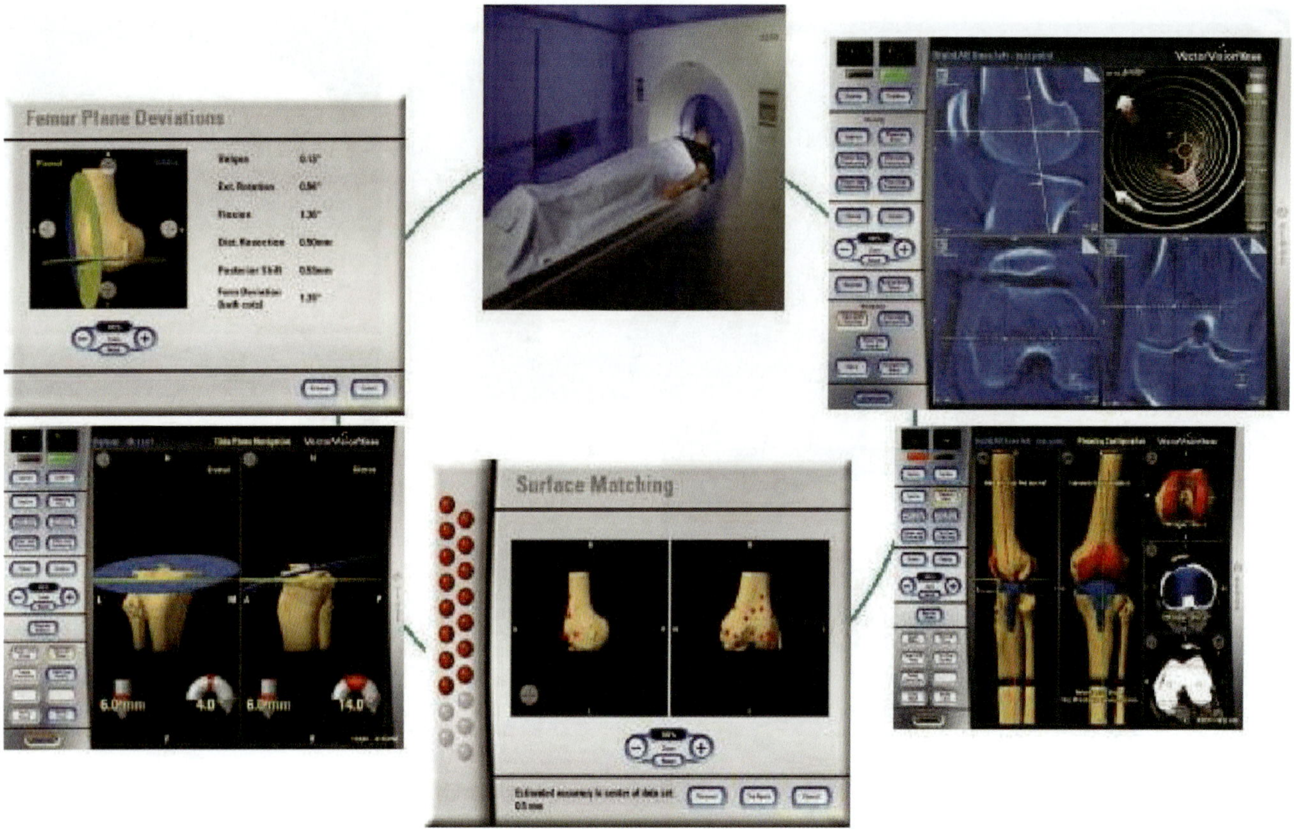

Fig. 10.4 Preoperative acquisition of skeletal information for image-based navigation system (Brainlab, Feldkirchen, Germany)

The advantage of the patient-specific templating system is that the technique is relatively easier to use, less invasive, time saving and accurate. The drawback of this system is that a longer time is required to create the positioning guide, it does not usually provide the intraoperative measurements, lack of information for soft tissue balancing, more chances of poor positioning of the guides due to an MRI alignment error, *and the surgeon should abandon the system in case the operation goes wrong*. While the navigation system is universally used for all patients, the patient-specific templating system is based on the skeletal information of each patient.

10.2.3.2 Classification According to the Method of Obtaining Images

Image-Based System (CT Scan or Fluoroscopy)

Image-based navigation system is used for osteotomy based on the information acquired from CT scan or fluoroscopy. In this system, either the information from the preoperative CT scan is registered or fluoroscopy is used during the operation to acquire the information (Fig. 10.4).

During the registration, the information acquired from the CT scan or fluoroscopy is stored in the computer system, and the kinematic information of the joint motion and bony information are matched with the input data (kinematic registration) (Fig. 10.5).

Kinematic registration is followed by surface registration which is obtained from the probe during the operation, and these are used to determine the position and direction of the cutting guide in real time for an accurate osteotomy. Therefore, *registration is the most important step* and the software is also as important as the hardware. If the registration is incorrect, the operation becomes inaccurate. The causes of incorrect registration are the presence of borderline blurs and when segmentation of images occurs. The operation also tends to be inaccurate when the soft tissues impinge between the probe and the bone, when the probe points to a different site because the bone is not perfectly spherical, the cortical screw that fixes the rigid body moves and the computer hardware and software are inaccurate.

The method of using fluoroscopy is the automatic registration system through fluoroscopy during the operation. This method is not convenient to perform the TKA as it requires the use of fluoroscopy. It is more helpful to insert pins in fracture surgery than in arthroplasty.

Image-Free System

Image-based system helps in the preoperative planning and postoperative evaluation, but it has been replaced by the image-free system because the image-based system is more time-consuming and it requires more effort since the acquisition of images before or during the operation is required.

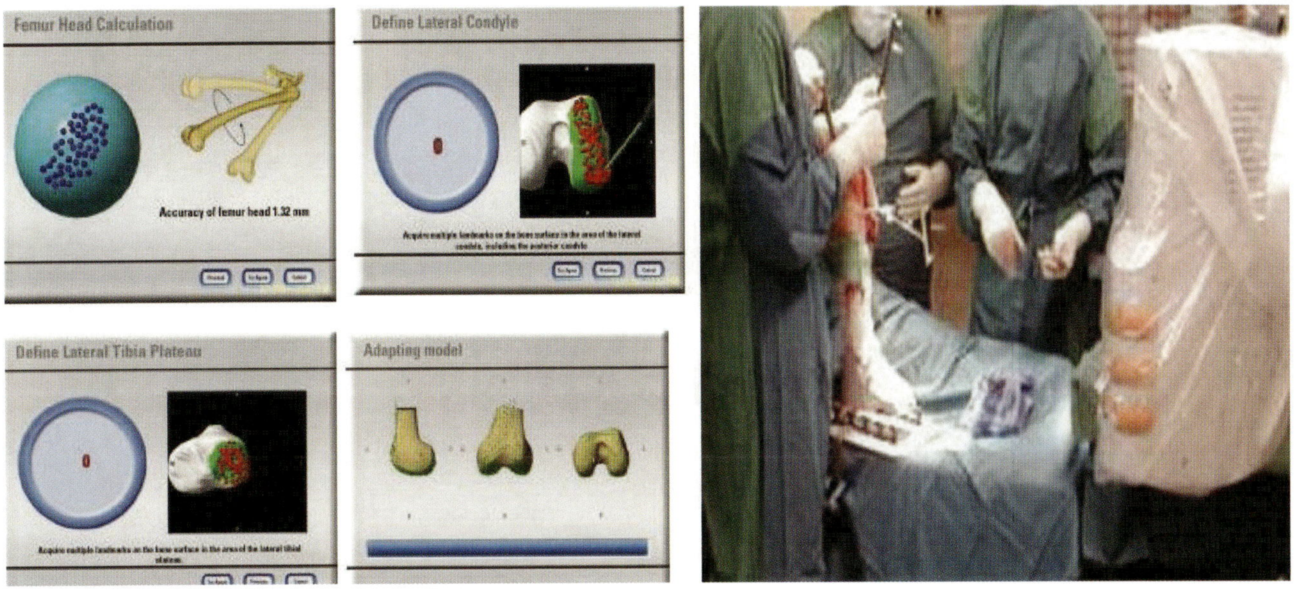

Fig. 10.5 Registration for image based navigation (Brainlab, Feldkirchen, Germany)

Image-free system does not need preoperative CT imaging or intraoperative fluoroscopy and it incorporates the standard cutting blocks and cutting guides from a preexisting instrument. *Currently, the image-free method for acquiring critical anatomic information has proved to be the most effective method for performing TKA. In this system, the standard skeletal structure is used as a basis to track and register the shape, position and axis of patient's anatomy during the operation, and an osteotomy is guided by the navigation system.* It identifies critical anatomic landmarks through both kinematic and surface registration.

For this method, a tracking camera and tracking marker (tracker) are required and this tracker is attached to the bone by a pin or a clamp (rigid body), which is fixed at more than three sites. Other trackers are attached to the surgical equipments and probe to guide the operation. *Also, the accuracy can be verified before performing the osteotomy in order to correct malalignment.* This system includes an optical system using the infrared light and an electromagnetic system using the electromagnets, and the method using the ultrasound is also being developed.

Optical System

Optical system comprises of an active type and a passive type; the active type has LEDs (light-emitting diodes) attached to the rigid body to emit infrared rays onto the camera and the passive type has reflecting spheres on the rigid body to reflect the light emitted from the LEDs onto the camera. By altering the degree of reflection from sphere to sphere, each set of information is received from each reflecting sphere without any confusion. Therefore in the active type, a cable or battery is required and in the passive type, there is a need to clean the reflecting spheres.

Operation begins by exposing the knee joint, *attaching the LEDs (light-emitting diodes) to the rigid body which is fixed onto the bone using special cortical screws and to the surgical tools.* The hip joint, knee joint, and ankle joint are moved in that order to *detect the center of the three joints and to calculate the three-dimensional motion for measuring the mechanical axis (kinematic registration).* The camera (optical localizer: Fig. 10.6) connected to the computer monitor receives the infrared rays emitted from the LEDs attached to the rigid body. When the *probe points towards the bony and articular landmarks* during the operation, the infrared rays emitted from the LEDs attached to the probe are recorded (surface registration) to *acquire the information needed for the operation i.e. the position and direction of the femur and the tibia.*

Based on this registration, the most ideal osteotomy line and direction are monitored in real time.

When a *tensioner is applied to check the tension of* the medial and lateral *collateral ligaments*, the medial/lateral joint space of the knee joint in extension and flexion can be *seen on the monitor as numerical values*, which is used for ligament balancing (Fig. 10.7). The degree of external rotation can be adjusted according to the extension and flexion gap while performing anterior-posterior osteotomy of the distal femur. Also, the ideal size and position of the prosthesis can be determined so as to perform arthroplasty that is appropriate for each patient.

The benefit of the optical system is that it is fast and accurate, and the drawbacks are that the position of the surgeon and the assistants must be selected carefully such that *the camera should not interfere the visual field*, and the results of surgery can be affected by illumination of the operation room.

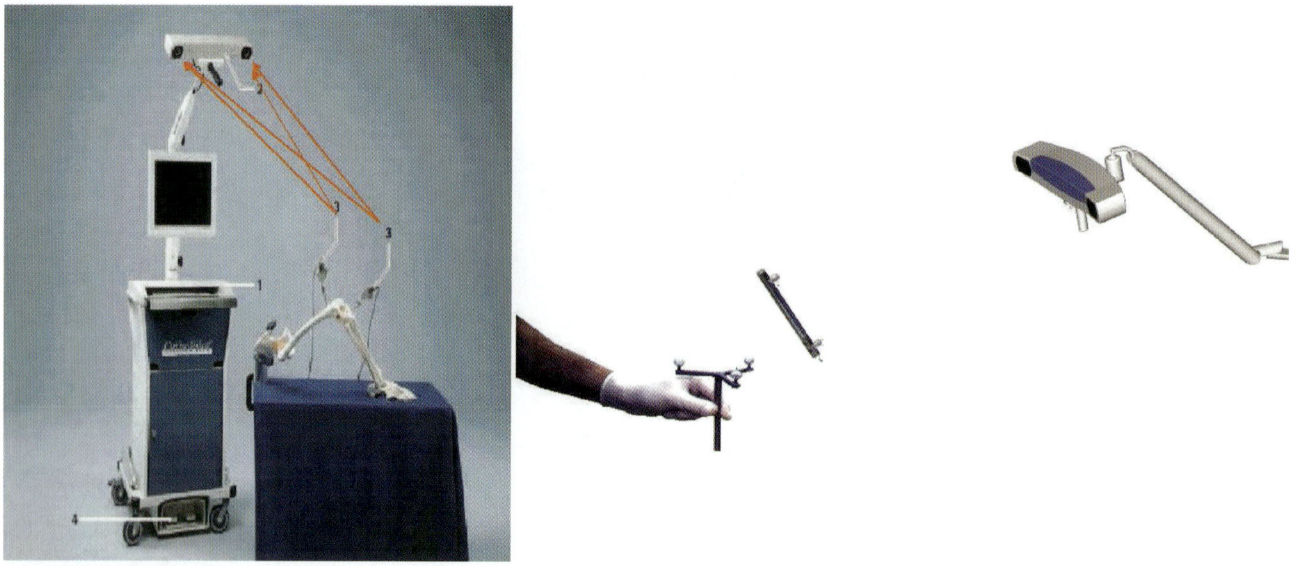

Fig. 10.6 Image-free optical navigation system (Otrhopilot; Aesculap, Tuttlingen, Germany)

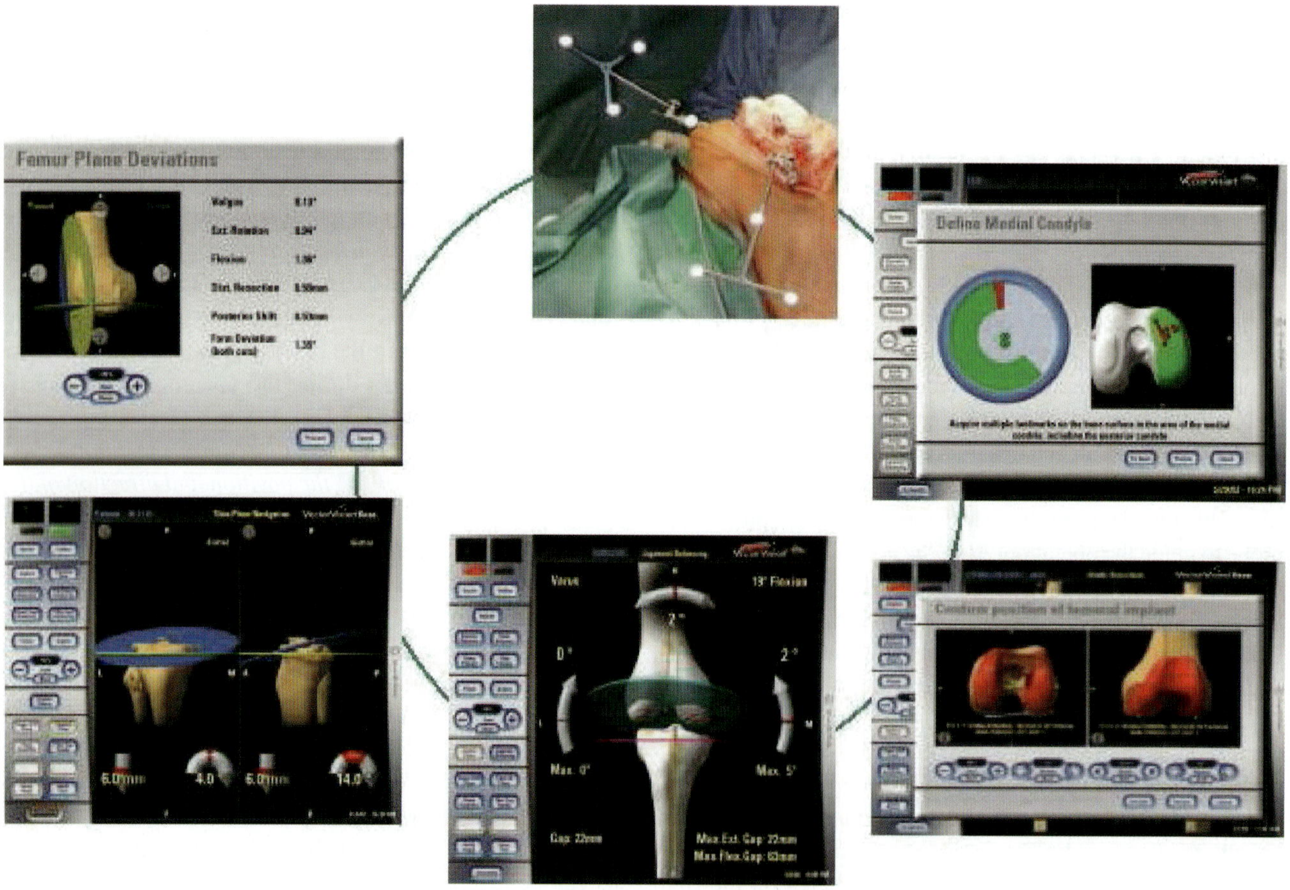

Fig. 10.7 Image-free navigation on the screen

Electromagnetic Computer System (EMC)

The navigation system that was used in the early stage had limitation of camera's visual field and it could only ensure up to 180° of visual field. And the tracker was fixed far away from the operation site using a pin, which caused sterilization problems, soft tissue damage or tethering, and projection

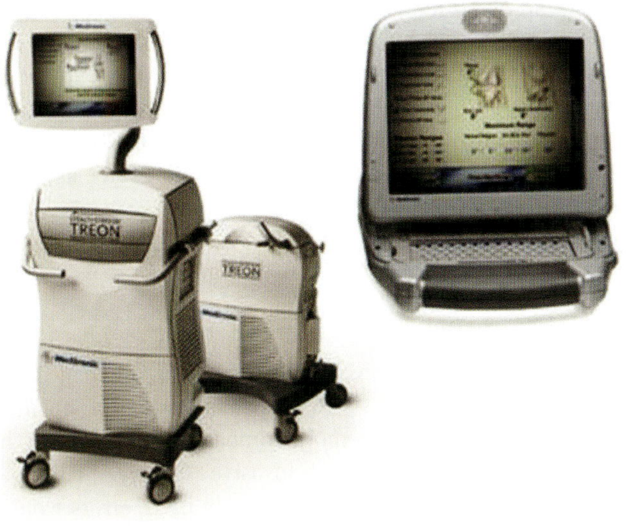

Fig. 10.8 Electromagnetic computer system (TREON; Medtronic, New York)

of large tools. To overcome these drawbacks, the EMC was developed *to obtain non-line-of-sight signal* which can pass through the soft tissues and is not related to the visual field.

Electromagnetic computer system *(EMC)* uses *a localizer that creates a weak intensity magnetic field to generate microvoltage and a sensor to detect its intensity*. The magnetic field is created by the localizer that can use either direct or alternating current, but alternating current can create a more consistent magnetic field. The localizer has three or more generator coils and the number of coils affects the performance level of the system. More number of coils contribute to more accurate and more diverse functions, but this requires a larger capacity computer. The sensor at a distance from the magnetic field can receive and transmit the information to the computer (Fig. 10.8). This system requires dynamic reference frames (DRFs) to be attached near the operation field, which serve as the tracker.

This system was first applied in pediatric neurosurgery and otorhinolaryngology due to instability of signals, metallic interference and slow response to positional change. Currently, it has become an additional option for the navigation system in the orthopedic field after increase in the number of generator coils which can be attached to the soft tissues.

The benefit of this system is that it is convenient to use since it is not affected by the position of the surgeon (non line of sight), the coils attached to the bones and tools are small and the accuracy is very good. Also, the gap balance can be achieved as it can show both the shape and the numerical values which allow for immediate correction when osteotomy is not performed correctly.

Its weakness is that distortion may occur and its safety in the human body is uncertain. It can also be *time consuming and expensive* as it uses disposable coils. *Distortion* is largely divided into *conduction distortion and ferrous interference. Conduction distortion is mostly caused by metals, aluminum or carbon* and not so much by titanium. *Ferrous distortion is more common when there is more iron in the metal.* In such cases, incorrect data may appear, the monitor may stop or show a message of "no reading." In order to prevent distortion, *it is important to create the operation field of a low-iron environment.* For example, it is recommended to use a fluoroscopy-compatible operation table, place the Mayo stand as far as possible and install the EMC equipment close to the operation field. Lionberger suggested the following for successful electromagnetic navigation: the distance between the localizer and the operative field should be between 15 and 25 cm, instrumentation selection of titanium or cobalt chrome and minimization of metals between the transmitter and the receiver coil. Also, the magnetic signals created by the localizer along with their receivers are sensitive to movement. Therefore, rigid or steady dampening movement during acquisition or measurement of data improves the speed of data registry.

The *EMC* is more advanced than the pre-existing navigation system since it is easier to achieve the gap balance, correct the improper osteotomy immediately and it is useful in minimally invasive surgery due to smaller tools. However, the operation room should be properly prepared as this can distort the information, it has a gradual learning curve and its safety in the human body should be ensured.

Ultrasonic System

This is a new system and is different from the other systems since the speed of sound is used to acquire information. However, its weakness is that the speed of sound changes according to the temperature and it is difficult to sterilize the tools.

10.2.4 Indication

The indications for computer assisted arthroplasty are the same as those for TKA. This technique can be more helpful in achieving alignment when there is a deformity. However, it is *not recommended in some patients* because it may prolong the operation time and cause errors. *In case of obese patients*, it may be difficult to find the accurate landmark. In case of patients with *severe osteoporosis*, a fracture may occur where the pin is inserted or at the rigid body fixation site, or rigid body may move.

Computer assisted arthroplasty can be performed with minimally invasive surgery (MIS), but MIS is not always indicated in computer assisted arthroplasty, and the possibility of errors increases when the osteotomy is done from the lateral side.

10.3 Result

Computer assisted TKA has not been used for an enough time for evaluating the clinical results of the long-term follow-up. However, there are many reports regarding the alignment.

In the evaluation of X-ray results, the concept of *outlier* is applied, which refers to *the number of degrees off the target alignment*, and *3° off the target alignment is most commonly used criteria for outlier*. In other words, an outlier is considered when the alignment is more than 3° off the neutral alignment.

There are many reports about the accuracy of coronal alignment, and its relationship with the clinical results. Mason et al. reported the results of meta-analysis of 29 articles which stated that 3° outliers were noted in 9 % of cases in which navigation surgery was performed and in 32 % of cases in which conventional surgery was performed. Whereas Kim et al. reported that there was no difference in radiological alignment between the two methods. Hernandez-Vaguero et al. compared the clinical results between the image-free navigation system and the conventional system. They concluded that there were no differences in the functional and clinical scores or implant survival at the 8-year follow-up, although more complications occurred in the conventional group. Ensini et al. and Dutton et al. reported that there was no difference in the clinical results between the conventional surgery and the computer assisted surgery, although radiological alignment was better with computer assisted surgery. Song et al. reported that *there was a decrease in the number of outliers, but there was no difference in the clinical results* at the short-term follow-up when navigation was applied for soft tissue balancing. Bauwens et al. reported the results of a meta-analysis of 3,423 patients, which suggested that computer assisted surgery does not affect the average alignment; there was not much difference between the two methods when the number of outliers was set at 5°, as opposed to the statistically significant difference when the number of outliers was set at 3°. Also, there was not much difference in the clinical results between the two methods. The results of rotational alignment and sagittal alignment were inconsistent.

Blood loss and the incidence of fat embolism can be decreased by avoiding the use of an intramedullary rod. However, the operation time may be prolonged.

To summarize, there are several advanges of CAOS. The first is that computer assisted surgery is a safe method. There are not many complications associated with the use of this technique. The incidence of deep vein thrombosis and bleeding can either be reduced or it can be the same. Wound healing is consistent with that using the conventional method and postoperative care is also the same as that after the conventional method. *Second*, the number of *outliers in the coronal plane is reduced* and the alignment is more accurate. However, the sagittal and rotational alignment is still unclear. *Third, the operation time may be prolonged by 15–30 min*, but this can be reduced with experience. The operation time varies according to the type of system used and the surgeons' experience with the conventional and computer assisted systems. Generally, practicing on more than 10–20 cases is needed for accurate performance of the computer assisted procedures.

10.3.1 Future of CAOS

Computer systems are developing day by day, and hence the future of the computer assisted surgical method is promising. The systems will become more compact thereby making it easier to perform minimally invasive surgery. With the advancement of the systems, the probability of errors would decrease and it would be easier to obtain more accurate and detailed information regarding soft tissue balancing and rotational alignment of the prosthesis.

Also, computer data storage would be helpful in arthroplasty research. A system or software that can perform TKA as well as other operations with the use of a single system will be developed. This would make the operation more convenient to perform, more accurate, more effective, less expensive, and allow more number of surgeons to perform computer assisted surgery. The use of robotic surgery will also increase with time.

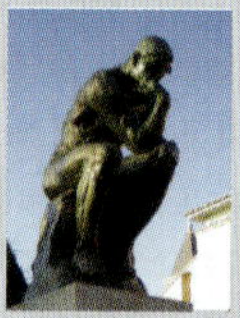

Author's Opinion

I do not have any experience of computer assisted surgery, and hence I am not in a position to evaluate it.

In terms of accuracy, it is clearly superior to the conventional methods. However, it is uncertain how the accuracy reflects in the clinical results. Theoretically, an accurate alignment leads to good results, but the conventional methods have shown satisfying results, and the results of well-aligned and well-balanced artificial joints can be affected by many other factors.

Although currently this method is expensive and time-consuming, it will become less expensive with the development of more advanced equipments. The operation time will decrease with the use of advanced systems and increase in the surgeon's experience.

The concept of computer assisted surgery should be understood as a type of surgical tool that helps the surgeons to perform the operation more accurately. So, it is important to comprehend and follow the basic principles of arthroplasty.

Computer assisted surgery cannot satisfy the surgeons who believe that surgery is an art. I believe that a beautiful painting can be more impressive than a photograph and a well-made handicraft can be better than the machinery products.

10.4 Minimally Invasive Surgery

10.4.1 Overview

Minimally invasive surgery is used to reduce the length of the skin incision and the arthrotomy without affecting the results of surgery. Choi et al. stated that minimally invasive surgery *not only refers to the length of the skin incision but also to the extent to which the important anatomical structures are involved* and that this technique must not be inferior to the conventional technique in terms of the results and complications. Bonutti et al. also stated that the purpose of MIS is not just to minimize the skin incision but also to minimize the soft tissue injury. In this respect, they emphasized that it is important to prevent trauma to the quadriceps tendon. They also stated that patellar eversion caused permanent damage to the quadriceps tendon and the conventional method of dislocating the tibiofemoral joint seriously damaged the joint capsule.

The main focus of debate in minimally invasive surgery is how beneficial is it in comparison to the conventional technique and what type of problems can it cause. It is generally believed that *this technique is beneficial for reducing pain and facilitating rehabilitation in the early stage, but it is not superior to the conventional technique at the long-term follow-up. It takes more time to perform the operation using this technique, which increases the risk of infection, and the incidence of malalignment may also be increased.*

10.4.2 History

Since Repicci and Eberte introduced a method for reducing the size of the incision for unicondylar knee arthroplasty (UK) in the 1990s, minimally invasive surgery has become popular for UK. After this, the possibility of its application to TKA was researched. Cook et al. applied this technique in TKA by performing osteotomy on the femoral side first and by using an extramedullary tibial guide which was used in UK. Tria applied his technique and developed a new tool for MIS to resect the distal femur from the medial to lateral side. Bonutti et al. also introduced a method of MIS while keeping the leg suspended. With this method, it became easier to widen the joint gap and establish ligament balance. Currently, smaller instruments are used for MIS so as to be able to follow a procedure similar to the conventional procedure. MIS can be used in combination with computer assisted surgery in order to improve the accuracy.

Some surgeons use the term "less invasive surgery (LIS)," which indicates that the size of the incision and arthrotomy is in between those of the conventional technique and MIS.

10.4.3 Indication

The indications for MIS are narrower than those for TKA. The patient should have more than 90° of joint motion (flexion contracture of not more than 10° and flexion of 90° or more), and a *varus deformity of not more than 15° and a valgus deformity of not more than 20°. This technique is not recommended in patients with osteopenia, inflammatory arthritis and patients who are heavier than 180 lbs. The knee circumference has a bigger impact than the obesity itself and this technique is not recommended when the thigh is too thick, quadriceps muscles are large or the patellar tendon is short. This technique should also not be used in cases when an operation has been performed previously on the knee joint. Since the operation time can be prolonged, MIS is still not recommended in patients who are too old or have medical problems and who cannot sustain a longer duration of surgery*. Tria et al. experienced the need for conversion to the conventional technique in two patients while performing MIS. One patient had rheumatoid arthritis, was very obese and had weak bones, and the other patient had excessive bleeding from the lateral side. Based on these criteria for the indications for MIS, Scuderi et al. demonstrated that minimally invasive surgery can be performed in about 58 % of patients who need a TKA.

10.4.4 Surgical Technique

10.4.4.1 Approach

A midline skin incision about 8–10 cm long is made from the superior pole of the patella to the tibial tuberosity, but it can be extended in obese patients and the site of the skin incision can vary from surgeon to surgeon (Fig. 10.9). *Arthrotomy is largely divided into four types and it is the key procedure in MIS* (Fig. 10.10). After arthrotomy, *the patella is not everted but it is retracted laterally in most cases. As a result, the strength of quadriceps muscles is maintained, incidence of patella baja is decreased and pain on flexion is reduced.*

However, excessive retraction while performing this technique *can cause wound healing problems and can increase the risk of infection.*

Limited Parapatellar Arthrotomy

This arthrotomy invades the quadriceps tendon by about 2–4 cm and it is used more commonly. It is simple, provides good exposure and is convenient to extend the arthrotomy with this method. The concept of a mobile window is used in this arthrotomy.

Quadriceps-Sparing Arthrotomy

This arthrotomy is nearly the same as the limited paramedial arthrotomy except that the quadriceps tendon is spared in this arthrotomy. The purpose of this arthrotomy is to maintain the muscle strength of the extensor mechanism without damaging the quadriceps tendon. For better exposure, patella can be resected first and cutting from the side is often required for execution of this arthrotomy. The arthrotomy can be extended like in the limited parapatellar arthrotomy for ensuring a better exposure.

However, Huang et al. reported that there were *more outliers with the quadriceps-sparing arthrotomy than with the conventional approach.*

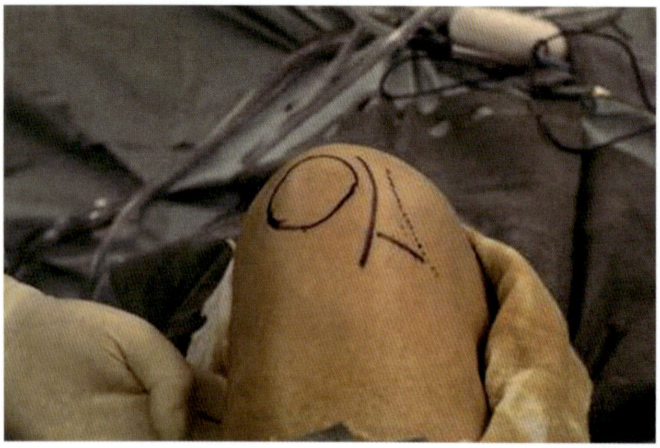

Fig. 10.9 Skin incision in minimally invasive surgery

Limited Subvastus Arthrotomy

The benefit of this arthrotomy is that it follows the natural planes of dissection and it does not invade the extensor mechanism. When this arthrotomy is used, it is important to protect the descending genicular artery, intermuscular septal artery and saphenous nerve.

This arthrotomy is not suitable for patients who are obese, have relatively shorter lower limbs and in muscular patients. Scuderi et al. stated that this arthrotomy is less painful than the limited parapatellar arthrotomy and ensures a more powerful extensor mechanism.

Limited Midvastus Arthrotomy

This arthrotomy has the benefits of the limited parapatellar arthrotomy in terms of exposure and those of the limited subvastus arthrotomy in terms of saving the extensor mechanism.

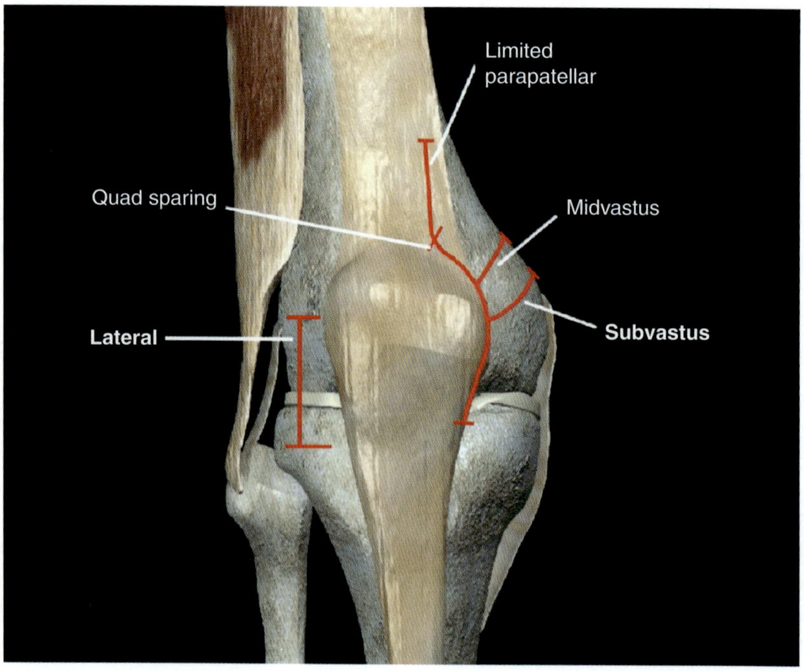

Fig. 10.10 Arthrotomy in MIS

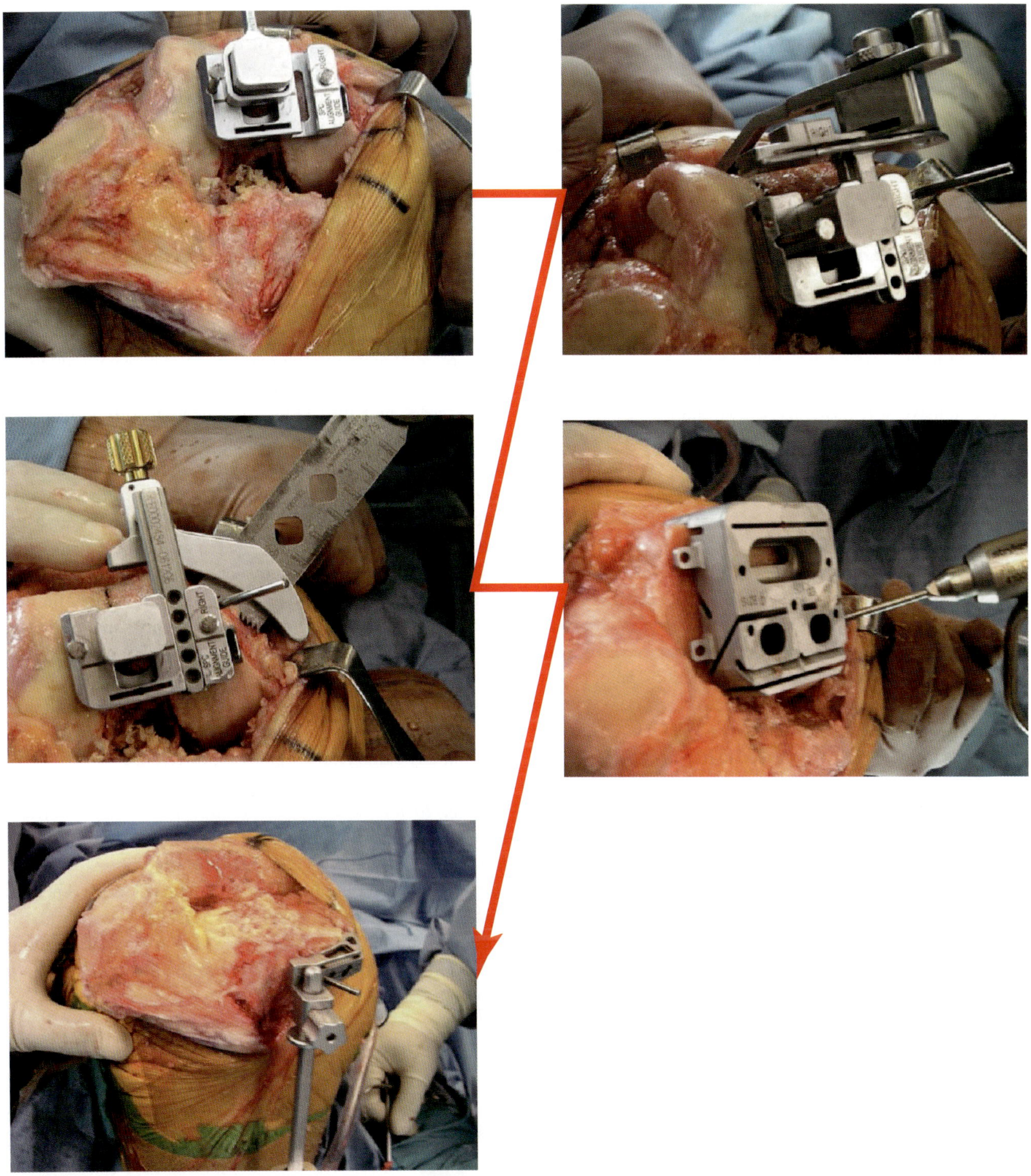

Fig. 10.11 Instruments used in minimally invasive surgery and the surgical procedure of femoral osteotomy

10.4.4.2 Osteotomy

In the early period, various types of surgical instruments were introduced for making a smaller incision. Currently, miniature forms of the conventional instruments that are used in TKA have been developed (Fig. 10.11). Computer assisted surgery has become necessary so as to recover poor visual references which are likely to be lost in MIS exposure and to increase the accuracy. So, some instruments have been designed to incorporate the tracker so as to make it possible to apply the navigation system. Electromagnetic computer assisted navigation system has more advantages than the other navigation systems in MIS, as even a small incision allows for the placement of DRFs (dynamic reference frames) without extending the incision.

Some surgeons perform osteotomy from the tibia first to ensure a better operation field, while other surgeons start osteotomy from the patella. Many surgeons prefer the Whiteside's line for determining the external rotation of the femur. *The basic techniques of osteotomy are the same as those in the conventional TKA.*

10.4.4.3 Balancing

Balancing technique is the same as that in the conventional TKA and many instruments have spacer blocks for establishing the balance. However in minimally invasive surgery, extensive soft-tissue release is impossible due to the limited exposure, and hence it is difficult to perform minimally invasive surgery in patients with a severe deformity.

10.4.4.4 Fixation

When cementing is done for fixation, it is *recommended to start from the tibia.* The modular design of the tibial stem is used in a certain product for easy insertion of tibial plate in MIS.

Since *it is not easy to remove the extruded cement around the prosthesis, it is not recommended to use too much cement.* Some surgeons prefer placing a gauze on the posterior side for removing the extruded cement easily. Romanowski and Repicci stated that all the technical issues found in patients who underwent MIS TKA and MIS UK were related to improper cementing.

10.4.5 Postoperative Care

Patients can begin ambulation 2 h after surgery if the patient's general condition is tolerable and can start walking when the conditions stabilize. Other rehabilitation programs are the same or can be started a little earlier than the conventional TKA.

10.5 Result

Arthroplasty with MIS *offers better results than the conventional techniques in the early stage.* This is because this technique does not violate the quadriceps tendon, and reduces postoperative pain and complications related to the extensor mechanism. *Factors affecting the prognosis include management of the blind area*, arteriolar and nerve injury on the lateral side, *alignment and positioning of the prosthesis, and cementing technique. The prognosis is also greatly affected by the surgeons' experience.* Tria et al. reported the results of their experience with 58 cases of MIS surgery stating that the average operation time was 110 min and the average amount of bleeding was 200 cm^3, and this amount of bleeding was still half of the conventional technique. Although the difference in the ROM after 6 weeks was not statistically significant, patients who underwent MIS achieved 126° of flexion, which was greater than 119° of flexion in the patients who were treated with the conventional technique. The postoperative varus angle was 2.5° in patients who underwent MIS, whereas the postoperative varus angle was only 1.0° in the patients who were treated with the conventional technique, and this difference was also not statistically significant. Bonutti et al. who are one of the pioneers of MIS observed 216 patients of MIS for 2 years and reported that 97 % of patients showed good results that are comparable to the results of the conventional technique. However, manipulation under anesthesia was needed in six cases and five cases required revision due to deep infection (two cases), chronic pain (two cases), and instability (one case). Yoo et al. reported that the early clinical results of MIS were good and there was no radiological difference, but the valgus angle tended to decrease during osteotomy of the distal femur. Despite the fact that the quadriceps tendon is spared in arthrotomy, Cook et al. reported that the incidence of a lateral retinacular release in the limited medial parapatellar arthrotomy was just the same as that in the conventional techniques. Seon and Song introduced computer assisted surgery in MIS in order to reduce the number of radiological outliers and reported that the number of outliers decreased in MIS computer assisted surgery without any statistically significant difference.

However, Whiteside emphasized that *MIS caused damage to the skin or muscles due to excessive retraction, which increased the risk of infection. Also the prolonged operation time caused problems associated with the long-term use of the tourniquet.* Barrack et al. reported that the incidence of early revision TKA was high in patients who had undergone MIS. Such discrepancies in the results may be mostly related to the level of surgeon's experience of MIS.

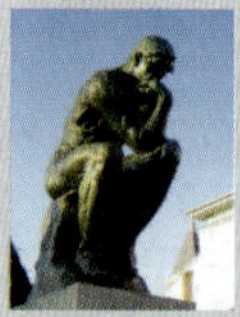

Author's Opinion

Although there are not many reports of long-term follow-up of MIS, I believe that the short-term results are very promising. In particular, this technique minimizes the incision to allow early activity and to reduce morbidity.

However, the indication needs to be selected more carefully. The surgical techniques used for reducing soft tissue injury and safe removal of extruded cement are closely related to the complications. Hence, a gradual learning curve is involved in mastering MIS.

I believe that MIS is not yet highly recommended as it may be inferior to the conventional techniques with respect to alignment and soft tissue balancing. And the clinical results are not any better than those of the conventional techniques at the long-term follow-up. In addition to this, MIS may cause wound problems due to excessive traction of the skin.

With the use of more advanced surgical instruments and surgical techniques along with the introduction of the latest computer systems, this technique would provide better results.

Bibliography

Aglietti P, Baldini A, Sensi L. Quadriceps-sparing versus mini-subvastus approach in total knee arthroplasty. Clin Orthop. 2006; 452:106–11.

Amiot LP, Poulin F. Computed tomography-based navigation for hip, knee, and spine surgery. Clin Orthop. 2004;421:77–86.

Anderson KC, Buehler KC, Markel DC. Computer assisted navigation in total knee arthroplasty: comparison with conventional methods. J Arthroplasty. 2005;20 Suppl 3:132–8.

Bargar WL. Robots in orthopaedic surgery: past, present, and future. Clin Orthop. 2007;463:31–6.

Barrack CM, Barnes CL, Burnett RS, et al. Minimal incision surgery as a risk factor for early failure of total knee arthroplasty. J Arthroplasty. 2009;24:489–98.

Bathis H, Perlick L, Tingart M, et al. Alignment in total knee arthroplasty. A comparison of computer assisted surgery with the conventional technique. J Bone Joint Surg. 2004;86-B:682–7.

Bauwens K, Matthes G, Wich M, et al. Navigated total knee replacement. A meta-analysis. J Bone Joint Surg. 2007;89-A:261–9.

Bellemans J, Vandenneucker H, Vanlauwe J. Robot-assisted total knee arthroplasty. Clin Orthop. 2007;464:111–6.

Bonutti P, Dethmers D, Stiehl JB. Case report: femoral shaft fracture resulting from femoral tracker placement in navigated TKA. Clin Orthop. 2008;466:1499–502.

Bonutti PM, Mont MA, McMahon M, et al. Minimally invasive total knee arthroplasty. J Bone Joint Surg. 2004;86-A Suppl 2:26–32.

Bonutti PM, Neal DJ, Kester MA. Minimal incision total knee arthroplasty using the suspended leg techinque. Orthopedics. 2003;26:899–903.

Chauhan SK, Scott RG, Breidahl W, et al. Computer-assisted knee arthroplasty versus a conventional jig-based technique. A randomized, prospective trial. J Bone Joint Surg. 2004;86-B:372–7.

Cheng T, Liu T, Zhang G, et al. Does minimally invasive surgery improve short-term recovery in total knee arthroplasty? Clin Orthop. 2010;468:1635–48.

Choi YJ, Tanavalee A, Pak AH, et al. Minimally invasive surgery for total knee arthroplasty. In: Scuderi GR, editor. MIS of the hip and the knee: a clinical perspective. 1st ed. New York: Springer; 2004. p. 187–98.

Chung BJ, Kang YG, Chang CB, et al. Differences between sagittal femoral mechanical and distal reference axes should be considered in navigated TKA. Clin Orthop. 2009;467:2403–13.

Clemens U, Miehlke RK. Experience using the latest OrthoPilot TKA software: a comparative study. Surg Technol Int. 2003;11:265–73.

Cook JL, Scuderi GR, Tenholder M. Incidence of lateral release in total knee arthroplasty in standard and mini-incision approaches. Clin Orthop. 2006;452:123–6.

Church JS, Scadden JE, Gupta RR, et al. Embolic phenomena during computer-assisted and conventional total knee replacement. J Bone Joint Surg. 2007;89-B:481–5.

Delp SL, Stulberg SD, Davies B, et al. Computer assisted knee replacement. Clin Orthop. 1998;354:49–56.

Dutton AQ, Yeo SJ, Yang KY, et al. Computer-assisted minimally invasive total knee arthroplasty compared with standard total knee arthroplasty. A prospective, randomized study. J Bone Joint Surg. 2008;90-A:2–9.

Ensini A, Catani F, Leardini A, et al. Alignments and clinical results in conventional and navigated total knee arthroplasty. Clin Orthop. 2007;457:156–62.

Fehring TK, Berend KR, Hofmann S, et al. Advanced technologies in performing total knee arthroplasty: roundtable discussion. In: Scott WN, editor. Surgery of the knee. 5th ed. Philadelphia: Churchill Livingstone; 2011. p. 1283–92.

Floren M, Davis J, Peterson MG, et al. A mini-midvastus capsular approach with patellar displacement decreases the prevalence of patella baja. J Arthroplasty. 2007;22:51–7.

Garg A, Walker PS. Prediction of total knee motion using a three-dimensional computer graphics model. J Biochem. 1988;3:67–72.

Haaker RG, Stockheim M, Kamp M, et al. Computer-assisted navigation increases precision of component placement in total knee arthroplasty. Clin Orthop. 2005;433:152–9.

Hafez M. Custom-made cutting guides for total knee arthroplasty. In: Scott WN, editor. Surgery of the knee. 5th ed. Philadelphia: Churchill Livingstone; 2011. p. 1240–54.

Hafez MA, Jaramaz B, Digioia III A. Computer-assisted knee surgery: an overview. In: Scott WN, editor. Surgery of the knee. 4th ed. Philadelphia: Churchill Livingstone; 2006. p. 1655–73.

Heal J, Blewitt N. Kinemax total knee arthroplasty: trial by template. J Arthroplasty. 2002;17:90–4.

Hernández-Vaquero D, Suarez-Vazquez A, Iglesias-Fernandez S. Can computer assistance improve the clinical and functional scores in total knee arthroplasty? Clin Orthop. 2011;469:3436–42.

Hofmann AA, McCandless J. Imageless computer navigation in total knee arthroplasty: the simpler wave of future. In: Scott WN, editor. Surgery of the knee. 5th ed. Philadelphia: Churchill Livingstone; 2011. p. 1217–22.

Huang HT, Su JY, Chang JK, et al. The early clinical outcome of minimally invasive quadriceps-sparing total knee arthroplasty: report of a 2-year follow-up. J Arthroplasty. 2007;22:1007–12.

Jenny JY, Clemens U, Kohler S, et al. Consistency of implantation of a total knee arthroplasty with a non-image-based navigation system: a case-control study of 235 cases compared with 235 conventionally implanted prostheses. J Arthroplasty. 2005;20:832–9.

Kalairajah Y, Cossey AJ, Verrrall GM, et al. Are systemic emboli reduced in computer-assisted knee surgery? A prospective, randomised, clinical trial. J Bone Joint Surg. 2006;88-B:198–202.

Kienzle III TC, Stulberg SD, Peshkin M, et al. A computer-assisted total knee replacement surgical system using a calibrated robot. In: Taylor RH, editor. Computer-integrated surgery. 1st ed. London: The MIT Press; 1996. p. 409–16.

Kim YH, Kim JS, Yoon SH. Alignment and orientation of the components in total knee replacement with and without navigation support: a prospective, randomised study. J Bone Joint Surg. 2007; 89-B:471–6.

Klein GR, Austin MS, Smith EB, et al. Total knee arthroplasty using computer-assisted navigation in patients with deformities of the femur and tibia. J Arthroplasty. 2006;21:284–8.
Krackow KA. Fine tuning your next total knee: computer assisted surgery. Orthopedics. 2003;26:971–2.
Krackow KA, Serpe L, Phillips MJ, et al. Operative technique: a new technique for determining proper mechanical axis alignment during total knee arthroplasty: progress toward computer-assisted TKR. Orthopedics. 1999;22:698–702.
Lionberger DR. Computer-assisted navigation: Minimally invasive surgery for total knee replacement. In: Scott WN, editor. Surgery of the knee. 5th ed. Philadelphia: Churchill Livingstone; 2011a. p. 1275–82.
Lionberger DR. Electromagnetic computer-assisted navigation. In: Scott WN, editor. Surgery of the knee. In: Scott WN ed. Surgery of the knee. 5th ed. Philadelphia: Churchill Livingstone; 2011b. p. 1223–31.
Lionberger DR. Electromagnetic computer assisted navigation in total knee replacement. In: Scott WN, editor. Surgery of the knee. 4th ed. Philadelphia: Churchill Livingstone; 2006. p. 1705–15.
Luring C, Hufner T, Perlick L, et al. The effectiveness of sequential medial soft tissue release on coronal alignment in total knee arthroplasty: using a computer navigation model. J Arthroplasty. 2006; 21:428–34.
Mai S, Siebert WE, Heeckt PF. Robotics in total knee arthroplasty. In: Scott WN, editor. Surgery of the knee. 5th ed. Philadelphia: Churchill Livingstone; 2011. p. 1269–74.
Martelli M, Mareacci M, Nofrini L, et al. Computer-and robot-assisted total knee replacement: analysis of a new surgical procedure. Ann Biomed Eng. 2000;28:1146–53.
Mason JB, Fehring TK, Estok R, et al. Meta-analysis of alignment outcomes in computer-assisted total knee arthroplasty surgery. J Arthroplasty. 2007;22:1097–106.
Matsen III FA, Garbini JL, Sidles JA, et al. Robotic assistance in orthopaedic surgery. A proof of principle using distal femoral arthroplasty. Clin Orthop. 1993;296:178–86.
Matsumoto T, Muratsu H, Tsumura N, et al. Soft tissue balance measurement in posterior-stabilized total knee arthroplasty with a navigation system. J Arthroplasty. 2009;24:358–64.
Matziolis G, Krocker D, Weiss U, et al. A prospective, randomized study of computer-assisted and conventional total knee arthroplasty. Three-dimensional evaluation of implant alignment and rotation. J Bone Joint Surg. 2007;89-A:236–43.
Nunley RM, Ellison BS, Zhu J, et al. Do patient-specific guides improve coronal alignment in total knee arthroplasty? Clin Orthop. 2012;470:895–902.
Patil N, Nett MP, Tria Jr A, et al. Surgical approaches in total knee arthroplasty: Standard and MIS techniques. In: Scott WN, editor. Surgery of the knee. 5th ed. Philadelphia: Churchill Livingstone; 2011. p. 1029–41.
Mihalko WM, Duquin T, Axelrod JR, et al. Location and number of cortical fixation points and the effect on reference base stability during computer-navigated total knee arthroplasty. J Arthroplasty. 2007;22:605–8.
Minoda Y, Kobayashi A, Iwaki H, et al. TKA sagittal alignment with navigation systems and conventional techniques vary only a few degrees. Clin Orthop. 2009;467:1000–6.
Moon YW, Seo JG, Lim SJ, et al. Variability in femoral component rotation reference axes measured during navigation-assisted total knee arthroplasty using gap technique. J Arthroplasty. 2010; 25:238–43.
Mullaji A, Shetty GM. Computer-assisted total knee arthroplasty for arthritis with extra-articular deformity. J Arthroplasty. 2009;24:1164-1169 e1161.
Munjal S, Krackow KA. Computer-assisted total knee replacement. In: Scott WN, editor. Surgery of the knee. 4th ed. Philadelphia: Churchill Livingstone; 2006. p. 1689–97.
Nabeyama R, Matsua S, Miura H, et al. The accuracy of image guided knee replacement based on computed tomography. J Bone Joint Surg. 2003;86-B:366–71.
Niki Y, Matsumoto H, Otani T, et al. Accuracy of implant positioning for minimally invasive total knee arthroplasty in patients with severe varus deformity. J Arthroplasty. 2010;25:381–6.
Nishihara S, Sugano N, Ikai M, et al. Accuracy evaluation of a shape-based registration method for a computer navigation system for total knee arthroplasty. J Knee Surgery. 2003;16:98–105.
Park SE, Lee CT. Comparison of robotic-assisted and conventional manual implantation of a primary total knee arthroplasty. J Arthroplasty. 2007;22:1054–9.
Perlick L, Bathis H, Tingart M, et al. Navigation in total-knee arthroplasty: CT-based implantation compared with the conventional technique. Acta Orthop Scand. 2004;75:464–70.
Picard F, Moody J, Jaramaz A, et al. A classification proposal for computer-assisted knee systems. In: Scott LD et al., editors. Medical image computing and computer-assisted intervention-MICCAI 2000, Lecture notes in computer science,1935; 2000.
Radermacher K, Portheine F, Anton M, et al. Computer assisted orthopaedic surgery with image based individual templates. Clin Orthop. 1998;354:28–38.
Repicci JA, Eberte RW. Minimally invasive surgical technique for unicondylar knee arthroplasty. J South Orthop Assoc. 1999;8:20–7.
Romanowski MR, Repicci JA. Minimally invasive unicondylar arthroplasty: eight-year follow up. J Knee Surg. 2002;15:17–22.
Romanowski MR, Repicci MR. Technical aspects of medial versus lateral minimally invasive unicondylar arthroplasty. Orthopedics. 2003;26:289–93.
Saragaglia D, Picard F, Chaussard C, et al. Computer-assisted knee arthroplasty: comparison with a conventional procedure. Results of 50 cases in a prospective randomized study. Rev Chir Orthop Reparatrice Appar Mot. 2001;87:18–28.
Schroer WC, Diesfeld PJ, Reedy ME, et al. Association of increased knee flexion and patella clunk syndrome after mini-subvastus total knee arthroplasty. J Arthroplasty. 2009;24:281–7.
Scuderi GR, Tenholder M, Capeci C. Surgical approaches in mini-incision total knee arthroplasty. Clin Orthop. 2004;428:61–7.
Scuderi GR, Tria AJ. Minimally invasive total knee arthroplasty. In: Scott WN, editor. Surgery of the knee. 4th ed. Philadelphia: Churchill Livingstone; 2006. p. 1631–9.
Seon JK, Song EK. Navigation-assisted less invasive total knee arthroplasty compared with conventional total knee arthroplasty: a randomized prospective trial. J Arthroplasty. 2006;21:777–82.
Siebert W, Mai S, Kober R, et al. Technique and first clinical results of robot-assisted total knee replacement. Knee. 2002;9:173–80.
Song EK, Seon JK, Yoon TR, et al. Comparative study of stability after total knee arthroplasties between navigation system and conventional techniques. J Arthroplasty. 2007;22:1107–11.
Sparmann M, Wolk B, Czupalla H, et al. Positioning of total knee arthroplasty with and without navigation support. A prospective, randomized study. J Bone Joint Surg. 2003;85-B:830–5.
Spencer JM, Chauhan SK, Sloan K, et al. Computer navigation versus conventional total knee replacement: no difference in functional results at two years. J Bone Joint Surg. 2007;89-B:477–80.
Stiehl JB. Computer navigation in primary total knee arthroplasty. In: Scott WN, editor. Surgery of the knee. 5th ed. Philadelphia: Churchill Livingstone; 2011. p. 1201–6.
Stockl B, Nogler M, Rosiek R, et al. Navigation improves accuracy of rotational alignment in total knee arthroplasty. Clin Orthop. 2004;426:180–6.

Stulburg SD. Computer-navigated total knee arthroplasty. In: Scott WN, editor. Surgery of the knee. 4th ed. Philadelphia: Churchill Livingstone; 2006. p. 1675–88.

Stulberg SD. Computer-navigated total knee arthroplasty. In: Scott WN, editor. Surgery of the knee. 5th ed. Philadelphia: Churchill Livingstone; 2011. p. 1207–16.

Stulberg SD, Loan P, Sarin V. Computer-assisted navigation in total knee replacement: results of an initial experience in thirty-five patients. J Bone Joint Surg. 2002;84-A:90–8.

Tanavalee A, Thiengwittayaporn S, Itiravivong P. Progressive quadriceps incision during minimally invasive surgery for total knee arthroplasty: the effect on early postoperative ambulation. J Arthroplasty. 2007;22:1013–8.

Teter KE, Bregman D, Colwell Jr CW. Accuracy of intramedullary versus extramedullary tibial alignment cutting systems in total knee arthroplasty. Clin Othrop. 1995;321:106–10.

Tria AJ. Advancements in minimally invasive total knee arthroplasty. Orthopedics. 2003;26:859–63.

Tria AJ. Minimally invasive total knee arthroplasty: the importance of instrumentation. Orthop Clin N Am. 2004;35: 227–34.

Tria AJ, Coon TM. Minimal incision total knee arthroplasty: early experience. Clin Orthop. 2003;416:185–90.

Victor J, Hoste D. Image-based computer-assisted total knee arthroplasty leads to lower variability in coronal alignment. Clin Orthop. 2004;428:131–9.

Whiteside LA. Mini incision: occasionally desirable, rarely necessary: in the affirmative. J Arthroplasty. 2006;21 Suppl 1: 16–8.

Yoo JH, Han DY, Han CD, et al. Radiological evaluation of quadriceps-sparing minimally invasive total knee arthroplasty. J Korean Orthop Assoc. 2006;41:454–60.

Yoshino N, Takai S, Ohtsuki Y, et al. Computed tomography measurement of the surgical and clinical transepicondylar axis of the distal femur in osteoarthritic knees. J Arthroplasty. 2001;16: 493–7.

About the Author

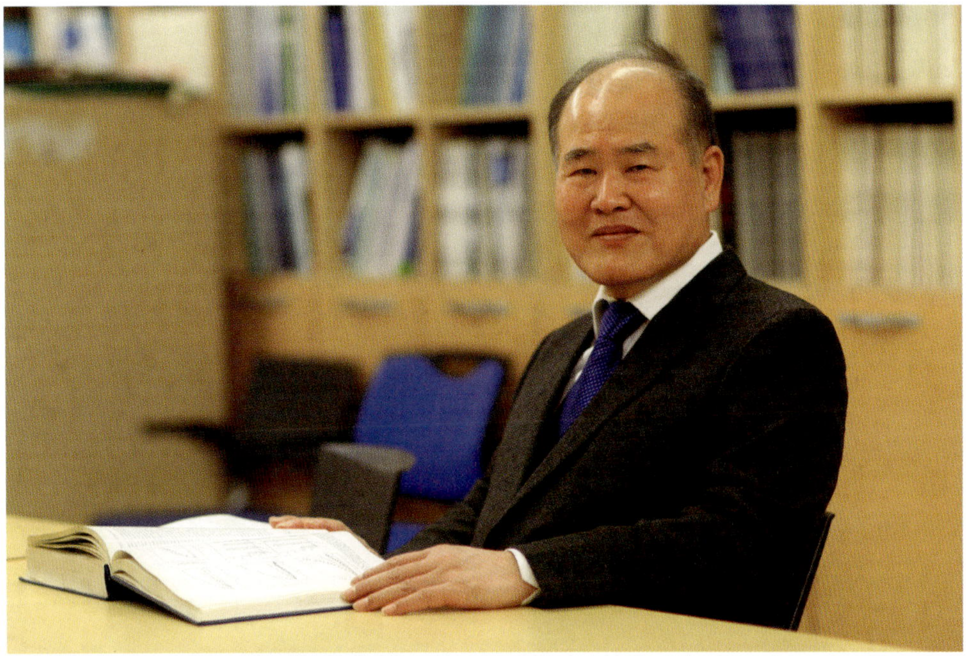

Wooshin Cho

Professor: Department of Orthopedic Surgery, Asan Medical Center, College of Medicine, University of Ulsan, Seoul, South Korea

1990–Present: Professor, College of Medicine, University of Ulsan

2001–2006: Chief Editor, Association of Korean Sports Medicine

2002: Chief Medical Staff, FIFA World Cup

2002–2006: AO Trustee

2001–2006: Chief Editor, Association of Korean Sports Medicine

2004–2007: Chief Editor, Journal of Korean Knee Society

2009–2010: Chairman, Korean Knee Society

2011–Present: Chairman, Association of Korean Sports Medicine

1995: "Wiring plate" was patented in Korea, Japan, England, Germany, and Switzerland

Has performed more than 5,000 total knee arthroplasties to date

Publications

Doctor! My Knee Hurts (2001): Dr. Research Group

Knee Joint Arthroplasty (Korean Edition), 2004 1st edition

Knee Joint Arthroplasty (Korean Edition), 2007 2nd edition

W. Cho, *Knee Joint Arthroplasty*,
DOI 10.1007/978-3-642-39389-1, © Springer-Verlag Berlin Heidelberg 2014

Index

W. Cho, *Knee Joint Arthroplasty*,
DOI 10.1007/978-3-642-39389-1, © Springer-Verlag Berlin Heidelberg 2014